Handbook of
Sports Injuries

Editor

R. Charles Bull, MD, BSc(MED), FRCS(C)
Active Staff, Orthopaedic Department, Humber River Hospital;
Consulting Staff, Orthopaedic and Arthritic Hospital;
Director, York University Sports Injuries Clinic,
Toronto, Ontario
Canada

McGraw-Hill
Health Professions Division

New York St. Louis San Francisco Auckland Bogotá Caracas
Lisbon London Madrid Mexico City Milan Montreal New Delhi
San Juan Singapore Sydney Tokyo Toronto

McGraw-Hill

A Division of The McGraw·Hill Companies

HANDBOOK OF SPORTS INJURIES

Copyright © 1999 by *The McGraw-Hill Companies*, Inc. All rights reserved. Printed in the United States of America. Except as permitted under the United States Copyright Act of 1976, no part of this publication may be reproduced or distributed in any form or by any means, or stored in a data base or retrieval system, without prior written permission of the publisher.

234567890 DOCDOC 99

ISBN 0-07-008993-0

This book was set in Times Roman by Better Graphics, Inc.
The editors were Martin Wonsiewicz, Susan R. Noujaim, and Steven Melvin;
the production supervisor was Richard Ruzycka.
The cover was designed by Marsha Cohen/Parallelogram
The index was prepared by Geraldine Beckford.

R.R. Donnelley and Sons Company was printer and binder

Library of Congress Cataloging-in-Publication Data
Handbook of sports injuries / editor, R. Charles Bull. — 1st ed.
    p. cm.
  Includes index.
  ISBN 0-07-008993-0
  1. Sports injuries—Handbooks, manuals, etc. I. Bull, R. Charles.
RD97.H36   1998
617.1′027—dc21   98-36208

Handbook of
Sports Injuries

Contents

Contributors

A. Amendola, MD, FRCS(C) [14]
Fowler Kennedy Sport Medicine Clinic, University of
Western Ontario, London, Ontario, Canada

Barry Bartlett, BPHE, MA, CAT(C) [21]
Professor, Sports Injury Management Program, Sheridan
College, Oakville, Ontario, Canada; MA, Exercise and
Conditioning; Consultant, National Hockey League
Conditioning and Performance; Consultant, National Hockey
League officials; and National Professional Lacrosse Player,
1975

David Bell, MD [14]
Fowler Kennedy Sport Medicine Clinic, University of
Western Ontario, London, Ontario, Canada

Wilma F. Bergfeld, MD [13]
Head, Dermatologic Research, The Cleveland Clinic
Educational Foundation, Cleveland, Ohio

R. Charles Bull, MD, BSc.(MED), FRCS(C) [8, 15, 21, 28,
29, 33]
Active Staff, Orthopaedic Department, Humber River
Hospital; Consulting Staff, Orthopaedic and Arthritic
Hospital; and Director, York University Sports Injuries Clinic,
Toronto, Ontario, Canada

Chris Broadhurst, CATA(C) [15]
Chief Therapist, Toronto Maple Leaf Hockey Club; Therapist,
Sports Medicine and High Performance Specialists, Toronto,
Ontario, Canada

Hugh Cameron [33]
National Running Coach, Newmarket, Ontario, Canada

Numbers in brackets refer to chapters written or cowritten by the contributors.

Wen Chao, MD [10]
Assistant Attending, Department of Orthopaedic Surgery,
St. Luke's-Roosevelt Hospital Center, and Assistant Clinical
Professor, Columbia University, New York, New York

Michael Clarfield, MD, CASM, ACSM [35]
Chief Physician, Toronto Maple Leaf Hockey Team; Director,
Sports Medicine and High Performance Specialists; Director,
Alan Eagleson Sports Clinic, York University; Physician,
National Ballet of Canada Company; and Assistant Professor,
University of Toronto, Toronto, Ontario, Canada

Richard G. Clarnette, MBBS, FRACS [18]
Wakefield Orthopaedic Clinic, Adelaide, South Australia,
Australia

Gloria C. Cohen, MD, CCFP, FACSM, Dip.Sport Med. [27]
Head Physician, Canadian Cycling Team, Sports Medicine
Consultant, Commonwealth Centre for Sport Development,
Victoria, British Columbia, Canada

Doreen Cress, CAT(C) [21]
Certified Athletic Therapist, Diploma of Sports Injury
Management, Mississauga, Ontario, Canada

Christopher T. Daley, MD, FRCS(C) [12]
Orthopaedic & Fracture Clinic, Faribault, Minnesota

R.Timothy Deakon, MD, FRCS(C) [34, 39]
Oakville, Ontario, Canada

Sandra Fielding, BSc(PT) [26]
Registered Physiotherapist, National Coaching Certification
Program, Level I Figure Skating Coach, Gold Level Ice
Dancer, Toronto, Ontario, Canada

Michael Ford, MD, FRCS(C), DABOS [5]
Orthopedic and Arthritic Hospital; Women's College
Hospital; Wellesley Hospital; Associate Director,
Spinal Instrumentation Learning Centre; Orthopedic
Consultant, Phantom of the Opera Company; Lecturer,
Faculty of Medicine, University of Toronto, Ontario,
Canada

Lorie Forwell, MSc(PT) [24]
Clinical and Research Coordinator, Physiotherapy, Fowler
Kennedy Sport Medicine Clinic, University of Western
Ontario, London, Ontario, Canada

Peter J. Fowler, MD [24]
Professor, Orthopaedic Surgery, University of Western
Ontario, Fowler Kennedy Sport Medicine Clinic, University
of Western Ontario, London, Ontario, Canada

Carol Gibson-Coyne, BSc(PT) [20]
Banff, Alberta, Canada

Rejean Grenier, MD [19]
Orthopaedic Surgeon, Laval University Medical Center,
Associate Clinical Professor, Department of Surgery, Laval
University, Quebec City, Quebec, Canada

William G. Hamilton, MD [10]
Senior Attending Orthopaedic Surgeon, St.Luke's-Roosevelt
Hospital Center, Clinical Professor, Orthopaedic Surgery,
Columbia University College of Physicians and Surgeons,
New York, New York

Anne Hartley, BPHE, CAT(C), Dip.ATM [32]
Professor and Clinical Therapist, Sheridan College, Sports
Injury Management Program, Oakville, Ontario, Canada

Mark Heard, MD, BPE, FRCS(C) [20]
Orthopedic Surgeon, Banff and Canmore, Alberta; Team
Physician, Canadian Alpine Ski Team; and Consultant,
Canadian Free Style Ski Team, Helicopter Skiing, and Alberta
Ski Team, Alberta, Canada

Thomas N. Helm, MD [13]
Assistant Clinical Professor of Dermatology, Buffalo Medical
Group, State University of New York at Buffalo,
Williamsville, New York

Simon Iu, MD [11]
General and Thoracic Surgeon, Willowdale, Ontario, Canada

Don Johnson, MD [17, 37]
Director, Sports Medicine Clinic, Carleton University,
Assistant Professor of Orthopaedic Surgery, University of
Ottawa, Ottawa, Ontario, Canada

Ben Kern [22]
PGA Golf Professional, Brampton, Ontario, Canada

Michael Kondracki, DDS [4]
Toronto, Ontario, Canada

Robert Lee, MD [26]
Waterloo, Ontario, Canada

Scott Livingston, BSc, CAT(C), CSCS [25]
Strength and Conditioning Coach, New York Islanders,
Uniondale, New York

Derek Mackesy, MD [41]
Associate Professor, Dept.of Family Practice, University of
Michigan, Ann Arbor, Orthopaedic Surgery Associates,
Ypsilanti, Michigan

Paul H. Marks, MD, BASc., FRCS(C) [16]
Lecturer, Department of Surgery, University of Toronto,
Head Team Physician & Orthopaedic Surgeon, Toronto
Raptors Basketball Club, NBA, Consulting Orthopaedic
Surgeon, National Women's Team Basketball Canada,
Varsity Blues Intercollegiate Athletics, University of Toronto,
Toronto, Ontario, Canada

Shauna Martiniuk, MD, CCFP [15]
Fellow in Emergency Medicine, University of Toronto,
Toronto, Ontario, Canada

J. Simon McGrail, MD, FRSC(C) [3]
Toronto Wellesley Hospital; Consultant, Ear, Nose, and
Throat, Toronto Maple Leaf Hockey Club, Toronto, Ontario,
Canada; Professional Soccer Player, Burmley, England; and
Team Physician, Hockey Canada, Canada Cups, and World
Hockey Teams

Craig McQueen, MD [31]
HCA St. Mark's Hospital; and Associate Clinical Professor,
University of Utah, Salt Lake City, Utah

Anthony Miniaci, MD [18]
Toronto Western Hospital, Toronto, Ontario, Canada

Lloyd Nesbitt, DPM [40]
North York, Ontario, Canada

Marlene Nobrega, BPT [28]
National Team Therapist, Tennis Canada; The Sports
Medicine Specialists, Toronto, Ontario, Canada

D.J. Ogilvie-Harris, MD, MSc, FRCS(C) [30]
Orthopedic Surgeon, Toronto Hospital; Associate Professor,
Orthopedic Surgery, University of Toronto; Orthopedic
Consultant, Toronto Maple Leaf Hockey Team and National
Ballet of Canada; Director, Sports Medicine Specialists,
Toronto, Ontario, Canada

Robert C. Pashby, MD [2]
Assistant Professor, Department of Ophthalmology, University of Toronto, Hospital for Sick Children; Mount Sinai Hospital, Toronto, Don Mills, Ontario, Canada

Thomas Pashby, MD [2]
Assistant Professor Emeritus, Department of Ophthalmology, University of Toronto; Honorary Consultant, Hospital for Sick Children; and Scarborough Centenary Hospital, Don Mills, Ontario, Canada

Andrew Pipe, MD, FACSM [36]
University of Ottawa Heart Institute, Ottawa Civic Hospital; Associate Professor, Department of Family Medicine, University of Ottawa; Chair, Canadian Centre for Drug-Free Sport, Ottawa, Ontario, Canada

Robert Quinn, MD [23]
Medical Director, Dominican Rehabilitation Center of Santa Cruz, Santa Cruz, California

Douglas W. Richards, MD, Dip.Sport Med. [16]
Medical Director, David L. MacIntosh Sport Medicine Clinic; Assistant Professor, Department of Family and Community Medicine, University of Toronto; Team Physician, Toronto Raptors Basketball Club, NBA, National Women's Basketball Canada; and Varsity Blues Intercollegiate Athletics, Bloor Medical Centre, Toronto, Ontario, Canada

Glen Richardson, MD [9]
Orthopaedic & Sport Medicine Clinic of Nova Scotia, Dalhousie University, Halifax, Nova Scotia, Canada

Joseph Rotella, MS, CAT(C) [32]
Professor and Clinical Therapist, Sheridan College, Sports Injury Management Program, Oakville, Ontario, Canada

Michael L. Schwartz, MD, MSc, FRCS(C) [1]
Professor, University of Toronto; Head, Neurosurgery,
Sunnybrook Hospital, Toronto, Ontario, Canada

Ato Sekyi-Out, MD, FRCS(C) [16]
Clinical Fellow, Orthopaedic Surgery, Department of Surgery,
Faculty of Medicine, University of Toronto, Toronto, Ontario,
Canada

William D. Stanish, MD, FRCS(C), FACS [9, 12]
Director, Orthopaedic & Sport Medicine Clinic of Nova
Scotia; Professor of Surgery, Dalhousie University, Halifax,
Nova Scotia, Canada

Kris D. Stowers, MD [38]
Tallahassee Orthopaedic Clinic, Tallahassee, Florida

Charles H. Tator, MD, PhD, FRCS(C) [1]
Professor and Chairman, Division of Neurosurgery, Toronto
Western Hospital, Toronto, Ontario, Canada

R. Peter Welsh, MD, ChB, FRCS(C), FACS [6, 22]
Associate Professor of Surgery, University of Toronto,
Toronto, Ontario, Canada; Orthopaedic Surgeon, Wakefield
Hospital, Wellington, New Zealand

C. Stewart Wright, MD, FRCS(C) [7]
Assistant Professor of Surgery, University of Toronto,
Orthopaedic and Arthritic Hospital, Toronto, Ontario, Canada

Rick Zarnett, MD, MSc, FRCS(C) [34, 39]
North York, Ontario, Canada

Foreword

Over the past 50 years, there have been significant changes in the practice of medicine, which have totally altered our lifestyles. In the days long past, when poliomyelitis, tuberculosis, and bacterial infections were common, there were relatively few people who were healthy enough to enjoy participating in sport. Along with the virtual elimination of these problems, arthroscopy, or minimally invasive surgery, has evolved and has played a major role in the treatment of joint injuries. Now, sports injuries are a significant part of our medical workload, with increasing numbers of people engaged in recreational and competitive activities for a much longer period of time. Also, our aging population is now physically able to participate in these endeavors. Therefore this handbook of sport injuries is a timely and useful guide to the treatment of sports injuries. It is noteworthy that practically all of the authors who have contributed to the book are recognized throughout the world as experts and leaders in their field. Dr. Bull deserves credit for bringing together such a group of knowledgeable people.

The content and organization of the handbook deserve mention. The first section deals with the injuries that affect each of the different areas of the body (e.g. knee, hand and wrist, dental). The second section deals with problems specific to each sport, and describes not only how to diagnose and treat the injuries, but also how to prevent, or at least minimize the severity of injuries in the various sports. The final section deals with the principles that cover all sporting activities, such as training, the use of drugs, orthotics, braces, and even computers.

This is a most comprehensive handbook and an excellent guide for any practitioner, whether he or she is a specialist or a primary care doctor, as all physicians are now seeing sport injuries in increasing numbers, due to the changing scene in medicine.

Robert W. Jackson, MD, OC, FRCSC
Chief, Department of Orthopaedic Surgery
Baylor University Medical Center
Dallas, Texas

Preface

Society has changed its emphasis on sports from the passive spectator to the active participant. Thus, far more sports injuries are occurring and different overuse complex injuries present themselves to the sports practitioner. There are more sports practitioners in many disciplines and varied ideas as to the ideal treatment.

The purpose of this book is to emphasize a practical approach in the care and prevention of these injuries. Actively practicing clinicians who are involved with specific teams have written each of the following chapters. Each chapter has been a team approach with very involved professionals. I am sure it took more time than they had anticipated, as they had to get together and work on the chapter as a team.

The audience includes the practicing medical clinician, physiotherapist, athletic trainer, and coach. Advanced students should find valuable information in this book. We would like to see a copy of the handbook in the doctor's and therapist's bag. There should be a place for it on the Phys.Ed. teacher's desk and in the team trainer's locker.

This book should give the reader an insight into the cause of the injury and a specific knowledge about the particular sport. Thus, treatment can be tailored to the individual from many different aspects, such as equipment alteration, bracing, exercise, physiotherapy, and when necessary, specific operations.

The first 14 chapters cover systemic anatomic injuries and emphasize the mechanism and physiology. They deal with emergency care and ongoing care of injuries to that area. They allow the practitioner to look up "Sprained Ankle," and spell out the latest management.

The second 17 chapters are written by active team doctors and trainers who are participating in the daily care of specific teams. Thus, there is a lot of practical advice regarding the sports themselves as well as the care of injuries. The practitioner can note the different methods of treating a sprained ankle in ballet dancers and gymnasts. There are guidelines regarding the return to participation and pitfalls.

The final 10 chapters are also written by authorities in the field of sports medicine who have done research or are actively participating in their chosen subjects. They are well illustrated and contain definitions and explanations of tests, weight training, physiotherapy modalities, the doctor's bag, references, groups (CATA, NATA) etc. Thus this book can be used as a quick reference by the family doctor who sees a basketball player with a sprained ankle, or as a resource that can be read from cover to cover. It is readable and it can be enjoyed by all types of sports medicine practitioners.

Acknowledgments

McGraw-Hill Staff especially: Susan Noujaim, Assistant Editor, and Martin Wonsiewicz, Publisher, Health Professions Division, New York; and David Moran, Manager, Medical Division, McGraw-Hill-Ryerson, Ltd. Canada.

Claire Bull, Typist, and Shelagh Bull, Secretary and Assistant.

Staff at the York Clinic, York University, who are always there to answer my questions and the questions of our dedicated patients.

Thanks to the individual authors who have provided me with so many clues over the years, which were incorporated into many chapters as well as their own chapters.

To my father, Alan Bull, M.D., who was one of the original sports medicine docs, and my mother, Mayme Bull, our team manager, secretary/treasurer, chauffeur, and bodyguard.

Finally, Ann Bull, my wife and motivator, who has supplied me with six children, who provided me with my own personal sports medicine lab.

R.Charles Bull, M.D., B.Sc.(MED), FRCS(C)

I | SYSTEMIC INJURIES

1 | Head Injuries and Concussions

Michael L. Schwartz   Charles H. Tator

Athletic injuries are determined by culture and location and vary widely in incidence and cause from one part of the world to another. In the province of Ontario, Canada, head injuries make up approximately 20 percent of all athletic injuries.[1] Motor sports are the most dangerous in this regard and account for more than 25 percent of the head injuries. Only slightly less dangerous is pedal bicycling, which accounts for just under 25 percent. The rest of the injuries occur with participation in a variety of other sports. Because head injuries, even apparently minor ones, are irrevocable and may be so devastating, people who are responsible for the safety of athletes must advocate safe practices and take measures that enhance prevention and the mitigation of brain injuries. They must be familiar with the mechanisms of brain injury and understand the pathophysiologic principles on which treatment is based.

PATHOPHYSIOLOGY

Most head injuries that occur in the context of athletic participation are caused by falls or collisions and, as a result, are blunt injuries. If the head is buttressed and acceleration of the brain is prevented, there is no significant injury to the brain unless a skull fracture occurs and a bone fragment is driven inward. In depressed skull fractures, there may be a focal injury to the underlying brain.

In most head injuries occurring during athletic activity, there is significant acceleration or deceleration imparted to the head. Although the brain floats in the cerebrospinal fluid, which tends to cushion impact, diffuse damage may occur even if the skull and the coverings of the brain are not broached. The brain is made up of delicate interconnected fibers named *axons* that may suffer damage with internal shear strains and distortions of cerebral tissue. There is also a fine network of blood vessels that has developed to satisfy the high metabolic requirement of neurons. Like the axons, these fine blood vessels may be torn easily because there is no tough internal framework to support the brain. As a result, a blow to the head or the impact when the head strikes the ground or other playing surface literally may tear the brain to pieces by the internal shearing forces that are generated on impact. This shearing injury is usually both diffuse and focal. The cranial cavity, because of its irregular shape, tends to limit rotation forces. Greater internal

3

shearing stress in the region of the sphenoid ridge characteristically causes damage to the adjacent frontal and temporal lobes.

Rotational forces of the brain that move it relative to the inner table of the skull may shear veins that conduct blood from the surface of the brain to the major venous sinuses. Under these circumstances, blood is released into the subdural space over the surface of the brain, resulting in a subdural hematoma. Intracranial blood clots also may be produced when a fracture in the temporal or parietal region crosses the middle meningeal artery and blood is released outside the dura to produce an extradural or epidural hematoma. In either case, the patient's level of consciousness declines as the hematoma enlarges, intracranial pressure rises, and the brain is increasingly distorted.

RELATIONSHIP BETWEEN THE LOCATION AND AMOUNT OF BRAIN INJURY AND THE SYMPTOMS AND SIGNS

In examining patients who have suffered head injuries, one must consider two aspects. There is the focal injury that is manifest by the loss of function of the injured part of the brain and the volume of brain diffusely damaged by the effects of deceleration. Injury to the motor strip that is located at the posterior edge of the frontal lobe produces contralateral weakness or paralysis of the arm, leg, or both. For virtually all right-handers and most left-handers, a left posterior frontal injury will interfere with the production of speech. Parietal injuries may cause contralateral impairment of sensation, and occipital injuries may cause hemianopia or loss of vision in one-half the visual field in both eyes. If the focal injury is caused by an indriven bone fragment or another penetrating object and there is no acceleration of the whole brain, there may be no loss of consciousness. On the other hand, there is a large range of severity of possible injury caused by acceleration of the whole brain that is brief and apparently completely reversible at the mild end of the spectrum and which is prolonged or even permanent when severe. Prolonged unconsciousness is invariably followed by measured changes in cognitive function or in overt neurologic signs.

Recent experience suggests that the least severe concussion can occur without any loss of consciousness, although such concussions usually cause a period of amnesia. However, even these concussions are accompanied by some tissue damage, such as tearing of axons. Because concussion is accompanied by subclinical tissue damage, its effect is cumulative and may result in progressive decline of cognitive and motor function when the blows are repeated, as they would be over a long career in boxing, football, or hockey.

THE ADDED EFFECT OF LOSS OF OXYGEN OR LOW BLOOD PRESSURE

Inadequate resuscitation that leads to hypoxia or arterial hypotension may cause inadequate cerebral perfusion and result in a "second injury."[2] Thus the priorities in resuscitation of the fallen athlete are the same as in resuscitation of patients with multiple injuries. The first three priorities are maintenance or establishment of an adequate airway; maintenance or provision of adequate breathing, even by mechanical ventilation if necessary; and maintenance or provision of adequate circulation.

EVALUATION

The person who cares for a fallen athlete must determine rapidly whether there is a condition requiring transfer to a neurosurgical unit, such as a traumatic intracranial hematoma. The probability of significant intracranial bleeding is determined by the mechanism of injury. An equestrian who falls from a horse and strikes his or her head is more likely to harbor an intracranial clot than a hockey player who was stopped by a hard body check and whose head never hit the ice. If the athlete is initially conscious and then his or her level of consciousness declines, or if initially he or she moved all limbs equally but is becoming weak on one side of the body, an expanding intracranial hematoma progressively distorting the brain and raising intracranial pressure should be suspected regardless of the mechanism of injury.

The Glasgow Coma Scale[3] is an essential adjunct in the management of patients with suspected brain injuries. The person evaluating the injured athlete is required to repeat, at intervals, a series of stereotyped observations as described by Teasdale and Jennett. One must determine whether the athlete opens his or her eyes to pain, to voice, or spontaneously; adopts an extensor posture or flexor posture in response to pain, localizes a painful stimulus, or follows simple instructions; or makes no sound, grunts, or answers questions inappropriately or appropriately. Therapeutic decisions may be based on improvement or decline in a 15-point scale.

RESUSCITATION

ABCs of Trauma Management

As stated earlier, the first priorities in resuscitation are *a*irway, *b*reathing, and *c*irculation.[4] In the provision of medical services for an organized athletic competition, there should be a prearranged emergency plan to provide personnel and specific procedures and equipment commensurate with the environmental conditions and the level of competition. A system of communication with local emergency services that can supply support personnel and additional equipment also should be established ahead of time. A physician in attendance at an athletic event should be equipped with a blood pressure cuff and a face mask that can be applied so as to provide positive-pressure ventilation should it be required. The remote possibility of having to intubate a patient or establish a surgical airway has to be considered. It should be decided in advance whether the responsible person will acquire the skills to perform endotracheal intubation or to place an intravenous line. Will a large-bore needle and cannula for emergency cricothyrotomy or a small tracheotomy kit be available? Since there is no blood loss in the vast majority of head injuries in sports, first aid will require maintenance of the airway and ventilation only. With airway and ventilation maintained, athletes who remain unconscious after an injury must be transferred immediately to the emergency department of a hospital with a neurosurgical service.

The Spine

Any person rendered unconscious has been hit hard enough to also have suffered a broken neck and should be treated accordingly. During resuscitation and transport of the unconscious athlete, precautions should be taken to stabilize the cervical spine in an anatomic position. In general, helmets and other protective equipment should only be removed in the hospital setting with gentle inline manual traction applied. Personnel in attendance at North American football or hockey games should be familiar with the disassembly of face masks and helmets and equipped with equipment such as screwdrivers, wire cutters, and bolt cutters. The proper technique requires the participation of several people to maintain gentle inline traction on the neck, support of the occiput, and removal and/or disassembly of the chin strap, mouthpiece, face mask, etc. The reason for these precautions with respect to helmet removal is that extension of the neck occurs when the helmet is removed, especially if the player is wearing shoulder pads, and this may worsen an unstable spinal injury. The design of newer helmets facilitates their removal without manipulation of the neck.

CONCUSSION

When there is significant acceleration of the whole brain, a period of cerebral dysfunction follows the impact. There is a continuum of severity of injury, with increasingly severe acceleration causing more severe signs and symptoms with slower and less complete recovery. Recent experience suggests that even the mildest injuries that cause only brief confusion and no other symptoms are significant. With more violent acceleration, in addition to confusion, there is a period of amnesia. When the most recent events prior to the impact are lost to memory, the phenomenon is called *retrograde amnesia* (RGA). The retrograde amnesia initially may be extensive but tends to shorten as time goes by. It is generally considered to be a less reliable measure of injury severity than the duration of *posttraumatic amnesia* (PTA), the period of memory loss that follows the injury. Some patients may appear normal following a blow to the head, but if questioned later about events surrounding their injury, they may have no recall, even though there was never any loss of consciousness. The mildest form of concussion, where there is confusion only, is termed grade 1 in the recently described Kelly and Rosenberg[5] classification if it lasts less than 15 min and grade 2 if it lasts longer. The original formulation that we derived[6] from the 1986 Cantu classification[7] of sports-related concussion relied on the presence or absence of PTA to assess the severity of concussion. At that time, PTA could only be assessed in retrospect. As a result, we did not allow the athlete to return to the contest in which he or she was injured. Another modification of the original Cantu classification, adopted by the Colorado Medical Society,[8] considers milder injuries causing confusion only and permits return to the game. Amnesia is taken as a criterion of grade 2 severity in the Colorado system.

The Kelly and Rosenberg system permits a real-time evaluation of concussion severity. In their system, concussion should be diagnosed when there is any of the following symptoms or signs: vacant stare, delayed verbal or motor responses, slurred speech, incoordination, distractibility, disorientation, inappropriate behavior, emotional instability, or memory deficit. A short, structured examination of any athlete suspected of having suffered a concussion should be undertaken as follows:

1. Mental status: orientation to person, place, and time.
2. Mental control: repeating short digit strings forward and backward, counting forward and backward, and repeating the months forward and backward.
3. Memory: recalling three words and three objects; recalling details of the game or prominent, current news events.
4. A very brief neurologic examination to detect asymmetry of sensory and motor function and balance should then be done. Visual fields tested by finger or hand movements with the subject facing the examiner are compared with the examiner's

visual fields. Having the athlete extend the arms forward with eyes closed assesses position sense and arm strength. Balance and lower limb function may be evaluated by having the athlete hop a few times on either foot.

Another feature of the Kelly and Rosenberg system is the application of exertional provocative tests. They recommend five push-ups, five sit-ups, five knee bends, and when appropriate, a 40-m sprint. The sprint may be adapted to match the athletic activity, for example, having a hockey player skate up and down the rink. Some athletes, who at rest have become asymptomatic after a concussion, will get headache, unsteadiness, or even a return of cognitive dysfunction after physical exertion. These new or recurrent symptoms probably are evoked by changes in cerebral blood flow induced by changes in cardiac output and systemic blood pressure.

SECOND IMPACT SYNDROME

In a very small number of reported cases, an athlete who had not completely recovered from an earlier concussion suffered a catastrophic outcome after what appeared to be a trivial second blow to the head. These individuals succumbed to a syndrome characterized by immediate, fulminating cerebral edema. The syndrome was given the name *second impact syndrome* by Saunders and Harbaugh.[9] Under normal circumstances, regional cerebral blood flow depends on the metabolic requirements of that particular region and is independent of systemic arterial pressure through a wide range of pressure. This phenomenon is called *autoregulation*.[10] We surmise that the cerebral edema develops as a result of increased cerebral blood flow (CBF) in an injured portion of the brain where autoregulation has been lost. When the arterial pressure is very high and exceeds the limits of autoregulation, for example, in hypertensive encephalopathy, or when the brain is injured and CBF varies with systemic arterial pressure, a sufficient rise in arterial pressure may induce cerebral edema. Physical exercise that sufficiently raises arterial pressure in a subject who has lost autoregulation may produce the headache, unsteadiness, and cognitive dysfunction described earlier that preclude a return to athletic activity or, when coupled with a blow to the head, the second impact syndrome. There is experimental evidence that autoregulation of CBF is restored in a matter of weeks.

RETURN-TO-PLAY GUIDELINES

It should be emphasized that there is no base of prospectively acquired evidence to validate these guidelines. In our view, the most important criterion for determining when it is safe for a player to return to play is the complete return of normal brain function as assessed by examination. A player should not return to training or competition until cognitive function is normal and all symptoms such as headache, unsteadiness, and cognitive dysfunction have subsided at rest and after exertion. Since there is evidence that subclinical permanent damage accumulates as repeated concussions occur, the required period of withdrawal from competition for a second concussion of a particular severity is increased as compared with that after the first. After a first grade 1 concussion, a player can return to the contest if after 20 min he or she is completely symptom free.[11] After a grade 2 concussion, the player is withdrawn from the contest and may play if well for 1 week, after passing an exertional provocative test. A player with a brief (seconds) loss of consciousness (grade 3 concussion) is suspended from play for 1 week but may then play if completely well at rest and after exertion. For a loss of consciousness lasting minutes, the athlete must be out for 2 weeks and pass the exertion test. Any athlete who remains drowsy or unconscious must be transported with appropriate airway protection and breathing and circulatory support to the emergency department of a hospital with a neurosurgical service. Neurosurgical consultation and, when indicated, brain imaging must be obtained. The consultant may wish to obtain a complete neuropsychological assessment of the athlete prior to return to competition. Any bruise (contusion) or blood clot (hematoma) or any other sign of recent trauma on computed tomography (CT) or magnetic resonance imaging (MRI) precludes return to play for the season. For second concussions, we recommend stiffer "penalties" and more stringent "hurdles" to get over, as indicated in Figs. 1-1 and 1-2 (pages 10–11), before return to play.

PREVENTION

Helmets have been of major importance in preventing brain injury in athletes. In certain sports, such as hockey and football, helmet use is mandatory. In these sports, major brain injury has been reduced but certainly not eliminated. Major brain injuries still occur in helmeted athletes, and repeated minor brain injuries, with their

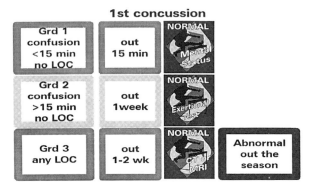

FIG. 1-1 The definitions of the grades[5] of severity of concussion are indicated in the left-hand column. Confusion only, without loss of consciousness (LOC), lasting less than 15 min is the least severe grade. Confusion lasting longer than 15 min is intermediate, and any loss of consciousness is considered the most severe grade. Column 2 indicates the "penalties" for a first concussion of the grades in column 1. Column 3 shows the "hurdle" that the athlete must get over to return to play. An athlete is sidelined for a minimum of 15 min but may return to play after a grade 1 concussion if his or her mental status returns completely to normal. If confusion persists for more than 15 min (grade 2), then the athlete is withdrawn from the contest but may return to competition on another day if the mental status is normal and the provocative exertional test evokes no symptoms. For grade 3 concussion lasting seconds, the athlete must be out 1 week and may return if completely normal. Neuroimaging and neurosurgical consultation are at the discretion of the treating physician. For more prolonged loss of consciousness, the athlete is sidelined for a minimum of 2 weeks, and neurosurgical consultation and possibly neuroimaging are advisable. Regardless of concussion grade, a contusion, hematoma, or any other sign of recent trauma on CT scan or MRI precludes return to play for the season.

cumulative and potentially irreversible effects, can occur in helmeted players. In other sports, such as competitive skiing, helmets may not be mandatory but are strongly recommended for all age groups. Bicyclists and equestrians of all ages should wear helmets. Helmets should be fitted properly, in good condition, and certified by one of the recognized testing associations such as the Canadian Standards Association, and the helmet strap must be secured.

Prevention should be a concern of all those involved in sports, including individual players and participants, parents, league officials, referees, coaches, and trainers. Respect for the opponent

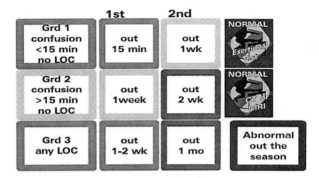

	1st	**2nd**	
Grd 1 **confusion** **<15 min** **no LOC**	**out** **15 min**	**out** **1wk**	NORMAL *Exertional*
Grd 2 **confusion** **>15 min** **no LOC**	**out** **1week**	**out** **2 wk**	NORMAL *CT or MRI*
Grd 3 **any LOC**	**out** **1-2 wk**	**out** **1 mo**	**Abnormal** **out the** **season**

FIG. 1-2   The definitions of the grades[5] of severity of concussion are indicated in the left-hand column. The "penalties," i.e., the required time out of competition after a first concussion, are indicated in column 2. In recognition of the cumulative effect of repeated concussions, the increased time of withdrawal from play for a second concussion is indicated in column 3. For example, after two grade 1 concussions suffered in the same contest, an athlete is withdrawn from competition and must not return for at least 1 week. The "hurdle" to get over prior to return to play is a symptom-free week, a normal mental status, and a normal provocative exertional test. Similarly, the "penalty" for two grade 2 concussions is a minimum of 2 weeks. The return-to-play "hurdle" is 2 symptom-free weeks, a normal mental status, and a normal provocative exertional test. Neurosurgical consultation and neuroimaging are advisable for any persistent symptoms. More than one grade 3 concussion requires withdrawal from play for at least 1 month. The return-to-play "hurdle" is 1 symptom-free month, a normal mental status, and a normal provocative exertional test. Neurosurgical consultation and neuroimaging are advised. Any persistent symptom at rest or after exertion precludes return to play. Regardless of concussion grade, a contusion, hematoma, or any other sign of recent trauma on CT scan or MRI precludes return to play for the season.

and the opponent's long-term health must be part of the psychology of competitive sports. In some sports, concussions could be reduced by eliminating fighting. Athletes should be ambassadors and supporters of brain injury prevention programs such as Think First.

REFERENCES

1. Tator CH, Edmonds V, Lapczak L: Analysis of 1594 cases of catastrophic injuries in sports and recreation with a view to prevention. *Can J Neurol Sci* 23(suppl 1):S31, 1996.

 2. Chesnut RM, Marshall LF, Klauber MR, et al: The role of secondary brain injury in determining outcome from severe head injury. *J Trauma* 34:216–222, 1993.

 3. Teasdale G, Jennett B: Assessment of impaired consciousness: A practical scale. *Lancet* 2:81–84, 1974.

 4. Committee on Trauma, American College of Surgeons: *Advanced Trauma Life Support Instructor Manual.* Chicago, American College of Surgeons, 1994.

 5. Kelly JP, Rosenberg JH: Diagnosis and management of concussion in sports. *Neurology* 48:575–580, 1997.

 6. Schwartz ML, Tator CH: Head injuries in athletics, in Harries M, Williams C, Stanish WD, Micheli LJ (eds): *Oxford Textbook of Sports Medicine.* New York, Oxford University Press, 1994, pp 698–705.

 7. Cantu RC: Guidelines for return to contact sports after a cerebral concussion. *Phys Sports Med* 14:75–83, 1986.

 8. Report of the Sports Medicine Committee: *Guidelines for the Management of Concussion in Sports.* Colorado Medical Society, Denver, 1990 (revised 1991).

 9. Saunders RL, Harbaugh RE: The second impact in catastrophic contact-sports head trauma. *JAMA* 252:538–539, 1984.

10. Lewelt W, Jenkins LW, Miller JD: Autoregulation of cerebral blood flow after experimental fluid percussion injury of the brain. *J Neurosurg* 53: 500–511, 1980.

11. Report of the Quality Standards Subcommittee: Practice parameter: The management of concussion in sports (summary statement). *Neurology* 48: 581–585, 1997.

2 | Eye Injuries and Eye Protection

Robert C. Pashby   Thomas J. Pashby

Although the eyes only account for 0.1 percent of the erect frontal silhouette, they account for 1 percent of sports injuries. An eye injury can end the career of a professional athlete and destroy the lifestyle and earning power of others. More than 90 percent of sports eye injuries are preventable, as proven in hockey, racquet sports, and paintball games.

Prevention is the key. Injured participants must be advised of the availability and need for protective eyewear. Tabulation of sports eye injuries is necessary to identify activities causing injury so that protective measures can be undertaken. Standards for protective equipment are essential. In Canada over the past 25 years, 4449 sports eye injuries have been reported by members of the Canadian Ophthalmological Society (COS), including 512 legally blind eyes. Dr. Paul Vinger, from Boston, in *Duane's Clinical Ophthalmology*, writes: "In 1980 U.S. dollars, the hockey face protector saves society $10,000,000 a year by preventing approximately 70,000 eye and face injuries in 1.2 million protected players."[1] Table 2-1 lists the sports causing the most eye injuries in various countries.

ASSESSING AN EYE INJURY

When an eye injury presents, a minimum amount of equipment should be in the hands of team physicians and trainers. This equipment should include a vision card, a penlight, sterile fluorescein strips, sterile eye pads, eye shields, tape, sterile cotton-tipped swabs, and sterile irrigation solution.

Injuries can be segregated into three groups:

1. Injuries that can be treated and the participant returned to action
2. Injuries that must be referred to an ophthalmologist but not on an emergency basis
3. Players that must be treated immediately and immediately sent to hospital for ophthalmologic care.

A routine eye examination must be made to determine the seriousness of the injury. The penlight is used to obtain an oblique illumination of the eye that will indicate damage to the conjunctiva, the cornea, the anterior chamber, the pupil, and the lens (Fig. 2-1).

The procedure to follow in eye examination is

1. Inspect the lids and brow for lacerations, bruising, and hematoma.

TABLE 2-1　The Sport Causing the Most Eye Injuries in
Various Countries

Country	Sport Causing Most Eye Injuries
Australia	Cricket
Canada	Hockey
England	Squash
Holland	Soccer
Ireland	Hurling
Japan	Baseball
New Zealand	Squash
Portugal	Soccer
Switzerland	Hockey
Sweden	Hockey
United States	Basketball
The Far East	Badminton

2. Look in the conjunctival sac for hemorrhage, lacerations, and
   foreign bodies. Evert the upper eyelid by using a cotton-tipped
   swab as a fulcrum at the superior tarsal border (8 mm from the
   lashes) and gently pulling the lashes out and up to expose a foreign body that can easily be brushed away. Such foreign bodies
   often lodge just inside the upper inner lid margin.
3. Examine the cornea for any foreign body, abrasion, or laceration. Abrasions are well outlined with fluorescein dye, which
   can be applied by pulling the lower lid downward and dipping

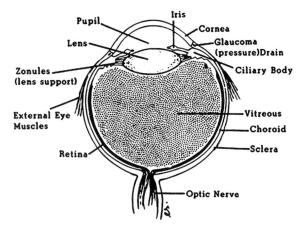

FIG. 2-1　Cross section of an eye.

tentially rather severe injury because it entails hemorrhaging into e anterior chamber of the eye. The person rendering first aid must e familiar with the appearance of a hyphema. A hyphema first appears as a haze in the anterior chamber (the area between the cornea nd the iris-lens diaphragm) (see Fig. 2-1). The iris appears somewhat muddy in color compared with the fellow eye, and the pupil is usually irregular in shape and sluggish in reaction to light. Vision is somewhat or extremely blurred. With rest, the blood usually settles down to form a level in the anterior chamber unless bleeding continues, in which case blood fills the anterior chamber to create a black "eight-ball" eye. Most hyphemas clear in a few days, but in about 15 percent of patients a secondary hemorrhage may occur usually between the second and fifth days after the initial injury. For this reason, all hyphemas demand ophthalmologic care and advice.

At this time, treatment continues to be controversial; bed rest and even hospitalization for children may be required. Aspirin (not used much at this time) or any drug that might cause further bleeding must be avoided. The blood usually settles down to form a level in the anterior chamber and absorbs in a matter of 5 or 6 days depending on the amount. The use of clot-lysing agents still remains controversial, and if the patient has increased risk factors, such as sickle cell disease, extra caution is needed in their use.

Secondary glaucoma and blood staining of the cornea are worrisome complications of hyphema and may result in prolonged or permanent disability. Antiglaucoma medical therapy and even surgical intervention may be necessary by the ophthalmologist to remove the blood and reduce the intraocular pressure.

Other Intraocular Injuries

Injuries to the posterior segment of the eye (see Fig. 2-1) are also common, occurring in 23 percent of reported patients in our study.

Choroidal Injuries

Choroidal injuries may result when a contrecoup force from a blow by a blunt object in the front of the eye produces a wave of pressure that forces the choroid against the sclera. A split may occur, and if this split involves the macular area, visual acuity is markedly reduced in the injured eye (see Fig. 2-1).

Choroidal hemorrhages may occur without rupture. Such hemorrhages may result in necrosis of the choroid and retina in that area. There is no specific treatment for those injuries, but they should be followed by an ophthalmologist.

Macular Injuries

Macular swelling often follows severe concussion of the globe with contrecoup force. Central vision is seriously affected. The macular a sterile fluorescein strip into the pool of tears in the lower fornix.

4. Assess the clarity and depth of the anterior chamber, and compare with the other eye.
5. Compare the size, shape, and light reaction of the pupil in the injured eye with the fellow eye.
6. Compare the iris colors of each eye.
7. Test the visual acuity using a reading card or a newspaper, and compare it with that of the uninjured eye. One should know the patient's vision in each eye with glasses or contact lenses before injury. If the vision after injury is less than 20/40, refer the patient to an ophthalmologist.
8. Test peripheral vision by the confrontation method. Have the patient fix on the examiner's nose, and after occluding the other eye, have the patient identify the number of fingers held up in all fields of gaze. A normal minimal visual field extends 85 degrees temporally, 65 degrees downward, 60 degrees nasally, and 45 degrees upward. Any loss of peripheral field must be referred for specialist's care immediately.
9. Assess the movements of the eye by asking the patient to look to the right, then up, then down. Similarly, look to the left, up, and down. These are the cardinal positions of gaze. Both eyes moving together should create no double vision when a light is held in the primary position and the six cardinal positions of gaze. Any double vision must be referred for ophthalmologic care.
10. Looking at the eyes, determine whether the injured eye is sunken (enophthalmos), making the palpebral aperture narrower, or proptosed (exophthalmos), in which case the aperture will be enlarged. A fracture of the orbital floor results in a sunken eye, whereas a retrobulbar hemorrhage causes a pushing forward of the eye. Of note in children, orbital floor fractures usually present with no ecchymosis, proptosis, or conjunctival hemorrhage, i.e., a quiet white eye, whereas adults are just the opposite.

One should be very careful not to force open an injured eye. If in doubt, it is better to apply a sterile pad and have the patient seen by an ophthalmologist. An exception to this is the case of a chemical burn, which demands immediate treatment by forcibly opening the eye, removing any particles, irrigating the eye with at least a liter of water, soda pop, or Gatorade, and then transporting patient to hospital with the eye uncovered.

In summary, injuries that can be treated immediately and the participant allowed to return to play include hematomas around the eye provided the eye functions normally, soft tissue injuries that can be sutured provided there is no loss of visual function and no lid margin involvement, and foreign bodies on the conjunctiva and cornea easily brushed off with no resulting visual complaints. Injuries that must be referred for ophthalmologic care are those causing loss of vision whether centrally or peripherally, discoloration of the iris, cloudiness of the anterior chamber, sluggish pupillary reaction to light, inequality of the pupils, diplopia in any field of gaze, a sunken or proptosed eye, or a painful eye. *If in doubt, refer to an ophthalmologist*!

TYPES OF EYE INJURIES AND THEIR MANAGEMENT

The percentages and types of 4400 serious injuries reported by Canadian Ophthalmological Society (COS) members are listed in Table 2-2. Of the total reported, 11.5 percent resulted in a legally blind eye. This seems a rather high percentage, but these injuries were those reported only by ophthalmologists and hence needed ophthalmologic care.

Soft Tissue Injuries

Orbital Hemorrhage

Orbital hemorrhages, or "black eyes," usually occur after blunt trauma to the orbital region. Proptosis of the eye may occur, and if severe, the eye is pushed forward out of the socket by hemorrhage into the orbit (the area behind the eye) and restricts ocular movements. If this retrobulbar hemorrhage is severe, the vascular supply to the optic nerve and retina may be interfered with, and this rarely results in visual loss. It is therefore urgent that ophthalmologic care be sought immediately. During transport, an ice pack should be applied and the head kept elevated.

Any soft tissue lid injury is not easily assessed before extreme swelling ensues, which can preclude a proper examination of the globe. Such an examination includes visual acuity and fields; pupillary size, shape, and reaction; iris color; and tests for double vision. Any foreign body in the eye must be identified and removed.

TABLE 2-2 Serious Eye Injuries

Type of Injuries	Percentage
Soft tissue	34
Hyphemas	27
Other intraocular injuries	23
Corneal injuries	9
Orbital fractures	4
Ruptured globes	3

Lid Lacerations

Lid lacerations may be caused by sharp objects, blunt tr
objects that catch the lid and actually tear it. Bleeding is co
by direct pressure, allowing the extent of the laceration to
sessed. Lacerations through the lid margin require met
surgical repair for proper cosmetic and functional results. L
tions or punctures of the upper or lower lids should be repair
an ophthalmologist, who will make anatomic closure of muscle
skin layers. A sterile eye pad should be applied prior to transpo
control bleeding and prevent infection.

Lacerations of the Lacrimal Apparatus

Medial lacerations of the upper or lower lid usually involve th
lacrimal drainage system. The canalicular laceration is best repaired by an ophthalmologist using a microscope. Rather than
simply repairing the lid laceration, refer the patient for canalicular
and lid laceration repair immediately.

In the case of severe eyelid trauma, the eyelids may become
disinserted from their attachment to the medial or lateral orbital
margins, causing a rounded appearance at the lateral canthus or a
widened appearance medially. Reattachment of the ligaments to
bone is necessary for good functional and cosmetic results. With lid
lacerations, as with any wound, control of bleeding (usually not severe) with sterile gauze is essential, and assessment of the globe
damage and visual function should be carried out before application of a sterile eye pad and transport for ophthalmologic care.
Tetanus prophylaxis is recommended as in any laceration. Moreover, a record should be kept of visual acuity, peripheral fields, and
presence or absence of diplopia, etc.

Conjunctival Injuries

In minor lacerations, suturing is not necessary. A search for foreign
bodies (as described previously), with removal, must be carried out,
antibiotic drops applied, and follow-up examination made in 24 h.
Foreign bodies often lodge just under the margin of the upper eyelid. Eversion of the eyelid (see above) will reveal their presence;
removal is achieved by wiping with a moist cotton-tipped swab.
The first aid attendant should be familiar with the procedure of
everting the upper eyelid. After removal of the foreign body, the
player usually can return to play.

Hyphema (Bleeding into the Anterior Chamber)

More than 1200 hyphemas have been reported associated with
sports injuries over the past 25 years. Hyphema is a common yet

swelling may result in the formation of a macular cyst that may rupture, causing a macular hole and potentially permanent visual impairment. At the present time, macular hole surgery may allow some hope for restored vision.

Retinal Injuries

Hemorrhages in the retina frequently follow blunt injuries to the eye. They are not incapacitating or noted unless they occur in the macular area. Retinal tears are not uncommon and may lead to retinal detachment. Detachment also may occur at the far periphery of the retina, the ora (the retina's most anterior attachment), and result in a dialysis of the ora. Early recognition and treatment of the tears and holes often will prevent retinal detachment. For this reason, eye injuries of even moderate degree deserve ophthalmoscopic examination. Testing of peripheral field may reveal the presence of a retinal detachment by the confrontation method described previously.

Detachments of the retina require immediate assessment and treatment. If the detachment is allowed to progress, as most do, to involve the macular area, normal central vision cannot be restored even though the retina is reattached successfully. Any loss of visual acuity accompanied by loss of field suggests retinal detachment. Follow-up examination is necessary, and the patient must be warned to report any loss of visual field. Over one-third of retinal detachments due to contusion are sports related. Successful recovery depends on early discovery and treatment by the ophthalmologist.

Rupture and Avulsion of the Optic Nerve

A severe direct blunt injury to the eye may rupture the optic nerve at its connection to the eye. One injury, seen by us, resulted in immediate blindness to an eye kicked by a boot. This is an unusual but very sickening injury for which there is no chance of visual recovery. The vision is totally absent in the injured eye (i.e., no light perception).

Corneal Injuries

Corneal injuries may cause lacrimation, photophobia, and blepharospasm. In all, there is sudden onset of sharp pain. Foreign bodies, if superficial, can be brushed off using a moist sterile cotton-tipped swab if they cannot be irrigated off using sterile irrigating solution. If not easily removed, a sterile eye pad should be applied and the patient referred for ophthalmologic care using the slit lamp and a sterile needle or spud. After removal of the foreign body, a topical antibiotic and a firm eye pad usually are applied for 24 h, at which time a follow-up examination is carried out.

Corneal abrasions produce similar symptoms and can be outlined with fluorescein, which stains the denuded epithelial area green, as seen with a cobalt blue filter. After determining that no other eye problem exists, a sterile eye pad is usually applied for 24 h, when a follow-up examination is done.

Corneal penetrating injuries are accompanied by severe pain with tearing, photophobia, and blepharospasm. If the eye can be opened easily, the pupil will be seen to be irregular, pointing to the area of laceration as the iris plugs the wound; the anterior chamber will seem shallow; and the iris will be adherent to or prolapsed outside the wound. If history suggests a potential penetrating injury, do not open the lids forcibly because this may cause further damage. Immediate ophthalmologic treatment is necessary. A sterile eye pad and shield should be gently taped in place; if these are not available, the bottom third of a disposable coffee or pop cup can be used as a shield and the patient transported to hospital for ophthalmologic assessment and repair.

In case of corneal injury or any other intraocular injury, if possible, a record must be kept of visual acuity, fields of vision, and diplopia (if present).

Injuries to the Lens

The lens can be injured by blunt trauma causing concussion that results in cataract formation. This may occur immediately or after a few days, weeks, or even months. In mild cases, the iris is driven forcibly against the anterior lens capsule, leaving a circular mark like that of a rubber stamp on the anterior lens capsule. This is readily seen as the pupil dilates. As a rule, this type of blow does not lead to cataract formation.

More severe blows rarely can cause a rupture of the lens capsule, allowing aqueous humor (the clear fluid in the anterior chamber of the eye) to enter and causing the lens to become opaque (see Fig. 2-1). Localized cataracts may develop after a blow without capsular rupture. Such opacities often take the form of a rosette in the subcapsular area of the lens. Blunt injury may cause the lens zonules, the fibers that support the lens in the eye, to rupture so that the lens loses its moorings. If all the zonules rupture, the lens becomes dislocated and may disappear back into the vitreous or even migrate forward to appear in the anterior chamber. If only some of the zonules rupture, subluxation occurs, and the lens may shift away from its central location.

Treatment of cataracts entails removal of the cataractous portion of the lens and restoration of visual function with an intraocular or contact lens. Some professional athletes have continued their careers under these circumstances. Direct injuries to the lens by penetrating wounds of the cornea are not uncommon. The cataractous lens material is removed at the time of corneal repair. Injuries to the lens must be recognized by the person rendering first aid and referred for ophthalmologic care. Decreased vision and pupillary and anterior chamber changes must be recognized (see Fig. 2-1).

Traumatic Glaucoma

Following blunt injury to the eye, the intraocular pressure may rise and fall, swinging between hypertension and hypotension for a few days before settling back to normal. In such cases there is usually no permanent structural damage within the eye. However, blunt injury may damage the anterior chamber angle, resulting in a split of the ciliary body with deepening of the angle and interference with aqueous outflow (see Fig. 2-1). Glaucoma develops in 10 percent of patients with split angle; it may occur soon after injury or even many years later. Problems of this type should be followed by an ophthalmologist, who can monitor intraocular tensions, because the development of glaucoma is usually insidious, causing damage to the optic nerve without the patient being aware of anything happening. Any loss of peripheral vision (field loss) resulting from glaucoma cannot be restored. A dislocated lens is another cause of secondary glaucoma. In this case it is necessary to remove the lens for control of intraocular pressure.

Secondary glaucoma is not uncommon with hyphema, especially with secondary hemorrhages. Irrigation of the anterior chamber and removal of the blood clot may be indicated if the intraocular pressure cannot be adequately controlled medically (i.e., with drugs). Should the intraocular pressure remain high with blood in the anterior chamber, not only is the optic nerve in danger, but blood staining of the cornea may occur. Even when the intraocular pressure is controlled, the blood staining rarely may remain, often taking years to absorb.

Orbital Fractures

There are two theories of orbital floor fracture. The first suggests that with blunt trauma the pressure within the orbit increases sufficiently to cause the "weak point," the orbital floor, to fracture and "decompress" into the maxillary sinus. The second theory, probably more likely, especially in children, is that the inferior orbital rim is pushed posteriorly, causing a buckling of the orbital floor bones and a "trapdoor" fracture with or without entrapment of tissues, including the inferior rectus muscle. Subsequently, limitation of ocular movement, especially on elevation, will ensue. Diplopia is commonly present, more marked on upward or downward gaze.

Ophthalmologic examination of the globe and investigation of the fracture with x-rays and computed tomography (CT), notably coronal views, are necessary, but not on an emergency basis. In addition, it may be necessary to free the entrapped muscle and insert a support along the orbital floor to cover the fracture.

Additional orbital fractures may occur in the maxilla or other portions of the orbital rim. They often can be recognized by direct palpation, an appropriate x-ray, and clinical evaluation. Fractures of the roof with potential cerebrospinal fluid leak necessitate neurosurgical assessment, with the ophthalmologist in the secondary position.

Fracture into any of the sinuses may leak air into the orbital cavity, producing crepitus (a crackling sound) when finger pressure is applied on the swollen area. The air and fracture are usually readily demonstrated on x-ray. Resolution without surgical intervention is usual unless a muscle is trapped. Systemic antibiotics are used often because a sinus cavity has direct connection with the orbit.

Ruptured Globe

Ruptured globes usually result from contact with an object such as a hockey stick or puck, a golf ball or club, a ski tip, a squash ball or racquet, a tennis ball, or a baseball. They are usually caused by high-velocity, low-mass missiles. Rupture also can occur when a slower-moving, high-mass object, such as a fist or large ball, strikes the eye with a glancing blow. This type of rupture usually occurs near the limbus, where the sclera is thinnest. Unfortunately, most of these injuries result in enucleation. A direct blow on the front of the cornea by an object larger than the orbital opening is more likely to produce a blowout fracture.

When ruptured, the globe often will appear soft or collapsed or sunken in the orbit. Such an eye must be gently covered with a sterile eye pad and shield, and the patient must be transported directly to hospital for ophthalmologic assessment and repair.

CONTACT LENSES

Because spectacles may present a problem when playing contact sports, many athletes in hockey, football, baseball, and other sports have found that contact lenses, when correction of refracting errors is necessary, are the answer to their problem. Historically, in the 1940s, large scleral contact lenses were custom made for proper fit and rested on the sclera. The central dome cleared the cornea and contained the refraction correction.

In the late 1940s, a young hockey player, future Hall of Famer, National Hockey League, Toronto Maple Leaf Tim Horton, turning professional, needed corrective glasses. Scleral contact lenses were fitted that were filled with normal saline solution and inserted underneath the lids to cover the front of the eyes. In the first preseason hockey game, Horton engaged in a fight with another player, and this caused concern. However, no damage occurred, and Horton continued to wear his contacts. The balanced salt solution in the contacts clouded over during play and had to be replaced with fresh normal saline between periods.

In the 1950s, hard corneal lenses became available. They were easier to fit and to insert but also more easily displaced after a blow. They might migrate off the cornea into the lower fornix or more commonly up under the upper lid. The displaced lens could be removed by irrigating the eye with sterile eye solution or could be lifted off by applying a small suction cup. We have seen a hard contact split in two halves from a blow in a hockey game with resulting corneal abrasion but, fortunately, no permanent visual defect. Both halves were found in the fornix and preserved as a trophy. At times, small foreign bodies could becomes trapped under these hard contacts, scratching the cornea, causing much pain, and preventing continuation of play.

In the 1960s, soft contact lenses became available. They were more comfortable but more fragile and required nightly disinfection and cleaning to prevent possible bacterial or fungal growth. They did not dislocate easily from the cornea and sealed out foreign bodies because of their larger size and snug-fitting edge. There was no spectacle blur on switching to regular glasses, as had commonly been the case with hard contacts. Soft contacts usually were replaced every 6 to 12 months because of the buildup of tear deposits.

Subsequently, a wide range of soft "hydrophilic" lens materials became available with higher water content and greater oxygen permeability. The very thin, high-water contact lenses were approved for extended wear, but ophthalmic experience showed that this regime could lead to a substantial increase in ocular infections.

Recently, disposable soft contact lenses have become available. They are available in powers up to 9 diopters of myopia and will compensate for up to 2 diopters of astigmatism. Because of their high water content, they are generally comfortable, and because they are discarded after 1 week of wear, there is less chance of a problem with protein deposits on the lens.

The advantage of contact lenses over regular glasses is an improved peripheral field of vision, less tendency to be displaced, and no fogging. It must be stressed, however, that they provide no protection against injury. Safety glasses or other types of eye protection must be worn where indicated.

PREVENTION

The old saying "prevention is better than a cure" sums up what has been proven in the effort toward the prevention of sports eye injuries, particularly in hockey, racquet sports, and war games. Paul Vinger, in *Duane's Clinical Ophthalmology*, writes: "Injury is probably the most unrecognized major health problem facing the nations today." He further states the impossibility of injury reduction without knowledge of injury incidence and severity.

In Canada since 1972, sports eye injuries have been reported by members of the Canadian Ophthalmological Society (COS). The data to date are listed in Table 2-3.

Hockey

Hockey is the sport causing most eye injuries in Canada, Sweden, and Switzerland. In Canada, 1860 hockey eye injuries were reported, including 298 legally blind eyes. Of the 298 blind eyes reported, none were suffered by players wearing Canadian Standards Association (CSA)–certified full face protectors, but 7 were suffered by players wearing CSA-certified half-shields (visors).

In the preprotector season (1974–1975), 258 eye injuries were recorded, including 43 blind eyes. This season to date (1996–1997), 12 hockey eye injuries have been recorded, including 3 blind eyes.

Because the face protectors available in 1972 were unsafe (the hockey stick blade could penetrate the wire mesh mask immediately over the eye areas), a standard was needed to eliminate unsafe products. A CSA standard was published, manufacturers produced safe products, the Canadian Hockey Association (CHA) demanded that all minor league players to wear CSA-certified protectors, and the Canadian government ruled that only certified protectors could be imported into or sold in Canada (see Fig. 2-2).

The percentage of hockey eye injuries treated at the Hospital for Sick Children in Toronto decreased from 11 percent in 1973 to 3 percent in 1978—a gratifying decrease. If all hockey players wear

TABLE 2-3 Sports Eye Injuries in Canada, 1972–1997

Sport	Years	Injuries	Blind Eyes
Hockey	23	1860	298
Racquet sports	21	1099	47
Baseball	21	490	31
Ball hockey	21	371	33
Football	21	189	9
War games	13	75	32
Golf	21	61	19
Basketball	21	48	1
Skiing (water and snow)	21	39	11
Volleyball	21	28	4
Lacrosse	21	19	0
Guns (BB)	21	19	4
Snowmobiling	21	11	5
Other sports	21	115	16
TOTAL		4424	510

CSA-certified protectors, and wear them properly, hockey eye injuries will cease to be a concern.

Racquet Sports

Over the past 10 years (1987–1997), the number of injuries reported in racquetball players has been greater than those reported in hockey players; in fact, 322 racquet sports eye injuries have been recorded compared with 282 hockey eye injuries. Racquet sports are presently the leading cause of sports eye injuries worldwide. Squash, racquetball, tennis, and badminton are included in our study.

Dr. Michael Easterbrook, of Toronto, discovered in the late 1970s that 17 percent of eye injuries reported in racquet sports were suffered by players wearing an open-type eye protector, one they had purchased believing that they were protected when, in fact, they were not. Subsequently, in 1982, a CSA standard for racquet sports eye protectors was published, and most racquetball and squash players began to wear CSA-certified protectors. Now badminton players, not wearing protectors, account for more racquet sports eye injuries than squash, racquetball, and tennis players combined (Table 2-4).

Of interest, the CSA-certified face protectors with polycarbonate lenses in a sturdy frame give protection from ball contact with the eye of the headform at speeds of 90 miles per hour.

TABLE 2-4 Racquet Sports Eye Injuries in Canada, 1976–1997 (1106 Injuries, 47 Blind Eyes)

Year	No. of Injuries	Racquetball and Squash (%)	Badminton (%)	Tennis (%)
1982[a]	90	73	13	14
1983	87	59	22	19
1984	115	58	16	26
1985	82	50	33	17
1986	83	39	33	28
1987	68	36	38	26
1988	46	39	46	15
1989	62	35	47	18
1990	40	35	55	10
1991	35	23	40	37
1992	33	24	52	24
1993	31	23	55	22
1994	27	26	56	18
1995	14	28	58	14
1996	19	21	68	11
1997	18	17	66	17

[a]CSA standard published.

Baseball

While baseball is the third leading eye injury sport in Canada, it is the leader in Japan and was the leader in the United States until recently overtaken by basketball. Of the 490 reported eye injuries in Canada, 31 were blinding injuries, and 90 percent of the injured players were injured by the baseball.

An American Standard for Testing and Materials (ASTM) standard for baseball face protectors has been established in the United States and gives protection with contact of the ball at speeds of 70 miles per hour. These protectors, made of polycarbonate or wire, are firmly attached to the batting helmet and are commonly worn in "Little League" baseball programs throughout the United States.

Ball Hockey

Ball hockey is a common sport in Canada, played on the streets and in school yards throughout the country. A ball, often an old tennis ball, is slapped at great speed with a hockey stick toward the net. To date (1997), Canadian records total 371 ball hockey eye injuries, including 33 blind eyes. Most blinding injuries are suffered by goaltenders not wearing eye or face protectors. They wear leg pads, belly pads, and goaltender gloves and hold a stick, but unfortunately, they usually have no protection above the neck. Ball hockey goalie masks are readily available and must be worn.

Soccer

Soccer is noted as causing the most sports eye injuries both in Holland and in Portugal. Fingers, elbows, and the ball are the usual injuring weapons. An underinflated ball can cause severe eye injury on contact.

Football

Many American football linemen are now attaching polycarbonate shields to the bars of their face protectors to prevent injury, mostly by opponents' fingers. In Canada, soccer and American football together have accounted for 189 reported eye injuries, including 9 blind eyes.

War Games (Paintball Games)

These games originated in New Hampshire in 1981 and by 1984 became popular in Canada, where 26 eye injuries were reported, including 14 blind eyes. To date (1997), 75 reported injuries have been recorded in Canada, including 32 blind eyes. None of the blind eyes were suffered by a player wearing appropriate eye protection.

Paintball games are usually comprised of two teams of 25 to 50 players in a playing field, and players are equipped with repeater guns with a carbon dioxide–powered muzzle capacity of 250 feet per second. The gun fires 14-mm colored gelatin bullets. When struck by a bullet, the opponent is "dead" and out of play.

Eye injuries occur when the eye protectors provided are not worn, either taken off because they are dirty or brushed off by trees or bushes. Dr. Paul Vinger, of Boston, has impacted paintballs on pigs' eyes. The eyes ruptured when fired on from a distance of 4 m. Dr. Vinger has been instrumental in establishment of the ASTM standard for paintball game eye protectors. Protectors must be worn by everyone in the environment of the games at all times, whether a participant or not. Eye injuries can be prevented.

Golf

Golf balls travel at speeds of up to 200 miles per hour with a club head speed up to 150 miles per hour. In 20 years (1960–1980), Dr. Vinger, at the Massachusetts Eye and Ear Infirmary in Boston, reports 8 eyes enucleated because of golf ball injuries and 3 eyes enucleated because of club head contact.

As a precaution, one-eyed golfers always should wear polycarbonate-lensed spectacles whether prescription or not. Golf eye injuries continue to occur even though it is a sport not highly associated with eye injury.

In Canada over the past 21 years, 61 eye injuries, including 19 blind eyes, have been reported. Some injuries have been club induced, but the majority are caused by a ball, often a ricochet from trees. Certainly one should never look to see who has called "fore."

Basketball

Basketball is presently the number one sport causing sport eye injuries in the United States, whereas in Canada it accounts for only 1 percent, likely due to the number of participants. One in 10 college basketball players in the United States (10 percent) sustains an eye injury each year, mostly corneal abrasions caused by fingers and elbows. Many players are now, wisely, wearing certified racquet sports eye protectors.

Skiing

Both snow and water skiers can suffer eye injuries. In fact, 39 such injuries have been recorded in Canada, including 11 blind eyes, caused by skis, ski poles, and even the ski lift. The types of eye injuries include corneal abrasions to cross-country skiers and ski pole injuries to both cross-country and downhill skiers. "Snow blindness" is also a concern; ultraviolet light–absorbing polycarbonate goggles should be worn. Water skiers must be aware of the ski tip when falling and a fellow skier's rope handle when he or she drops off. The boat driver and observer also must be alert to the skier's rope handle as it ricochets from the water.

Snowmobiling

Five blinding injuries among the 11 injuries reported by COS members resulted from contact with wire fences, tree branches, and the breaking or fracturing of nonpolycarbonate lensed goggles that shattered. Care must be taken on starting a dead machine battery. The proper way to connect battery cables when trying to recharge a discharged battery is available in the information book accompanying each machine.

Boxing

In Canada, boxing eye injuries have not been a serious problem; very few have been reported. Dr. Albert Cheskes, of Toronto, however, examined boxers for the local boxing commission and found several eye problems neither reported nor treated. Boxers may come from other areas seeking money for bouts, under assumed names, even if suspended in other areas.

In the United States, serious recorded boxing eye injuries also are few. There, also, boxers tend not to seek care because such injuries are considered part of the game. Even loss of vision in one eye may not be reported for fear of disqualification and loss of income.

Dr. Paul Vinger, in *Duane's Clinical Ophthalmology*,[1] reports the following:

1. Of 13 U.S. Olympic boxers examined, 3 had eyes with retinal holes and 1 was amblyopic with reduced vision to 20/400.
2. Another study of 23 eye injuries over a 10-year period included 1 retinal detachment and 1 eye that had been ruptured in a fight in a soldier at Westpoint. This eye had to be enucleated.
3. Among 70 boxers examined at the Manhattan Eye, Ear and Throat Hospital over a 2-year period (1984–1986), 43 had significant eye injuries; 2 of the boxers had 20/200 in the injured eye, and 24 percent had retinal tears.
4. In New Jersey, of 284 boxers examined, 19 percent had retinal tears and 15 percent had cataracts.

5. Another study of 505 boxers, all professionals, revealed that 18 percent had retinal tears, 39 percent had damaged anterior chamber angles, and 6 percent had cataracts.

The recommendation has been made that boxers wear thumbless gloves so that the glove thumb cannot be poked in the eye of the opponent. These gloves are also suggested for all nonchampionship bouts. In the 1930s, a Toronto boxer, Sammy Luftspring, fighting in New York for the world championship, was struck in the eye with his opponent's thumb. He subsequently lost the eye, ending his boxing career. An annual ophthalmologic examination is recommended, and perhaps one should be done before each scheduled fight. One-eyed boxers should not be allowed to perform owing to the obvious risk factor.

ONE-EYED ATHLETES

A person is functionally "one-eyed" when the loss of the better eye would result in a significant change in lifestyle owing to the poor vision in the remaining eye. Realistically, a person is considered one-eyed if vision in one eye is less than 20/40, because loss of the better eye would render him or her unable to drive an automobile in most areas.

Years ago, a patient, a young man name of Bailey, lost an eye in an accident. He was an outstanding hockey and football player at school. He was upset when he was told to not play hockey or football because of danger to his remaining eye. Subsequently, he became a track and field star, successfully representing Canada at the Olympic Games.

Presently, in the United States (because of better protection), one-eyed players are allowed to participate, providing racquet sports–certified eye protectors are worn under the other protection required in hockey, football, lacrosse, and baseball.

Finally, all one-eyed people (people who have useful vision in only one eye) must wear polycarbonate lenses, even in street wear glasses, whether they require prescription correction or not. The remaining functional eye must be protected.

Table 2-5 presents the COS survey results.

REFERENCE

1. Tassman, Jaeger (eds): *Duane's Clinical Ophthalmology*. Philadelphia, J.B. Lippincott, 1994.

TABLE 2-5 COS Survey: Eye Injuries in Canadian Sports, 1972–1997

Sport	1972–1973	1974–1975	1976–1977	1977–1978	1978–1979
Hockey	287(20)	258(43)	90(12)	52(8)	43(13)
Racquet sports			43(3)	12(1)	28(1)
Baseball			19(2)	2	2
Ball hockey			24(3)	8	9(2)
Football			13(1)	2	3
War games					
Golf			5(1)		1
Basketball				1	
Skiing			1(1)	1	3(2)
Volleyball			3(3)		
Broomball			2(2)		
Lacrosse			3	1	1
Hunting and BB guns					
Snowmobiling			2(1)		1
Other			6		1
TOTAL	287(20)	258(43)	211(29)	79(9)	92(18)

Note: Numbers in parentheses indicate numbers of blind eyes. Send injury reports to Dr. Tom Pashby, 20 Wynford Drive (215), Don Mills, ON (Canada) M3C IJ4;
Tel.: (416)441-1313; Fax: (416)441-6138.

TABLE 2-5 *(Continued)*

Sport	1986–1987	1987–1988	1988–1989	1989–1990	1990–1991
Hockey	93(18)	62(11)	37(6)	33(6)	21(3)
Racquet sports	66(3)	45(4)	62(3)	40(2)	35(1)
Baseball	34	16	24(2)	15(1)	14(1)
Ball hockey	18(1)	31	24(1)	14(1)	20(2)
Football	20(1)	12(1)	10(1)	8	6
War games	9(1)	2	6(4)	4(2)	4
Golf	4(1)	1	3	5(1)	4
Basketball	7		2	2	2
Skiing	6(1)	1		4	3(1)
Volleyball			3		1
Broomball	4	3	1	2	
Lacrosse				1	2
Hunting and BB guns			3(1)		1
Snowmobiling	1(1)	1(1)		1	
Other	5(1)	9(3)	7(1)	6(2)	5
TOTAL	267(28)	183(20)	182(19)	135(16)	118(8)

1979–1980	1980–1981	1981–1982	1982–1983	1983–1984	1984–1985	1985–1986
85(21)	68(20)	119(18)	115(13)	124(12)	121(18)	123(22)
58(1)	103(4)	100(3)	88(5)	115(6)	81(6)	83(1)
10	15	41(5)	68(3)	56(3)	43(2)	32(3)
27(2)	22(4)	10(2)	19(3)	25(2)	29(1)	28
1	8	4	27(1)	22(1)	15(1)	10
					26(14)	8(2)
1		5(4)	7(2)	3(2)	4(1)	5(2)
	2	4	3	5	1	2
		3(2)		2(1)	4	2(1)
6	3	2	3	4(1)		2
2	2	3	3	2		1
			3	4	1	1
	4(1)			1	5(2)	1
		1(1)		1	1	2(1)
7	3	6(1)	6(1)	9(2)	19(2)	7(1)
197(24)	230(29)	298(36)	342(28)	373(30)	350(47)	307(33)

1991–1992	1992–1993	1993–1994	1994–1995	1995–1996	1996–1997	Total
28(7)	32(5)	16(7)	19(5)	22(7)	12(3)	1860(298)
33	31(1)	27	14(1)	17	18(1)	1099(47)
18(1)	17(1)	23(2)	17(2)	11(2)	13(1)	490(31)
12(2)	16(2)	11(3)	7	4	13(1)	371(33)
6	3(1)	5(1)	4	2	8	189(8)
3(2)	1(1)	3(3)	2(1)	3(1)	4(1)	75(32)
4(1)	1(1)	2	1	1	4(3)	61(19)
2	4(1)	5	1	2	3	48(1)
1	2		3(1)	1	2(1)	39(11)
					1	28(4)
						25(2)
	1			1		19
1					3	19(4)
						11(5)
8(1)	2	3		2(1)	4	115(16)
116(14)	110(13)	95(16)	68(10)	66(11)	85(11)	4449(512)

| **Ear, Nose, and Throat Injuries**

J. Simon McGrail

The head and neck areas of the body are vulnerable to injury in sports involving bodily contact. The contact can be with an opponent's head, fist, or other part of his or her anatomy or with a foreign object held by the opponent such as a hockey or lacrosse stick. Injuries can be classified into soft tissue injuries with and without involvement of the underlying bone or cartilage.

SOFT TISSUE INJURIES

The types of soft tissue injuries are (1) contusions, (2) abrasions, (3) puncture wounds, and (4) lacerations.

Contusions

Most contusions are simple and require no specific treatment. The application of ice is always of comfort and value, and the ice can be held over the contused area for 5 to 10 min at a time. It is important not to make the skin waterlogged or to anesthetize it from the ice application. However, contusions also may result in the formation of a hematoma. Most hematomas will resorb spontaneously in a few weeks, but larger hematomas may require incision and drainage if they become encapsulated. If the decision is made to incise a hematoma, it should be done early rather than waiting for a few weeks, at which stage scar tissue and capsule formation can make recovery much more difficult. Hematomas of the external ear will be dealt with later.

Abrasions

Abrasions vary depending on the depth of injury. If just the epidermis has been abraded, a good simple cleaning is necessary, possibly with the application of an antibiotic cream for a few days. Deeper abrasions require much more careful attention. They must be cleaned thoroughly and particular attention paid to any foreign material that may have been embedded into the dermis. If foreign bodies are left in the wound, traumatic tattooing with or without infection may result. Foreign material becomes attached to the tissues in 10 to 12 h, so a good, careful cleaning before this saves a lot of aggravation.

Puncture Wounds

Any puncture wound should be probed to gauge its depth and to evaluate if there are any associated injuries to nerves and vessels.

This is one type of injury where x-ray examination may help if it is suspected that any foreign material has been driven through the skin. Puncture wounds often can be left to heal by secondary intention following irrigation with saline or hydrogen peroxide.

Perhaps the most important puncture wound is that caused by a human bite. This is not uncommon in rugby football and has recently gained significant publicity following a heavyweight boxing championship fight. Human bite wounds are invariably associated with infection and should be treated as a very serious entity. The wound should be cleansed thoroughly and probably is best left open to heal by secondary intention. If the bite has created a flap of skin, this can be placed loosely back in position and covered with a dry dressing. If a lip has been bitten, then it is probably best to very loosely close it, particularly to make sure the vermilion border is in continuity. In all human bites antibiotics are started immediately and penicillin with cloxacillin, with Cephalosporin as a substitute for penicillin in the case of allergies, seems to be the best combination. It is important to keep a close check on these wounds and take appropriate action if infection is supervening.

Lacerations

Lacerations are common in contact sports and can occur anywhere on the face or neck. They need to be cleansed thoroughly with an antiseptic solution and then irrigated thoroughly with saline. As with puncture wounds, examination for embedded foreign material and damage to vessels and nerves is mandatory. Some confusion and debate exist regarding the need for debridement in this type of injury. I believe that the less debridement the better. If there is a very obvious piece of nonviable tissue, then this can be removed, but the less the better. Simple facial lacerations can be repaired under local anesthetic and closed with 5-0 or 6-0 nylon sutures. If the laceration is deep, then a 3-0 or 4-0 subcuticular suture will give good support. Generally speaking, a simple laceration, whether requiring suturing or taping, should not prevent the player from returning to activity.

More extensive and deeper lacerations are a different matter. Lacerations involving the eyelids or the ears or through the alar cartilage of the nose and the lip should be dealt with in a hospital setting. In such a setting, careful cleansing, irrigation of the wounds, and a layer closure are the steps to take. In the case of a lip laceration, very careful attention must be paid to establishing continuity of the red line or vermilion border. This should be done first, and then the rest of the repair follows. In the case of a lacerated eyebrow, *never ever* shave the eyebrow prior to repairing the laceration. In the case of a torn eyelid, the free margin of the eyelid should be sutured first to establish good continuity. In a through-and-through nasal laceration, careful attention must be paid to the nasal mucosa, and then the rest of the laceration can be attended to. If this type of intranasal injury is neglected, adhesions will form causing nasal obstruction, which can be difficult to cure.

Deep lacerations to the face can be very significant if the facial nerve and/or the parotid duct are involved. It is a relatively simple matter to have the patient close the eyes tight, wrinkle up the forehead, screw up the nose, smile, and whistle, and these activities will reveal facial asymmetry. If there is injury of the facial nerve—and injuries such as this are not uncommon in motorcycle sporting accidents—then the facial nerve must be explored and repaired within a few hours of the injury. Similarly, the parotid duct needs to be repaired, usually over an indwelling stent.

Soft tissue injuries can be associated with damage to the deeper structures. These individual areas will now be reviewed.

The Neck

Injuries to the neck in sports are usually blunt injuries without laceration of the skin. The most important area in the neck is the airway. The larynx is susceptible to blunt trauma, such as a cross-check from a hockey stick or a karate chop or a forearm check in football or hockey. In laryngeal injuries, the head is usually extended, which brings the larynx closer to the surface, rendering it more vulnerable to the assault. In a significant injury, the player immediately will be aware of pain and discomfort in the neck, but more important, there can be varying degrees of airway obstruction. If there is an immediate hemoptysis, a mucosal tear is present, and the player must be removed from the field of activity and assessed thoroughly.

The major consideration is the adequacy of the airway. Provided the player can inflate and expand his or her chest well, even if his or her breathing is very noisy, there is still time to get the patient to a hospital for appropriate care. If, however, the breathing is such that the patient has gross airway obstruction, then an airway must be established immediately. Most laryngeal fractures involve the thyroid cartilage, and placing an airway into the cricothyroid membrane relieves the immediate danger. In the case of a laryngeal fracture, there is swelling in the neck, and it is possible usually to palpate the trachea and the cricoid cartilage immediately above the trachea, which is a very hard, solid rim of cartilage. Immediately above the cricoid cartilage there is a narrow groove, the cricothyroid membrane, and through this a needle can be placed or a stab incision can be made and any sort of tube, such as the outer casing of a ballpoint pen, can be placed. If there is a clinic setting available, then a Fisher tube, part of a standard intravenous set, is a useful cricothyrotomy tubing. Any time a cricothyrotomy is carried out, a tracheostomy must be done at a later stage, in a hospital setting, within 24 h. In 27 years of attending Toronto Maple Leaf games in the National Hockey League, I have diagnosed eight laryngeal fractures, which is a small number, but this still makes laryngeal fracture a highly significant clinical entity. Fortunately, most laryngeal injuries are hematomas or cracks in the thyroid cartilage and fall short of the badly smashed larynx that is fortunately only seen occasionally. In the case of the hematomas, or a crack in the cartilage, resolution with normal breathing is usually seen within a week of the injury, and players can then resume their normal activity. During this week, however, players should be excused from training as well as playing, and it is preferable to keep them in a hospital setting until the symptoms have subsided entirely. Most airway obstructive injuries settle down with rest, steam, and reassurance. I do not advocate sedatives because of their respiratory depressant action, and most patients will respond to a thorough explanation of why no sedation is being used. In the severe laryngeal fractures, which these days are associated with snowmobile or motorcycle accidents, a tracheostomy is often necessary, as mentioned earlier, and then a careful laryngoscopy is necessary to determine the extent of the injury. I do not recommend intubation of a patient with a suspected laryngeal fracture because this can compound the injury. It is much better to do a tracheostomy, establish a safe airway, and then thoroughly assess the larynx and repair it as necessary. Sharp injuries, such as those resulting from a skate blade, can cause significant and deep lacerations of the neck, and lacerations of the sternocleidomastoid muscle have been described, with or without laceration of the underlying jugular vein. Injury to the jugular vein can be very dramatic and very bloody, and it is necessary to exert pressure above and below the laceration to prevent any significant damage from occurring. Once the bleeding is controlled by pressure, this pressure must be maintained until the vein can be repaired surgically.

The Mouth

Injuries to the mouth include the lips, the teeth, and the tongue. Injuries to the lip were mentioned earlier, and again, it is important to stress that the continuity of the red line is critical in repairing such injuries. The lip has a very good blood supply, and the first aid personnel at sporting events should be taught to squeeze the lip tightly on both sides of the laceration until this can be repaired surgically. A similar principle applies to lacerations of the tongue, which are also very bloody and can be controlled by pressure. This type of injury occurs when a competitor, functioning with the mouth open and the tongue out, receives a blow under the chin that causes a self-inflicted bite. The main danger with a tongue laceration is swelling of the tongue, which may cause airway obstruction. In a significant tongue injury, observation of the patient in a hospital setting overnight to be sure that there is no airway obstruction is recommended.

It should be stressed that most mucosal injuries will heal spontaneously with minimal morbidity and often require either one or two loose sutures or no sutures at all. Injuries to the teeth may involve the teeth alone or the underlying bone. These will be discussed in the section on facial bone fractures.

The Nose

Because of its prominence, the nose is very easily injured and is said to be the most commonly fractured bone in the body. This is due to direct injury from a variety of sources and is usually easily diagnosed, as exemplified by Fig. 3-1, which shows a boxer who was struck on the side of the nose. The player often will be aware

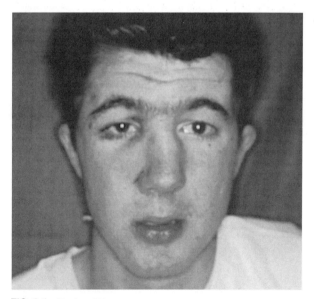

FIG. 3-1   Fractured nose.

when the nose has been broken, and in a number of sports, such as rugby and hockey, recurrent fractures are not uncommon and players easily recognize this when it happens. The player often will hear a crack, and this is commonly associated with an epistaxis that is often quite profuse. The clinical deformity is usually very clear, and the patient also will complain of an inability to breathe through one or both sides of his or her nose. I do not believe that x-rays of the nasal bones help in making the diagnosis, which can be done purely on clinical grounds. If the fractured nose is seen immediately, then often it can be replaced on the spot without anesthesia. This will reduce the bleeding, bruising, and edema that would otherwise follow.

By far the most important injury of the nose affects the nasal septum. Any time the nose is fractured, the nasal septum must be evaluated carefully. The chance of a septal hematoma forming is high in nasal fractures, and if it is overlooked, then absorption of the septal cartilage, with or without abscess formation, can occur. In children this is critical for the development of the nose, and if a septal hematoma, with or without an abscess, is neglected, then a snub nose will result that is incredibly difficult to repair from either a cosmetic or a functional point of view. Figure 3-2 shows a child

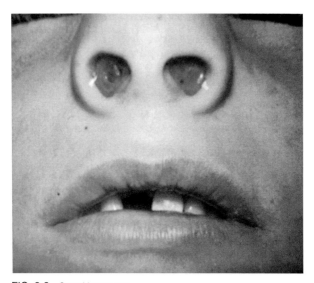

FIG. 3-2 Septal hematoma.

who suffered a hockey injury when not wearing a facial guard, and it is seen clearly that he has mucosal swelling in both nostrils. If swelling of the septum is observed, then the hematoma should be drained immediately. A sharp incision through the septal nasal mucosa is done, and the blood that is present is suctioned away. A small wick should then be placed through this incision, and the nose should be packed so that the septal mucosa can adhere to its underlying cartilage. If this injury is treated in such a manner, within 48 h the hematoma should resolve completely. This is one situation in which an antibiotic should be given in a nasal injury to prevent infection.

FACIAL BONE FRACTURES

The Nose

Nasal fractures have already been discussed, but it is stressed once again how important it is to rule out the possible associated septal hematoma. This has to be done by an intranasal examination using a good light source. It is further stressed that nasal fractures are invariably compound with an associated mucosal laceration and consequent nose bleeds. After any injury to the nose with epistaxis, the player is instructed to sit forward with the head down and to gently blow one nostril at a time. Most are very reluctant to do this, thinking it will aggravate the bleeding. In fact, by removing clots, the vessels are allowed to contract and retract, and this will stop a great many cases of epistaxis. If there is no associated fracture, the nose can be gently pinched, and this will stop most nose bleeds. If the bleeding stops quickly, there is no reason why the player cannot resume activity. If, however, there is an associated fracture, then applying ice to the back of the neck to cause reflex vasoconstriction often will help, together with a small amount of intranasal packing. If it is not possible to immediately manipulate the fractured nose back into its original position, then this can be done in a hospital setting either within the next 24 h or within the next 7 to 10 days depending on the amount of edema and bruising that may be present. After a nasal fracture has been reset, a splint should be applied to prevent further damage, and this is worn for at least 7 days. The player, unless he or she is a boxer, can resume his or her level of activity, but some form of nasal protection must be worn for at least 4 to 5 weeks. For a boxer, fighting should not be resumed for at least a month, but the athlete certainly can train during this waiting period.

The Zygoma and Orbit

Fractures of the zygoma result from a direct blow and usually result in a tripod fracture, with the zygoma being displaced medially and inferiorly. There may be an obvious flattening of the cheek, and the patient complains of pain locally and varying degrees of trismus due to the zygoma impinging on the coronoid process of the mandible and preventing the usual amount of mouth opening. If there is displacement of the lateral canthal ligament of the eye, which is attached to the zygoma, then diplopia also may be a complaint. There is significant tenderness over the fracture sites, and x-rays reveal the sites of the fractures usually with opacification of the maxillary sinus due to blood.

Most zygomatic fractures require surgical reduction. The majority can be repaired by the Gillies technique, with an incision made in the hairline through the temporalis fascia. The elevator is then placed below the zygomatic arch running between the temporalis muscle and its overlying fascia. Using this leverage technique, many zygomatic fractures can be reduced adequately. The player must then wear protection over this site for at least 1 month. It would be advisable to avoid further contact for a week to 10 days following the injury, but after this, the player should be able to resume activity with adequate protection. Blowout fractures of the orbit are not at all uncommon. This is usually due to a blow to the orbital rim that compresses the contents of the orbit, which breaks in its weakest point. This is usually the floor of the orbit and occasionally the medial wall or the lamina papyracea of the ethmoid sinuses. This invariably causes varying degrees of diplopia, with or without enophthalmus. The key to diagnosis is the inability of the eye to look upward, and this diagnosis is confirmed by radiologic investigations. Although a computed tomographic (CT) scan is very useful, I personally rely on tomograms of the orbital floor to give me detailed information as to its state. When there is obvious trapping of the orbital contents in the fracture site, then this must be repaired surgically. Many methods have been advocated, including a transconjunctival approach and an intraantral approach, but I prefer a direct approach through an external incision in the lower eyelid. This approach enables one to thoroughly inspect the orbital floor, free any trapped contents, and place a suitable graft to repair the bony defect found. The graft can be cartilage from the nasal septum or bone from the anterior antrum wall, or it can be a silicone implant. If the fracture is through the ethmoid sinuses, then the patient often will report that following blowing the nose, the eyelid swells up in an alarming manner, which is due to forcing air into the orbital area. No specific treatment is needed for this particular complication, and the player is simply instructed not to blow the nose for at least 2 weeks. If there is a large ethmoid fracture with herniation of orbital contents into this area, then an exploration through an external ethmoidectomy approach may be necessary. Again, the herniated trapped tissues can be released and placed back into the orbit, but repairing the defect is seldom necessary. However, occasionally there can be severe bleeding from the ethmoid fracture, and this usually involves the anterior ethmoid artery. Again, this is often seen with blunt injury in the area of the root of the nose, and the injuries that I have seen have mainly come from hockey pucks. If there is a brisk hemorrhage that is not controlled by packing, then the most expeditious course is to explore this through an external approach and clip the anterior ethmoidal artery. If this happens, the player should wear protection over this area for at least 2 weeks, and then normal activity can be resumed.

The Maxilla

Fractures of the maxilla are divided into three categories. LeFort type 1 fractures extend horizontally across the maxilla at the level of the floor of the nose and result in a mobile upper gingival area, together with varying amounts of mobility of the hard palate. LeFort type 2 fractures extend across the root of the nose on one or both sides and run down across the face of the maxilla to the gingiva. If both sides are involved, then the entire central upper jaw is mobile. In LeFort type 3 fractures, there is a separation of the facial bones from skull. This is usually caused by an anterior injury forcing the facial bones backward and downward, causing the classic "dish face" deformity.

Combinations of all three may occur, and the important areas to assess immediately are the state of the eyes and the teeth. If the eyes are moving well together without diplopia, and if the dental occlusion has not changed, then the fracture can be treated conservatively. However, if it is clear that there are problems with the eyes, teeth, or central face, then these patients must be dealt with in a hospital setting. X-rays of the facial bones invariably confirm the diagnosis, and various surgical techniques are necessary to realign the bones and hold them in position. Probably the most important step following a severe facial injury is to determine if there is any cerebrospinal fluid leakage. If there is, it is usually through the nose, and this should be documented and reported so that appropriate steps can be taken. In my practice, skiing injuries have accounted for most serious maxillary fractures associated with sporting activities. Great care must be taken before allowing the patient to resume the sporting activity, and it may be weeks to months before it is advisable for the patient to get back in action.

The Mandible

Fractures of the mandible are from some direct blow. The player may have heard the bone crack, and this is associated with considerable pain. The player will complain of some degree of malocclusion, and the simple clinical method to test if the mandible is fractured is to place the thumbs on the chin and the fingers on the angle of the mandible and press between the two, which will cause pain over the area of the fracture. If the blow sustained has been to the point of the chin, there may be no fracture of that area because such fractures are rare, but the forces can be transmitted up the mandible, and subcondylar fractures, either unilateral or bilateral, can occur. This may be associated with a hematympanum or even bleeding from the ear, so remember that all hematympanums are not caused by basal skull fractures. Some subcondylar neck fractures can be treated conservatively with a soft diet and staying out of trouble, but probably the majority of mandible fractures require some form of immobilization, whether this is by attaching the mandible to the maxilla or direct plating to the fracture site itself. Attention must be directed to the teeth. If there are obvious teeth missing and they cannot be found, a chest x-ray is mandatory to be sure they have not been aspirated.

Immobilization of mandibular fractures is for a 6- to 8-week period, and during this time, even with adequate protection, it is advisable for the player to refrain from contact sports. Training can continue, but actual playing should be discouraged.

It is possible that the mandible can become dislocated and not fractured due to an injury that occurs when the mouth is wide open. If this is the case, then it is advisable to reduce the dislocated mandible as quickly as possible before muscle spasm and edema prevent it. To reduce a dislocated mandible, sit behind the patient with his or her head against your chest. With the thumbs well protected, exert pressure just behind the last lower molars. The pressure exerted is downward and posteriorly, and at the same time, with the fingers under the mandible, roll the mandible upward and anteriorly, and the condyles will slip back into position. I usually suggest the use of diazepam to relax the muscles (and the patient) before attempting the reduction. If the dislocation can be reduced quickly, then normal activity can be resumed, usually in a day or two.

THE EAR

Injuries to the ear are common in wrestlers and more often in boxers. Unfortunately, we are all too familiar with the classic cauliflower ear of the wrestler and boxer, and this should be an entirely preventable result of injury. It is caused by a subperichondral hematoma that is not treated, which finally absorbs the underlying cartilage, resulting in the well-recognized, grotesque abnormality (Fig. 3-3). If a hematoma is recognized in the auricle, the correct treatment is immediate drainage. This can be done on the spot,

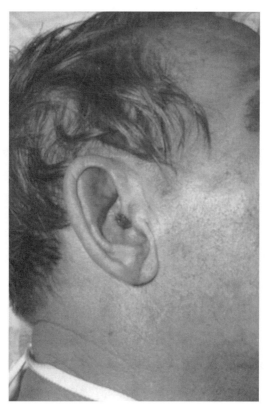

FIG. 3-3   Acute hematoma of the ear.

using a needle and syringe, and as much of the blood as possible should be removed using multiple stabs, following which careful pressure is applied to the ear using rolled up cotton so that all the little nooks and crannies of the ear can be under pressure. The hematoma should be inspected daily until it is clear that no further bleeding is occurring. An alternative to using a needle is to actually incise over the hematoma, and this gives very good drainage and is the technique that I personally prefer. The important aspects are to drain all the blood and to exert adequate pressure to prevent its recurrence. It is interesting that there have been a number of reports that even though wrestlers are wearing ear protection, it does not prevent this type of injury, which is often caused by rubbing of the forearm against the ear or the protection device over the ear. I suspect that this type of injury will continue to occur, but as mentioned earlier, if it is treated correctly, no residual deformity should result.

The use of antibiotic cream has been advocated, and this is usually done if the cotton pressure dressing is actually sutured into the auricle (Fig. 3-4). This is a worthwhile technique, but I prefer to see the patient on a daily basis to be absolutely certain that no hemorrhage is occurring that can loculate in different areas. I believe that

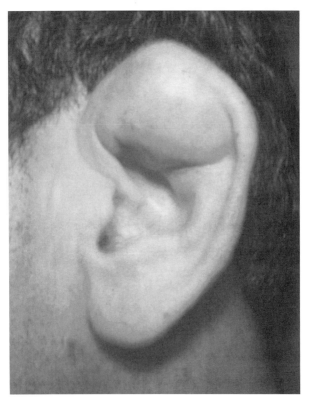

FIG. 3-4   Loculated hematoma of the ear.

antibiotics should be given to prevent perichondritis from supervening, which in itself can cause deformities. The antibiotics should continue for at least 7 days, and during this time, the player may continue to train but should not take part in contests until it is certain that the bleeding is fully controlled.

Apart from the preceding, most sporting ear injuries occur from diving. The association between diving barotrauma and perilymphatic fistula has been well recognized for the past 25 years. The diver will complain of hearing loss (which is neurosensory in nature), nausea, and vertigo, with or without vomiting. If the symptoms do not clear within 48 h and a fistula is suspected, then a tympanotomy approach by lifting the eardrum and looking into the middle ear is necessary. If a fistula is found, it can be plugged with fat or muscle; however, it should be stressed that although this will clear the vertigo, the hearing loss is permanent. Because of this, in a diver who has suffered this sort of injury, I would counsel that he or she give up diving on a permanent basis.

There are lesser degrees of barotrauma with varying degrees of hearing loss, and most of these will settle down conservatively with rest and decongestants. It is a difficult decision as to whether or not the diver should be counseled to stop diving. There is some evidence that further deterioration is not always the result of continuing to dive. Descriptions have been given of patients who have suffered inner ear barotrauma while diving but continued to dive against medical advice. Assessments made on some of these patients showed no further deterioration; however, I think that any diver who has had ear problems should be acutely aware of the possibility of losing ear function and probably should use a decongestant as a rule when diving. Anyone who has a significant upper respiratory tract infection with a great deal of nasal congestion should not dive, but if against all advice he or she do so, he or she should certainly use a strong decongestant to try to minimize any damage that may occur.

A significant number of traumatic perforations of the tympanic membrane are seen each year as a result of sporting activities. This usually occurs from scuba diving or diving into the water from a height or hitting the water with the side of the head while water skiing. It can occur from blows in boxing and wrestling, although these are unusual. If a perforation is recognized, it is vital to put nothing into the ear. A piece of cotton in the ear canal to prevent anything getting in is fine, but do not use ear drops or anything else. Make sure the patient is seen by an otologist as soon as possible. Most traumatic perforations will heal spontaneously if they are left alone, and the idea behind seeing an otologist immediately is that a small number of such perforations have a flap of tympanic membrane driven into the middle ear, and if this can be replaced immediately, it will heal extremely well.

Swimmers ear, or external otitis, is an extremely common occurrence. Although the exact cause of external otitis is not known, it is clear that getting water into the ears, whether from swimming, showering, or hair washing, causes flare-ups once the condition has become established. This is characterized by varying degrees of discomfort, swelling in the ear canal, and discharge. Swimmers should be counseled that this is a recurring problem that will continue throughout life. Steps should be taken to prevent water from getting into the ear canals, and whether this is by specially designed ear plugs or cotton wool smeared with petrolatum is an individual preference. If water does inadvertently get into the ears of such a patient, then ear drops should be instituted for 48 h to prevent a flare-up. Once external otitis has occurred, the most significant part of treatment is to debride and remove the discharge on a daily basis until the acute episode has subsided.

FIRST AID TIPS

1. For nose bleeds, with or without fracture, the patient should be instructed to gently blow the nose to remove clots, and this will hasten the cessation of bleeding. Remember to check the status of the septum to rule out a septal hematoma.
2. Any facial laceration that involves skin right through to mucosa definitely should be treated in a hospital setting. Loose sutures to close the skin laceration or simply covering it with a dry dressing is sufficient first aid care.
3. With a traumatic perforation of the eardrum, put *nothing* into the ear. No ear drops, no cotton-tipped swabs, just a piece of cotton in the outer ear canal.
4. In the case of a neck injury with an airway obstruction, place a large needle through the cricothyroid membrane as a lifesaving measure.
5. In a neck injury with significant bleeding, apply pressure above and below the laceration to compress the bleeding vessels.

It has been estimated that approximately 18 to 20 percent of sports-related accidents involve facial trauma and dental injury. About 50 percent of these involve the oral cavity and teeth.

A large number of injuries are due to involvement in high-risk contact sports such as boxing, football, hockey, lacrosse, rugby, soccer, and basketball. Accidents, however, also happen in medium-risk competitive sports such as diving, swimming, squash, water polo, baseball, skiing, and the martial arts.

DENTAL INJURIES

Teeth are somewhat unique and differ from any other body tissue. Bones will heal, and soft-tissue cuts, if sutured, also will heal. However, even though the enamel and dentin of a tooth are the hardest tissues in the body, they cannot heal or repair themselves. Once a tooth is fractured, the fractured or chipped portion is gone forever. Even though modern dentistry has many new and aesthetic materials, tooth fracture or loss means extensive and expensive treatment over many visits.

Dental injuries can be divided into two types: direct and indirect trauma. *Direct trauma* is usually the result of a "clean" blow to the teeth. A fractured tooth is usually the result of a direct blow from a stick, puck, ball, head, or fist. The mechanism also can be a direct blow from a diving board, golf club, and racquet, among others. *Indirect trauma* results from a blow to the lips, mouth, and jaw. The blow causes the lower jaw (mandibular teeth) to suddenly strike the upper (maxillary) teeth. This produces a sudden striking or crashing of the teeth together. The lips may cushion the impact somewhat. This mechanism can produce contusions, lacerations, and possible bone fracture. It also will increase the degree of luxation (loosening of a tooth or teeth).

Often indirect trauma is the result of a blow to the mouth, side of the head, or jaw. This can be from a stick, helmet, shoulder, knee, or elbow. In many cases it is the result of falling in such sports as football, hockey, lacrosse, and individual sports such as skiing, gymnastics, rollerblading, and figure skating.

ASSESSMENT OF ORAL AND DENTAL INJURIES

All dental injuries must be considered an emergency until properly assessed. The medical history must be reviewed, and if a medical emergency exists, it must be looked at and taken care of before the dental injury.

Clinical examination of the oral cavity, both the soft and hard tissues, must be done. Any soft tissue lacerations or cuts must be noted and, if necessary, debrided and sutured. The temporomandibular joint should be palpated, and the athlete should be asked to open and close the jaw slowly. Any pain or deviation to jaw movement should be investigated. The injured athlete should gently close the teeth together and note any pain to the teeth when the jaws are shut tight. The teeth should be examined for displacement, fracture, or mobility. Any sensitive teeth should be recorded.

As soon as possible the injured athlete should be seen in a dental operatory where proper dental x-rays can be taken. Any findings of fracture, mobility, chipped teeth, restorations, and percussion sensitivity must be noted. Proper recording is necessary because additional treatment (root canal treatment) may be necessary in months to come.

This assessment is usually done by the team dentist or athlete's own dentist. Since many teams, leagues, and individuals have dental and accident insurance, it is essential that proper examination, records, and dental x-rays be done to provide for the necessary treatment.

SOFT TISSUE INJURY

Soft tissue injuries of the mouth are usually the result of a direct blow from falling or the impact due to a stick, elbow, punch, or ball. The severity of the abrasion, laceration, or cut as a result of trauma must be assessed to see if sutures are necessary.

Identification of a dental injury such as a fractured tooth, a displaced tooth, or a possible jaw fracture can be compromised initially by the soft tissue injury (i.e., extensive bleeding). Therefore, it is important to fully examine the area after superficial treatment.

In cases of wounds that require closure, proper examination for fractured teeth and palpation of the wound site for any possible tooth fragments lodged in the soft tissue are paramount. Assessment of fractured teeth with pulp (nerve) exposure can be difficult in patients with profuse bleeding.

Control of any hemorrhage and cleansing of the wound of any foreign matter will help with proper assessment of the injury. Once the oral cavity has been assessed properly, closure of the laceration can be performed.

TOOTH FRACTURE

Once a dental injury involving the teeth and/or the jaw has been assessed, the athlete should see a dentist (team or personal dentist) as soon as possible. The dentist will then properly assess the injury using x-rays and provide necessary treatment.

Fractured teeth may range from simple chipped enamel to a severe coronal (crown) or root fracture. In all cases, dental x-rays should be taken to properly evaluate injury and proceed with treatment. The extent of root fracture will determine if the tooth can be saved. Severe fracture of the root will necessitate surgical removal of tooth and root. Temporization of the missing tooth would follow, and after a proper amount of time for healing of the extraction site, replacement of the missing tooth can be carried out. Replacement would be with crowns, fixed bridges, partial dentures, and more recently, possibly implants.

Enamel fracture or a broken restoration (filling) is examined by the dentist, and treatment usually involves repair and replacement of the area using current techniques (i.e., acid-etch, bonded composite restoration).

Root Fractures

Fractures to the crown of a tooth or to the root can occur. These are very painful, especially if the pulp (nerve) is exposed. Root fractures usually present hypermobility or displacement of the tooth. Many times the teeth will not occlude properly, and the injured athlete will notice that the bite does not seem right.

Tooth Fractures

Small Fractures

Chipped tooth enamel and cracks are seen; usually the tooth surface is rough, but the tooth is not loose. There is some sensitivity to air or cold. The athlete can continue to play but should see a dentist for x-rays and follow-up treatment within 24 h.

Large Fractures

In large fractures, there is usually a complete enamel layer fracture. The tooth is very sensitive because dentin is exposed. The tooth edges are very sharp and sometimes quite painful. Pulp (nerve) generally is exposed, and there is a visible area of bleeding in the fractured portion of the tooth. The athlete should see his or her dentist for emergency care because bacteria contaminate the pulp.

Displaced Teeth

Usually displaced teeth are very loose, and it is difficult to close the teeth together or bite down. It is also difficult to swallow because the teeth shut together causing pain. Frequently, there is accompanying numbness. The athlete should see his or her dentist for x-ray assessment and necessary emergency treatment.

AVULSION AND REPLANTATION OF TEETH

Avulsion of a tooth simply means that a tooth is cleanly knocked out of its socket. This occurs periodically, and the time lapse between avulsion and replantation is the most important factor. Usually it is the upper maxillary anterior teeth that can be knocked out, most frequently in children and young teenage athletes. Frequently, the athlete will remove the loose tooth and show it to the trainer or attending medical personnel

Ideal treatment is first to locate the tooth. The avulsed tooth should be picked up by the crown, trying not to touch the root surface, and gently cleansed of any debris by rinsing but not scrubbing. If possible, immediate proper repositioning of the tooth into the socket will aid in the future recovery of the avulsed tooth. If this is not possible, take the injured athlete and the avulsed tooth to a dentist immediately. If the athlete is seen within 30 min, he or she has an 80 percent chance that the tooth can be retained.

Never dry off the tooth completely. Storage of tooth during transport to the dentist should be in milk or sterile water. An alternative would be to wrap the washed tooth (not scrubbed) in a sterile gauze sponge moistened with water. Place the sponge in the athlete's cheek or under his or her tongue during transport to the dentist.

After proper evaluation of the tooth and socket, the dentist can reimplant the tooth, followed by internal splinting of the tooth to adjacent teeth with a stabilizing arch wire using bonding technique. The athlete should have periodic dental appointments to evaluate the "take" of the reimplanted tooth. Additional dental treatment may be required at a later date (i.e., root canal treatment).

TOOTH LUXATIONS

Trauma can cause displacement of teeth in a number of ways, varying from lateral to extrusive and intrusive displacement. The teeth will appear to be out of alignment, and the athlete will complain of not being able to close the mouth properly. Pain and numbness may be experienced. An extruded tooth is partially displaced out of its socket.

If the teeth do not align properly, then gentle realignment using finger pressure or a tongue depressor should be attempted. A dentist should be seen as soon as possible for dental x-rays and stabilization of the teeth.

Extruded and laterally luxated teeth are unstable, and they need to be repositioned carefully within their sockets using finger pressure. A gauze pad with gentle biting pressure will help stabilize teeth while the athlete is taken to the dentist. Since it may be quite painful to position the teeth properly, a dentist may have to use local anesthesia.

With an intruded displacement, the teeth can be driven into the tissues. This can happen in younger athletes when they are still in the mixed dentition stage. Manipulation of intruded teeth is difficult, and the athlete should be taken immediately to a dentist for x-rays and proper evaluation. The treatment may consist of partially repositioning the tooth and waiting for it to reerupt over a short period of time. The injured athlete should be monitored by the dentist for any further follow-up treatment.

With splinting of the teeth using a wire and acid-etch bonding technique, the athlete should be monitored with follow-up x-rays along with pulp vitality tests approximately every 3 to 6 months for several years. This is done to evaluate the teeth for any signs of root resorption, bone loss, or apical pathology.

Discoloration of teeth, swelling, and complaints of percussion pain also would be indications of possible nerve complications. Further treatment might involve root canal treatment and crowns.

MANDIBULAR FRACTURES

Fractures of the lower jaw (mandible) are common and comprise approximately 7 percent of injuries to this region. The fracture is usually a result of a direct trauma when falling or diving or due to a blow from an opponent's stick, elbow, or fist. Frequently the area fractured is the supracondylar region or the body of the mandible. The injured athlete usually has a malaligned bite and will complain of pain on biting and a loose tooth when closing the jaws together. When opening the mouth, the athlete will be limited, and the jaw usually will deviate to the side.

In cases of facial lacerations and cuts, intraoral examination for any fractured teeth or foreign material should be carried out to ensure that nothing can be swallowed. The athlete should be supported with a circumferential bandage from under the chin, wrapping up both sides to the top of his or her head. Gently tied on top, this will support the chin while the athlete is taken to have x-rays done that will determine the exact fracture site and whether any teeth have been fractured. This usually is done at a hospital by an oral and maxillofacial surgeon. The jaw is then wired for approximately 5 to 6 weeks.

MANDIBULAR DISLOCATIONS

Frequently the jaw can be dislocated as a result of a lateral blow while the athlete has the mouth wide open. This could be due to a blow from an elbow or a stick. With a dislocation, the athlete cannot close the mouth properly, and the jaw seems locked out of place. Immediate reduction of the dislocation should be attempted because over time the muscles can begin to spasm and increase the pain of delayed reduction of the dislocated mandible.

Reduction can be attempted by placing the hands on both sides of the mandible and gripping the chin. With a downward pressure first and then a posterior pressure, try to displace the mandible into its position. Another method would be to stand behind the athlete, and using the edge of a towel or gauze pads to cover the thumbs, place the thumbs bilaterally onto the athlete's lower side teeth, pushing the jaw gently downward and then pulling it gently back into position. Once the jaw has been repositioned, ice should be applied, and the athlete must see a dentist for follow-up treatment and observation of temporomandibular joint symptoms.

SPORTS DENTISTRY

Prevention

Dental injuries are the most common type of orofacial injury sustained. Most can be prevented or minimized by the use of properly made mouthguards. Mouthguards should be worn at all times during games, competition, and practice.

Purpose of the Mouthguard

1. To protect teeth and cushion any direct trauma that might cause tooth fracture or dislocation.
2. To hold the lips and cheeks away from the teeth, preventing lacerations.
3. To prevent the crashing of upper (maxillary) and lower (mandibular) teeth together, thus preventing fracture and chipping of teeth and enamel.
4. To act as a shock absorber and help prevent backward and upward displacement of mandible. This protection minimizes the chance of concussion or fracture of the mandibular condyles.

Types of Mouthguards

Stock Mouthguards

These come in several sizes and usually can be bought at sporting goods stores. They come ready to use. This type of mouthguard has many drawbacks. Usually such mouthguards are quite bulky and do not fit properly. They must be kept in by biting down. This makes breathing difficult. In younger athletes with erupting teeth, they can cause irritation, discomfort, and some pain. Sometimes such mouthguards are altered or cut to size by the athlete, which reduces protection. This type of mouthguard is not recommended.

Boil-and-Bite Mouthguards (Mouth-Formed)

This is a commonly used mouthguard. It is available commercially in limited sizes and is formed by placing it into boiling water and then fitting it in the mouth by biting on the material and using finger and cheek pressure to form the material around the teeth. Such mouthguards also tend to be bulky and do not fit properly. Their retention is somewhat poor, and they can cause a gagging effect. Athletes tend to cut them to reduce their bulkiness, thus lessening the protection. Again, this type of mouthguard is not recommended.

Custom-Made Mouthguards

This type of mouthguard is made by a dentist. The mouthguard is made after a custom impression has been taken by the dentist. Such mouthguards are comfortable, retentive, adapt to the teeth and ridge area, and allow the athlete to breathe in comfort. The mouthguard holds the lips and cheeks away from the teeth, thus helping to prevent lacerations. It distributes any direct trauma while protecting the anterior teeth. Covering all the occlusal (biting) surfaces of the upper teeth helps prevent fracture and chipping of the teeth when the teeth crash together on impact. The distribution of force helps minimize the chance of fracture of the angle and condyle of the mandible. This type of mouthguard is easily worn. It allows the athlete to breathe easily, drink water, and have normal speech.

A custom-made mouthguard by a dentist is the preferred choice. An athlete's own dentist or the team dentist can easily set up a program for making such mouthguards at minimal cost. Also, teams can contact the local dental society for the possibility of setting up a program for their respective leagues to have custom-fitted mouthguards made.

In the case of younger athletes wearing mouthguards, the dentist should continue to check proper fit because erupting permanent teeth can affect proper function of the guard. Custom mouthguards are still recommended for sports involving helmets with full face protection.

RECOMMENDED READING

Andreason JO: Treatment of fractured and avulsed teeth. *J Dent Child* 38:29, 1971.

Andreason JO: *Traumatic Injuries of the Teeth*, 2d ed. Philadelphia, WB Saunders, 1981.

Andreason JO, Andreason FM: *Essentials of Traumatic Injuries to the Teeth*. Copenhagen, Munksgaard, 1991, p 136.

Andreason JO, Andreason FM: *Essentials of Traumatic Injuries to the Teeth*. Copenhagen, Munksgaard, 1991, pp 11–12.

Camp JH: Diagnosis and management of sports-related injuries to the teeth. *Den Clin North Am* 35, 1991.

Greenberg MS, Springer PS: Diagnosis and management of oral injuries, in Torg JS (ed): *Athletic Injuries to the Head, Neck and Face*. St. Louis, Mosby–Year Book, 1991, chap 41.

Handler SD: Diagnosis and management of maxillofacial injuries, in Torg JS (ed): *Athletic Injuries to the Head, Neck and Face*. St. Louis, Mosby–Year Book, 1991, chap 40.

Kerr LI: Mouthguards for the prevention of injuries in contact sports. *Sports Med* 1986.

Lephart SM, Fu FH: Emergency treatment of athletic injuries. *Dent Clin North Am* 35, 1991.

Ranalli DN: Prevention of craniofacial injuries in football. *Dent Clin North Am* 35, 1991.

Torg JS: *Athletic Injuries to the Head, Neck, and Face*, 2d ed. St. Louis, Mosby–Year Book, 1991.

Wood AWS: Head protection: Cranial, facial and dental in contact sports. *Oral Health* 62, 1972.

Wood AWS: Mouth protectors: 11 years later. *J Am Dent Assoc* 86, 1973.

| **Neck, Spinal Cord, and Back**

Michael Ford

Recreational and elite-level sports are statistically safe endeavors compared with everyday activities such as driving a car. Nevertheless, injuries to the spine occur. These injuries range from the benign and brief discomfort of a paraspinal muscle strain to catastrophic quadriplegia.

Registries in Canada and the United States have been established to track the more catastrophic injuries.[1] These registries have allowed for early trend recognition and for efficacy assessment of specific interventions. Primary goals in the approach to spinal injury in sports are prevention, recognition and management of the acute injury, and rehabilitation.

EXTENT OF THE PROBLEM

A number of series clearly demonstrate that football contributes the greatest number of catastrophic injuries, followed by ice hockey, gymnastics, and wrestling.[2-4] A large series of college athletes demonstrated a back injury rate of 7 per 100 participants.[4] Eighty percent of the injuries occurred in practice, 6 percent occurred in competition, and 14 percent occurred during preseason conditioning. Muscle strains were the most common (59 percent), whereas 29 percent were associated with preexisting conditions.

In a study funded by the National Collegiate Athletic Association (NCAA) from 1977 through 1989, there were 128 cases of permanent cervical cord injuries as a result of football.[5] Defensive players were more at risk than offensive players.

An international registry established through Sport Smart Canada reported an average of 16.8 cases per year of major spinal injury as a result of hockey between 1982 and 1993.[1] Children younger than age 11 more often had ligamentous injuries of the upper cervical spine, whereas older children typically had adult patterns of injury involving the middle and more caudal cervical spine.[6]

ANATOMY AND BIOMECHANICS

The spine is a segmental structure comprised of 7 cervical, 12 thoracic, and 5 lumbar vertebrae. The caudal end of the spine consists of the sacrum and coccyx. The primary function of the spine is to house and protect the neural elements. It is capable of withstanding considerable forces before yielding. Injury occurs when the yield point of the tissues involved is exceeded. The forces required to

55

reach threshold are rate-dependent. Faster rates of application require less force to produce pathologic change.

Besides being a shock absorber, the intervertebral disk is also the primary stabilizer of the spine. The facet joints and interspinous ligaments further contribute to stability. The disk is relatively stiff in flexion and extension, as well as in lateral flexion. It is weakest when exposed to torsional forces. The outer annular fibers of the disk are firmly attached to the vertebral end plates. Suprathreshold forces result in yield at the level of the bone before disruption of the disk-bone interface occurs.

Two contiguous vertebrae and the intervening disk and ligamentous and muscular attachments constitute the *functional spinal unit* (FSU) (Fig. 5-1). Studying the biomechanics of one small section of the spine allows for a better understanding and for the validation of complex finite-element modeling studies.

The biomechanical properties of the FSU change with age. Postmortem studies have demonstrated the degenerative change in the intervertebral disk as we approach our late teens. At age 50, all of us have degenerative disks that typically are most advanced at L3–4, L4–5, and L5–S1.[7] Degeneration is a desiccation process, with the water content of the disk dropping from 90 to 63 percent

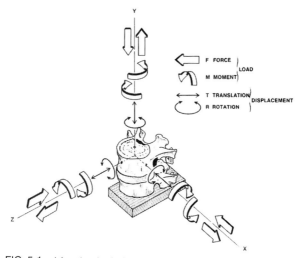

FIG. 5-1 A functional spinal unit or FSU demonstrating degrees of freedom and forces transmitted. (Reprinted with permission from White AA, Panjabi M: *Clinical Biomechanics of the Spine*, 2d ed.)

with aging. The disk becomes stiffer and stronger with age. This is the reason why disk herniations are relatively rare over age 50. Intradiscal pressures vary greatly depending on position, as illustrated in Fig. 5-2.

A disk herniation occurs when the outer annular fibers fail, allowing for migration of nuclear material (which has the textured appearance of crab meat), typically posterolaterally. This can cause secondary nerve compression and radiating limb pain. With greater

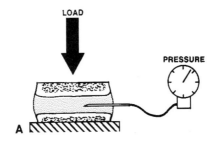

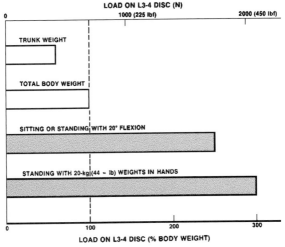

FIG. 5-2   Variation in intradisk pressure depending on position. *(Reprinted with permission from White AA, Panjabi M: Clinical Biomechanics of the Spine, 2d ed.)*

force applied to the FSU, components will fail, potentially leading to instability. *Instability* is defined as the lack of the ability to withstand normal physiologic forces, resulting in the potential for injury to the neural elements.

The first priority in the assessment of a spinal injury is the determination of stability. This can be difficult to do. Criteria have been established defining instability in the cervical and lumbar spine. These criteria are listed in Tables 5-1 and 5-2.

The presence of instability requires immobilization and bracing and/or surgery. A stable injury, however, can be treated with early mobilization. Missing an unstable injury can lead to permanent and catastrophic neurologic damage.

The spinal cord is the caudal extension of the brainstem, beginning at the level of the foramen magnum of the skull and extending down to approximately L1 or L2. Distal to this are peripheral nerve roots that make up the cauda equina. Therefore, injuries below L1

TABLE 5-1 Checklist for the Diagnosis of Clinical Instability in the Middle and Lower Cervical Spine

Element	Point Value
Anterior elements destroyed or unable to function	2
Posterior elements destroyed or unable to function	2
Positive stretch test	2
Radiographic criteria*	4
A. Flexion/extension x-rays	
1. Sagittal plane translation > 3.5 mm or 20% (2 pts)	
2. Sagittal plane rotation > 20° (2 pts)	
OR	
B. Resting x-rays	
1. Sagittal plane displacement > 3.5 mm or 20% (2 pts)	
2. Relative sagittal plane angulation > 11° (2 pts)	
Abnormal disc narrowing	1
Developmentally narrow spinal canal	1
1. Sagittal diameter < 13 mm	
OR	
2. Pavlov's ratio < 0.8†	
Spinal cord damage	2
Nerve root damage	1
Dangerous loading anticipated	1
Total of 5 or more = unstable	

SOURCE: Reprinted with permission from White AA, Panjabi M: *Clinical Biomechanics of the Spine,* 2d ed.

TABLE 5-2 Checklist for the Diagnosis of Clinical Instability
in the Lumbar Spine

Element	Point Value
Anterior elements destroyed or unable to function	2
Posterior elements destroyed or unable to function	2
Radiographic criteria*	4
A. Flexion/extension x-rays	
1. Sagittal plane translation > 4.5 mm or 15% (2 pts)	
2. Sagittal plane rotation	
> 15° at L1–L2, L2–L3 & L3–L4 (2 pts)	
> 20° at L4–L5 (2 pts)	
> 25° at L5–S1 (2 pts)	
OR	
B. Resting x-rays	
1. Sagittal plane displacement > 4.5 mm or 15% (2 pts)	
2. Relative sagittal plane angulation > 22° (2 pts)	
Cauda equina damage	3
Dangerous loading anticipated	1
Total of 5 or more = unstable	

SOURCE: Reprinted with permission from White AA, Panjabi M: *Clinical Biomechanics of the Spine*, 2d ed.

or L2 typically result in peripheral nerve or lower motor neuron injuries, whereas higher injuries result in cord or upper motor neuron damage. The spinal cord itself has no inherent resistance to injury. It has a very low yield point. The surrounding cerebrospinal fluid (CSF) and bony canal are instrumental in maintaining the integrity and function of the cord. Failure of the surrounding protective elements can result in a spectrum of injury to the cord ranging from transient edema, which results in temporary partial dysfunction, to cord transection, which is a permanent and complete injury.

PREVENTION OF SPINAL INJURIES

Screening

Routine x-ray screening of all sport participants is not a cost-effective approach to prevention. The very low yield does not justify this approach. There are, however, high-risk populations that warrant screening.

The growth of the Special Olympics has resulted in many individuals with Down syndrome participating in sports. Spinal hypermobility at C1–C2 has a prevalence rate of 25 percent, and 33 percent of these patients will demonstrate instability below

C1–C2 as they become adults. Only 3 percent, however, have neurologic deficits.[8]

Surgical stabilization and refraining from sporting activities are recommended in these individuals if the atlanto-dens interval (ADI) is greater than 9 mm on a standard lateral flexion view of the cervical spine. An ADI of 5 to 8 mm requires repeat x-rays every 3 to 5 years, with yearly neurologic assessments consisting of an accurate history and physical examination.

Pseudosubluxation in non-Down syndrome children is common. Typically, the child is less than 8 years old, and translations are seen at C2–3 and C3–4 of less than 4.0 mm. An ADI of less than 4.5 mm is normal.[9]

Congenital fusion of segments of the cervical spine is known as *Klippel-Feil syndrome*. Stresses applied to the spine are concentrated above and below the fused segment. When congenital fusion of C2–C3 is combined with occipitalization of the atlas, 75 percent will develop instability at C1–C2. These individuals require careful assessment prior to playing contact sports. A significant percentage also will have unilateral absence of the renal system, which has obvious significance in the event of a renal injury.

Routine lateral x-rays of the cervical spine should be carried out in all adults playing football. Radiologic features consistent with "spear tackler's spine" are a contraindication to continued play[10] (Fig. 5-3). Spinal canal stenosis with a Pavlov ratio of less than 0.8 is a predictor of probable frequent "burners" or "stingers" but is not a contraindication to play.[11] In the older athlete, degenerative changes may be present. In the absence of spear tackler's spine changes, there is no contraindication to play. These changes may be a predictor of an increased probability of mechanical neck pain, however.

Spondylolysis, or a defect in the pars interarticularis, typically at L5, is common in the athlete (Fig. 5-4). Prevalence rates of 6 to 47 percent have been demonstrated. This lesion is not a contraindication to play. A grade I or grade II spondylolisthesis (Fig. 5-5) is not a contraindication to play. Higher-grade slips, however, typically are symptomatic and may prevent participation in sports on the basis of the functional limitations this condition typically imparts.

Education

Education programs such as the Spinal Awareness and Prevention Program in Australia demonstrated a 20 percent reduction in spinal cord injuries.[12] Spearing in football (head-first tackling) is illegal and has been the single most important intervention in the reduction of spinal cord injuries in football.

Checking from behind in ice hockey should not be tolerated, since this has been recognized as a common spine injury mecha-

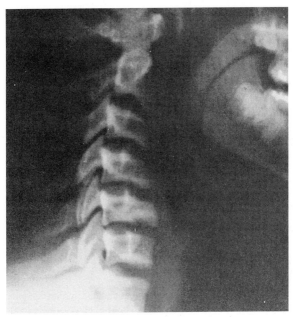

FIG. 5-3   Spear tackler's spine. Note the flattened cervical lordosis with secondary degenerative changes and narrowed cervical canal indicative of congenital stenosis with secondary acquired changes. (Reprinted with permission from Joseph S. Torg.)

nism. Helmets and face masks have virtually eliminated facial and ocular injuries but, unfortunately, have been linked to an increase in spinal injuries. This has occurred not because of biomechanical reasons but because of a false sense of security among players, leading to excessive and unwarranted risks.[13]

Equipment and Training

Over the years, recognition of hazardous field conditions has resulted in simple modifications to on-field equipment that are directly responsible for reductions in serious injuries. In football, a switch to a single padded-pole goal post reduced the frequency and injury severity of collisions. The break-away hockey net has done the same.

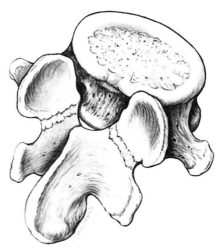

FIG. 5-4 Spondylolysis.

There is no evidence at present that the modern-day equipment worn by players has reduced spinal injury frequency and severity, however. Given that a large percentage of injuries occur during practice, the advisability of high-intensity, full-contact practices is brought into question.

The frequency of injuries associated with the use of the trampoline and minitrampoline has prompted Torg[14] to state that these devices have no place in gymnastics. The use of harness suspension devices in gymnastics and the development of aerated water landings in free-style aerial skiing are certainly training steps in the right direction. Moreover, there has been a call to eliminate some of the more dangerous head holds in wrestling, but to my knowledge, this has not been done.[15]

Factors have been identified that predispose the athlete to accelerated degenerative change. A too-early start at ages younger than 10 years and high-intensity training in gymnastics are associated with an increased incidence of juvenile osteochondroses and subsequent magnetic resonance imaging (MRI) changes associated with degeneration.[16] Given the permanence of many spinal injuries, prevention is the most important first step in the care of the athlete.

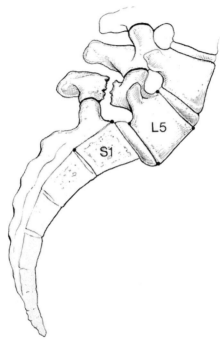

FIG. 5-5 Spondylolisthesis.

RECOGNITION AND MANAGEMENT OF ACUTE SPINAL INJURY

For the athletic trainer and physician involved in the care of athletes in football, ice hockey, wrestling, and gymnastics, an organized approach to the seriously injured athlete is a must. The first step is ensuring that proper equipment is available. The following is a list of the bare essentials:

1. Equipment for face mask removal, i.e., screwdriver and heavy bolt cutters
2. Oropharyngeal airway
3. Intubation equipment
4. Tracheostomy equipment
5. Semirigid cervical orthosis, that is, Philadelphia collar

6. Back board
7. Heavy scissors
8. Cellular phone

An organized team approach is mandatory. There must be a team leader coordinating efforts. The leader should be designated well in advance. Serious consideration should be given to practice drills. This will go a long way toward eliminating the panic that invariably permeates the air around the motionless, unconscious athlete who is not breathing.

Management of the acutely injured athlete is no different from management of the multiple-trauma patient. It is strongly recommended that the team leader be advanced trauma life support (ATLS) qualified. Worst-case scenarios should be practiced, i.e., the motionless, unconscious athlete lying face down and not breathing, wearing a tight-fitting helmet and full-face mask, with full equipment.

The team leader takes charge. The team members know who they are. A maximum of four individuals is recommended. Those not on the team should stay clear. The athlete is log-rolled as a unit onto his or her back. The team leader supports the head and shoulders as a unit (Fig. 5-6). Equipment personnel remove the face mask. The

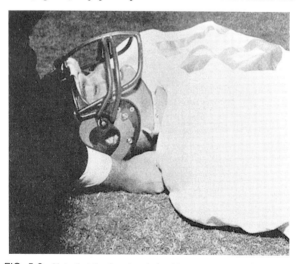

FIG. 5-6 Note that the head and shoulders are supported as a unit. (Reprinted with permission from Hochschuler SH (ed): *Spinal Injuries in Sports.*)

helmet should not be removed. Removal of equipment is an "all or none" procedure. Shoulder pads must be removed at the same time as the helmet is removed. Failure to do so forces the neck into hyperextension.[17]

The team leader then proceeds through the ABCs of trauma management. The unconscious athlete is assumed to have a serious cervical spine injury until proven otherwise. The head and shoulders are stabilized. An airway is established and maintained by whatever means required:

1. Jaw thrust
2. Oropharyngeal airway
3. Orotracheal mask
4. Nasotracheal tube
5. Endotracheal tube
6. Cricothyroidotomy
7. Tracheostomy

Care must be taken to ensure that the neck is stabilized throughout any of these procedures. Ventilation is required if the athlete is not breathing. Cardiopulmonary resuscitation (CPR) is initiated if there is no palpable carotid pulse. The athlete is then rolled to one side, the back board is placed behind, and the athlete is rolled back. The head is taped to the board. Transport by ambulance to the nearest appropriate facility should be done expediently. The cell phone is required to call for ambulance services and to notify the receiving hospital. The appropriate phone numbers should be taped to the phone.

Causing further neurologic injury to the athlete because of an ill-conceived and ill-equipped approach to the problem is totally preventable. In the conscious patient complaining of spinal pain and altered sensation or loss of movement, the emphasis on stability and preventing further harm remains. A brief description of mechanism should be obtained. Tender sites should be established. A quick neurologic examination assessing gross active motor power and a rough assessment of sensory level should be sought. Quick transport should be accomplished. Checking reflexes and posterior column function on the field is not necessary and only delays transport.

The athlete complaining of neck pain with no neurologic symptoms can provoke a difficult on-field judgment process. The presence of marked tenderness along the posterior spine should be treated as a serious injury until proven otherwise. Erring on the side of caution is the appropriate approach.

At the hospital, appropriate imaging (plain x-ray, CT, MRI) will be carried out. Treatment will be established, dictated by the presence or absence of stability.

MANAGEMENT OF BENIGN SPINAL PATHOLOGIES

Statistically, the athlete is far more likely to experience pain and functional limitations from benign spinal pathology than from a serious fracture/dislocation. The serious injuries are associated with a uniform and widely accepted approach to the problem. Ironically, it is the larger and more benign group of spinal problems that is associated with a controversial and heterogeneous approach.

Spondylolysis and Spondylolisthesis

The bridge of bone between the superior and inferior articular facets is the pars interarticularis. In the general population, approximately 6 percent of individuals have a genetically weakened pars that can fracture with everyday normal use. It is typically a slow-onset, fatigue-type fracture and is evident usually by age 5 or 6. Most such fractures are asymptomatic in children. The pars defect typically involves L5, but other levels can be affected.

During the growth spurt, a spondylolysis can result in the development of a spondylolisthesis, or forward slip of L5 on the sacrum. The grading of spondylolisthesis reflects the percentage of the anteroposterior (AP) dimension of the vertebral body of L5 that has slipped in relation to the sacrum. A slip of up to 25 percent of L5 on S1 is a grade I spondylolisthesis. A slip of 25 to 50 percent is grade II, 50 to 75 percent is grade III, and 75 to 100 percent is a grade IV.

Many of the lower-grade slips are asymptomatic. They may be responsible for an acceleration of degenerative change and the onset of back pain in adulthood, however. Higher-grade slips are more likely to be symptomatic at a younger age and often undergo stabilization surgery with reliable outcomes.

Spondylolysis without a slip can be occult, acute, or chronic. The adolescent athlete who experiences sudden-onset low back pain should be investigated for the presence of a spondylolysis. Oblique plain films usually demonstrate the lesion, although in 14 percent it is seen only on the lateral x-ray. In many cases, plain x-rays are normal. The lesion is reliably demonstrated in single photon emission computed tomographic (SPECT) scans. Planar technetium-99m bone scans are not as sensitive.[18] Acute lesions may heal with bracing in a lumbosacral orthosis for 6 to 12 weeks. Many will not heal, however.

Chronic, well-defined pars defects are unlikely to heal with bracing. In the adolescent with persistent pain secondary to a pars defect, elective repair may relieve many of the symptoms. In the symptomatic adult, elective fusion surgery is usually the surgical treatment of choice.

It should be made clear, however, that spondylolysis with or without a slip is a benign condition. Slip progression is rare in the adolescent and does not occur in the adult. Intermittent radicular symptoms are common, but neurologic injury does not occur. Therefore, the medical imposition of activity restriction is not justified. The acute spondylolysis lesion is the only exception.

Adolescent Idiopathic Scoliosis

This is a female-predominant genetic condition. Significant curves should be followed by a spine specialist to monitor progression. The presence of scoliosis, however, should not preclude full participation in sports.

Thoracic and Lumbar Scheuermann's Kyphosis

Abnormalities in the vertebral end plates in adolescence can result in contiguous wedging of vertebrae and herniation of disk material into the vertebral bodies. This can result in an accentuated thoracic kyphosis or flattened lumbar lordosis. This can be associated with the development of large, misshapen lumbar vertebrae, with disk height reduction. Again, however, despite dramatic x-ray changes, these are totally benign conditions. Scheuermann's kyphosis may cause some deformity as well as low back pain. Nevertheless, surgery is rarely indicated. Correction of severe thoracic deformities is primarily a cosmetic procedure. Once again, there is no need to impose activity restriction.

Mechanical/Degenerative Causes of Neck and Back Pain

This is the most common cause of neck and back pain and has been demonstrated to be very prevalent among even adolescent athletes.[19] The incidence increases with age, with a peak between the ages of 29 and 39 years.

The natural history is extremely variable, and the pain can last days to years. Between 70 and 80 percent of patients experience resolution within 2 to 3 months, however. In the acute phase, this problem can be virtually indistinguishable from a muscle strain clinically. The diagnosis is clinical, with a typical pattern of aggravation of symptomatology with activity and some relief with rest. The physical examination may be relatively noncontributory. The adolescent should have a SPECT scan if symptoms persist to rule out a potentially treatable pars lesion.

Imaging studies of any kind (x-ray, CT, MRI) in the adult rarely yield information that dramatically changes management. Treatment is typically conservative. Rest beyond 2 to 3 days is detrimental and does not improve the natural history. Muscle loss and bone density reduction occur at an alarming rate with protracted bed rest. Early mobilization is the key to preventing secondary changes of disuse. Treatment should be an active program that is exercise based, with functional restoration as the intended goal of treatment. Accompanying this is an education program to reassure the athlete that ongoing symptomatology does not mean further structural damage (hurt versus harm concept). Therapeutic modalities [i.e., transcutaneous electrical stimulation (TENS), interferential current (IF or IFC), laser, ultrasound, massage, traction, and VAX-D] are widely used, but efficacy has never been demonstrated in the peer-review literature.[20–24]

More invasive therapeutic modalities, such as epidural steroids, facet blocks, and rhizolysis, are also of limited benefit when compared with placebo or natural history. In the small minority of individuals with chronic, persistent, disabling, mechanical neck or low back pain, surgery *may* be indicated. Management is typically an *elective* stabilization or fusion procedure. This is somewhat controversial with variable outcomes. Return to sports is rarely a reasonable expectation.

Disk Herniation

A herniated nucleus pulposus (HNP) in the cervical or lumbar spine typically results in arm- and leg-dominant pain, respectively. This may be associated with a conduction deficit (altered or decreased sensation, motor power reduction or loss). In the absence of severe cord compromise causing myelopathic symptoms or a central lumbar HNP causing a cauda equina syndrome, treatment is always conservative initially.

In the individual who has continued severe pain 6 to 12 weeks after onset, appropriate imaging studies are indicated, with an aim toward elective surgical decompression. The individual who experiences urinary retention with or without overflow or bowel incontinence should be managed surgically emergently. The prognosis postoperatively is dictated by the speed of onset. Rapid-onset cauda equina syndrome is associated with a poor prognosis regardless of timing of surgery.

Conservative treatment of an HNP is again an active exercise-oriented approach to avoid the secondary changes of disuse. The McKenzie approach is used commonly and may help centralize the pain. Between 60 and 70 percent of disk herniations resolve within 6 to 12 weeks. Those which are still painful and functionally limiting are appropriately imaged.

In the cervical spine, the imaging modality of choice is the MRI or CT myelogram. Plain CT is not sensitive enough. In the lumbar spine, however, plain CT and MRI are close to being equivalent with respect to sensitivity and specificity. If there is a history of previous surgery of the spinal canal, a gadolinium-enhanced MRI is the imaging tool of choice.

The surgically managed cervical HNP is typically an anterior decompression and fusion, whereas a simple discectomy is all that is required in the lumbar spine. Thoracic disk herniations are very rare. Those which cause an intercostal radiculopathy only are managed conservatively. Thoracic cord compression, however, is dealt with surgically.

Burners and Stingers

A "burner" or "stinger" is very common in football. It is typically initiated by a tackle. It is felt to be due to a C6 root traction injury secondary to flexion and lateral deviation of the neck.[25] These injuries are typically transient and self-limiting. The existence of congenital and/or secondary acquired cervical canal stenosis increases the probability of experiencing these symptoms.

REHABILITATION

After stability has been established through whatever means, rehabilitation can begin. The benign conditions typically are stable, so there is no reason for delay. Treatment is a program of functional restoration. Stiffness is addressed with an exercise program aimed at regaining range of motion, and weakness is treated with a resistive strengthening program. This always should be combined with an education program. Any program that emphasizes the use of passive modalities is to be discouraged.

PROGNOSIS AND RETURN TO SPORT

Spinal cord concussion secondary to transient edema of the cord typically results in very early and often complete return of neurologic function. The incomplete lesion will have varying degrees of recovery, but in many instances the return is not functional. The individual who still has complete or profound loss of function beyond the period of spinal shock (return of the bulbocavernosus reflex) typically does not experience any return of useful function.

The benign spinal pathologies statistically are associated with a good prognosis and ultimate return to sport without restriction. Athletes with spondylolysis or spondylolisthesis treated surgically can in some cases return to sport, but this is not a reasonable expectation. The individual with a surgically treated HNP of the lumbar spine has a high probability of returning to sport without significant functional limitation.

A patient with a cervical HNP treated with an anterior decompression and fusion, however, is an individual who is at risk for injury of adjacent levels. There are no well-established guidelines, but I would be somewhat reluctant to allow someone who has had a surgical fusion to return to contact sports such as football.

Prior to clearing an athlete to return to sport, two important questions must be answered:

1. Is there a significant potential for further structural harm?
2. Is performance going to be significantly hampered by residual symptoms?

These questions must be answered by careful clinical assessment that includes a history, physical examination, and possible imaging studies. Question 1 usually can be answered objectively by establishing the presence of clinical and radiologic stability. Question 2 is a decision between the medical personnel and the athlete based on functional capacity assessments during practice sessions. These are best done in a stepwise fashion.

SUMMARY

The medical team's responsibility is to the athlete and athlete only. Prevention is the prime goal, followed by ensuring that no further harm is done to the injured athlete. Recognition of significant injury is extremely important, and a tendency to err on the side of caution should be adopted. Subsequent rehabilitation should be evidence based, avoiding the adoption of useless treatment.

REFERENCES

1. Tator CH, Carson JD, Edmonds VE: New spinal injuries in hockey. *Clin J Sports Med* 7:17–21, 1997.
2. Mueller FO, Cantu RC: Catastrophic injuries and fatalities in high school and college sports, fall 1982–spring 1988. *Med Sci Sports Exerc* 22:737–741, 1990.
3. Bruce DA, Schut L, Sutton LN: Brain and cervical spine injuries occurring during organized sports activities in children and adolescents. *Prim Care* 11:175–194, 1984.
4. Keene JS, Albert MJ, Springer SL, et al: Back injuries in college athletes. *J Spinal Disord* 2:190–195, 1989.
5. Cantu RC, Mueller FO: Catastrophic spine injuries in football (1977–1989). *J Spinal Disord* 3:227–231, 1990.
6. McGrory BJ, Klassen RA, Chao EY, et al: Acute fractures and dislocations of the cervical spine in children and adolescents. *J Bone Joint Surg* 75A:988–995, 1993.
7. Miller JAA, Schmatz C, Schultz AB: Lumbar disc degeneration: Correlation with age, sex, and spine level in 600 autopsy specimens. *Spine* 13(2):173, 1988.

8. Pizzutillo P: Spinal considerations in the young athlete, in *Instructional Course Lectures*, vol 41. Park Ridge, IL, American Academy of Orthopaedic Surgeons, 1993, chap 46, p 463.

9. Cattell HS, Filtzer DL: Pseudosubluxation and other normal variations in the cervical spine in children. *J Bone Joint Surg* 47A:1295–1309, 1965.

10. Torg JS, Sennett B, Pavlov H, et al: Spear tackler's spine: An entity precluding participation in tackle football and collision activities that expose the cervical spine to axial energy inputs. *Am J Sports Med* 21:640–649, 1993.

11. Meyer SA, Schulte KR, Callaghan JJ, et al: Cervical spine stenosis and stingers in collegiate football players. *Am J Sports Med* 22:158–166, 1994.

12. Yeo JD: Prevention of spinal cord injuries in an Australian study (New South Wales). *Paraplegia* 31:759–763, 1993.

13. Murray TM, Livingston LA: Hockey helmets, face masks, and injurious behavior. *Pediatrics* 95:419–421, 1995.

14. Torg JS: Epidemiology, pathomechanics, and prevention of athletic injuries to the cervical spine. *Med Sci Sports Exerc* 17:295–303, 1985.

15. Wu WQ, Lewis RC: Injuries of the cervical spine in high school wrestling. *Surg Neurol* 23:143–147, 1985.

16. Pollähne W, Teichmüller HJ, Ahrendt E: Spinal injuries from the radiologic point of view in children in intensive training for competitive sports. *Radiol Diagn (Berl)* 31:479–487, 1990.

17. Palumbo MA, Hulstyn MJ, Fadale PD, et al: The effect of protective football equipment on alignment of the injured cervical spine: Radiographic analysis in a cadaveric model. *Am J Sports Med* 24:446–453, 1996.

18. Read MT: Single photon emission computed tomography (SPECT) scanning for adolescent back pain: A sine qua non? *Br J Sports Med* 28:56–57, 1994.

19. Kujala UM, Taimela S, Erkintalo M, et al: Low-back pain in adolescent athletes. *Med Sci Sports Exerc* 28:165–170, 1996.

20. Griffin LY: Introduction: Applications of rehabilitation modalities in the treatment of acute injuries, in *Instructional Course Lectures*, vol 41. Park Ridge, IL, American Academy of Orthopaedic Surgeons, 1993, chap 42, p 437.

21. Basford JR: Low-intensity laser therapy: Still not an established clinical tool. *Lasers Surg Med* 16(4):331–342, 1995.

22. van der Heijden GJ, van der Windt DA, de Winter AF: Physiotherapy for patients with soft tissue shoulder disorders: A systematic review of randomised clinical trials. *Br Med J* 315(7099):25–30, 1997.

23. Deyo RA, Walsh NE, Martin DC, et al: A controlled trial of transcutaneous electrical nerve stimulation (TENS) and exercise for chronic low back pain. *N Engl J Med* 322(23):1627–1634, 1990.

24. Sawyer M, Zbieranek CK: The treatment of soft tissue after spinal injury. *Clin Sports Med* 5:387–405, 1986.

25. Rockett FX: Observations on the "burner": Traumatic cervical radiculopathy. *Clin Orthop* 164:18–19, 1982.

6 | The Shoulder in Sports

R. Peter Welsh   Stefan Jacobs

The shoulder is an extraordinary joint complex enveloped in muscle capable of propelling the body, supporting its weight, and projecting a missile. Its wide movement range enables the precise positioning and placement of the hand, facilitating the finest of human motor function.

Shoulder movement can be explosive, as in pitching a baseball; repetitious, as in propelling the body swimming; or static, as in sustaining loads when weightlifting.

The shoulder is a complex interaction of four joint systems; the glenohumeral, acromioclavicular, sternoclavicular, and scapulothoracic articulation; it is subject to injury from direct trauma or overuse in repetitious activity.

The glenohumeral joint, by virtue of the disparity in size and shape of the humeral head and its articulating glenoid fossa, is inherently unstable. It relies on strong muscle support; therefore, the shoulder may be vulnerable not only in terms of injury to the joints but also to the supporting musculature as well.

In the younger age group, heavy use and overstrain injuries are common from the loads and demands of training; in the older athlete degeneration starts to take its toll, affecting the rotator cuff as well as the articulations themselves.

It must be remembered that shoulder pain may reflect not only local pathology from the shoulder itself but also may be the site of referred pain from cardiac ischemia, cervical spine, thoracic outlet source, or, on remote occasions, from an intraabdominal disorder. Therefore, it is important to define accurately the source of shoulder pain and to identify the precise pathology, if one is to manage the athlete with shoulder dysfunction.

As in all areas of medicine, the history of injury and origin of symptom complaint is of prime importance. Specific clinical features may be confirmed by clinical examination with newer scanning techniques, such as computed tomography (CT) and magnetic resonance imaging (MRI). The advent of arthroscopy has offered an opportunity to both define and deal with intraarticular pathologies previously unrecognized. Rehabilitation of shoulder injuries above all involves the training and reconditioning of muscle support and is the mainstay of all efforts in recovery of the shoulder-injured athlete.

SHOULDER GIRDLE FRACTURES

Clavicle Fracture

It is said that the most common bone broken is the collarbone. Certainly in sports, fracture of the clavicle is a common injury, usually resulting from a fall on an outstretched arm or by direct impact on the point of the shoulder. Less commonly, it may arise from direct trauma.

Generally, the fracture occurs in the midshaft at the junction of the inner two-thirds and outer third, where the muscle attachments of the pectoralis below and the trapezius above converge. This results in a displacement of the fracture, which may unite with bayonet apposition with overlap without ultimate disability to the athlete. A clavicle fracture is at least temporarily a disabling injury, particularly to those involved in contact sports, because the fracture must completely consolidate before an athlete returns to sports such as hockey or rugby.

Most uncomplicated fractures can be handled by a simple figure eight truss. Such a commercially available brace support offers a measure of immobilization and comfort for the initial 3 weeks postinjury, but it need not be sustained on a protracted basis, as immobilization is a relative expression.

The fracture must be allowed to consolidate before upper extremity activity is resumed. Contact sports may require 4 months before the activity is resumed, because the risk of refracture is otherwise high.

Fractures of the distal clavicle involving the acromioclavicular (AC) joint pose a particular problem and may necessitate open reduction and internal fixation. Otherwise only fractures threatening to become compound or those breaching the clavipectoral fascia could be considered for open reduction. Nonunion can result from overzealous return to early activity, and open reduction with bone grafting may be demanded if this happens. Such an injury may be career threatening, because an athlete cannot return to contact sports with a plate in place. The plate must subsequently be removed, but this leaves a resultant focus of potential weakness from the screw holes for many months thereafter. Thus open reduction is to be avoided unless absolutely required.

Fractures of the Proximal Humerus

Avulsion fractures of the greater tuberosity result from direct falls in young active athletes. The tendon bone junction is strong and the tuberosity may avulse. This can occur also in association with dislocation of the shoulder. A closed reduction of the shoulder may reduce the fragment, but if there should be malreduction with the tuberosity remaining prominent by more than 5 mm, open surgery should be considered. Late impingement is likely to be a problem otherwise.

Surgical Neck Fracture

Surgical neck fractures can occur in contact sports. Their significance lies in the possibility of growth plate injury in the adolescent with unfused epiphysis. In the older age group, overzealous early therapy can delay union and in some circumstances even promote a nonunion. There must be time allowed for adequate consolidation recognizing the risk of frozen shoulder development.

SHOULDER INSTABILITY

The shoulder joint is inherently unstable by virtue of the disparity in size and shape of the humeral head and the glenoid fossa. Shoulder stability is provided by capsular containment with ligamentous reinforcement via its attachment to the glenoid labrum. More than this, however, the shoulder relies for its stability on coordinated muscle control from the cuff stabilizers, the supra- and infraspinatus as well as the subscapularis. The deltoid plays a pivotal role also in controlling the relationship of the humeral head with the glenoid fossa.

ACUTE DISLOCATION

Direct trauma to the shoulder or indirect transmission of force through the outstretched upper extremity can result in dislocation of the shoulder anteriorly or posteriorly.

ANTERIOR DISLOCATION

Anterior dislocation commonly follows a fall on the outstretched extremity that drives the shoulder anteriorly to lie in a subcoracoid location. This may strip the glenoid labrum, producing a so-called Bankhart lesion. An impression fracture of the superior paraarticular surface of the humerus, a Hill Sach's lesion, may also be produced.

The shoulder contour becomes squared off, and clinical examination should confirm intact function in the axillary nerve supply in the deltoid, the muscular cutaneous nerve to the biceps, as well as to the more distal upper extremity function.

Wherever possible, it is helpful to obtain x-rays of the shoulder in two planes with an AP and an axillary lateral confirming the true location of the shoulder and excluding the possibility of an associated fracture. Early reduction may be performed, minimizing the possibility of neurovascular compromise. Adequate sedation may be offered, followed by gentle longitudinal traction with some countertraction. The traditional Hippocratic method offers gentle counterresistance with the use of a stocking foot in the axilla. This has the effect of helping lateralize the humerus, and provided this is carried out gently, it can be a most effective technique.

Traction applied with the individual lying prone on the table with the arm downward can also reduce the shoulder. It is important to be gentle and produce adequate relaxation. After reduction neurovascular function should be retested and confirmatory x-rays obtained.

Postreduction management in the younger individual traditionally employed the sling and swath for a number of weeks before initiating an active rehabilitation program. It is now recognized that in the younger individual there is a high risk of recurrence. Therefore, there has been a recent tendency to consider early arthroscopic stabilization in those competitively inclined in this age group. However, generally sling support is offered for 3 weeks, during which time isometric exercises are initiated. Active rehabilitation starts at 3 weeks, emphasizing exercise to achieve range but avoiding the provocative abduction and externally rotated position for 3 months.

POSTERIOR DISLOCATION

A direct fall on the outstretched arm may induce a posterior dislocation of the shoulder and can direct impaction injury to the shoulder.

A posterior dislocation results in a shoulder compromised in its movement; however, in contrast to the athlete with an anterior dislocation, the contour may appear normal. Therefore, it may not be immediately apparent that the shoulder has been dislocated. It is most important that such injuries be recognized, for the late effect of unrecognized dislocation is premature arthritis and a permanently compromised shoulder. X-rays in two planes readily confirm the location of the shoulder, with the transcapular or axillary lateral an essential part of the x-ray evaluation.

Closed reduction may be achieved under intravenous sedation, as with an anterior dislocation; in refractory cases general anesthetic may be required. Simple traction with compression from behind generally achieves reduction. A simple sling support should be offered and isometric exercises initiated. The provocative position that potentiates redislocation—that of forward flexion in internal rotation and adduction—must be avoided.

RECURRENT SHOULDER DISLOCATION

Recurrent anterior dislocation of the shoulder is a common outcome following an acute dislocation. Predisposing factors include detachment of the glenoid labral ligament complex, capsular stretching, or on occasion fracture of the glenoid rim itself. When obtaining a history of recurrent dislocation, it is important to establish whether the individual's problems arose from an originating trauma or whether they developed spontaneously. X-ray review will determine whether there is a lesion of the humeral head, a Hill Sach's lesion, or a glenoid rim lesion. Confirmation of the direction of dislocation is essential, with the position in which the arm is unstable usually one of abduction and external rotation. The frequency and ease of dislocation determines the requirement or otherwise for formal stabilization. If an individual is hampered in day-to-day activity, at work, or in his or her sport such that participation becomes impossible, then stabilization should be considered. If harm may accrue from continued sports participation, as in contact sports, or activities such as skydiving or scuba diving, then surgery must be undertaken.

In the clinical examination one should evaluate the state of general joint laxity of the individual as well as clinically confirm the direction of instability. Specifically, the *apprehension test* is of value (Fig. 6-1). With the patient lying supine and the arm abducted to 90 degrees and externally rotated, forward pressure is exerted by leverage over the examiner's hand placed under the proximal humerus. Distinct apprehension may be elicited with the sensation relieved when the arm is eased into slight internal rotation and the examining hand behind the shoulder removed. Pressure backward on the upper arm induces relocation of the shoulder and easing of discomfort and apprehension.

A positive sulcus sign may be induced by downward traction on the arm inducing a gapping or sulcus between the acromion and the humeral head. This may indicate a state of generalized ligamentous laxity, or a tendency to multidirectional instability. Deltoid function in controlling the sulcus should be assessed by isometric review with correction of the tendency demonstrated.

A trial of full rehabilitation should be undertaken in all individuals presenting with episodes of recurrent instability. This should aim at stabilizing the internal and external rotators, as well as strengthening the supportive muscles of the shoulder girdle, the trapezius, and the latissimus. The deltoid is of prime importance and should be trained to work synchronously. If there is uncoordination in its contraction then the shoulder may be squeezed in and out of joint. Those individuals with voluntary capability to dislocate the shoulder are not candidates for surgical treatment.

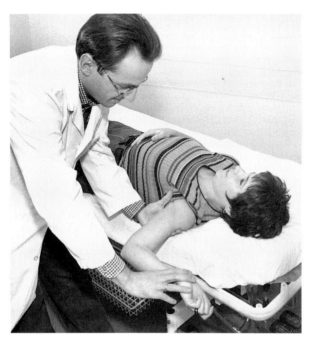

FIG. 6-1   Apprehension test for anterior instability.

Operative treatment may be resorted to in individuals unable to participate in their sport without risk of redislocation. It must be remembered though that episodes of recurrent dislocation in their own right do not predispose necessarily to premature arthritis of the shoulder. Indeed, there is a greater incidence of arthritis of the shoulder in those overzealously tightened surgically rather than from the effects of the recurrent dislocation itself.

In the younger individual suffering traumatic dislocation, arthroscopic stabilization has a clear role to play. The high rate of recurrence in this age group makes surgical consideration reasonable and, if treated early before there is capsular distortion, is accompanied by a high rate of success. In the more mature individual or one who has had multiple episodes of dislocation over a longer period of time, the capsular and ligament structures become stretched and open surgery is preferred.

The surgical techniques employed today set the objective of achieving optimal stabilization without zealous overtightening.

Earlier procedures, such as the Putti-Platt and Magnuson-Stack, have fallen from favor because they tighten the shoulder too much. In some instances this induces a tendency to posterior subluxation and limited external rotation, grossly compromising performance with the tightened shoulder predisposed to arthritis. The technique preferred today includes reattachment of the glenoid labrum by means of direct suture, the Bankhart repair, or the use of suture anchors (Fig. 6-2). Some individuals can be stabilized by the judicious use of an arthroscopic staple or resorbable pegs applied extraarticularly.

In individuals in whom the ligaments are reattached directly by closure of the Bankhart lesion, early rehabilitation may be initiated following a short period of sling support, usually around 3 weeks. During this time, emphasis is placed on maintaining cardiorespiratory fitness, allowing for the limitations imposed by being sling restrained.

Following the period of immobilization the emphasis should be on general conditioning for a further 3 weeks, with initiation of formal strengthening exercises and range of motion exercises starting 6 weeks postsurgery. There should be no forcing of abduction and external rotation for 3 months, but in general if overall fitness is maintained at the same time as the shoulder is rehabilitated, resumption of contact sports such as hockey can be allowed 4 months

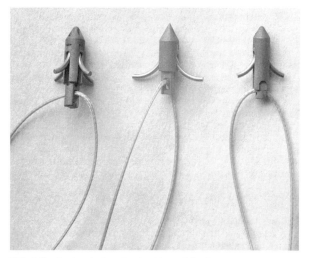

FIG. 6-2   Anchor devices for shoulder stabilization surgery.

postsurgery. Over the course of 9 months, in about 80 percent of cases, close to normal range of motion is achieved. Earlier techniques were more restrictive than this.

For those who have a Bankhart lesion, the success of stabilization is in excess of 90 percent. The shoulder should remain stable in the long term with regard to any dislocation tendency. However, almost 30 percent of dislocators may present without a Bankhart lesion or anatomic deficit in the ligament support. These individuals have sustained a stretching of the capsule and are predisposed to a multidirectional tendency to instability, although the predominant position of instability may well be one of an anterior–inferior dislocation.

A capsular shift repair should be initiated when the capsular laxity is overlapped, inferior redundancy is drawn upward, and capsule is oversewn. In these instances, the muscle may also be overlapped somewhat to try to tighten the shoulder more comprehensively. These patients have a higher propensity to stretch out their repair, with success rates only in the order of 80 to 85 percent overall in terms of a recurrent subluxation or dislocation tendency.

SHOULDER SUBLUXATION

It is recognized that many individuals have an element of incipient instability. Indeed, the competitive athlete may ride on the cutting edge with regard to maintaining optimal flexibility and sustaining stability of the joint structure. The lax-jointed athlete who excels in gymnastics and diving, and participates commonly in high-level throwing sports, manifests an indication of subluxability on clinical examination. An instability tendency in its own right may not necessarily imply a state of disability requiring treatment.

However, other athletes may describe a dead arm phenomenon in the course of their throwing activity. As they cock to throw there may be an anterior subluxation of the shoulder, and as they follow through there may be almost a release of the arm and with it a sensation of weakness and paresthesia in the arm and hand. These individuals, although not frank dislocators, do bear consideration of surgical repair with capsulolabral plication. In the competitive thrower, however, the balance is so fine that to undertake surgical treatment on this group of individuals invites disaster. Overzealous tightening can result in loss of function from a reduction in the range of motion and flexibility of the shoulder such that the fine performance edge that makes an athlete elite may be lost. In general, this group of individuals should be extensively rehabilitated with appropriate strengthening regimens that emphasize total balance in the rehabilitation of the shoulder girdle muscles, both the stabilizers and power groups.

MULTIDIRECTIONAL INSTABILITY

Multidirectional instability is more common in the individual with generalized joint laxity. In determining the predominant direction of instability, one must recognize the position in which the shoulder is most vulnerable. A shoulder may be unstable in multiple planes, that is anteriorly or posteriorly, or it may tend to sag inferiorly. The anteriorly unstable shoulder can be dealt with by a capsular shift repair, which also deals with the inferior redundancy. The patient with posterior instability is more problematic. If the shoulder slips backward in simple activities with the arm held in adduction and internal rotation, there is probably no stabilizing procedure that will allow the patient to return to competitive athletics. Posterior capsular shift surgery may be undertaken, or on rare occasions a humeral osteotomy may be performed. This contains the shoulder for normal lifestyle activities but not for strong athletic endeavor. Similarly, it must be recognized that those who have a tendency for the shoulder to slip inferiorly on an involuntary or voluntary basis cannot be helped by any surgical repair.

VOLUNTARY DISLOCATION

Voluntary dislocation is a form of multidirectional instability whereby the individual can control the dislocation. The patient can selectively displace the humerus from the joint, either anteriorly or posteriorly by muscle contraction, and then relocate the shoulder by selective contraction of the deltoid. Sometimes this is coupled with a dyskinetic pseudowinging tendency of the scapula, which further exaggerates the disability. Unfortunately, there is no surgical treatment that satisfactorily meets the demands of this group of individuals. Muscle retraining is to be encouraged, and to this end biofeedback has a place in trying to reeducate the appropriate muscles to respond in a coordinated manner.

ACROMIOCLAVICULAR DISLOCATION

Injury to the acromioclavicular joint is one of the more common injuries sustained in contact sports such as ice hockey, rugby, soccer, and football. A fall on the point of the shoulder can spring the acromioclavicular joint, with consequent descent of the shoulder. Classified as grade 1 dislocations when there is contact maintained between the end of the clavicle, in the young athlete this may result at times in an osteolysis of the articular cartilage and outer end of the clavicle. In grade 5 the whole scapula is displaced downward. Grade 2 subluxations maintain partial contact and paradoxically can lead sometimes to greater long-term problems than those where there is a complete separation. Late arthritis may occasionally require surgical consideration in grades 1 and 2 situations. Grade 3 dislocations are relatively common. There is a springing upward of the clavicle and loss of continuity with the acromion. Not only may there be instability in an up–down plane, but also in a forward–backward plane. This may necessitate late repair in up to 30 percent of instances. Grade 4 dislocations are associated with a gross posterior displacement of the outer end of the clavicle. Grade 5 dislocations are rare and require surgical treatment, as do the grade 5 when there is gross inferior subacromial or subcoracoid displacement of the clavicle.

Management of the acromioclavicular joint should, wherever possible, remain conservative other than for the rare grades 4 and 5 injuries. Grade 3 injuries are perhaps somewhat controversial in that in years past there was a tendency to recommend surgical repair. However, problems with failure of internal fixation to maintain the reduction and the prolonged disability (in terms of time away from sports participation) associated with surgical intervention led more and more to a conservative approach. In most instances simple treatment with sling support until comfortable is initiated, followed by a graduated program of exercises, isometric at first, then progressing to resisted strengthening and mobilization of the shoulder as comfort allows.

Treated conservatively one can return an athlete with an AC joint to sports participation in 4 to 6 weeks. Treated surgically with internal fixation and the need subsequently for removal of any screws or pins, return to sports in 4 to 6 months is the norm. Quite clearly, the conservative route is preferred wherever possible (see Fig. 27-4).

For those patients requiring late surgery because of disabling instability, reconstruction of the ruptured coracoclavicular ligaments by transplantation of the coracoacromion ligament is recommended. The repair must be protected with some form of internal fixation. Even so, the failure of such device may be upward of 20 percent. For this reason, sometimes a simple beveling of the outer end of the clavicle and capsuloplasty is recommended unless the instability is major.

STERNOCLAVICULAR DISLOCATION

Sternoclavicular dislocation may occur in contact sports or from heavy falls. More commonly the sternoclavicular joint subluxates anteriorly. In such a location, it may remain stable and not cause problems. If it dislocates posteriorly, however, then serious compromise of the airway can occur.

Management of the acute posterior dislocation requires the individual to be laid flat on the back over a small roll placed between the shoulder blades and the shoulders braced backward. In the emergency room a towel clip clamped around the collarbone with the patient suitably anesthetized can facilitate the reduction. Bracing in a figure eight truss is then necessary for 4 weeks to allow the joint to stabilize.

Chronic instability of the sternoclavicular joint is a problematic condition. The sternoclavicular joint should never be excised. One cannot treat this joint with the "impunity" that can be applied to the acromioclavicular joint in terms of resection. Uncontrollable instability can result from such an undertaking, with compromise of shoulder function and possible respiratory compromise. The joint must be stabilized without pin or screw fixation. A cottony Dacron 4-mm tape is preferred to secure the joint, although a fascialata graft may be used.

GRINDING SCAPULAR SYNDROME

Sometimes individuals develop a penchant for grinding their shoulder blades after injury to the shoulder. These individuals become troubled by the feeling of crepitus. This causes them to asynchronously contract the serratus posterior, levator, and rhomboid muscles so that the shoulder blade protracts and retracts across the chest wall, which results in friction in the scapulothoracic bursal plane. These individuals have to be properly reeducated in the control of their shoulder musculature, or the habit can become entrenched and difficult to eradicate.

MUSCLE RUPTURES AROUND THE SHOULDER

Subscapularis rupture is an uncommon but important injury, which may go undetected (Fig. 6-3). It follows trauma in which an individual, in adducting and internally rotating the arm, meets an opposing force or resistance, thus snapping the subscapularis. It can also be associated with anterior dislocation of the shoulder on occasion.

Following an acute trauma to the shoulder in which there is failure to progress, the injury is identified by a positive lift-off test (Fig. 6-4). The arm is held in internal rotation with the back of the hand against the spine. Next, an attempt is made to lift the hand away from the spine. If the palm cannot be brought outward from the spine 3 to 5 in., then a rupture of the subscapularis must be suspected. It can of course be defined by MRI study. Surgical repair of the subscapularis is required to restore function to the shoulder.

PECTORALIS MUSCLE RUPTURE

The pectoralis major arises in a broad sheet as two distinct heads, an upper clavicular head and a lower sternal costal head. This pro-

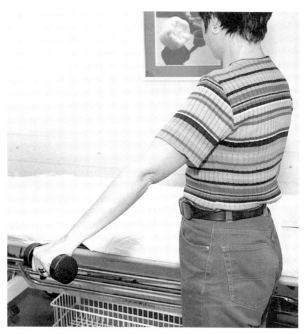

FIG. 6-3 Subscapularis rupture—supraspinatus strengthening in the plane of the scapula.

duces the round appearance of the anterior axillary fold. Contusion sprains are relatively common and are managed as other soft tissue injuries with RICE followed by graduated mobilization and gentle strengthening stretching exercises.

Excessive muscle stress, a direct blow, or a tearing against resistance can induce partial or complete rupture in the substance of the muscle. Ruptures may occur in the muscle belly, at the musculotendinous junction, or at the insertion. Excessive muscle tension is the most common mechanism, and rupture of such a muscle is more common in those who have used androgenic steroid in their muscle-building program. Complete rupture of the pectoralis major demands early surgical treatment in the active athlete. Tendon avulsion can be repaired directly and is more satisfactory than when the tear occurs at the musculotendinous junction where the tissue tends to shred.

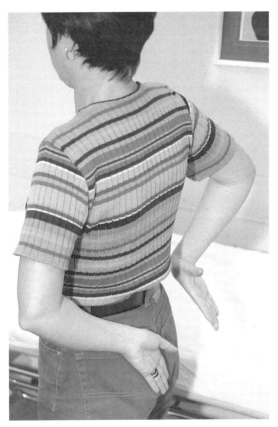

FIG. 6-4   Positive lift-off test.

RUPTURE OF BICEPS

Biceps Tendon Rupture

Rupture of the long head of the biceps is not uncommon in the middle-aged and older athlete. It is associated with an element of degeneration of the long head where it passes between the transverse-humeral ligament in the bicipital groove. This may occur spontaneously or in the course of an activity such as throwing or lifting.

There is immediate pain in the shoulder and retraction of the long head with the characteristic Popeye muscle deformity in the upper arm. Management is generally symptomatic except when the injury occurs traumatically in the younger individual, as it can in wrestling or weight lifting. If treated within the first week, surgical tenodesis of the tendon in the biceps groove can be achieved. However, the results of long head biceps tendon rupture in the older age group are generally satisfactory other than for the deformity induced. Strength is regained over the course of 6 weeks to 3 months, and normalization of activity can be achieved during this time.

Rarely, contraction of the muscle belly in the upper arm is associated with a cramping and tightness. Late fascial release and modified tenodesis may be considered under these circumstances. On occasion the retained intraarticular portion of the ruptured biceps tendon can cause an internal derangement in the shoulder that is amenable to arthroscopic resection.

Biceps Muscle Rupture

Relatively uncommonly the biceps muscle can be ruptured by direct trauma, as with a hockey stick slash on the arm. There is an obvious separation of the biceps muscle in midsubstance before hematoma and swelling may obscure this defect. The hematoma should be aspirated and the arm immobilized with the elbow in flexion for 6 weeks. Rehabilitation thereafter is slow, but without such treatment a major deficit in function can accrue.

ROTATOR CUFF DISORDERS

Rotator cuff dysfunction has probably been the most intensively addressed aspect of shoulder injury management in recent years. The rotator cuff comprises the stabilizing enveloping muscles and tendons arising from the shoulder blade. They embrace the humeral head, inserting circumferentially with the subscapularis in front, the supraspinatus above, and the infraspinatus and teres minor behind. The rotator interval is bridged by the biceps tendon in the space where the subscapularis passes inferiorly to and the supraspinatus superior to the coracoid process.

The rotator cuff and biceps tendon mechanism therefore come in intimate contact with the undersurface of the overhanging acromion and the coracoacromial arch formed by the coracoacromial ligament bridging from the coracoid process to the acromion and the outer end of the clavicle at the AC joint.

Interposing between the coracoacromial arch and the cuff complex below is the subacromial bursa, which is subject to reactive change in response to trauma and tendon degeneration involving the cuff structures. In addition to the subacromial bursa the shoulder is invested by numerous bursi, notably the subdeltoid bursa and the subscapularis bursi, investing the gliding planes around the shoulder.

THE IMPINGEMENT SYNDROME

In recent years much has been made of the term "impingement." It has come to be accepted almost as a diagnosis. Rather, impingement is a symptom, it is pain from catching of the rotator cuff tendons under the coracoacromial arch; and it is a sign, manifest in the demonstration of a painful arc. The painful catching of the shoulder may be elicited by careful examination in different positions of flexion, rotation, and abduction. Although a plethora of eponymous tests have been described, first and foremost when examining the shoulder one must bear in mind that the objective of the exercise is to define exactly the site and source of the pain.

Examination of the shoulder should be carried out palpating for the area of specific tenderness as the arm is carefully flexed, partially abducted, and rotated. This may be defined "what" structure is impinging against "what," enabling a specific diagnosis to be formulated. Comparison should always be made with the opposite side with the examination completed by adduction stress testing for AC joint involvement.

ROTATOR CUFF
TENDINITIS/SUBACROMIAL BURSITIS

Overuse is the most provocative cause of rotator cuff dysfunction in the throwing athlete. Passage of the rotator cuff tendons beneath the coracoacromial arch produces reaction in the subacromial bursa with strain on the tendon insertion, as well as impingement of the tuberosity. It must be remembered that in the younger individual most situations of impingement come from overstrain, overuse, and muscle imbalance. Therefore, the rotator cuff, particularly the supraspinatus, must be specifically strengthened. The exercise is relatively simple—forward elevation to 90 degrees in a 30-degree forward position, not in abduction to the side as it is commonly practiced but in the plane of the scapula and held at 90 degrees with 1.5-kg weight for a matter of 7 to 10 s. A series of repetitions repeated in frequent sessions on a daily basis over a course of 3 to 4 weeks selectively strengthen the supraspinatus and restore balance to the musculature that controls the shoulder.

Indeed, selective strengthening of the external rotator creates steady improvement in performance and amelioration of impingement symptoms. Above all the provocative activity must be modified in terms of the intensity and duration of practice. Careful attention to technique in throwers and swimmers plays a vital part in reducing recurrence. However, in the acute instance, non-steroidal medication may be employed as well as a subacromial injection of corticosteroid into the bursa along with the generous installation of 8 to 10 mL of Xylocaine to disperse the agent through the bursa and not just deposit the active agent locally (where it might induce tendinous degeneration). Single injections are not a problem—if one injection is effective, further injections should not be required. If there is a recurrence some months later, then the injection might be repeated two to three times. Refractory cases may then be considered for surgical management.

It must be remembered also that an athlete may manifest features of impingement when there is muscular imbalance around the shoulders. When there is shoulder imbalance, there may be an element of incipient instability; therefore, rehabilitation should emphasize stabilizing the shoulder with a strengthening program while maintaining appropriate flexibility.

SURGERY FOR IMPINGEMENT

One must remember that impingement is not a diagnosis. It is a symptom and a sign. One must always consider "what" is being impinged by "what." In any individual with chronic refractory impingement, one must consider whether there is an underlying injury to the rotator cuff. In the athlete who is over the age of 50, attrition takes its toll, and degenerative tears of the rotator cuff are relatively common by the age of 60. In the younger athlete there is impingement of the tuberosity in the supraspinatus insertion beneath the coracoacromial ligament. There is a traction on the ligament attachment to the acromion, and spur development can lead to beaking that produces chronic impingement with mechanical obstruction. An impingement of the cuff insertion or biceps tendon may occur, with the subacromial bursa itself becoming thickened and "inflamed."

The subacromial bursa is subject to trauma in direct falls on the shoulder with hemorrhage into the bursal sac with a subsequent reactive bursitis. Such injury usually responds to conservative treatment, and settles with steroid injection, but if the acromion and coracoacromial ligaments continue to offer obstruction, then surgical release may be considered.

In the older individual, imaging studies of the rotator cuff should be made to determine its integrity, either by ultrasonography, MRI, or arthrography. In all cases likely to be benefited by surgery, one should be able to obtain relief from the impingement feature elicited clinically by the subacromial injection of local anesthetic. The installation of 10 to 15 mL of 1% Xylocaine into the subacromial bursa should take away the individual's pain for the duration of the anesthetic, approximately 1 h. If relief does not occur, then one must suspect an underlying internal derangement of the shoulder, as it might affect the biceps tendon, or the biceps labral mechanism. Incipient instability should be considered, as well as the reason why the individual does not respond to the local anesthetic challenge.

Arthroscopic decompression has been shown to be efficacious in the hands of the true arthroscopic specialist. The release of the coracoacromial ligament and the beveling of the anterior edge of the acromion can be very effectively accomplished. Interestingly, in controlled studies the recovery time and the morbidity of the procedure by either open or closed technique have not been shown to be substantively different. The open procedure can be done with a mini-deltoid splitting approach yet enable wide visualization of the cuff and readily confirmed decompression of the subacromial space. In general this has proven to be a more reliable approach in cases of chronic refractory impingement.

FAILED SURGERY

Results of decompression of the cuff in general terms are quoted in the nonathletic group in the 80 percent category. However, in reality, in the elite or competitive athlete, rotator cuff decompression surgery has a far lesser incidence of success. It should be undertaken with due recognition that the individual may not return to the elite competitive level enjoyed prior to injury.

Two causes of failure may be noted: nonrecognition of incipient instability or internal derangement that affects the biceps labral mechanism, both of which clearly require treatment other than acromioplasty.

In the middle-aged athlete, adhesive capsulitis may masquerade as impingement. Indeed, an individual with impingement may have an element of adhesive capsulitis. The mistake commonly made in this group is undertaking surgery on these individuals who may afterward develop a full-blown frozen shoulder syndrome.

ROTATOR CUFF PATHOLOGY

Undoubtedly, impingement comes to play an important part in the genesis of the syndrome of impingement owing to rotator cuff tendinitis with compression of the rotator cuff tendons between the humerus and the overlying coracoacromial ligament and anterior acromion. However, it is too simplistic to attribute all cases of tendinitis to impingement alone. A hypovascular "critical zone," where the blood supply to the rotator cuff is deficient (about a centimeter from its insertion), leads to an "A zone" of relative hypovascularity. There are undoubtedly individual predisposition factors, such as genetic background to tendinitis or enthesopathy at the bone tendon junction.

Calcific tendinitis is an entity unto itself. Calcific deposits develop in the rotator cuff tendon just proximal to their insertion. They may remain asymptomatic for years, becoming acutely evident with an episode of acute bursitis or tendinitis. Under such circumstances, aspiration may be attempted with needling of the lesion and a steroid injection to control the reaction. If there are repeated episodes of acute tendinitis with flare-ups, or persistent tendinitis that does not settle, then excision of the calcium deposit may be carried out arthroscopically or by open surgery.

Rotator Cuff Tears

Acute rotator cuff tears may occur in the younger athlete with normal tendon structure when the arm, moving in abduction and external rotation, is met by an opposing force that violently changes the direction of the arm movement tearing the tendon. In the younger athlete, it is perhaps more likely to actually avulse the tuberosity with the tendon attachment. X-ray clearly identifies such injuries.

The acute tear of the rotator cuff itself is actually uncommon in the younger individual, but is important when the appropriate history is elicited to identify the exact nature of the shoulder pathology by ultrasonography, arthrography, or MRI. Acute tears in the younger individual and tuberosity fractures with displacement clearly require surgical treatment.

Chronic Rotator Cuff Tear

The majority of rotator cuff tears occur in the middle-aged and older athlete. With aging, the tendon structure undergoes degeneration. It may be owing to a combination of factors, as noted from impingement as well as primary degeneration of the tendon itself.

Confusion sometimes exists with regard to a definition of rotator cuff tears. A partial-thickness rotator cuff tear refers to a strain, a breakdown of the intracapsular attachments of the tendon leaving the tuberosity attachment still intact. Most tears start in this manner, with few tears in fact being caused by direct attrition to the superficial or bursal surface.

A complete rotator cuff tear refers to a through-and-through defect in the cuff substance so there is communication between the shoulder joint and the subacromial space. It does not relate to the size of the lesion. Thus, an individual with a complete rotator cuff tear, a full-thickness tear, may exhibit full range of motion and excellent strength in the shoulder. The patient may also demonstrate an impingement sign and obviously present with impingement symptoms. Thus, an individual in the older age group who presents with an impingement syndrome must be considered as having a rotator cuff tear until proven otherwise.

Investigation of the integrity of the rotator cuff can be evaluated by arthrography, which has long been the benchmark standard and is the most easily available and least expensive technique. Ultrasonography has become more reliable in recent years, and MRI has become the standard evaluation.

An individual presenting with an impingement associated with a rotator cuff tear can be managed conservatively at the outset. Many are able to cope with a modified approach to the sport, but if not then surgical repair should be considered.

The surgery endeavors to reattach the rotator cuff tendon, and the repair must be protected for the first month to 6 weeks from any resisted strengthening. The initial recovery should focus on regaining gentle assisted range of motion, with recognition that it will take 6 to 9 months to rehabilitate an individual with a rotator cuff tear. Even so, there may be some continuing limitation experienced in overhead reach and in return to throwing sports and some long-term limitation, although the expected outcome in 70 percent of instances is certainly better than with nonintervention.

The problem in the older age group is with regard to the size of the tear, the quality of the tendon, and the mobility of the cuff in terms of being able to achieve a successful reattachment, with the added factor, a biological one, that is the repair process itself. With long-standing tears there is no value in attempting reattachment if on CT scan there is shown to be atrophy from musculature with fatty fibrous infiltration. In undertaking rotator cuff repair, the primary goal is control of pain; the reduction of the impingement catching that limits regaining of strength, and full mobility is not necessarily an expected outcome.

INTERNAL DERANGEMENT OF THE SHOULDER

Prior to the availability of the newer imaging techniques and the advent of arthroscopy as a diagnostic tool, some athletes showed a persistent indication of catching pain in the shoulder but did not fit the category of impingement or instability. Many of course were treated for impingement or on occasion even for shoulder subluxators. In reality they had injury to the biceps tendon and the biceps labral mechanism.

When the shoulder is forced into abduction, the tuberosity may be impacted against the superior glenoid margin. This can result in a separation of the biceps tendon and its labral attachments. An MRI or CT arthrography can help define the so-called SLAP lesion, which is positively identified at arthroscopy (Fig. 6-5). Unfortunately, although some of these lesions are amenable to arthroscopic techniques, some are not, and the mainstay of treatment in these cases must remain the general rehabilitation of the shoulder musculature. These injuries may indeed prove career-threatening to the elite athlete.

The biceps tendon itself may be subject to subluxation from its groove. Rupture of the transverse humeral ligament, although rare on its own, can occur, but may be seen in association with a rotator cuff tear. Under these circumstances the checkrein effect of the biceps is lost with a consequent presentation of impingement.

FROZEN SHOULDER

One of the most perplexing conditions seen around the shoulder is the spontaneous development of a tightening of the capsule of the shoulder, adhesive capsulitis. It can, of course, also complicate trauma to the shoulder, including fracture, dislocation, or cuff trauma. Paradoxically, a completely frozen shoulder is almost never seen in the presence of a complete rotator cuff tear. In spontaneously developing frozen shoulder there is a 25 percent incidence of bilaterality. The middle-aged athlete, following overuse of

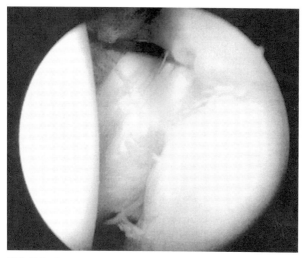

FIG. 6-5   Slap lesion with separation of biceps labral mechanism.

the arm, even without such provocation, may develop pain in the shoulder that becomes associated with an ever-increasing tightening of the shoulder over the course of a week or two. The key to recognition is that there is a global restriction in shoulder movement. There is limitation in flexion and external rotation, but the giveaway sign is the limited internal rotation as demonstrated when the hand will not turn behind the back. Abduction and external rotation are clearly compromised as well. Under these circumstances, it is important to recognize that this is not a situation of impingement, that the x-rays of the shoulder are invariably normal, and that the rotator cuff itself is intact. It is not an arthritis. Indeed, it is its own entity, and although it appears that it should demand aggressive therapy, such is not the case. Although exercise is to be encouraged, gentle flexibility drills are the only effective means of maintaining range. Unfortunately, the condition often runs its own natural course and is remarkably refractory to medications, including nonsteroidal medication and injected corticosteroid. Authors have related that the use of oral prednisone in short course helps to deal with the severe pain that may sometimes be associated with this condition.

On occasion those who are persistently tight may benefit from a manipulation under anesthetic. This may be very useful in helping regain some mobility, which can then be capitalized on by a physiotherapy program. Recently there has been a vogue for consideration of arthroscopic release but there is no proof that this offers materially greater benefit than a gentle manipulation alone. It should be noted that the diabetic, for reasons unknown, seems to be particularly refractory to treatment.

It used to be believed that all cases of frozen shoulder would resolve in 2 years or so; unfortunately, that is not so and even up to 7 years later one may see residuum of tightness with some shoulder restriction in up to 30 percent of individuals.

DEGENERATIVE ARTHRITIS

Acromioclavicular Arthritis

The acromioclavicular joint is the most commonly damaged joint around the shoulder, with injury to the articular cartilage and to the meniscus leading to a breakdown of the joint surfaces. As noted, in the younger individual there may even be an osteolysis of the outer end of the clavicle. In the older athlete the development of spurs and cystic change in the joint are seen.

Most cases can be handled conservatively with a generalized exercise program. The condition tends to be episodic, with flare-ups and long remissions. However, if it proves refractory and corticosteroid injection is not effective, then joint debridement by arthroscopic surgery or open technique may be required.

Glenohumeral Arthritis

In the active athlete, degenerative arthritis of the shoulder is not common. However, to those who have been subject to overzealous tightening or anterior stabilization surgery devastating arthritis may develop. Scapularis release and debridement may be considered in such individuals. Occasionally, arthroscopic surgery may help; however, in extreme cases there may be no other outcome to consider but joint replacement.

NEUROVASCULAR DYSFUNCTION AROUND THE SHOULDER

Brachial Plexus Injury

There is no more devastating injury to the upper extremity than trauma to the brachial plexus. The level of involvement depends on the type of injury sustained, but if the neck is forcefully laterally flexed to the opposite side and the shoulder is forced down, then there may be avulsion of the plexus proximally at the nerve root level. Such injury clearly requires neurosurgical review.

Local injury to the brachial plexus can occur with dislocation of the shoulder. Certainly, the longer a dislocation is unreduced and chronic, the more prolonged will be any neurologic deficit encountered. Obvious management includes the avoidance of such a calamity and early treatment of the condition.

It is well to remember one's basic methodology and the salient features of upper limb enervation in all instances of major trauma to the shoulder. The axillary nerve supplies the deltoid muscle with a sensory area on the lateral aspect of the deltoid. The musculocutaneous nerve supplies the biceps, and its cutaneous distribution is on the lateral side of the forearm. The radial nerve is the motor for thumb extension, with an area of sensory supply in the anatomic snuff box. The median nerve is responsible for thumb tip flexion and supplies the enervation to the index and middle fingers. The ulnar nerve supplies the finger abductors, and its sensory supply supplies the ulnar side of the fourth finger and all of the fifth finger.

OTHER NEUROLOGIC PROBLEMS

Quadralateral Space Syndrome

The compression of the axillary nerve by a fibrous band in the quadralateral space has been described. This may account for posterior shoulder pain in the throwing athlete who, when he or she abducts and externally rotates the arm in the cocking motion of throwing, induces the compression of the axillary nerve. The difficulty in trying to confirm a diagnosis on neurologic examination is normal; EMG studies are likewise sound. There could only be arteriography of the subclavian artery that one would visualize the impact on the posterohumeral circumflex artery. This must be considered a rare cause of posterior shoulder pain.

Suprascapular Nerve Entrapment

Suprascapular nerve entrapment can present in the suprascapular notch area or can be entrapped more distally as it passes around the base of the acromion to enervate the infraspinatus. The supraspinatus muscle is spared in these instances. This condition may masquerade as tendinitis and requires bipolar EMG study evaluation.

The problem in the competitive athlete who may develop this condition is that even with surgical release recovery is not very satisfactory. It is more important perhaps if the infraspinatus is functioning to rehabilitate this muscle group, recognizing the deficiency, which may linger in the infraspinatus.

In an individual with gross wasting of both spinatii one has to consider the differential diagnosis of a rotator cuff tear. Occasionally, there may also be a ganglion in the notch causing nerve compression. This clearly requires MRI definition.

VASCULAR PROBLEMS

Vascular problems have been described in individuals presenting with symptoms of fatigue, muscle ache, and lack of endurance, as well as intermittent paresthesia. An element of axillary artery occlusion occurs during the throwing action. This can be caused by a thoracic outlet syndrome.

Axillary Vein Thrombosis

"Effort thrombosis" has been described in active athletic individuals following strenuous effort or repetitive action. This masquerades as a thoracic outlet syndrome, a condition requiring venogram for definition.

Thoracic Outlet Syndrome

Individuals may present with paresthesia in the extremity, pain in the shoulder and arm, and normal neurologic review on examination; however, on Wright's test, obliteration of the pulse occurs when the head is turned to the opposite side (side flexed) and the arm is abducted overhead. The pulse returns on lowering the arm to the side. The classic Adson's maneuver is similar, except the head is rotated to the involved side (Fig. 6-6). X-rays may reveal a cervical rib as a predisposing factor.

In most instances, an exercise regime working on shoulder retraction and shoulder girdle muscle strength should be the mainstay of treatment. Surgery for thoracic outlet is not generally rewarding in athletes. Thoracic outlet syndrome can be confused with shoulder "burners" or "stingers." They commonly occur in football,

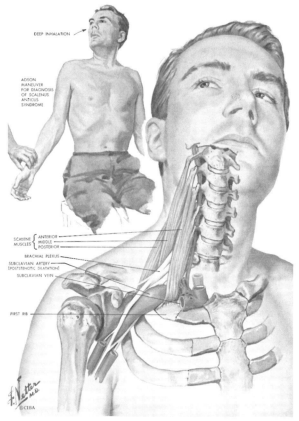

DEEP INHALATION

ADSON
MANEUVER
FOR DIAGNOSIS
OF SCALENUS
ANTICUS
SYNDROME

SCALENE ⎰ ANTERIOR
MUSCLES ⎱ MIDDLE
          POSTERIOR
BRACHIAL PLEXUS
SUBCLAVIAN ARTERY
(POSTSTENOTIC DILATATION)
SUBCLAVIAN VEIN

FIRST RIB

FIG. 6-6   Adson's maneuver.

hockey, wrestling, and so on, with direct forceful head, neck, and shoulder contact. The athlete gets a very hot feeling like a blow torch. This can radiate down the arm to the hand with neuresthesia of the whole hand. Symptoms usually subside in a few minutes. If a neurologic examination is normal, the athlete can return to play. A player who receives multiple burns should be seen by a neurologist for EMG and nerve conduction studies. Etiologic theories vary (cord contusion, C5-6 nerve root compression, brachial plexus stretch).

CONCLUSION

This chapter has sought to outline some of the more common problems seen in the athlete's shoulder. Whatever the pathology identified, the mainstay of rehabilitation must remain the full development of strength and flexibility in all muscle groups investing the shoulder girdle.

Wrist and Hand Injuries

C. Stewart Wright

These are very common sports injuries and may be bony or soft tissue in nature. We see fractures, dislocations, and epiphyseal injuries. Ligaments and tendons may be strained or torn. There are numerous mechanisms of injury, especially falling on the outstretched hand (FOOSH). This may be made worse if the player is holding something like a stick, racquet, or ski pole when he or she hits the ground. Injuries also occur when the hand is on the receiving end of a blocked shot, a kick, or fingers being hit end on by a ball. Hand and wrist injuries may prove frustrating for players, trainers, and physicians owing to difficulties in making a diagnosis and obtaining a successful outcome.

THE WRIST

Bony injuries of the distal radius and ulna are usually secondary to considerable force, such as taking a fall, flying off a speeding vehicle, or being struck with a stick. These may be extraarticular, the so-called Colles' fracture, or enter the joint. A high index of clinical suspicion is necessary, and point tenderness over the distal radius is a fracture until proven otherwise. Impacted or undisplaced fractures may be amenable to functional bracing for 2 to 3 weeks. Whether intra- or extraarticular, these injuries require accurate reduction. If a reduction cannot be maintained by closed means then percutaneous pins or an open reduction may be necessary. Occasionally, external fixation may be needed and can be used alone or in conjunction with open means. These injuries usually require up to 6 weeks in a cast. Although the fracture may heal in 6 weeks, full recovery may be protracted and often requires considerable therapy. It is not uncommon to see patients continue to gain range of motion and strength for 12 to 18 months.

Fracture-dislocations of the wrist may occur with a volar lip (Barton's fracture), dorsal lip (reverse Barton's), or radial styloid fracture (chauffeur's fracture). Closed reduction is usually possible, but maintenance of reduction often requires pins or plate fixation.

Distal radioulnar joint (DRUJ) injuries usually occur with rotational forces through the forearm. One should always examine the joint above (elbow) looking for injuries to the radial head or proximal radioulnar joint. DRUJ injuries may result in subluxation or dislocation in either a dorsal or volar direction. This may be associated with a number of fractures, including Colles', radial shaft, radial head, ulnar, and radial epiphyseal injuries. The joint itself may be involved with a variety of injuries, including fractures of the sigmoid notch of the radius, ulnar head fractures, cartilage injuries of the ulnar head, and ulnar styloid fractures. Also at risk to damage is the triangular fibrocartilage complex (TFCC) including the articular disk or meniscus, dorsal and volar ligaments, and the ulnar collateral ligament.

DRUJ instability usually requires a long arm cast for 4 to 6 weeks. Dorsal displacement is managed in full supination, and volar instability is held in neutral rotation. Pin fixation across the DRUJ may occasionally be necessary. Once the acute injury has settled there may be concern about damage to the TFCC. The pain is localized to the fossa just distal to the end of the ulna. Symptoms are usually provoked by forearm rotation as well as radial and ulnar deviation. A wrist arthrogram is helpful in diagnosing a full-thickness tear. If symptoms persist after a reasonable period of time (8 to 12 weeks) then wrist arthroscopy may be considered. As in the knee the meniscus may be arthroscopically debrided and occasionally repaired. Players may usually return to sport in 2 to 3 weeks using a wrist support as necessary.

Carpal injuries represent a wide spectrum. Sprains, strains, flake fractures, and undisplaced carpal bone fractures are at one end. The dorsum of the triquetrum is the most common flake fracture. There are reported cases of fractures to each one of the carpal bones, including the pisiform. Displaced scaphoid fractures and scapholunate dissociation with rotatory subluxation of the scaphoid are more severe injuries (Fig. 7-1). The worst injuries have a perilunate component. This represents an injury to the intrinsic and extrinsic ligaments that hold the scaphoid, lunate, triquetrum, and capitate together. These injuries may be a pure perilunate dislocation, or they may be associated with a bony injury. The three most common injuries are transscaphoid, transcapitate, or transradioulnar. These usually require open reduction and should be referred to a hand surgeon.

An often missed diagnosis is a fracture of the hook of the hamate. This is usually from a direct blow or load through a bat, golf club, hockey stick, or racquet. There is localized tenderness 2.5 cm distal to the pisiform on a line from the pisiform to the second metacarpophalangeal joint. Like undisplaced scaphoid fractures, this injury may not be appreciated on plain x-rays. A specific hamate view may show the fracture (Figs. 7-2 and 7-3*A*). It may also be seen on a carpal tunnel view (Fig. 7-3*B*). If necessary, additional studies are used, including bone scan, tomograms, or CT scans.

Hamate hook fractures are slow to settle and are not aided by a cast. They should be treated expectantly as there are reported cases taking up to 2 years to settle. Additional padding in the area may

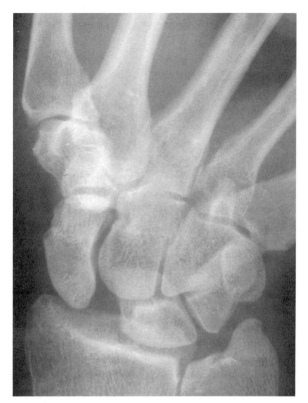

FIG. 7-1 Scapholunate dissociation.

allow the athlete to return to competition once the acute pain has settled. Bicycle gloves are often a useful adjunct. If pain persists the hook fragment may be excised, but there is a risk of damage to the motor branch of the ulnar nerve.

Scaphoid fractures require special mention because they are frequently missed and they have a nonunion tendency. They are the second most common wrist injury, behind only fractures of the distal radius. The typical patient is a young adult male who has fallen on his hand. This may initially be dismissed as a sprain or strain and not fully evaluated. Any athlete with pain in the anatomic snuff box or over the scaphoid tubercle requires radiologic evaluation.

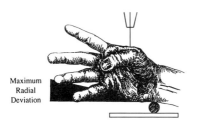
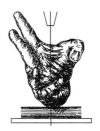

Maximum
Radial
Deviation

FIG. 7-2   The forearm is in the neutral position. The wrist is maximally deviated. The thumb is maximally opposed.

Routine wrist x-rays may miss the fracture, and scaphoid views must be ordered (Fig. 7-4). If these are normal and clinical suspicion persists, then other studies are needed. A nuclear bone scan or tomograms usually help in the diagnosis. If the initial studies are normal but the athlete is very sore, then a splint is used for 2 weeks and the studies repeated.

The most common site of scaphoid fracture is through the middle third of the bone ("waist fracture"). The more proximal the fracture, the more likely it is that the blood supply has been disrupted to the proximal pole (Figs. 7-5 and 7-6). The fracture may also be associated with an unrecognized carpal instability.

Undisplaced fractures of the scaphoid can be managed in a scaphoid cast but may take 3 to 4 months to heal. If there is no sign of union by 3 months or if the fracture is displaced initially then open reduction and internal fixation should be employed. As with wrist fractures there is a long period of rehabilitation to regain motion and strength. The athlete may need to use a scaphoid splint on return to sports until good function has been restored.

With long-standing nonunion of the scaphoid there is a high likelihood of osteoarthritis of the wrist. This may take 10 to 15 years but occurs in a predictable manner. It begins at the radioscaphoid joint initially and then at the capitolunate joint. This long-term complication can hopefully be avoided with increased vigilance in assessing the painful wrist in an athlete.

In the adolescent one needs to be aware of epiphyseal injuries of the distal radius and ulna. These are Salter type I injuries and are normal radiographically. It is a clinical diagnosis with tenderness just proximal to the radial or ulnar styloid. A splint or cast may be necessary as dictated by the severity of symptoms.

When one encounters a bony injury around the wrist care must be taken to assess for any associated neurologic damage. The radial

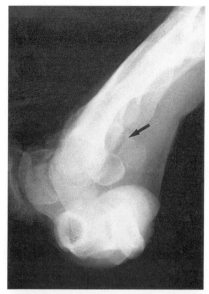

A

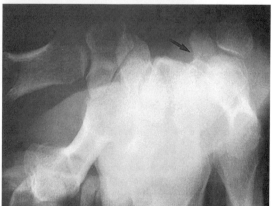

B

FIG. 7-3   *A.* Hook of the hamate fracture. *B.* Carpal tunnel view with hamate hook fracture.

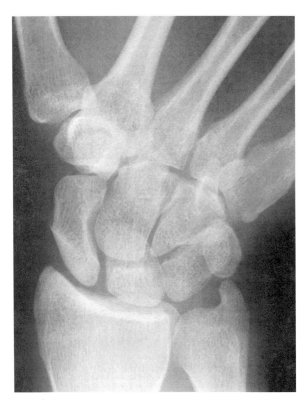

FIG. 7-4   Scaphoid view with wrist in ulnar deviation.

sensory nerve is at risk with direct trauma on the radial side of the wrist from contact with a stick, as in hockey or lacrosse. Median nerve dysfunction with an acute carpal tunnel syndrome may occur even with an undisplaced distal radius fracture. There may be damage to the ulnar nerve with injuries to the elbow or ulnar side of the wrist such as hamate fractures. If there is neurologic injury associated with dislocation then this should be reduced as expeditiously as possible. Prophylactic median nerve release may be needed with the severe carpal injuries as there can be considerable swelling in the first 24 h after injury. The carpel tunnel is usually released open but can be done with arthroscopic assist. The complication rate is

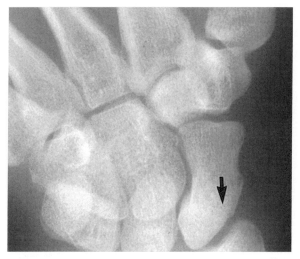

FIG. 7-5   Fracture of the proximal pole of the scaphoid.

slightly higher with the closed techniques (neurologic and vascular), but it is purported to have less downtime for the patient.

Tendon injuries at the level of the wrist are uncommon. More common is a posttraumatic tendinitis of the flexor carpi radialis, flexor carpi ulnaris, the first extensor compartment (de Quervain's), the radial wrist extensors, or extensor carpi ulnaris. These often prove slow to settle but usually respond to a combination of splinting, oral nonsteroidal anti-inflammatory drugs (NSAIDs), therapeutic modalities, stretches, and corticosteroid injections. Functional braces may allow athletes to continue playing while these conditions settle. A small percentage of patients may require surgical release of a tendinitis at the wrist.

The retinaculum surrounding the extensor carpi ulnaris may be disrupted when rotational force is applied to the wrist. This may happen with a shanked golf shot when the club strikes a root or rock (watch out for the hook of the hamate fracture as well). If this results in subluxation of the tendon then reconstruction of the retinaculum may be necessary. Again, a functional brace may be needed on return to sports.

Over the last 10 years wrist arthroscopy has been playing an increasingly larger role in managing athletic injuries. It allows patients to return to sport more quickly than when open procedures

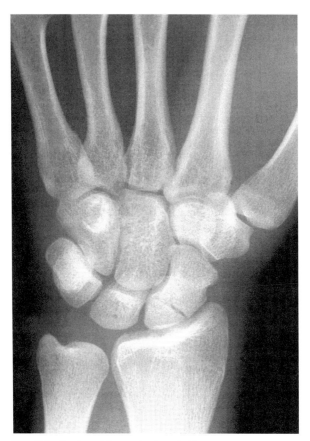

FIG. 7-6 Fracture of the proximal scaphoid.

are performed. Arthroscopy is used for both diagnosis and in treatment. It can be used as an adjunct to limited open reduction of a wrist fracture. TFCC debridement or repair has become possible arthroscopically.

It is not uncommon to see normal wrist x-rays and yet find pathology arthroscopically. Partial ligament tears, chondromalacia of articular surfaces, and synovitis of the joint can be diagnosed and debrided with use of the arthroscope. As in the knee, osteoarthritis of the wrist can also be treated arthroscopically with patients returning to sports in 2 to 3 weeks. A wrist support or taping may be necessary for the first few weeks and range of motion exercises may begin the day of surgery.

THE HAND

The vast majority of hand fractures seen in the athlete (up to 90 percent) can be handled by closed means. The goal is for early unloaded range of motion of the digits within 1 week of the injury. This helps to lessen swelling and prevent joint and tendon adhesions. Extension block splinting, buddy taping (adjacent finger strapping), and the use of Coban and range of motion exercises are used to achieve these objectives.

Fractures in the hand may be oblique, transverse, or comminuted (Fig. 7-7). Excessive shortening must be avoided (especially with the proximal phalanx), or the extensor mechanism will not function properly. Malrotation and excessive angulation must also be corrected (Fig. 7-8). With the metacarpophalangeal (MCP) and proximal interphalangeal (PIP) joints in flexion, rotation is checked by ensuring that the nail plate points toward the scaphoid tubercle. When obvious malalignment of a digit is seen on the playing field it should be gently realigned and taped to the adjacent digit.

With metacarpal neck fractures (Boxers' fracture) up to 35 to 40 degrees of volar angulation may be accepted in the fourth and fifth metacarpals. This relates to mobility of the subjacent carpometacarpal (CMC) joints. Less angulation is acceptable as the fracture becomes more proximal in the metacarpal. No more than 15 to 20 degrees is acceptable with the second and third metacarpals. Many metacarpal neck fractures are stable and can be managed with early motion, buddy taping, and a compressive bandage to help with the swelling. Unstable fractures may need pin fixation and a gutter splint.

Many phalangeal fractures are stable in flexion and unstable in extension. If a stable range can be established then extension block splinting using buddy taping allows motion through that range. Position of the fracture should be checked weekly with an x-ray over the first 3 weeks. A fracture that is unstable through all ranges or has an intraarticular component may require operative fixation. Range of motion is started once stability has been obtained.

Most displaced hand fractures can be reduced under a digital or metacarpal block. Gentle traction usually allows correction of the deformity. If successful reduction cannot be either obtained or maintained, then open reduction or percutaneous pinning may be necessary.

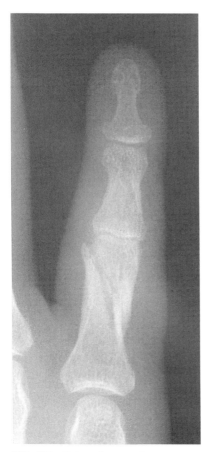

FIG. 7-7   Oblique fracture of the proximal phalanx.

Crush injuries of the fingertip are often associated with a fracture, and most are amenable to a splint. If the nail is avulsed it can be replaced to act as a splint. A laceration of the nail bed with a bony injury represents a compound fracture. This should be managed with a thorough debridement and antibiotic coverage. The nail

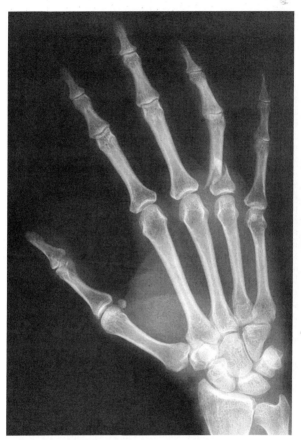

FIG. 7-8 Proximal phalanx fracture with malrotation.

bed may also require repair with a fine absorbable suture. The nail may be replaced to splint the nail bed while it heals.

Dislocation may occur in any of the joints in the hand. They are usually in a dorsal direction and can often be reduced on the playing field by applying traction to the digit. Occasionally soft tissue becomes interposed in the joint, making reduction difficult. This can occur at the MCP level with the flexor tendons or at the interphalangeal level with a volar plate caught in the joint. Dislocations are also managed with early unloaded range of motion employing buddy taping and occasionally extension block splinting. CMC joint dislocations may be unstable and require pin fixation.

Ligament injuries are very common at both the MCP and interphalangeal joint level. It is useful to think of these joints as a box with four sides. These sides include the volar plate, radial and ulnar collateral ligaments, and the extensor mechanism. Each structure can be palpated and stressed in turn to assess for injuries. If sore enough, a digital block may be necessary for this examination. At the MCP joint the collateral ligaments are in maximum tension in flexion and are tested in this position as well as in extension.

MCP injuries to the collateral ligaments and volar plate are often slow to heal and may require long-term use of buddy taping. Volar plate injuries may need extension block splinting. The thumb MCP ulnar collateral ligament (UCL) injury is referred to as a "ski-pole" or "gamekeeper's" thumb. Ski poles with strap bindings are a common source of this injury, although it can occur with any "FOOSH" injury.

Sprains of the UCL of the thumb are managed with a removable splint and early unloaded range of motion. The splint is discontinued once local discomfort has settled. Much of the hand surgery literature suggests that complete UCL tears require surgery. My experience has been that many of these can be treated by closed means. This would include 3 to 4 weeks in a short scaphoid-type cast followed by a removable splint. The exceptions are the grossly unstable joint that was likely a dislocation and represents damage to more than the UCL. A large bony fragment usually renders the joint unstable and requires repair. Whether ski-pole thumbs are treated operatively or not the athlete may need to use prophylactic splinting or taping once they resume their sporting activities.

Boutonniere injuries occur at the PIP level with a disruption of the central slip of the extensor tendon mechanism. They are often the result of longitudinal force to the finger such as catching a basketball. Once the central slip is disrupted, the lateral bands may sublux volarly and result in a PIP flexion deformity. There may also be a secondary hyperextension deformity of the distal interphalangeal joint (DIP). If the injury is appreciated initially, the PIP joint is splinted in extension for 6 to 8 weeks and the DIP joint left free for motion. Often this injury is overlooked or does not fully develop for 10 to 14 days. If the athlete presents with a PIP flexion contracture then dynamic splinting is used during the day and static splinting at night. Prophylactic splinting is used at sport until the injury has completely resolved, which may be 6 months or longer.

A late boutonniere may not respond to splinting alone and may require surgical repair. This involves release of the collateral ligaments and volar plate. The lateral bands are released and moved dorsally, and the central slip of the extensor is reconstructed. Six months of splinting and therapy may be needed for a successful outcome.

At the DIP joint, injury to the extensor mechanism results in a mallet finger. This may be an injury to the tendon alone, involve a bony fragment, or go through the epiphysis in the adolescent athlete. Most of these are managed with splinting unless the bony fragment renders the DIP joint unstable. Full-time splinting for 6 weeks results in a successful outcome in the vast majority of cases. Night splinting is continued for a further 3 to 4 weeks. A delay in treatment for up to 6 weeks may still result in a favorable outcome as long as there is still an inflammatory reaction over the DIP joint when the splinting is commenced. A late mallet finger can be reconstructed by removal of an ellipse of skin and tendon dorsally (tenodermatodesis). The defect is closed to correct the flexion deformity and the DIP joint pinned for 6 weeks. A protective splint is employed for a further 6 weeks for sports.

A further tendon injury is the "rugger jersey" finger. This is an avulsion of the profundus tendon from the distal phalanx. The ring finger is most commonly involved, and the injury usually occurs when something being tightly gripped (the opponent's sweater) is forcibly pulled away. This results in forced extension of the digit while the flexor profundus is maximally contracted. The tendon may be avulsed or a fragment pulled off of the distal phalanx. Commonly, the tendon retracts to the PIP level but may end up in the palm. The significance of this injury is often not initially appreciated. Ideally, it is repaired within 10 days, although success is possible up to 8 weeks postinjury. If seen several months later, the profundus stump may be excised and the DIP joint fused if unstable. Restoration of tendon function at that time often requires a two-stage tendon reconstruction with significant downtime from sport.

The extensor expansion is a retinaculum that stabilizes the extensor tendon over the MCP joint. This structure may be forcibly disrupted (typically the radial side) with subluxation or dislocation of the tendon in an ulnar direction. These occur most commonly in the index and long fingers. Patients present with swelling, pain, and complaints of weakness. They may also be aware of the tendon snapping over the metacarpal head. A minor disruption is managed by buddy taping and may be slow to settle. Most require surgical reconstruction of the radial sagittal band.

Ring avulsion injuries occur when a ring catches on something while the athlete is pulling away or falling. They run a spectrum from a crush of the soft tissues to amputation. Any suggestion of circulatory compromise should be referred to a hand surgeon. An athlete who insists on wearing rings while competing should be encouraged to purchase a breakaway-type ring to minimize the occurrence of this injury.

One final mention is made of human bites. These can happen when the hand ends up in an opponent's face or mouth. The typical injury is over the dorsum of the MCP joints. These wounds require thorough debridement, should be left open, and need antibiotic treatment.

RECOMMENDED READINGS

1. Green DP: *Operative Hand Surgery*, 3d ed. New York, Churchill Livingstone.
2. American Society for Surgery of the Hand: *Hand Surgery Update*. Park Ridge, IL, American Academy of Orthopaedic Surgeons.

8 | Knee Injuries

Charles Bull

Knee injuries are the most frequent problem in most sports clinics. Orthopaedic sports medicine specialists often end up doing 60 to 70 percent of their elective surgery on knees. Recently, the diagnosis and treatment of knee injuries has made great advances. The treatment of anterior cruciate tears has been revolutionized by advances in arthroscopic equipment and techniques.

ANATOMY

The knee is an inherently unstable joint held together by ligaments, cushioned by menisci, and covered by muscles. The quadriceps muscle extends the knee, and the medial and lateral hamstring muscles (semitendinosus, semimembranosus, and the two heads of biceps femoris) flex the knee.

The femur and tibia are hinged by four fibroelastic ligaments—the anterior and posterior cruciate ligaments cross in the center of the joint and the medial and lateral collateral ligaments are attached to the sides of the joint. The medial and lateral menisci cushion the tibia against the femoral condyles and provide some additional internal stability. The patella functions as a sesamoid bone in the quadriceps muscle over the femur (Fig. 8-1).

The patella has three facets (medial, lateral, and odd) that articulate with the distal femur. When the knee is in full extension, the patella articulates with the suprapatellar pouch (bursa). In 10 to 20 degrees of flexion, the patella articulates with the hyaline cartilage of the most proximal femoral trochlea. This groove between the femoral condyles allows the patella to track with flexion and extension.

In midflexion the articulation is at the medial and lateral facets. In full flexion the peripheral portions of the medial and lateral facets and the odd facet are involved. Thus as flexion progresses past 45 degrees (1/4 squat), weight-bearing load increases on the patella and femoral groove.

DIAGNOSIS

Normal movement of the knee allows flexion and extension, internal and external rotation, and sliding movements of the femur on the tibia. When the joint is forced beyond its normal excursion, ten-

113

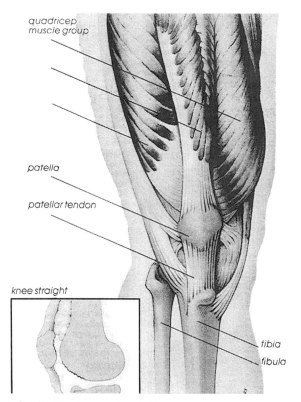

quadricep
muscle group

patella

patellar tendon

knee straight

tibia

fibula

FIG. 8-1   Muscles around front of the knee.

sion failure occurs in the surrounding muscles, fibrous capsule, and ligaments. The description of the mechanism of the injury combined with a careful and complete physical examination usually lead to an accurate diagnosis.

HISTORY

The injury may have occurred through crouching or twisting, or the knee may have given out while landing after jumping. Valgus injuries are produced by direct force to the lateral aspect of the knee, and contusions are caused by direct blows or falling on the flexed knee. An audible or palpable popping sensation usually indicates a severe ligament or bone injury. In severe injuries the knee gives way on weight bearing or weight bearing is too painful to continue playing sports or working. Generalized swelling that develops within 24 h indicates serious injury with blood in the joint (hemarthrosis). Localized swelling or swelling that develops after 24 h is usually caused by increased synovial fluid in less severe injuries (effusion).

EXAMINATION

Both knees should always be examined with pants, shoes, and socks removed. Observe the ability of the patient to bear weight on the injured leg and any limp or difficulty walking. Is swelling of the knee localized or generalized? Identify localized tenderness and note any limitation of full extension or flexion.

Test the collateral ligaments with valgus and varus stresses with the knee in full extension and 30- and 60-degree flexion. Note the amount of laxity and pain with each test compared to the uninjured side. Always examine the anterior cruciate ligament using the Lachman test. Note any posterior displacement of the tibia on the femur indicating an injury to the posterior cruciate ligament. Pressure applied to the medial border of the patella with the knee in extension produces pain and apprehension after subluxation or dislocation of the patella. We were taught to always x-ray all knee injuries, but owing to the extreme financial crisis in medical care, the Ottawa Knee Rule is suggested.

The Ottawa Knee Rule, a guideline to avoid unnecessary x-rays for knee injuries in adults, apparently works well in clinical practice, according to an article in *The Journal of the American Medical Association* (JAMA).[1] Ian Stiell and colleagues, from the University of Ottawa, assessed the impact of the Ottawa Knee Rule at two teaching and two community hospitals in Ottawa over two 12-month periods. "Implementation of the Ottawa Knee Rule led to a decrease in use of knee radiography without patient dissatisfaction or missed fractures and was associated with reduced waiting times and costs," they wrote. "Widespread use of the rule could lead to important health care savings without jeopardizing patient care." The researchers examined data on the treatment of 3907 adults with acute knee injuries who sought help in the emergency department. After the first 12-month period, attending physicians at one teaching and one community hospital were taught the Ottawa Knee Rule.

When compared with the first 12-month period, the researchers found a *26.4 percent reduction* in the proportion of patients referred for knee radiography at the hospitals using the Ottawa Knee Rule and only 1.3 percent reduction at the hospitals not taught the Ottawa Knee Rule. No patient discharged without radiography was subsequently found to have a fracture. In addition, among patients who did not have knee fractures, the researchers found that those who were discharged without radiography spent less time (about 33 minutes less) in the emergency department and incurred lower medical charges (about $133 less) than patients who underwent radiography. Of the patients successfully reached for follow-up, nearly all (95.7 percent not receiving radiography and 98 percent receiving radiography) said they were satisfied with their care.

"We believe that the health economic implications of the study are important," the researchers wrote. Approximately 13.5 million extremity radiographic series are ordered each year in U.S. emergency departments. These high-volume, little-ticket items may add as much to rising health care costs as more expensive, but low-volume, high-technology items. As the researchers noted, "We estimate that more than $1 billion may be spent annually in the United States and Canada on outpatient knee radiography. We believe that widespread implementation of the Ottawa Knee Rule would lead to significant societal health care savings." Under the Ottawa Knee Rule, a knee x-ray series is required for knee injury patients with at least one of the following:

Age 55 years or older
Isolated tenderness of the patella (kneecap)
Tenderness at the head of the fibula (calf bone)
Inability to flex the knee 90 degrees
Inability to bear weight both immediately and in the emergency department

Instruction in use of the Ottawa Knee Rule included a brief lecture, a pocket card, and several posters mounted in the emergency department. The rule has not been tested on patients under the age of 18 years. The rules have been endorsed and modified by the Buffalo, New York Group.[2]

Remember that anterior pain in the knee can be referred pain from the hip in a child (articular synovitis, slipped capital femoral epiphysis, Legg-Perthes Disease) or in an adult (osteoarthritis of the hip). Occasionally, posterior pain in the knee can be referred pain along the lumbosacral nerves related to sciatica.

TREATMENT OF KNEE INJURIES

Early accurate diagnosis is the key to successful treatment of knee injuries. Once fractures and neurovascular injuries have been ruled out, general treatment of the more common injuries is begun. If a specific diagnosis cannot be made or there has not been significant reduction in the pain and swelling after 48 h, orthopaedic consultation is necessary.

Torn Meniscus

The menisci are the most frequently injured structures in the knee. Autopsy studies have reported an incidence of 54 percent torn menisci. In the United States one person per thousand has arthroscopic surgery every year. Therefore, many patients with a torn meniscus do not require surgery.

There is usually point tenderness over the torn meniscus that is aggravated by crouching or compression (Figs. 8-2 and 8-3). There is frequently an effusion and atrophy of the thigh. Occasionally the knee is locked in partial flexion (Table 8-1; Fig. 8-4).

A careful examination leads to an accurate diagnosis in 90 percent of torn menisci. An MRI study increases the diagnostic accuracy to over 95 percent. The MRI should be compared with the clinical examination since treatment is still a clinical decision. When a patient can squat without difficulty, arthroscopic surgery is *not* usually necessary even though the MRI shows a torn meniscus.

The final decision regarding surgery is made by the patient according to his or her symptoms and the physical requirements of his or her lifestyle. When surgery is necessary, arthroscopic partial meniscectomy is the standard procedure. Peripheral tears of the menisci in young people can be sutured arthroscopically.

A meniscus repair is most likely to succeed within the first 6 weeks postinjury. Thus, the knee can be scoped at 2 weeks. If there is a lack of extension and swelling, the arthroscopy is better done at 3 or 4 weeks. The anterior cruciate repair is easier at about 6 weeks.

Anterior and midportion medial meniscus repairs can be done well arthroscopically. Posteromedial and lateral repairs usually require a small incision as well as arthroscopy. Bucket handle tears are only repaired in teenagers, but smaller peripheral repairs can be done up until the age of 40.

MENISCAL CYSTS

Lateral Meniscal Cyst

When a horizontal cleavage tear of the lateral meniscus develops, fluid may extrude from the joint into the soft tissues through the defect in the meniscus. This collection of fluid, which varies with activity, is caused by the valvelike effect of the horizontal split in the lateral meniscus, which allows fluid to escape from the knee joint and traps the fluid. When the torn segment of the lateral

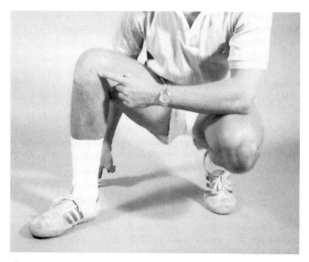

A

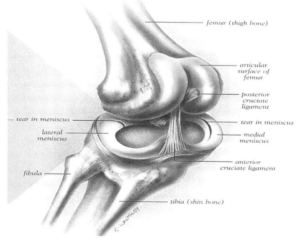

B

FIG. 8-2 Incomplete crouching and point tenderness over torn meniscus.

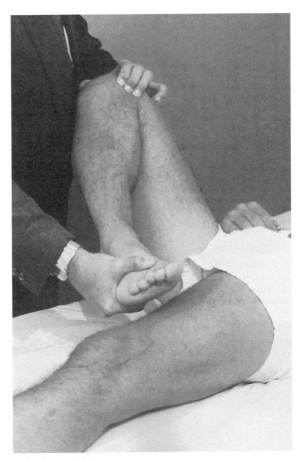

FIG. 8-3 Compression produces pain over torn meniscus.

meniscus is removed, the flap valve is obliterated, marsupializing the cyst. This procedure can usually be performed arthroscopically.

Medial Meniscal Cyst

In the degenerative tears of the medial meniscus a horizontal cleavage tear may allow fluid from the knee joint to extrude out of the

TABLE 8-1 Differential Diagnosis of a Locked Knee

Displaced meniscal tear
Loose body
Intraarticular fracture
Displaced intraarticular ligament (anterior cruciate ligament)

joint producing a cystlike collection of fluid. This collection of fluid usually communicates with the medial meniscus on an MRI study. Clinically the medial meniscus cyst is small and discrete with a firm rubbery texture adjacent to the posterior horn of the medial meniscus.

The treatment is combined arthroscopic excision of the medial meniscus tear and open excision of the medial meniscal cyst. The communication between the tear of the medial meniscus and the medial meniscal cyst is not usually found at arthroscopy, and open excision is usually necessary. This differs from lateral meniscal cysts where the lateral meniscal tear is usually readily visible and the cyst can be exposed arthroscopically.

Knee Ligament Injuries

Medial collateral and anterior cruciate injuries comprise over 95 percent of all knee ligament injuries. Injuries to the posterior cruciate ligament account for less than 5 percent, and lateral collateral injuries are rare.

Medial Collateral Ligament Injuries

The medial collateral ligament is torn when a valgus force is applied to the lateral aspect of the knee—usually while the knee is

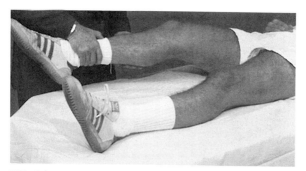

FIG. 8-4   Incomplete extension when knee is locked due to torn meniscus.

partially flexed. The ligament is examined by applying a valgus stress on the knee in full extension and 30- and 60-degree flexion.

A partial tear is described as a grade 1 (first-degree) *sprain* when there is <5-mm opening of the medial side of the joint at 0 degrees flexion on valgus stress compared to the opposite normal knee. This is a microscopic tear; the fibers are stretched and there is some microscopic hemorrhage. There is *no* abnormal joint laxity.

A grade 2 (second-degree) *tear* is also partial, but tissues are macroscopically torn. There is loss of function, more swelling, and pain. There is more laxity, up to 10 mm, a definite endpoint is noted.

A grade 3 (third-degree) *tear* is a complete ligament tear with loss of joint stability. A very soft endpoint, or no endpoint, is felt on testing. The joint opens 1.0 to 1.5 cm. The anterior cruciate is usually involved. *Beware*: This injury can occur on some occasions with only a minimal effusion (Fig. 8-5A, B).

Treatment

Surgery is not necessary for partial or complete tears of the medial collateral ligament. The knee is initially rested in an immobilizer for comfort, and active protected motion is begun while wearing a hinged brace. Grade 1 sprains usually heal sufficiently for return to sports within 3 to 4 weeks. Grade 2 tears heal within 6 to 8 weeks. Grade 3 tears take at least 3 months to return to full competition.

An MRI study is not usually necessary for isolated medial collateral ligament sprains. Peripheral tears of the medial meniscus often accompany medial collateral ligament tears and heal completely as the ligament heals.

Anterior Cruciate Ligament Injuries

A torn anterior cruciate ligament is the most common serious knee injury in sports. The anterior cruciate can be torn by an external rotation injury while the foot is planted, by suddenly falling with the knee fully flexed, or by landing with the knee in hyperextension after jumping. The patient frequently hears and feels a "pop" and notices immediate pain and a feeling of instability. The athlete is unable to continue the game, and the knee usually swells within 12 h (hemarthrosis) (Tables 8-2 and 8-3).

TABLE 8-2 Differential Diagnosis of Hemarthrosis

Anterior cruciate ligament tear
Patellar subluxation
Intraarticular fracture
Meniscal tear

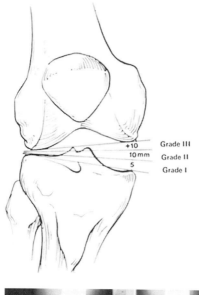

A

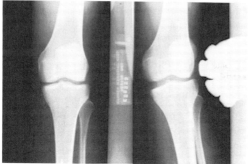

B

FIG. 8-5 Complete tear of medial collateral ligament (grade 3 sprain).

Examination

The majority of anterior cruciate ligament tears are missed on the first examination. Since a neglected anterior cruciate ligament injury leads to instability, torn menisci, and eventually arthritis, early

TABLE 8-3 The Usual Features of a Torn Anterior Cruciate Ligament

Audible pop
Giving way
Immediate swelling
Unable to continue

accurate diagnosis is essential for definitive treatment and preservation of the knee (Fig. 8-6).

There are two important tests in diagnosing a torn anterior cruciate: The Lachman test and the Pivot Shift test. The Lachman test, which is more than 85 percent accurate, is the most important test for a torn anterior cruciate. With the patient supine the knee is held in 20-degree flexion. While the hamstring muscles are relaxed, the tibia is pulled gently forward with the femur stabilized (Fig. 8-7). Comparison with the other knee reveals the normal knee has a definite endpoint as the tibia is pulled forward. When the anterior cruciate ligament is torn the endpoint is indefinite. This is graded as: first, second, and third, with third the most severe laxity.

In some cases where your hand is too small or the thigh is too big to properly relax the hamstring, a two-handed Lachman test can be done. This is done with both of the examiner's hands on the tibia. It is best to have an assistant hold the femur and relax the hamstrings or strap the femur to an exercise bench. This can also be accomplished by placing the examiner's thigh beneath the knee, and the upper hand can stabilize the femur on the thigh.

MacIntosh Lateral Pivot Shift Test

The patient is supine and relaxed. The foot is internally rotated and allowed to sag into extension. The heel of the examiner's hand is placed on the proximal lateral tibia with a strong valgus stress. As

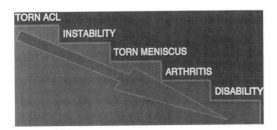

FIG. 8-6 Gradual deterioration of the knee in active individual with unrepaired torn anterior cruciate ligament.

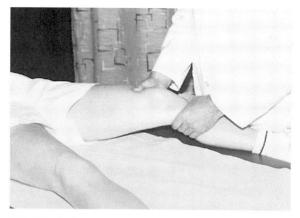

FIG. 8-7   Lachman test is the most reliable test for a torn anterior cruciate ligament.

the leg is flexed from full extension to 10 degrees of flexion, the tibia partially dislocates. This is graded: one a slide, two a shift, and three a real "clunk." According to Reid's *Sports Injury Assessment and Rehabilitation,*[3] this grade 3 is a shift of 15 mm medial and 22 mm lateral of the tibial plateaus. This is equivalent to a Lachman test of more than 15 mm. The sports practitioner can perfect these tests after a few instruction sessions at the sports clinic.

Testing the ligament with the knee flexed to 90 degrees (Drawer test) is unreliable. If the initial Lachman test or Pivot Shift test is unsatisfactory owing to swelling or muscle spasm the knee should be carefully reexamined after 48 h. Occasionally, examination under anesthesia is necessary. Arthroscopic examination is helpful, but a torn ligament can appear intact at arthroscopy if the sheath is intact. Therefore, arthroscopic examination must be accompanied by examination of the ligament under anesthesia.

An MRI study may be helpful but it is not always diagnostic for complete acute tears. An MRI is unreliable in long-standing tears because fibrosis owing to scar tissue may give the appearance of an intact ligament. The final determination of a torn anterior cruciate ligament is made on clinical examination.

When the anterior cruciate ligament is torn there is a 70 percent chance of associated articular cartilage and bone injury (bone bruises). An associated tear of a meniscus is found in 50 percent of acute anterior cruciate ligament injuries. If the anterior cruciate ligament tear is not treated in an active person there is an 80 percent chance of developing a torn meniscus within 1 year. Therefore, early diagnosis and treatment is essential to avoid irreversible damage to the joint.

Treatment

X-rays are necessary to rule out an avulsion of the tibial attachment of the anterior cruciate ligament that can be immediately treated surgically with open reduction and internal fixation.

Initially isolated anterior cruciate ligament tears are treated with RICE and crutches followed by protected active motion as the swelling subsides. It is usually not necessary to aspirate the knee unless the effusion is quite tense. If the medial collateral and anterior cruciate ligaments are both torn, a hinged brace should be worn to protect the medial collateral ligament. The anterior cruciate ligament does not heal and needs to be replaced by surgical reconstruction for a stable functional knee in an active individual.

When full motion has been recovered and swelling is minimal, surgical reconstruction of the anterior cruciate ligament is planned. Associated medial collateral ligament tears do not require surgical repair.

The torn anterior cruciate ligament (ACL) is replaced by a bone–patellar tendon–bone graft inserted under arthroscopic control or through a miniarthrotomy. More recently an arthroscopic anterior cruciate ligament repair using hamstrings has been advocated by many knee surgeons. This avoids postoperative patellar tendinitis, and the patient is rehabilitated more quickly with less stiffness.

Studies according to Don Johnson show semi-T and gracilus composite graft is equal to 11-mm patellar tendon graft.[4] The four-bundle tensioned graft is 250 percent the strength of the normal ACL (4300 newtons compared to 1750 newtons for the normal ACL).

Complete graft healing takes 10 to 12 weeks. There is no hamstring weakness after graft harvest. Other graft possibilities are allografts and quads tendon grafts. Synthetic (Gortex) grafts were not successful. Presently, biological tissue must be used for cruciate ligament repairs. These repairs are followed by immediate full motion and early weight-bearing using crutches.

Posterior Cruciate Ligament

The posterior cruciate ligament (PCL) is usually torn by a hyperextension injury (stepping into a hole) or a direct blow to the front of the tibia while the knee is flexed at 90 degrees. This injury occurs when the tibia strikes a goal post while the knee is flexed or a dashboard in a head-on collision. Swelling and pain may not be as severe as in anterior cruciate ligament injuries, and the patient may be able to bear full weight on the injured leg. The diagnosis is made by flexing the knee to 90 degrees while the patient is supine and comparing the injured knee to the unaffected knee. The prominence of the anteromedial tibia is lost in posterior cruciate ligament tears, and anterior pressure on the tibia produces posterior displacement of the tibia (posterior Drawer sign). X-rays should be obtained to rule out an avulsion of the tibial attachment of the posterior cruciate, which can be treated surgically.

The posterior cruciate ligament does not heal and reconstructive replacement with bone–patellar tendon–bone graft or semitendinosus (hamstrings) is necessary if significant functional instability develops.

Lateral Collateral

Injuries of the lateral collateral ligament are occasionally seen in sports injuries but more frequently occur following severe motor vehicle trauma. Careful examination of the peroneal nerve should be carried out in all cases of lateral collateral ligament injuries. This "lateral corner injury" can require urgent surgery.

Posterolateral Injuries

Posterolateral injuries are occasionally seen following sports-related injuries and may occur as an isolated injury or in combination with posterior cruciate ligament injuries. Increased external rotation of the tibia compared to the noninjured knee while the knee is flexed to 90 degrees is usually diagnostic.

Dislocations of the Knee

Dislocations of the knee are usually posterior and follow severe direct trauma. Frequently more than one ligament is torn—usually the anterior and posterior cruciate ligaments. Knee dislocations are frequently accompanied by vascular and nerve injuries. Therefore, careful neurovascular examination of the leg and frequently angiography are indicated following knee dislocations.

The popliteal artery is injured in 32 percent of cases.[5] If the blood supply is not restored in 6 to 8 hours, there is an 86 percent amputation rate.

Peroneal nerve injury occurs in 14 to 35 percent of cases. Spontaneous recovery occurs in some cases of nerve stretch. Late cable grafting may be necessary at 3 months with transection. Surgical reconstruction should be done within 2 weeks and reconstruction of the ACL and PCL is recommended, to be done by an experienced knee ligament team.

Dislocation of the Patella

The patella is dislocated by an external rotation force on the tibia while the foot is planted and the knee is in valgus. The injury usually occurs in adolescence, the patella dislocates laterally and often reduces spontaneously. The patient often hears a pop, notices a sensation of giving way, and develops swelling within 12 h. These clinical features are similar to tears of the anterior cruciate ligament, and a torn anterior cruciate ligament must be ruled out before the definite diagnosis of patellar dislocation is made. The injury occurs when the knee is in partial flexion, and when the knee is fully extended while taking an x-ray the patella may spontaneously relocate.

In acute dislocation of the patella there is a definite endpoint on the Lachman test indicating an intact anterior cruciate ligament. The patellar apprehension test produced by pressure on the medial border of the patella while the knee is extended produces pain and an immediate reaction (apprehension) in the patient (Fig. 8-8).

X-rays may show a small avulsion fracture off the medial border of the patella. An intraarticular loose body is occasionally seen caused by an osteochondral fracture resulting from the patella shearing the anterolateral corner off the lateral femoral condyle as it forcibly relocates.

Acute patellar dislocations are treated with protected active motion using a knee support with a patellar pad within a few days of the injury after the initial pain and swelling have subsided. If recurrent dislocations or subluxation of the patella occur, each

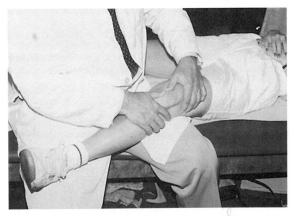

FIG. 8-8   Patellar apprehension test.

episode produces further articular cartilage damage to the patellofemoral surfaces. In recurrent dislocations of the patella surgical realignment of the patella is indicated to prevent severe traumatic patellofemoral arthritis.

Injuries of Knee Extension Mechanism

The extensor mechanism of the knee can be interrupted by avulsion of the patellar tendon from the tibial tuberosity, rupture of the patellar tendon, fracture of the patella, or rupture of the quadriceps muscle and tendon. Ruptures of the patellar tendon usually occur in young adults following severe acute flexion injuries. Ruptures of the quadriceps muscle more frequently occur in patients over 40 following sudden weight bearing on the flexed knee, such as missing a step. When the extensor mechanism is interrupted, active extension of the knee is not possible. When extension of the knee is not possible against gravity, interruption of the extensor mechanism must be suspected and orthopaedic consultation obtained.

Clinically, a defect can be felt in the patellar tendon below the knee or in the quadriceps tendon above the knee when a complete rupture of the tendon or muscle has occurred. When extension is possible against gravity even with marked difficulty, the lesion is probably a partial rupture and it will heal conservatively. An MRI is helpful in the operative decision. At operation, restoration of full extension is mandatory. Thus postoperative prolonged rehabilitation is necessary to regain full flexion.

KNEE INJURIES IN CHILDREN

In the growing child the distal femoral and proximal tibial physeal plates are more vulnerable to injury than the ligaments of the knee. Therefore, every knee injury in children should be x-rayed with comparison views of the uninjured knee, keeping a high index of suspicion for epiphyseal fractures or separations.

Osteochondritis Dissecans

Separation of osteochondral fragments from the medial and lateral femoral condyles may be developmental or related to trauma. This condition must be suspected in growing children or young adults who complain of recurrent knee pain without specific trauma. X-rays of the knee show the lesion that most frequently occurs on the lateral aspect of the medial femoral condyle.

The lesions are graded 1 to 4:

Stage 1 (in situ) in 10- to 13-year-olds with the articular surface intact.

Stage 2 (separating) articular surface intact but softened. Occurs in 13- to 15-year-olds with more pain and effusion.

Stage 3 (loose lesion) ages 14 to 20. These can be pinned, although results are inconsistent.

Stage 4 (displaced lesion) usually over age 15 years. The loose body is removed and bed debrided. Initial good results can usually be obtained, but the knee is prone to future osteoarthritis.

The key to prognosis of this avascular necrosis problem is epiphyseal closure. Prior to closure it is called juvenile osteochondritis, and this usually heals. However, if it has not healed before closure of the distal femoral epiphysis, the adult osteochondritis results, which has a much poorer prognosis.

Sports participation depends on symptoms, but in all cases, cutting, jumping, and pivoting sports should be discouraged. This condition is similar to Legg-Perthes disease of the hip and Panner's disease of the capitulum of the elbow.

COMMON PAINFUL KNEE CONDITIONS

Patellofemoral Pain Syndrome (Chondromalacia)

Studies have shown that patellofemoral pain syndrome comprises up to 50 percent of all overuse injuries. The pain is frequently seen in adolescents and young adults following repetitive jumping activities. The syndrome is caused by an irritation of the undersurface of the patella. The pain is usually a dull pain that seems to come from deep in the knee. It is worst with deep knee bend–type sports. Usually there is pain climbing stairs and after sitting for a prolonged period of time. The pain is caused by compression of the patella against the femur that increases as the knee is bent.

Basically, the irritation of the patella causes an inflammation that causes the pain. *This is not arthritis.* It is most common in children and adolescents who almost always grow out of this problem.

Predisposing Factors

1. Maltracking. When the patella is not symmetrical in the femoral groove it is said to be maltracking, which causes increased compression between the patella and the femur. Maltracking is most common in people who have wide hips, knock knees, or tibial torsion (rotation of the lower leg).
2. Flat, pronated feet
3. Overuse ("too much, too soon" syndrome)
4. Weak inner thigh muscles
5. Tight outer knee structures
6. Muscle inflexibilities
7. Previous or repetitive trauma to the knee

Examination

Frequently, the exact location of the pain is difficult to find but there is usually painful crepitus on compressing the patella against the underlying femur. There is frequently tenderness under the medial border of the patella. Kneeling is uncomfortable and rising from a kneeling position leading with the affected leg produces pain.

If an effusion is found, a thorough examination should be carried out for a significant chondral abnormality or arthritis.

X-rays are usually negative in chronic patellofemoral pain unless arthritis is present. Conservative treatment emphasizes patellar sparing quadriceps stretching and strengthening. It is important to avoid open chain extension exercises using weights or machines that aggravate the irritation on the patellofemoral joint. Short-range closed chain exercises, using pain as a guide are suggested (see Chap. 33), as are the following.

EXERCISES

The key to treating this problem is an exercise program to help control the patella in the femoral groove. When the exercises are done regularly and properly, this problem is almost always dramatically improved.

Stretches

Flexibility is an important part of injury treatment and prevention. For stretching to be effective it must be done on a regular basis. Always stretch when you are warmed up. It is important to stretch before and after activity. Stretching should not be painful. All stretches should be done in a slow static manner with *no* bouncing. Hold stretches for at least 30 to 60 s and repeat several times. For difficult problems, a therapist may have to assist you to improve your flexibility.

Single Quadricep Stretch

Standing with your back straight, pull your foot back. Push down and back with your knee until you feel a stretch in your quadriceps (thigh) muscle. If this causes knee pain, then do not do this stretch until your knee is improved.

Hamstring Stretch

Sit on the floor with your injured leg straight and the opposite leg curled in. Bend forward from the hips and reach toward your toes. You will feel a stretch in your hamstring muscle.

Hip Flexor Stretch

The sore knee is resting on a pillow. With your back straight push your hip through until you feel a stretch in the front of the hip. Place opposite hand on your thigh for balance.

STRENGTHENING EXERCISES

There is very little pressure in the patellofemoral joint in the first 25 to 30 degrees of knee flexion. These two exercises strengthen the knee without aggravating the condition. Do these exercises daily. Discontinue if they cause pain.

Static Quads

Sit on the floor with a towel roll or pillow under your knee. Pull your toes toward you and compress the towel roll with your knee. Hold 10 to 15 s. Repeat 30 times.

Quarter Squat

Squeeze a towel roll or pillow between your knees. Slowly lower down into a quarter squat. Keep your knees pointing straight with your knees directly over your second toe. Do three sets of 15 repetitions. This can progress to a single leg quarter squat with your injured knee. Remember to keep your knee pointing straight ahead.

The following is a guide to sports participation for patellofemoral syndrome.

SPORTS

Quarter Squat Principle

There is very little pressure between the patella and the femur when the leg is straight or only slightly bent. The best activities are ones that limit the knee to a range between 0 degrees (straight) and 45 degrees (1/4 squat).

Good Sports

These sports are easiest on the knee.
1. Swimming (flutter kick, knees straight)
2. Slow jogging, walking
3. Skating
4. Cross-country skiing
5. Roller blading

Moderately Good Sports

These sports can be performed by some, but could cause problems for others.

1. Easy cycling (seat high, low gears, and high cadence—pedal at 85 to 95 rpm)
2. Soccer
3. Baseball
4. Hockey
5. Skiing (downhill, avoid moguls)
6. Aerobics

Aggravating Sports

These sports can be hardest on your knees, as they include deep, lunging knee actions. These sports are most likely to aggravate your condition.

1. Volleyball
2. Basketball
3. Running (sprints, downhill)
4. Football
5. Racquetball
6. Squash

Use your judgment. When your knees hurt, avoid all but the good sports. Total rest may be required. When your knees get better after treatment, you should be able to enjoy all sports.

Always warm up well before you play.

REPETITIVE OVERUSE SYNDROMES

Such syndromes include patellar tendinitis (jumper's knee), pre-patellar bursitis (housemaid's knee), and tibial tubercle apophysitis (Osgood-Schlatter's disease).

These conditions are frequently seen in the physician's office and although trauma is frequently claimed as the instigating factor, it is usually related to overuse in sports that require constant squatting, kneeling, or jumping.

Examination locates the point of tenderness over the inferior pole of the patella in patellar tendinitis and over the tibial tuberosity in apophysitis. Soft tissue swelling between the shin and the patellar tendon is found in prepatellar bursitis.

These extraarticular conditions subside with time and symptomatic treatment while reducing the activities that aggravate the problem. Temporary reduction of athletic activities is recommended in apophysitis until the tibial tubercle softening and fragmentation heal, at approximately age 15 years.

Jumper's knee can be operated on in rare cases. This requires the use of a tourniquet and thus a general anesthetic. A small incision is made at the junction of the patella and the patellar tendon. The tendon is split longitudinally. Usually an area of necrotic tissue is found and excised. A portion of the lower pole of the patella is removed. The patellar tendon originates anterior to this and is not compromised. This procedure has good results and allows a return to jumping sports in the persistent cases that have not responded to all other modes of treatment.

POPLITEAL CYSTS (BAKER'S CYST)

Popliteal cysts in children present as a swelling over the postero-medial aspect of the knee. The cyst is a transient collection of fluid between the medial head of the biceps and the joint that does not require treatment and usually resolves spontaneously and disappears.

Popliteal cysts in adults are usually not true cysts but rather a posterior extension of an effusion secondary to degenerative arthritis or a torn medial meniscus. Treatment of the cause with anti-inflammatory medication is the first option. Arthroscopic surgery is occasionally indicated if conservative measures are not successful. Excision of the cyst is rarely necessary.

Popliteal cysts in patients with rheumatoid arthritis represent extension of the synovial disease into the posterior compartment of the knee and may produce pressure on the neurovascular structures. If conservative treatment of the arthritis does not reduce the swelling or pressure of the symptoms, then surgical removal is indicated. A total synovectomy of the knee is usually recommended at the time of surgery.

SYNVISC

Dr. Tim Deakon, Oakville, Ontario (*Practical Arthroscopy* 2:2–224, February 1998)

Viscosupplementation for Osteoarthritis of the Knee

When people ask about "gel" injections in the knee for osteoarthritis, I assume they are asking about the use of hyaluronic acid derivatives that are just now becoming available for use in the United States. Hylan GF-20 has been available as an intraarticular injectable since 1993 in Canada.

The products currently approved for use include Synvisc and Suplasyn. There are a couple of other agents that have recently become available as well, but I have little experience with these. Synvisc has been available in Sweden since 1995.

The combined Canadian and Swedish sales totaled U.S. $6.2 million in 1996. I have used both Synvisc and Suplasyn for the past 3 years, completing about 350 courses of the injections. Synvisc consists of three prepackaged syringes containing 2 cc each of Hylan GF-20. These are injected weekly for 3 weeks. The hyaluronic acid derivative is extracted from rooster combs and is polymerized and crosslinked. Allergy to eggs or chicken is a contraindication to treatment.

Synvisc works best in early osteoarthritis or in knees that fail to improve after arthroscopy. It also seems to work in some cases of more advanced OA.

It is unlikely to work where a significant malalignment exists or where the OA is full compartment bone on bone. I have had some good results in severe patellofemoral chondromalacia although the company does not promote this use. The injections *must* be intraarticular. Intrasynovial or extraarticular injections do not work and are much more likely to produce inflammatory reactions. These reactions still occur with intraarticular injections in an incidence of about 1 to 2 percent. I have changed my injection technique to ensure it gets in the joint.

The response rate in good candidates appears to be about 65 to 70 percent. Some responses are more dramatic than cortisone, and their effect can last 6 to 18 months. I have one patient (a physician) who has had five courses of Synvisc and he swears by it. The key is to use it on knees that are not yet too bad.

REFERENCES

1. Stiell I et al: *JAMA* 1997.
2. Leddy JJ: *Am J Sports Med* 26(2):158–165, 1998.
3. Reid DC: *Sports Injury Assessment and Rehabilitation.* New York, Churchill Livingstone, 1992.
4. Johnson D: *Pract Arthroscop* 5(2):175, 1997.
5. Johnson D: *Pract Arthroscop* 7(2):206, 1997.
6. Adams ME, Atkinson MH, Lussier AJ, et al: The role of hylan (Synvisc) in osteoarthritis of the knee. *Osteoarthritis and Cartilage* 3:213–226, 1995.
7. Deakon T.: *Pract Arthroscop* 2:2–224, 1998.

9 | **The Athlete's Arthritic Knee**

Glen Richardson   Bill Stanish

Athletics are an integral part of life for many people. It is well known that physical activity confers longevity and a sedentary lifestyle is associated with an increased mortality rate. With increased societal awareness of the benefits of physical activity, a new group of athletes with unique problems is beginning to emerge, the masters athlete.* One of the medical problems that aging athletes must face is osteoarthrosis of the knee. This condition can be very disabling, thus discouraging a healthy physical lifestyle. Unfortunately, osteoarthrosis of the knee is a chronic disease affecting the social and psychological well-being of an athlete. Therefore, it is imperative that the sports medicine physician be adept at diagnosing and treating osteoarthrosis of the knee.

BASIC SCIENCE

The knee is often thought of as a simple hinge joint, but it is really an unconstrained joint with a number of complex movements. There are many structures that support the knee joint, and any abnormalities of these structures can result in disability. In osteoarthrosis, the soft tissues of the knee joint are involved, but the key pathologic process is loss of articular cartilage. To fully understand the pathologic process occurring in osteoarthrosis, it is necessary to know about normal articular cartilage.

Articular cartilage is connective tissue with unique mechanical properties created by its biologic structure. Basically, articular cartilage consists of two components, cells and extracellular matrix. Chondrocytes are the cell type found in articular cartilage. They are responsible for the formation and maintenance of the extracellular matrix that forms the articular cartilage. Since the articular cartilage is a relatively avascular environment, the chondrocytes receive most of their metabolic requirements from the synovial fluid. The low oxygen tension of the articular cartilage forces the chondrocytes to rely mostly on anaerobic metabolism. Chondrocytes have been shown to replace degraded matrix and remodel the articular surface. Chondrocytes have a number of important functions in growing children, but in the aging athlete the function is restricted to the degradation and synthesis of the extracellular matrix. The interactions between chondrocytes and the articular cartilage are

*Senior runners: over 35 years; masters runners: over 40 years. This varies from sport to sport.

controlled in part by cytokines such as IL-1, TGFb, and insulin-dependent growth factor one. Science has shown that with aging, the ability of chondrocytes to synthesize certain proteoglycans and respond to stimuli such as growth factor decreases. The inability of the chondrocytes to maintain the homeostasis of the articular cartilage leads to degeneration.

The extracellular matrix is composed of fluid and various macromolecules. Approximately 80 percent of articular cartilage is water. It is the interaction of water with the macromolecules that determines the structure and properties of articular cartilage. The structural macromolecules of articular cartilage include: collagen, proteoglycans, and noncollagenous proteins. Collagen is the main structural element of articular cartilage. Type II collagen forms 90 to 95 percent of collagen found in articular cartilage. Type IX collagen is felt to form covalent bonds in the extracellular matrix. Type XI collagen also forms covalent bonds to type II collagen. Both of these collagens are thought to provide stabilizing cross-links within the extracellular matrix. Type VI collagen is found concentrated around chondrocytes and may help their attachment to the matrix.

Proteoglycans are another important component of articular cartilage. It consists of a protein core that is attached to glycosaminoglycan chains. The most common glycosaminoglycan chains include hyaluronic acid, chondroitin sulfate, and dermaton sulfate. The two main classes of proteoglycans are the large aggregating proteoglycan monomers called aggrecans and the small proteoglycans, such as decorin, biglycan, and fibromodulin. There is not much information on noncollagenous proteins. Research suggests that they along with glycoproteins help to stabilize the extracellular matrix.

Articular cartilage is not a homogenous layer of extracellular matrix and chondrocytes but has distinct zones. There are four histologically different layers in articular cartilage. *Zone 1* is the superficial layer. This very thin layer is relatively acellular and its composition allows its resistance to shear forces of joint motion. In addition, it may also filter the influx of fluid from the synovium, thereby shielding the articular cartilage from the immune system. *Zone 2* is the transitional zone. The tide mark separates the middle, or *Zone 3*, from the fourth zone of calcified cartilage. *Zone 4* is a thin zone of calcified cartilage, which separates the uncalcified zones from the subchondral bone.

There is an important interrelationship between chondrocytes and the matrix. The matrix filters nutrients, waste products, cytokines, and synthesized molecules that all have effects on chondrocytes. Thus any stimulus that affects the matrix will have indirect effects on chondrocytes, thereby allowing the chondrocytes to respond to stimuli affecting the matrix.

DEVELOPMENT OF OSTEOARTHROSIS

The primary derangement of osteoarthrosis of the knee is the degradation of articular cartilage. The loss of articular cartilage leads to changes in the subchondral bone with sclerosis, osteophyte, and cyst formation. Furthermore, all tissues that act on the knee are involved in osteoarthrosis including the synovium, ligaments, capsule, and muscle. The soft tissue contractures and muscle weakness from inactivity result in the clinical picture of osteoarthrosis with pain and loss of function.

The earliest histologic changes in articular cartilage is the fraying or fibrillation of the superficial zone. With time and further degeneration of the matrix, the formation of clefts develop in the articular cartilage. These eventually extend through the transitional zone to the subchondral bone. The formation of clefts and fibrillation causes instability of the articular cartilage. Consequently, fragments of the cartilage are liberated into the joint. Eventually all the articular cartilage is removed, leaving eburnated bone.

This progression of articular cartilage failure occurs at the molecular level. It can be divided into three stages. The first stage involves an increase in the water content of the matrix with a decrease in the aggrecan concentration. There is also a decrease in the length of the glucosaminoglycans. At this point there is no change in the collagen composition. It is felt that the increase in water content decreases articular cartilage stiffness and thus is more likely to fail. The second stage involves the chondrocyte response to stress on the matrix. The increased anabolic and metabolic activity of the chondrocytes in the second stage allows the matrix to withstand the forces of degradation. Eventually, the chondrocytes fail to respond to the changes in the matrix and the third stage develops. The chondrocytes are unable to maintain homeostasis, and the balance shifts in favor of matrix destruction.

Hyaline cartilage becomes degenerative under principally two conditions. The first is hyaline cartilage overload. In situations of disturbed joint mechanics, such as genu varum, hyaline cartilage degeneration can occur depending on the degree of exogenous demand. Following the initial blistering, the joint surface progresses to frank erosion with eburnation if the mechanical disturbance is not rectified. The second condition is hyaline cartilage underloading. Although unusual, the situation of persistent underload can offer an unfavorable situation for hyaline cartilage survival. This situation occurs far less frequently than overload but does require the same type of mechanical adjustment.

PRIMARY AND SECONDARY OSTEOARTHROSIS

The classification of osteoarthrosis is based on the presumed etiology. Primary osteoarthrosis is the most common, where the condition is idiopathic with no known cause. Quite often inflammation is not an important component of primary osteoarthrosis. Secondary osteoarthrosis occurs when the etiology can be identified. The secondary causes of osteoarthrosis are varied and should be addressed in the athlete. Intraarticular fracture, high intensity impact joint loading, ligament injuries, dysplasia of the joint, and aseptic necrosis, to name a few, have been identified as causes of osteoarthrosis. Identification of a secondary cause may initiate treatment before the development of end-stage osteoarthrosis.

EVALUATION OF THE MASTERS ATHLETE

As always a thorough history is necessary evaluating the aging athlete. The physician must be aware of the secondary causes of osteoarthrosis, other causes of a painful knee, and any comorbid medical conditions. A careful history helps to discriminate conditions such as rheumatoid arthritis, seronegative arthropathies, or crystaloid disease. Typically the patient with osteoarthrosis of the knee will complain of pain with activity and decreased range of motion. Quite often, patients will complain of pain localized to one particular region of the knee, often the medial joint. There may be a history of knee effusions, but not to the extent found in other inflammatory conditions.

The physical exam of the painful knee provides invaluable information for diagnosis and treatment. It is important to determine the alignment of the knee as altered joint mechanics play a significant role in the development of osteoarthrosis. Furthermore, treatment options may depend on the alignment of the knee. For example with genu varum, the medial compartment of the knee must be unloaded. The physical exam should identify any ligamentous instability, which may be found in the masters athlete with a chronic anterior cruciate ligament deficiency. The presence of a significant effusion may suggest inflammatory disease or infection. A sterile aspiration of the effusion should be performed if there is any doubt in a diagnosis.

Plain x-ray films of both knees in the standing position provides additional information. The amount of articular cartilage can be evaluated by measuring the joint space. The standing films convincingly demonstrate this. Bony changes of osteoarthrosis are evident, such as sclerosis, cysts, and osteophytes.

NONINVASIVE THERAPY

Nonsteroidal Anti-Inflammatory Drugs (NSAIDs)

Certainly osteoarthritis of the knee in an athlete can be quite painful and relief of this pain is one of the chief reasons for seeking medical attention. For many years, the first line of medical analgesia has been the nonsteroidal anti-inflammatory drugs (NSAIDs). This family of drugs is very effective in reducing inflammation and pyrexia. This is accomplished through its interference with cyclooxygenase. This enzyme catalyzes the reaction that synthesizes cyclic endoperoxidases from arachidonic acid. These are the precursors to prostaglandin.

Prostaglandins

D_2, E_1, E_2, and F_2 are major components in the acute inflammatory response to trauma. This causes dilation of blood vessels and leakage of fluid into the surrounding tissues. This is usually much greater than the body needs for healing, and that results in significant pain. NSAIDs have an antiprostaglandin effect.

A number of studies have demonstrated the effectiveness of NSAIDs in the symptomatic treatment of osteoarthrosis of the knee. In a systematic review of randomized controlled trials of NSAIDs for treatment of osteoarthrosis, they were found to be superior to placebo in all short-term studies. Although there are greater than 50 different brands of NSAIDs on the market, only 5 of 32 studies demonstrated any clinically significant difference between NSAIDs in osteoarthritis.

Despite the obvious effectiveness of NSAIDs for the treatment of the symptoms of osteoarthrosis, there are serious side effects associated with NSAID use. The most common complication is the frequent gastrointestinal (GI) problems. This can range from simple dyspepsia to severe bleeding or perforation. The symptoms of GI upset are often masked with further medications, including H_2 blockers, hydrogen ion pump blockers, or misoprostol. Other toxic side effects of NSAIDs include intestinal nephritis, hepatic dysfunction, allergic reactions, and drug interactions. It is important for physicians to remember that the cost-effectiveness of NSAIDs may be too narrow for less affluent athletes. Ironically, certain NSAIDs may have deleterious effects on articular cartilage. In a randomized controlled study, indomethacin was shown to cause a significant decrease in joint space compared to placebo.

Some investigators have suggested the use of local NSAIDs gel instead of oral agents to avoid the common side effects. In a randomized controlled clinical trial with 290 patients with osteoarthritis of the knee there was no statistical difference between the active treatment groups and placebo. However, in patients with more painful osteoarthritis prior to treatment, both active intervention groups were statistically more effective than the placebo. The authors also found that GI reactions were three times higher with oral NSAIDs. Based on this evidence, certain athletes with painful osteoarthrosis of the knee may benefit from an NSAID gel.

Dimethylsulfoxide (DMSO) is a chemical solvent that is rapidly absorbed through the skin. Thus other chemicals can be transported into tissues adjacent to the knee joint, such as NSAIDs, local anesthetics, or corticosteroids.

A 70% solution of DMSO has its own anti-inflammatory action. This is enhanced by the addition of Voltaren (diclofenac) and is available commercially as Dimethaide-D or Pennsaid. A daily or twice-daily application of six or eight drops on the arthritic joint usually relieves pain and decreases swelling.

Acetaminophen

An important alternative to NSAIDs for alleviation of pain is acetaminophen. This class of drugs has a safer toxicity profile as compared to the NSAIDs. There have been a number of studies comparing the efficacy of acetaminophen to NSAIDs. Acetaminophen has consistently been shown to be superior to placebo. Furthermore, at a dose of 4 g per day, acetaminophen is equally effective as an analgesic dose of ibuprofen. A prospective randomized, controlled study found after 6 weeks of treatment, acetaminophen and naproxen both caused a modest improvement in pain. The difference between groups was not significant. There was also a high drop rate in the study suggesting that the long-term use of either drug for osteoarthrosis is not very successful.

Ultrasound

The high-frequency sound waves of ultrasound are felt to penetrate into the soft tissues surrounding the knee joint and facilitate pain relief and increased mobility. A randomized clinical trial was performed to examine this effect on patients with osteoarthritis of the knee. In this study patients were subjected to an exercise regime, and a randomly selected group received ultrasound while the other group received a sham treatment. Although the treatment group did experience an improvement in pain, gait velocity, and range of motion, there was no statistical difference between treatments and sham groups. The effect of the exercise program may have masked any benefits provided by ultrasound. Further research into ultrasound may prove it to be a useful modality.

Exercise

For the masters athlete with osteoarthrosis of the knee, continued participation in exercise may be perceived as worsening the condition. Research has not supported this opinion in all cases. There is evidence that repetitive, high-impact loading of the knee is a risk factor for the development and progression of osteoarthrosis of the knee. However, low-impact exercise may be beneficial. In a randomized controlled study examining the effect of exercise in 102 patients with osteoarthritis, the treatment group reported statistically significant improvements in pain and physical activity based on the AIMS tests. Walking distance improved in the treatment group compared to control group as well. The benefits of aerobic activity for patients with osteoarthrosis have been reported elsewhere. This data would suggest that the aging athlete should not stop physical activities but may have to change to low-impact exercises to maintain physical and mental health.

Another important benefit of exercise is the maintenance of an appropriate body weight. There is evidence that an increased body mass index (BMI) above normal can increase the risk for development of osteoarthrosis of the knee. Furthermore, weight loss may help decrease the symptoms of osteoarthrosis. Unfortunately, the once active aging athlete can be trapped in the vicious circle of osteoarthrosis and decreased activity that leads to weight gain, which worsens arthritic symptoms.

Capsaicin Cream

Capsaicin is an extract from chili peppers that is used in a cream base and rubbed into the affected joint. The effect of capsaicin is felt to be its inhibition of substance P. In a randomized, blinded study, 70 patients with osteoarthritis of the knee with moderate to severe pain were given 0.025% capsaicin cream or placebo every 4 h. After 4 weeks there was significant improvement in visual analogue pain scores as well as the physician's global assessment of pain. The most bothersome side effect is the burning sensation that occurs.

Laser Therapy

The use of laser therapy has been investigated for the treatment of osteoarthritis. Researchers found that patients receiving red and infrared radiation applied to the affected knee did better than placebo on visual analogue pain scales and the short-form McGill pain questionnaire. How laser therapy exerts its effect is unknown.

Acupuncture

Once considered an exotic therapy from the orient, acupuncture has gained considerable acceptance as a legitimate therapy. In a study of 40 patients with osteoarthritis, researchers compared the effect of acupuncture versus a sham acupuncture. All patients improved after 3 weeks, but none could be attributable to the traditional acupuncture.

Transcutaneous Nerve Stimulation

Transcutaneous nerve stimulation (TENS) has been used in the treatment of various chronic pain conditions, including osteoarthrosis of the knee. There are some theoretical advantages of using TENS as opposed to medical therapy for pain because of its lack of toxic side effects. Published research has been divided on the benefits of TENS for osteoarthrosis of the knee. In one randomized study of 30 patients with a 12-month history of osteoarthrosis of the knee, both the TENS and sham groups reported pain relief. There was no significant difference between the two groups. Another study did find a clinically significant improvement in pain control; however, most of the pain relief occurred only when using the device. Researchers have compared TENS to naproxen in a clinical trial. There appeared to be no difference in the ability of TENS or naproxen to relieve pain. Nevertheless, a large placebo effect was found to be just as effective. There may be an effect, but there has not been a study with enough statistical power to demonstrate it.

Bracing and Wedged Insoles

Often the disease process in osteoarthrosis in the masters athlete involves only one compartment of the knee. Therefore, any physical modalities that facilitate unloading of the involved compartment should improve pain and function. Both bracing and wedged insoles have been used to address the problem of mechanical malalignment in osteoarthrosis of the knee. The use of the Generation II knee brace was evaluated in 20 patients with medial compartment disease. Nineteen of 20 patients experienced pain relief and 17 of 20 had an increase in quadriceps muscle strength. Conclusions drawn from case series should be analyzed critically, but the use of proper bracing could provide enough relief to allow the aging athlete to continue active exercise. Lateral heel wedges have been evaluated as a treatment for medial osteoarthrosis of the knee. Theoretically the lateral heel wedge imparts a valgus stress across the knee joint, thus reducing the pressure through the medial compartment. In a study of 149 patients with medial osteoarthrosis, lateral heel wedges were more effective in patients with mild to moderate osteoarthrosis than in those with advanced changes.

INVASIVE THERAPIES

Intraarticular Corticosteroid Injections

Unlike diseases such as rheumatoid arthritis, osteoarthrosis often is not associated with significant inflammation. It is not surprising that the use of intraarticular steroid injections is associated with some debate. Deciding which patient should receive an injection can be difficult, as many predictors of inflammation are not predictors of a patient's response to the injection. Intraarticular methyl prednisolone acetate has demonstrated significant reduction in visual analogue pain scores at 3 weeks in a randomized study. It is important to note that research into steroid injections is associated with a large placebo effect. In a randomized controlled study of triamcinolone hexacetonide (THA) intraarticular injections in patients with osteoarthrosis, a statistically significant improvement was found only at 1 week and thereafter placebo was just as efficacious. Based on these results, the sports medicine practitioner should use intraarticular steroids carefully as complications such as septic arthritis may be difficult to justify in a healthy athlete.

Intraarticular Hyaluronan Injections

In articular cartilage, aggrecan molecules bind to a chain of hyaluronate-forming macromolecular complexes that are immobilized within the articular cartilage. In osteoarthrosis it is hypothesized that the hyaluronate synthesized is abnormal preventing aggregation or there is rapid degradation of hyaluronate. The effect of injecting hyaluronan (Hyaluronic acid derivative) into the knee joint is unknown. It is described as viscosupplementation and is thought to improve arthritic knees by increasing the viscosity of synovial fluid. A randomized placebo-controlled study of intraarticular hyaluronan injections found no difference between treatment and placebo groups at 20 weeks as both groups had improvement above baseline. Stratification of their results found a clinically significant improvement in pain in patients over 60 years old with a number of symptoms. Although no significant side effects were reported in the study, the sports medicine physician should choose patients carefully for this treatment. The cost and multiple injections required may be inappropriate for most aging athletes.

ARTHROSCOPIC SURGERY

Surgical interventions often begin with arthroscopy in the masters athlete with osteoarthritis of the knee. The indications for arthroscopy in the older athlete include failure of conservative treatment or clinical suspicion of a mechanical derangement that is correctable with arthroscopy, such as a meniscal tear. Studies have shown patients with short duration of symptoms or mechanical symptoms of unstable meniscal tears or loose bodies will do better after arthroscopy. It is essential to have a candid discussion with older athletes about what can reasonably be expected from arthroscopy. Patients may have unrealistic goals for surgical result. Arthroscopy can help alleviate the symptoms of osteoarthrosis through a number of mechanisms. The first effect is attributed to the washout of the knee. It is felt that lavage removes debris and inflammatory mediators from the joint. Studies have demonstrated 86 percent good results in 1 year and 81 percent good results in 2 years with washout alone. It is important to note that the effects of lavage decrease with time. Arthroscopic partial meniscectomy in the degenerative joint can produce good results. This effect is especially true with acute tears. Degenerative tears are not as rewarding. A review of the arthroscopic debridement studies found an average 68 percent good results and 32 percent poor outcomes at a mean follow-up of 35 months. Clearly, the results of meniscectomy deteriorate with time.

Finally, arthroscopic debridement of the osteoarthritic knee can provide pain relief for the older athlete. The best results occur in patients with obvious fibrillation of the articular cartilage with unstable edges. It is apparent that patients who have significant varus or valgus malalignment with medial or lateral compartment osteoarthritis have a worse response to arthroscopic debridement. The use of arthroscopy in osteoarthrosis of the knee is a purely palliative procedure, before more definitive surgery is required.

ARTHROSCOPIC DEBRIDEMENT OF THE OSTEOARTHRITIC KNEE[1]

Robert Jackson recently presented his results of arthroscopic debridement of the osteoarthritic knee. He considers a debridement to be removal of all loose flaps of articular cartilage, trimming of a degenerative meniscus, and removal of symptomatic spurs. He feels that if in doubt, you should err on the conservative side of surgical excision.

The patients were divided into four categories (Table 9-1).

The patients in stages 1 and 2 had good results and were improved in the short term in 85 percent. At 3 years 60 percent of the

TABLE 9-1 Four Categories of Arthroscopic Debridement

	Symptoms	X-Ray Findings	Arthroscopic Findings
Stage 1	Postexercise pain	Normal	Softening
Stage 2	Activity pain Taking NSAIDs	Decreased joint space	Fibrillation
Stage 3	Rest pain	Angular deformity	Fragmented
Stage 4	Limited function Decreased ROM	Severe changes Osteophytes	Erosion to bone

patients were still good. This makes it a reasonable procedure to offer patients. In stage 3, patients had only fair results and took a long time to rehabilitate. The patients in stage 4 had poor results. The message is, there is no benefit in arthroscopic debridement in the severe stage 4 patient. He found that abrasion arthroplasty was no better than joint lavage. Beware of the laser. Bob has expressed concern over the use of the laser. There have been several cases of massive loss of articular cartilage and avascular necrosis of the femoral condyle as the result of laser debridement.

Don Johnson says, "Some of my most unhappy patients in the past have been the middle-aged jocks with unrealistic expectations for an arthritic knee."

OSTEOTOMY

In patients over 30 and under 60 with a varus deformity between 2 and 15 degrees, an osteotomy should be considered. The medial compartment collapse creates a varus (bowlegged) knee with constant medial pain and effusion. A valgus osteotomy is indicated when relief cannot be obtained by NSAIDs and physiotherapy and the patient's job is compromised, and if there is severe limitation in sports then this is a good operation. The osteotomy is usually high tibial (HTO), but a low femoral procedure can be done when the deformity is in the femur. A small incision is used, and an oscillating saw removes a wedge from the bone. The lower tibia is straightened, closing the wedge against a medial periosteal hinge. Thus the weight-bearing forces are swung into the lateral compartment, unweighting the medial compartment. Then this can be held with staples or a plate and screws. Care is taken to avoid putting the knee into valgus. Results usually give the patient a good 5 to 10 years of comfort, prior to a total joint replacement.

The procedure allows more vigorous sports and impacting than after a total joint, because the natural femoral and tibial surfaces are still intact.

Operative complications should be discussed realistically with the patient.[2]

11 percent need revision at 7.5 years[3]
Nonunion occurs in 8 percent
Vascular injury
Intraarticular fracture occurs in 5 to 10 percent
Peroneal nerve injury occurs in 6 to 10 percent
Section
Compartment syndrome
Deep venous thrombosis (DVT)

TOTAL KNEE ARTHROPLASTY

This procedure basically gives the patient a *new knee*. The patient
ends up with a metal cap on the femur, a metal and polyethylene replacement of the proximal tibia, and a polyethylene cap on the
patella. It is a good, well-engineered operation. The indications are
the same as an osteotomy: inability to function well in the job or
sports.

1. Usually the patients have to be over age 60 because the prosthesis only lasts 10 to 15 years (depending on the abuse heaped on
   it).
2. Often the opposite or good knee and hip become painful from
   overuse and this provokes the patient to seek the surgery.
3. The procedure, hospitalization, and physiotherapy are all much
   more prolonged than with an HTO.

The patient is hospitalized for 7 to 10 days on anticoagulants and
antibiotics. A continuous passive motion machine (CPM) is used
although scientific results do not indicate significant long-term
benefit. The first 2 days are quite painful in spite of a nerve block
and use of an on-demand intravenous pain pump. Complications
are the same as HTO plus loss of implant fixation and chronic pain
and swelling of the leg.

Postoperative manipulation under anesthesia is required in 15 to
21 percent of cases up to 8 weeks postoperatively. Indications: less
than 75-degree flexion in 10 days and less than 110-degree flexion
in 6 weeks. Patients can return to sedentary work in 6 weeks, moderately hard work in 10 weeks (i.e., orthopaedic surgery), and
heavier work in 12 weeks.

The ultimate goal with activity is mild pain, mild swelling, no
NSAIDs, no bracing, and range of flexion of 100 to 130 degrees
with a normal knee (good leg) flexion of 140 degrees.

Patients with arthroplasty should be given antibiotics for all dental and surgical procedures, similar to prosthetic heart valve
patients. Physiotherapy in a clinic or at home should be done for
6 months. Strength improves up to 1 year. Home programs are ef-

fective up to 48 months after THA or TKA. Return to sports depends on the preoperative fitness level of the patient. Principles to avoid are:

Overload of joint
Repetitive strain
Impact more than body weight
Lack of conditioning

Thus, no running and jumping are allowed, because the load on the joint above the impact strength of the polyethylene leads to increased wear. Stress analyses say as thick a polyethylene component as possible (Tables 9-2 to 9-4).

TABLE 9-2 Very Good, Good, Skilled Sports, Bad, and Extreme

Very good	**With care—ask doctor**
Stationary bike	Low impact aerobics
Golf	Weight lifting (free or
Dancing	machines)
Walking	Stair master (quick short
Swimming	steps)
Good	Tennis doubles
Bowling	**Bad**
Cross-country skiing	All contact sports
Speed walking (4 miles,	Baseball—basketball
1 hour)	Football—hockey
No jogging or running	Soccer—squash
Skilled sports	**Extreme**
Bicycling (street)	Mountain bike riding
Ice skating	Ski racing
In-line rollerskating	Horse jumping
Horseback riding	Dog sled racing
	Marathon cycling

TABLE 9-3 Painful Arthroplasty

Intrinsic	**Principles: Avoid**
Loosening	Overload of joint
Sepsis	Repetitive strain
Occult fracture	Impact more than body
Prosthesis failure	weight
Extrinsic	Lack of conditioning
Spine pathology	**Failure**
Bursitis tendinitis	Loss of implant fixation
Nonunion of osteotomy	Chronic pain
Neurologic lesions	Swelling of leg

TABLE 9-4 Keys to Successful Arthroplasty

Personal Physiotherapy	Hugh U. Cameron
Muscle stim. At home for 6 weeks	Avoid impact loading
6 Months, 2 hours daily— 3 × per week	No running and jumping
Bilat. quads atrophy	Load on joint above impact strength of polyethylene
Slow and steady wins the race	leads to increased wear

REFERENCES

1. Jackson R: What works and what doesn't. *Pract Arthroscop* 1(6): 33, 1995.
2. Petrie D: *Pract Arthroscop* 2(6):60, 1996.
3. Simurda, 1991.
4. Stiehl JB, de Amdrade JR: Activities after replacement of the hip and knee. *Ortho Spec Ed* 1.1:32, 1995.

10 | Ankle and Foot

Wen Chao   William G. Hamilton

ANATOMY

The ankle joint, which is shaped like a carpenter's mortise, is formed by the distal end of the tibia (tibial plafond and the medial malleolus), the distal end of the fibula (lateral malleolus), and the dome of the talus. The anterior tibiofibular ligament and the posterior tibiofibular ligament hold the fibula securely in the sigmoid notch of the tibia. The dome of the talus is held under the mortise by the deltoid ligament medially, and anterior talofibular ligament, calcaneofibular ligament, and posterior talofibular ligament laterally. Because the dome of the talus is shaped like a segment of a cone with its apex on the medial side, and the dome is wider anteriorly than posteriorly, the ankle joint is a complex joint with multiple planes of rotation. In general, it has approximately 15 to 20 degrees of dorsiflexion and 35 to 40 degrees of plantarflexion. With normal walking, the ankle joint has an arc of motion ranges from 20 to 36 degrees, with an average of 24 degrees.[1,2]

The joint beneath the ankle joint is the subtalar joint. It is formed by the talus and the calcaneus. These two bones are held together by several ligaments: cervical, interosseous, lateral talocalcaneal, posterior talocalcaneal, and medial talocalcaneal.[3] The subtalar joint is one of the most important joints of the foot and ankle because it acts like a mitered hinge. It converts rotation of the vertical axis (ankle joint) into rotation of the horizontal axis (calcaneocuboid and talonavicular joints). The total arc of motion from inversion to eversion can vary from 20 to 60 degrees.[4]

The talonavicular and calcaneocuboid joints together are also known as the transverse tarsal joint. The significance of the transverse tarsal joint is that it transmits the motion that occurs in the subtalar joint into the forefoot. When the subtalar joint is in an everted position, the transverse tarsal joint is unlocked and the forefoot is supple, ready to make contact with the ground. When the subtalar joint is in an inverted position, the transverse tarsal joint is locked and the forefoot becomes a rigid lever arm ready for powerful push-off.

The navicular articulates with the three cuneiforms (medial, middle, and lateral). Each of the cuneiform bones, in turn, articulates with a metatarsal bone (first, second, and third). Usually, minimal motion occurs between the navicular-cuneiform articulation and between the cuneiform-metatarsal articulation. Occasionally, there is an increased laxity in the navicular-medial cuneiform joint and medial cuneiform-first metatarsal joint, which can lead to problems in these joints. The cuboid articulates with both the fourth and the fifth metatarsal. These two joints are more mobile compared to the three medial tarsometatarsal joints. Most commonly, there are three phalanges (proximal, middle, and distal) in each toe except for the great toe, where there are two phalanges (proximal and distal).

The tendons around the ankle joint can be divided into four compartments. The medial compartment contains posterior tibial tendon, flexor digitorum longus, and flexor hallucis longus. The lateral compartment includes peroneus brevis and longus tendons. The Achilles tendon and the plantaris tendon, if present, are in the posterior compartment. Finally, tibialis anterior, extensor hallucis longus, extensor digitorum longus, and the peroneus tertius are located in the anterior compartment. The tendons in the foot include: extensor digitorum brevis, extensor hallucis brevis, flexor digitorum brevis, flexor hallucis brevis, abductor hallucis, adductor hallucis, abductor digiti minimi, flexor digiti minimi brevis, quadratus plantae, interossei, and lumbricals.

There are five major nerves that are located in the foot and ankle: posterior tibial, saphenous, superficial peroneal, deep peroneal, and sural. The posterior tibial nerve divides into two main branches while coursing through the tarsal tunnel: medial plantar nerve and lateral plantar nerve. Prior to entering the tarsal tunnel, posterior tibial nerve gives off the medial calcaneal nerve, which provides sensation to the posterior heel. The medial and lateral plantar nerves innervate the muscles that originate in the foot and provide sensation on the plantar aspect of the foot. The first branch of the lateral plantar nerve (also known as Baxter's nerve) travels under the heel to supply motor function of abductor digiti minimi. The saphenous nerve supplies sensation to the medial side of the ankle and foot. Superficial peroneal nerve innervates peroneus longus and brevis muscles in the lower leg. It then divides into two branches in the distal leg: intermediate cutaneous and dorsal medial. Dorsal medial branch provides sensation to the medial aspect of the great toe and lateral aspect of the second toe. The intermediate cutaneous branch supplies sensation to the medial and lateral aspects of the third and fourth toes. Deep peroneal nerve innervates extensor hallucis longus, tibialis anterior, extensor digitorum longus, peroneus tertius, extensor digitorum brevis muscles, and sensation to the first web space.

DIAGNOSIS

Making the diagnosis of a sports-related injury frequently requires the following: some understanding of the sport and the mechanism of the injury, performing a detailed physical examination, and obtaining the appropriate diagnostic studies, if necessary. The foot and ankle injuries that are discussed in this chapter include:

Lateral ankle sprain
Medial ankle sprain
Syndesmosis sprain
Ankle instability
Subtalar sprain
Midfoot sprain
Forefoot sprain
Achilles tendinitis
Achilles tendon rupture
Peroneal tendinitis and rupture
Peroneal tendon subluxation and dislocation
Posterior tibial tendinitis/rupture and tarsal coalition
Flexor hallucis longus tendinitis
Posterior ankle impingement
Anterior ankle impingement
Osteochondral lesions of the talus

Each injury is reviewed in detail, along with mechanism of injury, physical findings, diagnostic studies, and treatment.

Lateral Ankle Sprain

The most common injury in sports that involve running and jumping is the ankle sprain. Ankle sprains account for approximately 25 to 50 percent of injuries in running sports.[5] The incidence of ankle sprains in general is 1 per 10,000 people per day. Ninety percent of all ankle sprains are lateral and only 10 percent are medial. "Sprains" occur when a ligament has been injured. There are several classification systems to grade the severity of the ligament injury. The grading system that is the simplest to use and easiest for patients to understand is the following: grade 1, ligament stretched; grade 2, ligament partially torn; grade 3, ligament completely torn.

The majority of the lateral ankle sprains occur when the foot and ankle are in a plantarflexed position. Because the anterior talofibular ligament is under tension when the foot and ankle are in a plantarflexed position, the most commonly injured lateral ankle ligament is the anterior talofibular ligament. If the inversion is severe enough, calcaneofibular ligament becomes injured after the anterior talofibular ligament. Rarely, when the inversion stress occurs with the ankle in a dorsiflexed position, an isolated tear of the calcaneofibular ligament may happen.

To get a sense of the severity of the sprain, several questions should be asked. Did the ankle swell immediately? Were you able to resume playing or did you have to stop? If you stopped playing, were you able to walk on your own or did you require someone's help? What treatment was given so far? Was this a first time sprain or one of many?

On physical examination, there will be swelling and tenderness around the lateral malleolus. If the sprain occurred several days ago, ecchymosis (laterally mostly, but can be medially or distally) may be present. When examining the lateral ligaments, each ligament (anterior talofibular, calcaneofibular, and posterior talofibular) should be palpated individually to determine which ligament has been injured. To rule out other injuries:

Palpate the head of the proximal fibula to look for Maisonneuve fracture (injury of the interosseus membrane).

Squeeze test at the midfibula and tibia and palpate the anterior tibiofibular ligament to rule out a syndesmosis injury (high ankle sprain).

Palpate the tip of the distal fibula to rule out an avulsion fracture.

Palpate the posterior malleolus for trigonal process fracture (Shepherd's fracture) or peroneal subluxation.

Palpate the anterior process of the calcaneus for an avulsion fracture.

Palpate the base of the fifth metatarsal for a tuberosity fracture.

The anterior drawer test is performed with the ankle in 10 to 15 degrees of plantarflexion. The anterior drawer test of the injured ankle should be compared to the uninjured ankle in order to determine the severity of ligamentous laxity.

Standard anteroposterior, mortise, and lateral radiographs of the injured ankle should be obtained. Most of the time after a lateral ankle sprain, the plain radiographs of the ankle will be normal. However, the plain radiographs of the ankle will reveal fractures of the distal fibula, anterior process of the calcaneus, tuberosity of the fifth metatarsal, talar dome, and a widening of the syndesmosis.

The initial management of an acute sprain is rest, ice, compression, and elevation (RICE) for at least the first 48 h followed by warm, moist heat or contrast baths (*i*ce for *i*njury and *h*eat for *h*ealing). Most of the time, the injured athlete will be able to bear weight as tolerated with a rigid or semirigid ankle brace using a cane or crutches. Occasionally, cast immobilization is used to treat grade 3 sprains. As soon as the pain improves, physical therapy should begin. Instead of using a cookbook approach, the rehabilitation program should be tailored according to the individual athlete's level of pain and discomfort. It usually initiates with ankle range of motion exercises and isometric peroneal strengthening. When most of the range of motion has been restored, ankle strengthening exercises (especially aggressive peroneal tendon strengthening) should begin. The injured athlete may return to sports when pain and swelling have mostly resolved and the peroneal tendons are strong. For "the sprained ankle that won't heal" after 3 months, look for the following:

Residual peroneal weakness
Posterior impingement on the trigonal process
Shepherd's fracture (fracture of the trigonal process)
Peroneal tendon tear or subluxation
Fracture of the lateral process of the talus
Fracture of the tip of the fibula or symptomatic os subfibulare
Fracture of the anterior process of the calcaneus
Sinus tarsi syndrome
Osteochondral lesion of the talar dome

Medial Ankle Sprain

Isolated medial ankle sprains are rare compared to lateral ones. This is because the medial ankle ligament (deltoid ligament) is much stronger than the lateral ankle ligaments. Deltoid injuries usually occur in conjunction with lateral ligamentous injuries or bony injuries. The mechanism of an isolated deltoid injury is usually a pronation-eversion injury. For example, landing from a triple jump or a broad jump onto an abducted foot with the heel in valgus may cause a medial ankle sprain.

On physical examination, there is usually pain and swelling around the deltoid ligament. More importantly, other injuries, such as syndesmosis injury, lateral ligamentous injury, high ankle sprain, high fibula fracture, or Maisonneuve fracture, must be excluded. Because the neurovascular bundle courses around the medial malleolus, a careful neurovascular exam of the foot should be made.

Standard mortise, anteroposterior, and lateral radiographs of the ankle should be obtained to rule out fractures. If no fractures are detected and an isolated rupture of the deltoid ligament is suspected, a valgus stress anteroposterior radiograph of the ankle can be performed to show if there is significant instability.

The treatment for an isolated medial ankle sprain is similar to lateral ankle sprain. Again, on rare occasions, cast immobilization is used to treat grade 3 sprains. If there are other associated injuries, then the treatment depends on the associated injuries. Medial ankle sprains usually heal more slowly than lateral sprains. For "the medial injuries that won't heal," you need to rule out osteochondral lesion of the talar dome, posterior tibial tendon tears, flexor hallucis longus tendinitis, or medial malleolar pathology.

Syndesmosis Sprain

Syndesmosis sprains represent a spectrum of injury from minor sprains to frank separation of the distal ends of the tibia and fibula. The most important mechanism of injury is external rotation. For example, when a skier falls, the internal ski may be forced into external rotation, which can lead to either a knee injury or a syndesmosis injury with or without a fibula fracture. Oftentimes, the athlete is unable to describe the mechanism of injury, but he or she will comment that it was different from a typical ankle sprain.

On physical examination, there is pain and swelling localized to the anterior tibiofibular ligament. The lateral ankle ligaments are usually not tender. The "West Point test," also known as the "squeeze test," is helpful in making this diagnosis. This test is performed with squeezing the fibula and tibia together at midcalf level. If pain is reproduced at the syndesmosis, then the diagnosis is confirmed. Another helpful test is the presence of pain in the syndesmosis on external rotation of the tibia with the ankle in dorsiflexion.

Standard radiographs of the ankle should be obtained to rule out fractures and to determine if there is any widening at the syndesmosis. If x-rays of the ankle are normal, and there is a high index of suspicion for a syndesmotic injury, stress radiographs of the ankle with the ankle in dorsiflexion, external rotation, and abduction may reveal a diastasis between the fibula and tibia. This is opposite to the usual maneuvers for the stress x-rays to determine anterior talofibular ligamentous laxity. Other diagnostic studies that may be helpful in making the diagnosis are arthrography of the ankle, bone scan, CT scan, and MRI. Bone scan, arthrogram of the ankle (used more often prior to the advent of MRI), and MRI are more helpful in detecting a rupture of the syndesmotic ligament without radiographic diastasis between the fibula and tibia. CT scan is the study of choice to determine the rotational relationship between the fibula and tibia.

The treatment for acute syndesmosis sprain without diastasis is very similar to a grade 3 ankle sprain. The athlete should be warned that this injury almost doubles the time to return to play in comparison with a grade 3 ankle sprain. If frank diastasis is present, then surgical stabilization is required.

Ankle Instability

Chronic and recurrent ankle sprains require careful evaluation to rule out other associated injuries. Athletes with recurrent lateral ankle sprains usually present to the office with either "functional instability" or "mechanical instability." Functional instability is a subjective feeling of the ankle giving way, but objectively, the range of motion is still within normal limits. Mechanical instability is when there is an objective finding of ankle instability. More than 50 percent of the patients with functional instability also have mechanical instability.

On physical examination, there may or may not be pain over the lateral ankle ligaments. The anterior drawer test and the inversion stress will be positive. It is very important to test the strength of the peroneal tendons (peroneal weakness is a common cause of functional instability) and to rule out other ankle problems (cartilaginous, bony, and tendinous).

Standard radiographs of the ankle are obtained to rule out any bony pathology. Then stress views of the ankle joint (talar tilt and anterior drawer) and subtalar joint are helpful in making the definitive diagnosis of ankle instability. CT scan and MRI of the ankle are useful in ruling out other concomitant problems, such as osteochondral lesion of the talus and peroneal tendon tear.

Treatment usually starts with aggressive physical therapy. Frequently, after improvements in proprioception, strength, and flexibility are made, the symptoms of instability resolve. The studies on the effectiveness of a lace-up type of ankle brace in providing stability of the ankle has not been conclusive. Therefore, if an athlete feels more secure with the use of a comfortable ankle brace and especially if it helps with his or her performance, then the ankle brace may be used. Biomechanical studies have demonstrated that taping really does not provide significant support to prevent ankle instability.[6] After failing nonoperative treatment, surgical stabilization of the lateral ligaments may be necessary to correct the ankle instability.

Subtalar Sprain

It is difficult to distinguish between ankle and subtalar instability based on the history of the injury. The mechanism of subtalar sprains is similar to that for ankle sprains. In most of ankle sprains, the inversion occurs with the foot in plantarflexion. Therefore, the anterior talofibular ligament tears first and then the calcaneofibular ligament, if the injury is severe enough. However, if the inversion happens with the foot in dorsiflexion, then the calcaneofibular ligament can be injured without injuring the anterior talofibular ligament resulting in an isolated subtalar instability. Athletes with a subtalar sprain often have a hard time with running or walking on uneven surfaces.

It is important to remember that subtalar instability may coexist with ankle instability. On physical exam, there is more inversion of the subtalar joint on the injured side compared to the normal side. There may be tenderness in the area of the sinus tarsi. Standard radiographs of the ankle should be obtained to rule out other bony pathology. Stress radiographs of the subtalar joint are helpful in making the diagnosis. This is performed with a 40-degree Broden's view of the subtalar joint while applying inversion stress to the lateral aspect of the calcaneus and fifth metatarsal while stabilizing the distal tibia. The diagnosis of subtalar instability is made if there is any widening of the posterior facet.

Acute treatment of subtalar instability is similar to the acute treatment of ankle sprain or instability. The treatment of chronic subtalar instability is similar to the treatment of chronic ankle instability: Peroneal strengthening and proprioceptive training are extremely important in the treatment of both acute and chronic subtalar instability. The use of a lace-up type of ankle brace may be helpful. However, biomechanical studies on its efficacy in providing subtaler joint stability have not been conclusive. Surgical stabilization is indicated only if nonoperative treatment fails.

Midfoot Sprain

It is extremely difficult to estimate the incidence of midfoot sprains in sports because of the lack of specificity in the reporting of the injuries. In general, some sports have very low rates of injuries to the foot, such as swimming and skiing, and other sports, such as running, ballet, basketball, and football, have higher incidences of foot injuries.[7] The most common mechanism of injuries is twisting of the foot.

Patients usually complain of pain in the midfoot region. The degree of pain on palpation depends on the severity of the injury. Each of the articulations in the midfoot should be tested: transverse tarsal (calcaneocuboid and talonavicular), intertarsal (navicular-cuneiforms), and tarsometatarsal joints. If the pain is too severe to be examined in the emergency room or the office, then examination under anesthesia with possible stress radiographs should be performed.

Standard radiographs of both feet are obtained to evaluate the bony alignment. The anatomy of the midfoot has greater variation. Therefore, often it can be helpful to compare the x-rays of the injured foot to the other side. If avulsion fractures are present, then the ligamentous injury may be more serious than expected. Stress radiographs of the foot should be performed when the suspicion of tarsometatarsal instability is high. Computed tomography can further delineate the bony injury, especially if surgical treatment may be required. Finally, MRI can be used to better define the extent of soft tissue trauma to the midfoot.

The acute treatment of a "minor" sprain without any evidence of instability is RICE, weight bearing as tolerated with crutches or cane, and stiff-soled shoe or a wooden postop shoe. As the symptoms improve, gradual increase in activities and rehabilitation program should begin. It may take 4 to 6 weeks before the patient may return to sports. If there is midfoot instability, stabilization using a non-weight-bearing cast, insertion of percutaneous pins, or internal fixation may be required. The recovery time is much longer and could take up to 3 to 6 months before a return to sports.

Forefoot Sprain

Like the midfoot sprains, the true incidence of forefoot sprains in athletes is difficult to define. Since the introduction of artificial playing surfaces, much more attention has been made to the injuries of the foot, especially the sprain of the first metatarsophalangeal joint (also known as "turf toe"). The common mechanism of injury of the sprained first metatarsophalangeal joint is hyperextension at that joint.[8] Although sprains of the lesser toes are not well described in the literature, many patients and athletes have "stubbed" their toe(s).

On physical examination, there is usually pain and swelling in the area of the affected joint. The dorsal joint capsule, plantar plate, and medial and lateral collateral ligaments of the affected joint should be palpated for identification of the specific injured structure. For the hyperextension injury at the first metatarsophalangeal joint, the severity of pain and swelling is based on the severity of the sprain. For example, a grade 3 sprain can present with pain and swelling both on dorsal and plantar aspects of the first metatarsophalangeal joint. Occasionally, there may be a concomitant fracture of the sesamoid or separation of a bipartite sesamoid. Standard radiographs of the foot should be obtained to rule out any bony pathology.

The acute treatment of a sprained toe is RICE and the use of stiff-soled shoes until symptoms improve. The use of crutches may be required for the first few days for some grade 3 sprains because of pain with weight bearing. For a sprained lesser toe, buddy-taping to the adjacent toe may provide some support. It usually takes 3 to 4 weeks before resume playing for grades 1 and 2 sprains, and 6 weeks for grade 3 sprains. Surgical treatment is rarely required for this injury. Most of the surgeries are performed to treat chronic problems, such as nonunion of sesamoid fracture, loose bodies in the joint, or osteochondral lesions of the articular surface.

Achilles Tendinitis

Achilles tendinitis is usually caused by an overusage of the tendon, especially for younger athletes (under 25 years of age), for example, a runner running too many miles early in the training schedule. For those athletes who are over 25 years of age, Achilles tendinitis may be owing to degeneration within the substance of the tendon. In athletes with cavus feet, they can be more susceptible to Achilles tendinitis. When an athlete presents with posterior heel pain, differentiation must be made between superficial adventitious bursitis ("pump bumps"), retrocalcaneal bursitis, Achilles tendinitis, or insertional Achilles tendinitis. Oftentimes, the pain is caused by a combination of the preceding problems.

The retrocalcaneal bursa is located between the superior tuberosity of the calcaneus and the Achilles tendon. In athletes, especially runners, with a relative prominent superior tuberosity, retrocalcaneal bursitis can form owing to chronic irritation. The superficial adventitious bursa is located between skin and the Achilles tendon; therefore, inflammation is usually caused by pressure from a shoe counter. Achilles tendinitis may occur either within the substance of the tendon or at its insertion.

On physical examination, the best method to exam the Achilles tendon is to squeeze the substance of the tendon between the thumb and index (or middle) finger. The area of inflammation will be identified by the presence of pain when the tendon is being squeezed. With chronic tendinitis, the substance of the tendon will feel enlarged and irregular. For insertional tendinitis, the pain is located at the Achilles insertion. Superficial adventitious bursitis can be identified by an area of swelling superficial to the tendon corresponding to the top of the shoe counter. Retrocalcaneal bursitis can be diagnosed by pain and swelling when the retrocalcaneal bursa that is anterior to the tendon is squeezed between thumb and index (or middle) fingers.

Diagnosis of Achilles tendinitis and bursitis are made clinically, therefore, no diagnostic studies are required to make the diagnosis. A lateral radiograph of the foot can be obtained to look for posterior heel spurs that may be present in chronic insertional tendinitis or to assess the size and shape of the superior tuberosity of the calcaneus. Keep in mind that many people have posterior heel spurs without having any symptoms in the Achilles tendon. To further evaluate the extent of degeneration of the tendon, MRI is the study of choice.

The initial treatment of Achilles tendinitis is rest. Depending on the severity of the symptoms, rest can mean using heel cups or shoes with an elevated heel or using a short leg cast or brace. The heel cups, pads, or shoes with an elevated heel are extremely helpful for the treatment of superficial adventitious bursitis and retro-calcaneal bursitis by lifting the inflamed bursa away from the pressure of the heel counter or by increasing the retrocalcaneal space. Physical therapy needs to be started as soon as the pain has improved enough. The rehabilitation program should be administered by the physician along with the supervision and guidance of a physical therapist. In general, the program emphasizes Achilles stretching and gastroc-soleus strengthening. The athlete may resume training when the pain in the Achilles tendon resolves. Corticosteroid injection into the Achilles tendon should be avoided since rupture of the tendon has been reported after injections. However, corticosteroid injections can be very effective in the treatment of retrocalcaneal bursitis. Nonsteroidal anti-inflammatory medication may be used for a short period of time but never to mask the symptoms. Orthotic devices usually are not helpful in the treatment of this problem unless the athlete has pronated feet. Surgical management is only indicated for Achilles tendinitis, insertional tendinitis, or retrocalcaneal bursitis that have failed nonoperative treatment for 6 to 12 months. At the time of surgery, each of the problems that is present needs to be addressed. Superficial adventitious bursitis alone rarely requires surgical treatment.

Achilles Tendon Rupture

Rupture of the Achilles tendon is a devastating injury to the athlete. This injury usually occurs in recreational athletes who are over 30 years of age. The rupture often occurs during the routine playing of tennis or basketball without any specific event of injury. The mechanism of rupture is a strong dorsiflexion force on a contracted gastrocnemius-soleus muscle complex.

On physical examination, a palpable defect is present at the site of rupture. Thompson's test (spontaneous plantarflexion of the foot with squeezing of the calf muscle) produces no plantarflexion of the foot. The Thompson's test is best performed with the patient lying prone on the examination table with both feet hanging off the end of the table.

The acute treatment is to immobilize the foot and ankle in a maximum plantarflexed position to bring the two ends of the tendon as close together as possible. If closed treatment is elected, then the foot and ankle need to be immobilized in a plantarflexed position for a total of 8 weeks in a short leg cast, followed by a removable brace with a heel lift for an additional 4 weeks. Rehabilitation can be started in the removable brace. There is a higher risk of rerupture with this method of treatment.[9] If open surgical repair is elected, the recovery period is similar to the closed treatment, but there is a smaller risk of rerupture. However, wound complication can develop after surgery.[9] The advantage of surgical treatment is that the natural resting length of the tendon will be restored intra-operatively. The restoration of the natural resting length of the tendon is crucial in restoring the strength in the powerful gastroc-nemius-soleus complex. The long recovery period and the complication of rerupture with closed treatment and wound problems with surgical treatment make this a devastating injury for the athlete. Nevertheless, open surgical repair of the ruptured Achilles tendon is the recommended treatment for a quality athlete.

Peroneal Tendinitis and Rupture

In athletes, peroneal tendinitis is usually caused by an overuse problem. Occasionally, it may be associated with a history of trauma (e.g., ankle sprain) or an anatomic problem, such as chronic abrasion against the fibular groove. Frank ruptures of the peroneal tendons are extremely rare. More commonly, longitudinal tears can occur within the substance of the tendon from chronic tendinitis or after a lateral ankle sprain.

On physical examination, there is usually tenderness and swelling along the course of the peroneal tendons on the lateral aspect of the ankle. Pain may be present along the peroneal tendons when testing the strength of the tendons against resistance with the foot in maximum plantarflexion and eversion. To detect subtle weakness in the peroneal tendons, the foot is tested against resistance going from a supinated position to an everted position. Diagnosis can be confirmed by injection of 1 to 2 mL of lidocaine (not mixed with corticosteroids) into the tendon sheath. It is very difficult to distinguish between tendinitis, longitudinal tear, or frank rupture of the tendon on physical exam.

Standard radiographs of the ankle are obtained to rule out other bony pathology. A ruptured peroneus longus can be detected by a proximal displacement of the os peroneum (Fig. 10-1). MRI of the ankle may be used to evaluate the integrity of the peroneal tendons. Unfortunately, there can be false-positive and false-negative results.

The acute treatment for peroneal tendinitis is initially RICE and anti-inflammatory medication and then physical therapy for peroneal strengthening. Occasionally, some form of immobilization may be helpful in reducing the symptoms. For chronic peroneal tendinitis, the persistence of symptoms is usually owing to an inadequate resting period for the tendon to heal. Therefore, it is very important to educate the athlete concerning the pathophysiology of the disease process so that he or she can participate in the treatment of the problem.

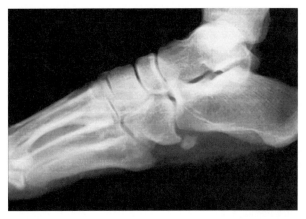

FIG. 10-1   Radiograph of proximal displacement of os peroneum indicating a ruptured peroneus longus tendon.

For chronic peroneal tendinitis, longitudinal tears, and frank ruptures of the tendon, surgical treatment may be indicated after failing conservative treatment. For chronic tenosynovitis, the tendon sheath and the tendon are both debrided. If there are degenerations within the substance of the tendon or longitudinal tears, then side-to-side repair of the tendon can be made. If the diseased tendon is too degenerated for debridement and repair, then tenodesis of the proximal end of the tendon to the other tendon can be performed. This can also be done for the treatment of a frank rupture of the tendon, and a primary repair of the tendon is impossible.

Peroneal Tendon Subluxation and Dislocation

Acute subluxation or dislocation of the peroneal tendons are usually owing to trauma. The sport that causes most of the traumatic subluxation or dislocation of the peroneal tendons is skiing.[10,11] The most common mechanism of injury is a forced dorsiflexion of the ankle with a sudden contraction of the peroneal tendon. In some people, they can voluntarily sublux the peroneal tendons out of the fibular groove, probably because of a shallow retrofibular groove or deficiencies in the superior peroneal retinaculum.

In an acute injury, it can be difficult to distinguish between lateral ankle sprain and peroneal subluxation. In both conditions, there is pain and swelling along the lateral aspect of the ankle.

However, in peroneal subluxation, the maximum area of tenderness is at the posterior border of the fibula, whereas the maximum area of tenderness for an ankle sprain is usually in the anterior talofibular ligament region. Also, athletes with peroneal subluxation usually have some apprehension with attempted eversion of the foot.

In chronic subluxation or dislocation of the peroneal tendons, usually there is no pain or swelling along the lateral border of the ankle. The chief complaint may be a popping noise on the lateral aspect of the ankle. The diagnosis can be made by subluxation of the peroneal tendons when the foot is brought into maximum dorsiflexion and eversion.

Standard radiographs of the ankle are important for detecting a rim fracture of the fibula. This is indicative of an avulsion of the superior peroneal retinaculum. More commonly, the radiographs of the ankle will be normal. Since subluxation or dislocation of peroneal tendons is a clinical diagnosis, it is unnecessary to obtain other diagnostic studies. However, CT scan and MRI may be helpful in making the diagnosis.

After an acute injury, the foot and ankle can be immobilized in a non-weight-bearing cast for 6 weeks in order for the superior retinaculum to heal. Since there is a high rate of recurrence, surgical treatment after an acute injury is often recommended. For an athlete who wishes to return to sports as quickly as possible, surgical treatment is the preferred treatment. For chronic dislocated peroneal tendons, patients are often asymptomatic. These patients are best left alone.

There are numerous methods of surgical treatment for subluxing peroneal tendons. They include: (1) direct repair, reattachment, or reconstruction of the peroneal retinaculum; (2) bone block procedures; (3) groove deepening procedures; and (4) rerouting of the peroneal tendons. Since there are many surgical ways to address this problem and the results are similar, the best procedure is one with which the surgeon is most familiar and experienced. If the retinaculum can not be repaired for some reason, the bone block fractures, or the groove deepening fails, then rerouting of the peroneal tendons under the calcaneofibular ligament is a good "bail out" procedure.

Posterior Tibial Tendinitis/Rupture and Tarsal Coalition

The majority of posterior tibial tendon disorders are chronic, progressive problems that mostly occur in older people. In athletes, posterior tibial tendinitis can develop because of overusage. Most patients have idiopathic flat feet or flat feet owing to accessory navicular. Occasionally, painful flat feet in a young athlete can be caused by tarsal coalition (peroneal spastic flat feet). Tarsal coalition may be bony, cartilaginous, or fibrous. The two most common types are calcaneonavicular and talocalcaneal coalitions. Very rarely, an injury can lead to an acute avulsion of the insertion of the posterior tibial tendon at the navicular.

On physical examination, there is pain and swelling along the course of the tendon around the medial aspect of the ankle. The most common area of the tendon to be affected is between the tip of the medial malleolus and the insertion site at the navicular. Subtle weakness in the tendon can be detected when the foot is tested against resistance from an everted position to a plantarflexed and inverted position. Also, observation of both feet bearing weight should be made to determine whether both feet are flat (pronated) and if they are symmetrical. If one foot is more pronated than the other, tarsal coalition or a unilateral accessory navicular may be present. Therefore, the range of motion of the subtalar joint should always be examined in athletes with painful flat feet.

Posterior tibial tendinitis is a clinical diagnosis; therefore, no other diagnostic tests are necessary. However, standard radiographs of the foot are necessary to make the diagnosis of acute avulsion of the navicular at the insertion site of the tendon, tarsal coalition, and accessory navicular. If tarsal coalition is suspected, calcaneonavicular coalition is best detected on an oblique view of the foot, and a Harris view (axial view) of the calcaneus is best to show a talocalcaneal coalition. A CT scan can further evaluate the extent of the coalition.

For acute posterior tibial tendinitis, RICE, anti-inflammatory medication, and occasionally, immobilization in a walking cast or boot are recommended. After resolution of the symptoms, if the athlete has bilateral flat feet, arch supports and custom orthotic devices may prevent future problems. For chronic posterior tibial tendinitis, after failing 6 months of conservative treatment, surgical treatment may be indicated. Frequently during surgery, intratendinous degeneration or longitudinal tears of the tendon are present. Surgery usually involves debridement of the tendon and sheath, excision of degenerated tendon, and repair of the tendon, if necessary.

Immobilization in a walking cast or boot may be helpful in alleviating the acute symptoms of tarsal coalition. However, oftentimes, the coalition needs to be excised surgically in order to get rid of the symptoms. In older patients or those who fail resection of the coalition, fusion of the affected joint may be necessary.

Flexor Hallucis Longus Tendinitis

This is a problem that almost exclusively occurs in ballet dancers.[12] Flexor hallucis tendon travels through a fibro-osseous tunnel on the posterior aspect of talus. It then passes through the sustentaculum tali. Because of the frequent gliding motion of the tendon passing through this bony structure, it can become inflamed. This then starts a vicious cycle of more irritation and inflammation around the tendon as it glides through the fibro-osseous tunnel. It is analogous to de Quervain's disease in the wrist.

On physical examination, there is usually pain and swelling along the course of the tendon around the posteromedial aspect of the ankle. If it is inflamed enough, it can cause pain or triggering of the tendon at the fibro-osseous tunnel with passive range of motion of the great toe. Frequently, this problem is mistaken for posterior tibial tendinitis. Lateral view of the ankle with the ankle in neutral position and a forced plantarflexion lateral view of the ankle are useful in ruling out a concomitant os trigonum or a trigonal process fracture.

The initial treatment is RICE, anti-inflammatory medication, and physical therapy. When the symptoms persist despite aggressive conservative treatment, surgery may be indicated. Surgery usually involves the release of the tendon sheath, debridement of the tendon and the sheath, and repair of the tendon if necessary. If there is also a posterior impingement problem, then it should also be explored to remove any scar tissue and bony pathology.

Posterior Ankle Impingement

Posterior ankle impingement is also a problem frequently seen in ballet dancers.[12] This is caused by repetitive trauma in the soft tissue, trigonal process, or the os trigonum with releve, frappe, or tendu.

On physical examination, the diagnosis of posterior ankle impingement is made based on the plantarflexion test. This test is performed by placing the foot into a maximum plantarflexed position. This maneuver forces the bone or soft tissue to be pinched between the posterior lip of the tibia and posterior lip of the calcaneus. If the plantarflexion test reproduces the pain, then the diagnosis is confirmed.

A lateral radiograph of the ankle in a neutral position and a lateral radiograph of the ankle in maximum plantarflexion should be obtained. The forced plantarflexion view of the ankle can demonstrate the pinching of the trigonal process or os trigonum in between the tibia and calcaneus (Fig. 10-2). Other diagnostic studies are usually not necessary.

The initial treatment is similar to the treatment for flexor hallucis tendinitis: RICE, anti-inflammatory medication, and physical therapy. Occasionally, a corticosteroid injection may be helpful in decreasing swelling and inflammation around the posterior soft tis-

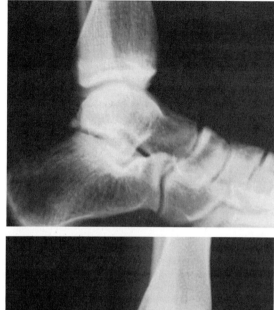

A

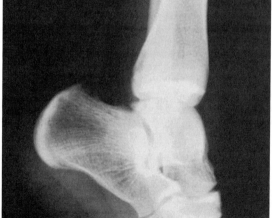

B

FIG. 10-2   Lateral radiographs of the ankle in neutral (*A*) and in forced (*B*) plantarflexion for posterior ankle impingement.

sue. If the dancer has failed conservative treatment, then surgical excision of the bony prominence or the pinched soft tissue is indicated.

Anterior Ankle Impingement

Osteophytes can form on the anterior aspect of the ankle joint with repetitive impingement of the tibia and the neck of the talus. As the spurs build up, more impingement occurs on the anterior aspect of the ankle. The spurs may be located on the tibia only, talus only, or both.

On physical examination, there is tenderness to palpation across the anterior aspect of the ankle. The dorsiflexion of the affected ankle will be decreased. A lateral radiograph of the ankle in neutral position and a lateral radiograph with the ankle in maximum dorsiflexion should be obtained to confirm the diagnosis of anterior ankle impingement and to determine the location of the osteophytes (Fig. 10-3): anterior tibia only, neck of the talus only, or both.

Conservative treatment includes the use of a heel lift to open up the front of the ankle in an attempt to decrease impingement of the spurs. If the symptoms are severe and debilitating, then excision of the anterior ankle osteophytes is indicated. This procedure can be done either using an ankle arthroscope, if the osteophytes are on the anterior tibia only, or through a small arthrotomy, if the osteophytes are on the neck of the talus only or both the tibia and talar neck.

Osteochondral Lesions of the Talus

Osteochondral lesions of the talus can occur either spontaneously or after a lateral ankle sprain. For those that form spontaneously, there may be a vascular etiology. The osteochondral lesions are mostly located on either the anterolateral or posteromedial aspect of the talar dome. The anterolateral lesions tend to be shallower and more waferlike in shape. Also, they are more likely to be associated with a traumatic etiology. The posteromedial lesions tend to be deeper and more cuplike in shape. Out of the lesions that do not have a traumatic etiology, more of them are located in the posteromedial than the anterolateral aspect of the talar dome. The symptoms are similar to lateral ankle sprain. This problem is one of the reasons why an ankle sprain may not heal after adequate treatment.

On physical examination, there is usually mild pain to palpation either at the anterolateral or posteromedial aspect of the ankle. Mild effusion may be present in the ankle joint. If there is concomitant

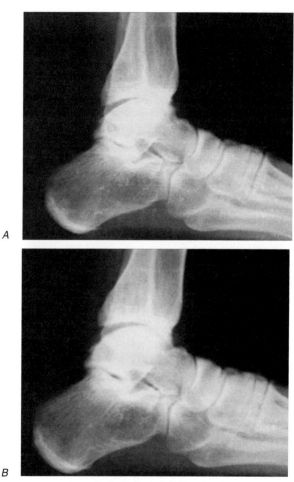

A

B

FIG. 10-3 Lateral radiographs of the ankle in neutral (*A*) and in forced (*B*) dorsiflexion for anterior ankle impingement.

ankle instability, anterior drawer and talar tilt test will be positive and peroneal tendon strength should be checked.

Standard radiographs of the ankle should be obtained. If the radiographs are normal and the suspicion for this problem is high, then MRI is the study of choice to further evaluate the talar dome. If the radiographs reveal an osteochondral lesion of the talus, a CT scan can be helpful to further delineate the extent of the lesion. Several classification systems are available to stage osteochondral lesion of the talar dome: Berndt and Harty, MRI, CT, and arthroscopic (Fig. 10-4).[13–16] In general, the grading system of the lesion is very similar in all of the classification systems, except for the arthroscopic system: grade 1 is subchondral compression; grade 2 is partial separation of the fragment; grade 3 is complete separation of the fragment without displacement; and grade 4 is complete separation of the fragment with displacement.

If the osteochondral lesion of the talar dome is detected after an acute injury, the treatment is to immobilize the ankle with a cast or brace for 6 weeks, usually non-weight-bearing. Most of the time, these lesions are not discovered until many months after the injury when they continue to be symptomatic. At this time, conservative treatment usually is not effective. The surgical treatment of these

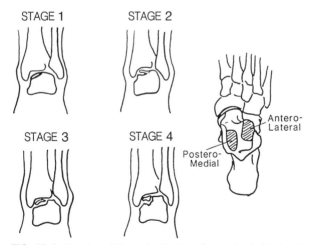

FIG. 10-4   Berndt and Harty classification of osteochondral lesion of the talus. (Reprinted with permission from Reid DC: Ankle region, in: *Sports Injury Assessment and Rehabilitation.* New York, Churchill Livingstone, 1992, p. 257.)

lesions involves debridement, curettage, and drilling of the lesions. For the large cystic lesions with an intact articular surface, curettage and bone grafting may be necessary to fill the defect. The anterolateral lesions are easier to approach with an arthroscope or anterior arthrotomy. The posteromedial lesions may require a medial malleolar osteotomy in order to gain exposure since they are usually deeper, larger, and posterior in location. After the surgery, depending on the size and location of the lesion, a period of non-weight-bearing in a cast or a brace followed by a period of weight bearing in a brace is the general postoperative care.

REFERENCES

1. Ryker NJ Jr: Glass walkway studies of normal subjects during normal walking. *Univ Calif Prosthet Device Res Rep* 11(20), 1952.
2. Berry FR Jr: Angle variation patterns of normal hip, knee and ankle in different operations. *Univ Calif Prosthet Devices Res Rep* 11(21), 1952.
3. Sarrafian SK: *Anatomy of the Foot and Ankle: Descriptive, Topographical and Functional*, 2d ed. Philadelphia, Lippincott, 1993.
4. Isman RE, Inman VT: Anthropometric studies of the human foot and ankle. *Bull Prosthet Res* 97:10–11, 1969.
5. Garrick JG: The frequency of injury, mechanism of injury, and epidemiology of ankle sprains. *Am J Sports Med* 5:241–242, 1977.
6. Rovere GD, Clarke TJ, Yates CS, et al: Retrospective comparison of taping and ankle stabilizers in preventing ankle injuries. *Am J Sport Med* 16:228–233, 1988.
7. Clanton TO, Schon LC: Athletic injuries to the soft tissues of the foot and ankle, in Mann RA, Coughlin MJ (eds): *Surgery of the Foot and Ankle*, 6th ed. St. Louis, Mosby, 1993, p. 1095.
8. Clanton TO, Butler JE, Eggert A: Injuries to the metatarsophalangeal joints in athletes. *Foot Ankle* 7:162–176, 1986.
9. Nistor L: Surgical and non-surgical treatment of Achilles tendon rupture. *J Bone Joint Surg* 63A:394–399, 1981.
10. Murr S: Dislocation of the peroneal tendons with marginal fracture of the lateral malleolus. *J Bone Joint Surg* 43B:563–565, 1961.
11. Stover CN, Bryan DR: Traumatic dislocation of the peroneal tendons. *Am J Surg* 103:180–186, 1962.
12. Hamilton WG: Foot and ankle injuries in dancers, in Mann RA, Coughlin MJ (eds): *Surgery of the Foot and Ankle*, 6th ed. St. Louis, Mosby, 1993, p. 1241.
13. Berndt AL, Harty M: Transchondral fractures (osteochondritis dissecans) of the talus. *J Bone Joint Surg* 41A:988–1020, 1959.
14. Anderson IF, Crichton KJ, Grattan-Smith T, et al: Osteochondral fractures of the talus. *J Bone Joint Surg* 71A:1143–1151, 1989.
15. Ferkel RD, Sgaglione NA: Arthroscopic treatment of osteochondral lesions of the talus: Long-term results. *Orthop Trans* 17:1011, 1993–1994.
16. Ferkel RD: Articular surface defects, loose bodies, and osteophytes, in Ferkel RD (ed): *Arthroscopic Surgery: The Foot and Ankle*. Philadelphia, Lippincott-Raven, 1996, p. 151.

Serious injuries of the chest and abdomen requiring hospital care are rare in sports. We have all witnessed "heart stopping" body checks in hockey and football games, yet we may not recall any incidence of a chest or abdominal emergency. The reason is that this type of trauma is low velocity. However, when injured, these compartments provide some of the most difficult diagnostic challenges.

The chest and abdomen are cavities with potential spaces that house our vital organs. Life-threatening injuries can have occurred while the patient exhibits minimal initial symptoms or signs.[1] For example, hemorrhage of more than 1 L of blood in the abdominal cavity produces no distension or visible evidence. Further, complete disruption of the thoracic aorta from a high-speed deceleration injury, such as in motor sport racing, presents with normal vital signs.[2] The aortic adventitia remains intact and contains the disruption. Ultimately, with each heartbeat, the adventitia tears, and death occurs suddenly from exsanguination.

The decision as to which athlete may be treated on the grounds and which must be sent to the emergency department is one of the toughest calls to make. In the end, if there is no obvious evidence for significant trauma to the chest or abdomen, we must rely on our index of suspicion.[3] The following information may help sharpen that index of suspicion.

CLASSIFICATION

Penetrating versus Blunt Trauma

Penetrating wounds in sports are usually superficial. Management depends on location and depth of the injury. This is as opposed to a gunshot wound, where the path of the missile is often unpredictable. Furthermore, tissue damage from high-velocity ballistics far exceeds the path itself.

The question here is whether the protective chest cage or abdominal wall muscles have been transgressed. Superficial wounds are sutured on the premises. In those wounds which appear deeper, simple digital exploration with aseptic technique can be very diagnostic. If the examining finger hits solid muscular fascia, suturing of the skin and subcutaneous tissue is sufficient. This is done under sterile conditions with healthy tissue and all foreign material removed. If there is a suggestion of a hole in the fascia, no matter how small, surgical consultation is required.

171

Suturing of surface wounds in the chest and abdomen is generally safe. Two areas require extra caution. Wounds above the clavicle and in the groin region may be in close proximity to underlying neurovascular bundles.

Blunt injury can be divided into two types: In the first type, the athlete is relatively stationary, and he or she is hit by a blow such as from a puck or an elbow. In the second type, the athlete sustains what is known as deceleration injury. Here the athlete is moving and is brought to an abrupt stop, such as a downhill skier slamming into the barricades. While these two types of blunt injuries are not mutually exclusive, the former tends to cause damage locally, and the deceleration type of injury can produce catastrophic injury distant from the site of impact.

In the stationary athlete, the depth of injury varies with the magnitude of the blow. Damage is first seen in the skin and subcutaneous tissue. With increasing force, muscle and then the specific underlying organ is injured. Deceleration forces may cause complete disruption of deep organs while showing very few superficial signs. For example, in motor sports, the point of impact may be the driver's sternum, but the fatal injury is in the descending portion of the thoracic aorta next to the vertebral column.[2]

Low versus High Velocity

Although this classification seems redundant, it is important to emphasize the profound effect that high-speed deceleration injury has on the chest and abdominal viscera. This type of injury is not seen in the extremities and musculoskeletal system.

The chest cavity with its bony protection generally comes to an abrupt stop as a whole. The abdominal cavity is far less predictable. Here, unusual or even potentially fatal injury can occur at lower velocities. For instance, motor vehicle accidents involving the lap seatbelt show that injuries can range from rupture of the diaphragm to localized fracture of the pancreas over vertebral body L1.[1] This same injury may be seen in bicycle racing when the falling athlete lands on the handlebar.

Chest versus Abdominal Injury

These two cavities should be considered as one. Note the anatomic relationship. The dome of the diaphragm, and hence the liver, comes as high as the level of the nipples across the chest. The costal margin of the middle to lower ribs covers over the upper abdominal contents. Sensory pathways from these two cavities are often intermingled, creating what is known as *referred pain*. For example, pain in the shoulder or lung apex may be referred from blood irritation under the ipsilateral diaphragm from splenic rupture (Kehr's sign).[4]

ANATOMY OF CHEST AND ABDOMINAL INJURY

The chest viscera is protected by bony structures all around. It has weak points. No great force is required to break a rib in the middle to lower section. This has been seen to occur with a sneeze or a blow by an elbow. It is not the rib fracture that should send the athlete to the hospital but rather what else may be injured secondarily. As mentioned earlier, fracture of left lower ribs may be associated with splenic rupture.

Fracture of ribs 1, 2, and 3 requires great force. Any symptoms or signs such as crepitus or exquisite localized tenderness that suggest fracture here must be managed in hospital to examine for concomitant internal injury.[2] The same is true for fracture of the sternum and vertebral body. Rupture of the diaphragm may occur with injury seemingly localized to the abdomen.

The abdomen is less well protected, and it has "sides," with the liver on the right and the spleen on the left. Ancient warriors knew to hit their opponents under the left costal margin because ruptured spleen in those days meant certain death. The liver is more resilient and may be managed conservatively when injured.[1]

Age may be the most important factor in the treatment of splenic injury. Studies have shown that in the pediatric age group, rupture of this organ is managed successfully without surgery.[5,6] It seems that the adult spleen is friable, particularly in the diseased state, such as in infectious mononucleosis.[4] Treatment for the adult ruptured spleen is splenectomy. In a few instances, nonsurgical treatment may be indicated, such as when the diagnosis is made days after the injury. Very close monitoring is then required for signs of delayed rerupture.

The retroperitoneum is like the mediastinum. These are two well-protected potential spaces. A severe blow to the retroperitoneum causing renal hemorrhage is well tolerated and usually treated conservatively. However, trauma enough to cause disruption to any mediastinal organ is associated with a high fatality rate.[1,2]

SPECIFIC INJURIES

When the physician has, per chance, the opportunity to witness how the injury was caused, the speed of deceleration, the point of body contact, and whether the athlete was prepared should be noted.

"Wind Knocked Out"

This is perhaps the most common chest/abdominal sports injury. It is caused by an acute reflex that stops diaphragmatic movement momentarily as a result of sudden stretch of that organ.[7] Common examples are hockey boarding checks that compress the anteroposterior diameter of the chest and helmet contact with the epigastrium in the football running back. Physical examination reveals an athlete in acute respiratory distress who recovers within seconds; minutes later, the athlete is completely asymptomatic, and his or her chest and abdomen are normal. No treatment is required. Note that this injury is low velocity and recovery is rapid.

Rib Fracture

Rib fracture is not uncommon in contact sports. Many athletes may have sustained this injury and are capable of continuing play. The diagnosis is often made after the event. Physical examination alone is very accurate. If the athlete has an exquisitely tender rib and this finding is reproducible, the diagnosis is made. Note that subtle, nondisplaced rib fracture or fracture of the rib across the cartilage portion might not show on plain x-ray or even with special "rib views." Bone scan will demonstrate a "hot spot."

Chest x-ray is helpful in diagnosing associated injury. A fractured rib may cause bleeding from tearing of its neurovascular bundle.[8] If the inner lining of the ribs (i.e., parietal pleura) is intact, the extravasated blood remains "extrapleural." The result is an inner chest wall hematoma, and the treatment is conservative with repeat chest x-ray to rule out expansion or complications.

Pneumothorax/Hemothorax

Fractured ribs that tear through the parietal pleura may cause bleeding into the chest cavity, i.e., a *hemothorax*. More seriously, laceration of the underlying lung with leakage of air and blood results in *hemopneumothorax*. Often, bleeding stops but air leak persists. As the pneumothorax expands, the lung collapses. Air is trapped within the chest cavity. The injured person experiences shortness of breath and compensates by an increase in respiratory effort. This may result in a ball-valve effect. Air is drawn from the punctured lung into the chest cavity, but no air escapes. The result is *tension pneumothorax*. Such a person is desperately ill, gasping for air and feeling faint. He or she is hypoxic and hypotensive. The latter is due to tension pneumothorax shifting the mediastinum to the opposite chest. Venous return to the heart is mechanically obstructed. Pulses are faint with paradoxical fluctuation to respiration, air entry is absent in the affected side, and neck veins are distended. Immediate treatment is indicated: needle aspiration to the affected side, second intercostal space, or midclavicular line. This may not resolve the entire pneumothorax, but tension and, therefore, impending cardiovascular collapse are averted. The stabilized athlete then requires an intercostal chest drain.

Simple pneumothorax causes symptoms of shortness of breath and pain. The degree of shortness of breath varies with the percentage of pneumothorax. Pain, however, can be highly variable. Unusual pain may occur in the subscapular region, in the shoulder tip, or in the base of the neck with minimal pneumothorax. Intervention with chest drainage is indicated for a "significant sized" pneumothorax and for an expanding pneumothorax. Note that an untreated pneumothorax reabsorbs at the rate of 1.25 percent per day.[8] Therefore, a 25 percent pneumothorax requires 20 days to resolve, assuming no further air leak. This formula may help in deciding whether to aspirate a stable pneumothorax.

Hemothorax causes more pain than pneumothorax. Blood irritates the sensitive pleura. The injury splints the affected side, narrowing the rib space and thus making chest tube insertion difficult. Blood reabsorption in the pleural space is not as complete as air. Healing often leads to scar tissue formation and a "trapped" lung. Hemothoraces should be assessed, monitored, and treated in hospital.

Lung Contusion

Blunt trauma to the chest may result in lung contusion,[9,10] with or without rib fracture, bleeding, or air leak. This diagnosis is difficult to make initially. Chest x-ray abnormalities may not show for 1 to 2 days. Changes in oxygenation appear much earlier. The athlete develops "unexplained" shortness of breath, cough, and rarely, hemoptysis. Most lung contusions resolve spontaneously. Follow-up observation is required.

Sternal Fracture

Unlike motor vehicle accidents involving the steering wheel,[10] in sports, fracture of the sternum is uncommon. It requires a high-speed blow to the anterior chest wall. The chief complaint is pain at the exact site of fracture. As in rib fracture, the associated shortness of breath may be secondary to splinting or to deep organ injury. On examination, there is reproducible tenderness. There may be palpable crepitus with each breath. The finding of a sternal "step" suggests displacement. Bruising may or may not be visible. All sternal injuries require vital signs monitoring, chest x-ray, electrocardiogram (ECG), and serial cardiac enzyme determinations. This injury should be treated as cardiac contusion or myocardial infarction.[11] The fractured sternum, however, will heal without reduction or fixation, even with displacement.

Rarely, chronic nonunion of sternal fracture is encountered. Surgery is indicated for symptoms of pain from rubbing of the fractured ends. The operative procedure involves debridement of the fibrous tissue that has built up between the fracture. This is followed by bone grafting and wire stabilization.

Abdominal Wall (Fig. 11-1)

Injury to the abdominal wall must be differentiated from intraabdominal injury. Common blows to the abdomen in contact sports rarely cause significant injury, especially if the athlete is prepared. When abdominal pain persists after such a blow, specific findings on physical examination may help clarify the diagnosis.

Injury to the abdominal wall may cause disruption to the muscle fibers and/or fascia. Muscle fiber injury may bleed locally and tamponade with hematoma formation. Pain and tenderness are specific to the site of injury. There should be no gastrointestinal symptoms. Physical examination shows visible or palpable hematoma with local guarding. The abdomen is benign. Straight-leg raising or head raising exaggerates the hematoma and physical findings. The contrary is seen in intraabdominal injury. Tensing of the abdominal muscles by these maneuvers protects against irritation of intraabdominal structures and thereby lessens the symptoms and signs.

Injuries to the abdominal wall and abdominal contents are not mutually exclusive. Initial examination may be confusing. An abdominal wall hematoma is self-limiting; intraabdominal bleeding does not exhibit the same tamponade effect, and thus tenderness here may be localized at first and then becomes generalized. Repeat examination is necessary to guard against a missed diagnosis.

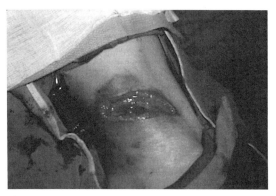

FIG. 11-1   Serious abdominal wall injury.

Abdominal Cavity

There are two sensory pathways in the abdomen: visceral and somatic.[12] *Visceral* sensations are carried by the splanchnic nerves. They respond to distension or displacement of the internal organs. The result is poorly localized pain in the abdominal midline and almost always associated with nausea, cramps, and/or vomiting. Contusion and hematoma of the gut and mesentery both present with visceral symptoms. Physical examination shows minimal findings of mild, poorly localized tenderness. Accurate diagnosis may not be possible. Note that a cut or rupture in the intestine does not always evoke this response. The secondary leakage of blood and intestinal contents activates a different sensory pathway known as somatic.

Somatic sensations are carried by nerves in the abdominal wall and are responsible for the symptoms and signs of peritonitis.[12] Almost all bodily fluids leaked from disrupted abdominal organs will cause peritonitis. The fluid may be blood from a laceration of liver, spleen, or mesentery; it may be bile, gut contents, or acid from the stomach or urine from a bladder rupture. The injured person exhibits all the deep visceral sensations described earlier in addition to the somatic manifestations.

Peritonitis

Peritonitis must be recognized. Irritation of the peritoneum causes reflex tensing of the abdominal wall musculature. This reflex may be unilateral initially. Irritation of the left upper quadrant by a bleeding spleen causes localized rigidity. The athlete has no control over this rigidity. He or she is reluctant to move. Any displacement of the abdomen increases pain. Even breathing is made shallow. Head or leg elevation improves tenderness as further contraction of the abdominal muscles protect against movement. This is completely opposite to muscular injury such as hematoma formation in the abdominal wall. Tenderness is recognized on palpation over the injured organ with maximal guarding. Rebound and/or referred tenderness is seen while examining quadrants of the abdomen remote from the site of injury.

Liver/Spleen Injury (Fig. 11-2)

Liver lacerations always bleed. This causes irritation to the right hemidiaphragm. Pain is experienced both in the right upper quadrant and referred to the right shoulder. Splenic injuries are associated with pain in the left upper quadrant and referred to the left shoulder. Fracture of the lower ribs, particularly along the anterior

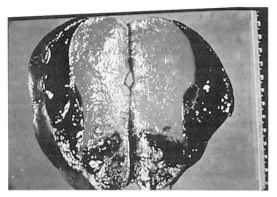

FIG. 11-2   Subcapsular splenic rupture.

axillary line, will cause pain and tenderness to extend to the upper quadrants of the respective side of the abdomen. The diagnosis of any intraabdominal injury is made difficult by referred pain. In these circumstances, assume that an intraabdominal injury has occurred until proven otherwise.

Small Intestine, Mesentery, Urinary Bladder Injury

Peritonitis originating from the lower abdominal viscera may be limited to the lower quadrants by the transverse colon and its over-hanging omentum.[12] For instance, rupture of the urinary bladder may cause peritonitis in the lower quadrants only. Similarly, shearing of the small intestine and its mesentery in high-speed deceleration injury causes spillage of blood and gut contents posterior to the omentum and inferior to the transverse colon. Peritonitis may be "localized." The injured person appears sicker than suggested by the initial physical signs. In time, full-blown generalized peritonitis is seen. Early referral to hospital care based on a high index of suspicion is warranted.

Retroperitoneal Injury

The hallmark of retroperitoneal injury is back pain. This has to be differentiated from musculoskeletal-disk injury. Great vessels in the retroperitoneum are well protected and are almost never disrupted.[1] Injury to the pancreas and the retroperitoneal portion of the duodenum may result from a direct blow. These injuries produce symptoms that originate from the back and radiate bilaterally to the front. Visceral symptoms are present with colic, nausea, and/or vomiting. These gastrointestinal symptoms are not pronounced in injuries involving only the musculoskeletal system. Peritonitis is very late in the course of retroperitoneal trauma. Examination will show an athlete whose symptoms are out of proportion to the minimal physical findings and who appears sicker than from a back strain. There is tachycardia from significant fluid and blood loss. Some books have described Cullen's sign, which is periumbilical discoloration, and Grey-Turner's sign, which is flank discoloration from retroperitoneal bleeding.[13] The presence of these signs confirm large bleeds. Absence of these signs does not exclude retroperitoneal injury. Palpation of the abdomen reveals tenderness across the upper quadrants. There are no obvious peritoneal signs. Percussion of the vertebral column produces little findings. However, stretching of the psoas muscle by hip extension and external rotation will demonstrate pain and spasm indicative of a retroperitoneal process. Hospital management with computed tomographic (CT) scanning is required.

CHRONIC AND RECURRENT INJURIES

Like most major injuries, full recovery from chest and abdominal conditions takes 8 weeks, after which time there are no particular restrictions to training other than that it be progressive and reasonable. Certain injuries may run a chronic course, such as pancreatic trauma and abscess formation. Ongoing treatment by a specialist is required. Splenic injuries treated by splenectomy require pneumococcal vaccination and, in the pediatric age group, prolonged antibiotic coverage.

Nonunion of a fractured rib or costochondral cartilage junction may cause chronic pain, and surgical consultation for definitive treatment is indicated. Fracture of a rib across its bony portion heals far better than the junction between bone and cartilage. Recurrent fracture across bone is distinctly uncommon, whereas fracture across rib cartilage requires little force. Extra protective equipment may be helpful.

Herniation in the chest is almost unheard of. The exception is in the hiatus and diaphragm, and this may present as a chronic gastrointestinal complaint such as postprandial bloating and pain.

Inguinal Hernia

In contrast to the chest, abdominal wall or inguinal hernias are very common. An athlete who complains of recurrent pain in the groin must be examined for herniation before the diagnosis of groin injury is made.[14] Males are affected far more than females, and bilaterality is also common. The athlete should be examined while standing. A bulge in the inguinal region may be visible. Palpation finds a reducible and reproducible hernia. In the absence of any bulge in the male, the examining index finger is passed by the loose skin of the scrotum to the external inguinal ring. The athlete is asked to cough. Reproducible pain and impulse at the fingertip confirm the diagnosis of inguinal hernia. Both sides should be examined as well as the testicles.

Abdominal wall hernias are seen most commonly in the umbilical region. Examination should be carried out in both the standing and supine positions. While standing, the hernia may be visible. While supine, the hernia may reduce spontaneously or may require reduction. Also, the size of the musculofascial defect should be noted.

Not all hernias are easy to diagnose. Inguinal hernias may present initially with localized pain and tenderness on digital examination; however, no bulge or impulse is detected. The posterior inguinal canal musculature may be stretched without producing herniation. Time will tell if there are any sequelae. In the athlete with bilateral inguinal symptoms but no obvious findings, particularly in the female, laparoscopy has been beneficial in diagnosis and treatment.

FINAL NOTE

Significant sports-related injury to the chest and abdomen is rare. However, injuries here may be life-threatening. Diagnosis is often difficult and requires a high index of suspicion. Simple x-rays, chest x-rays, and routine blood work may give a false sense of security.

Acute blood loss of 500 cc or more from splenic rupture may present with mild tachycardia, normal blood pressure, and a normal hemoglobin level. A loss of 1000 cc or more blood may produce orthostatic hypotension and a normal hemoglobin level. The reason for this has to do with how the measurement of hemoglobin concentration is done. When there is acute blood loss and a contracted intravascular volume, hemoglobin concentration remains the same. The body also compensates with vasocontraction and tachycardia to maintain blood pressure. Several hours later, with redistribution of bodily fluids, the hemoglobin concentration then falls to reveal the real picture.

In the same light, a normal chest x-ray initially does not preclude fractured rib, punctured lung, lung contusion, or an intrathoracic bleed. These conditions may present radiographically with time. Chest x-ray findings of lung contusion usually show 24 h after injury. A widened mediastinum from disruption of the great vessels is present immediately.[2] Despite the fact that the athlete may be entirely stable or perhaps even hypertensive, the finding of a widened mediastinum, blurring of the aortic knob, or opacification of the left lung apex is an ominous chest x-ray sign of an aortic tear. The attending physician should always bear this point in mind.

Unlike orthopaedic injuries, which may be apparent on plain x-rays, the diagnosis of chest and abdominal injuries begins with an astute clinician. There will always exist controversies as to the best diagnostic tool for these areas of trauma. Studies have compared the accuracies of ultrasound, CT, peritoneal lavage, laparoscopy, and laparotomy.[3,15,16] These debates are beyond the scope of this chapter. The objective here is to guide the primary physician in the treatment of sports-related injuries to the chest and abdomen.

REFERENCES

1. Boulanger BR, et al: Blunt abdominal trauma. *Emerg Med Clin North Am* 14(1):151–171, 1996.
2. Pretre R, et al: Blunt trauma to the heart and great vessels. *N Engl J Med* 336(9):626–632, 1997.
3. Colucciello SA: Blunt abdominal trauma. *Emerg Med Clin North Am* 11(1):107–123, 1993.
4. Hohn DC: Spleen, in Way et al (eds): *Current Surgical Diagnosis and Treatment,* 8th ed. 1988, chap 29.
5. Tepas JJ: Blunt trauma in children. *Curr Opin Pediatr* 5(3):317–324, 1993.
6. Stylianos S: Controversies in abdominal trauma. *Semin Pediatr Surg* 4(2):116–119, 1995.
7. Birrer RB: Abdominal injuries, in Birrer RB (ed): *Sports Medicine for the Primary Care Physician,* 2d ed. 1994, chap 42.
8. Fullerton GA, et al: Blunt trauma: Trauma to the chest wall, in Pearson FG, et al (eds): *Thoracic Surgery.* 1995.
9. Demling RH, et al: Blunt chest trauma. *New Horizons* 1(3):402–421, 1993.
10. Jackimczyk K: Blunt chest trauma. *Emerg Med Clin North Am* 11(1):81–96, 1993.
11. Schick EC Jr: Nonpenetrating cardiac trauma. *Cardiol Clin* 13(2):241–247, 1995.
12. Anderson JE: *Grant's Anatomy,* 7th ed. 1978.
13. Schwartz SI, et al: Manifestations of gastrointestinal disease, in Schwartz SI, et al (eds): *Principles of Surgery,* 3d ed. 1979.
14. Lovell G: The diagnosis of chronic groin pain in athletes: A review of 189 cases. *Aust J Sci Med Sport* 27(3):76–79, 1995.
15. Leppaniemi AK, et al: The role of laparoscopy in blunt abdominal trauma. *Ann Med* 28(6):483–489, 1996.
16. Catre MG: Diagnostic peritoneal lavage versus abdominal computed tomography in blunt abdominal trauma: A review of prospective studies. *Can J Surg* 38(2):117–122, 1995.

Soft Tissue Injuries: Overuse Syndromes

Christopher T. Daley   *William D. Stanish*

Overuse injuries of soft tissue are common in the athlete and nonathlete alike. In our fitness-conscious society, individuals seem motivated by a heightened awareness of the beneficial aspects of exercise. This has resulted in more people than ever exercising regularly and participating in sports. While individuals seem aware of the cardiorespiratory and associated health benefits of exercise, they also need to be aware that these activities also bring problems with injury.

Regardless of whether the sporting individual is an elite world-class competitor, a weekend novice, or an "aging warrior," tendinitis and other overuse injuries can and do occur. While the incidence of overuse injuries is not exactly known, they have been estimated to account for 35 to 65 percent of all sports injuries.[1]

It is difficult, if not impossible, to determine the true incidence because frequently overuse injuries are never brought to the attention of a physician. Despite this, such injuries account for over 50 percent of the injuries seen in a primary care setting[2] and are the most frequently encountered athletic injury.

Independent of whether muscle, tendon, cartilage, or hard tissue is involved, injury results from a simple mismatch between stress on a given tissue and the ability of that tissue to withstand the stress. There are two basic mechanisms behind tissue trauma: single-impact macrotrauma and repetitive microtrauma (damage at the microscopic or molecular level). *Overuse* therefore can be defined as the level of repetitive microtrauma sufficient to overwhelm the tissue's ability to adapt[1] or, in other words, its healing capacity. Overuse injuries of soft tissue include damage to tendons (from paratenonitis to tendinosis), muscles, bursa, and nerves. They include impingement and snapping syndromes, apophysitis, friction syndromes, and compartment syndromes.

When one looks back through the literature, it appears that the term *overuse injury* was first coined by Slocum in 1968.[3] These types of injuries received recognition years before, and several examples are cited in other major texts.[1,4] In the past, treatment regimens included mandatory rest and/or immobilization, which resulted in predictable musculoskeletal atrophy with impaired function. In addition, the treatment and rehabilitation programs were aimed at the acute problem without much emphasis on the etiology of the injury. The result was methods of treatment that often fell short of the athlete's expectations. Many experienced sports medicine physicians can no doubt cite a post–steroid injection tendon rupture as evidence of another pitfall of the treatment regimens of the past.

In the past several decades, much greater emphasis has been placed on basic research of the pathophysiology and etiology of overuse injuries. We do know that these maladies most frequently result from repetitive microtrauma and overload secondary to extrinsic factors (such as training errors) and intrinsic factors (such as decreased flexibility). We know that relative rest with early movement, not forced immobilization, with later emphasis on a graduated exercise program is more physiologic and will likely return the athlete to his or her premorbid activity level sooner. We are also aware that this group of disorders remains a great diagnostic and therapeutic challenge for sports medicine clinicians because our understanding of overuse problems is still somewhat limited.

PATHOLOGY AND PATHOMECHANICS

Pathomechanics of Microtrauma

Prior to exploring specific overuse injuries, it is necessary to have an adequate understanding of how repetitive microtrauma affects tissues. The most basic principle in the etiology of an overuse injury is that tissue is exposed to a force that can provoke damage.[5] A single episode of excessive stress may cause microtrauma, but usually it results from repetitive loading at a force well within the physiologic range.[1] Injury from overuse results from a mismatch between stress on a given tissue and the ability of that tissue to withstand the stress. The failure pattern of tendons is representative of the disruption observed in most tissues with a high collagen content and serves as an excellent model for demonstrating microtrauma.[1] As a tendon is elongated, its collagen fibers are stretched from a relaxed, resting configuration to a taut, straight cord. If the tensile force causing elongation is removed after the initial 4 percent of elongation, then the fibers return to their natural resting state. If, however, sufficient tension is maintained to achieve 4 to 8 percent elongation, microtrauma occurs as the molecular bonds and crosslinks are disrupted, allowing the collagen fibers to deform. Beyond this degree of elongation, individual collagen fibers eventually fail along with the remaining structural elements, leading to complete macroscopic failure of the tendon.[5]

Inflammatory Healing Response to Injury

The response to the microtrauma sustained in overuse is usually in the form of inflammation that progresses through distinct pathologic phases.[6] Immediately after injury, the inflammatory cascade is activated, and vasoactive substances (including prostaglandins synthesized from arachidonic acid) are released, resulting in increased capillary permeability and fluid transudation. These, in turn, activate the complement system. Neutrophils, monocytes, and eosinophils are attracted to the injured area, where these cells release degradative enzymes that can destroy tissue. Fibroblasts and endothelial cells migrate to the area to aid in the healing process. If no further injury occurs, the inflammatory phase will run its course in 48 h to 6 days.[7] If further injury occurs, this phase can last much longer and be more intense. Pain, swelling, and tenderness are hallmarks of this stage. Tissues adjacent to the injured tissue can become enveloped by this process so that localizing the exact site of injury is difficult. It becomes obvious that even though inflammation is necessary for healing to occur, treatment needs to minimize this inflammatory process to avoid a chronic situation leading to tissue destruction and eventual fibrosis. Nonsteroidal anti-inflammatory drugs (NSAIDs) are important because they are able to block the synthesis of the vasoactive prostaglandins via the cyclooxygenase-mediated pathway. This will help to control the whole inflammatory cascade at a very early step. Ice, elevation, and compression help limit inflammation, but relative rest with avoidance of the provocative activity remains the most important treatment modality.

The second, or proliferative, phase begins the third day after injury and usually lasts 1 to 2 weeks, producing collagen and ground substance. At this stage these early products of repair are immature and disorganized, so applied stress must be low enough to avoid disruption and triggering of another inflammatory response. Gradual introduction of stress allows collagen cross-linking and fibril size to increase while preventing progressive musculoskeletal atrophy.

Beginning at approximately 20 days after injury, the remodeling and maturation stage occurs, during which collagen cross-linking continues, slowly returning the damaged structure to its preinjury strength.[1] It is during this phase that the healing of tendons and ligaments will be increased if progressive controlled stress is applied on the tissues. If excessive stress is applied, resulting in injury, the inflammatory response will be restarted.

These three stages are a continuum and are essentially occurring in waves at about the same time. In addition to these three pathologic stages, the pathway common to all tissues likely involves a direct or indirect effect on the microvasculature with subsequent oxygen deprivation.[8]

Effects of Disuse

It is well established that all musculoskeletal tissues atrophy under conditions of deprivation load.[9] The tissues become weaker both structurally and materially as collagen degradation exceeds synthesis, resulting in a net decrease in collagen. In athletes undergoing strength and endurance training who receive proper rest and nutrition, the vascularization of the white (fast-twitch) muscle fibers and the reversion to red (slow-twitch) fibers gradually improve, which increase strength and endurance of the muscle. In prolonged disuse, the fiber conversion is reversed, and the muscle loses strength and endurance with resulting atrophies. The effects of disuse are shown in Table 12-1.

Since most musculoskeletal tissues adapt to increased loads by becoming larger or stronger, the concept of using early motion with gradual stress application has been used in treating overuse injuries.[5]

ETIOLOGY

Given that repetitive stress can traumatize tissue, the potential for injury is enhanced by a wide variety of predisposing factors. These risk factors can be divided into extrinsic and intrinsic factors (Table 12-2). Exercise and the challenge of sport expose even the most subtle anatomic imperfections.

Extrinsic Risk Factors

Extrinsic factors play a large part in preventing many runners from participating fully in their sport because they predispose the athlete to injury. Of these injuries, 60 to 80 percent are associated with extrinsic factors such as training errors and changes in running activities.[10] The most important risk factor for injury is a training error such as excessive mileage, sudden change in intensity, and running on sloped surfaces. In track and field athletes, overuse injuries are more common in middle- and long-distance runners than in sprinters, hurdlers, and jumpers,[11] presumably because they are associated more with endurance training. Hill work, especially

TABLE 12-1 Effects of Exercise and Disuse

Exercise		Disuse
↑	Collagen synthesis	↓
↓	Collagen degradation	↑
↑	Collagen cross-linking	↓
↑	Metabolic enzymes	↓
↑	Collagen fibril size	↓
↑	Collagen tensile strength	↓
↑	White muscle fiber vascularization and conversion	↓
↑	Tissue strength and endurance	↓

TABLE 12-2 Risk Factors Associated with Overuse Injury in Sports

Intrinsic
    Malalignment: foot pronation, cavus foot, arthritis, femoral neck
        anteversion, genu valgum/varum, previous malunion fractures
    Leg-length discrepancy
    Poor flexibility
    Muscle weakness and imbalance
    Neuromuscular coordination defect
    Ligamentous laxity
    Female gender
    Youth/elderly
    Obesity
    Type O blood group
Extrinsic
    Training errors: distance, intensity, frequency, hill work,
        technique, slope running
    Playing surface
    Footwear: improper fit, inadequate cushioning,
        excessively stiff sole, poor heel counter
    Environmental conditions
    Poor equipment

downhill running, can give rise to patellofemoral disorders, popliteus tendinitis, and iliotibial band friction syndrome. Running on banked surfaces can lead to the "short-long syndrome," and the athlete may suffer from iliotibial band friction syndrome or trochanteric bursitis. For cyclists, riding with too much pedal resistance is a major cause of injury, illustrating poor technique as a cause for overuse problems. Tennis players who perform on surfaces such as all-weather concrete suffer more commonly from injury than do those who play on a less rigid, lower-friction clay surface. Overuse injuries are more common in soccer played on artificial turf than in that played on grass or gravel. Proper footwear including insoles has been shown to decrease the incidence of overuse injuries in military recruits and in running athletes.

Most injuries that occur during cold weather are due to rigorous exercise without warm-up. Under such conditions, as found in fall football and winter skiing, the muscle and connective tissue viscosity is not optimal (increased tissue stiffness and intertissue resistance), thus predisposing to injury on muscle contraction because the elastic component cannot absorb the forces. An increase in temperature of about 8 to 10°F is observed for optimal muscle functioning. Excessive elevation in muscle temperature, however, also needs to be avoided because it impairs circulatory thermoregulation and contributes to the destruction of tissue proteins with water loss.

Intrinsic Risk Factors

Intrinsic factors are also common in running athletes, especially malalignments such as excessive pronation and cavus foot deformity.[10] Excessive pronation is associated with injuries such as medial tibial stress syndrome, Achilles tendinitis, tibialis posterior tendinitis, plantar fasciitis, patellofemoral disorders, and iliotibial band friction syndrome. Factors such as leg-length discrepancy, poor flexibility, muscle weakness and imbalance, deficit in neuromuscular coordination, and ligamentous laxity also can cause running injuries.[10] While pronation of the foot can lead to medial injuries, a cavus foot predisposes to injuries of the lateral side of the lower extremities such as iliotibial band friction syndrome, trochanteric bursitis, Achilles tendinitis, metatarsalgia, and stress fractures.

Some athletes can manifest malalignments known as "miserable malalignment syndrome" that predisposes to significant risk in activities such as distance running. The combination of malalignments includes excess femoral neck anteversion, genu valgum, squinting patellae, excessive Q angle, functional equinus, and foot pronation.[1] The clinician therefore needs to assess the lower extremity as a complete functional unit. Posture has been shown to be important in patients with shoulder overuse problems.

Age itself is a risk factor, since the elderly have been reported to have an increased incidence of overuse injuries. Increasing age in track and field[11] and other running activities predisposes to Achilles tendinitis and other overuse syndromes. Young athletes also are at increased risk. All too frequently promising young athletes are being exposed to high-intensity training at a very young age without awareness by coaches and parents that the immature musculoskeletal system is unable to cope with excessive repetitive biomechanical stress. Sites of overuse injury reflect the sites of rapid musculoskeletal development, as evidenced by such injuries as Osgood-Schlatter's disease and Little Leaguer's elbow. The risk of injury in adolescents is most pronounced during the rapid growth spurt when other factors, such as muscle tightness, also become important in the etiology of sports injury.[12]

Gender may be a factor, because there seems to be a higher incidence of overuse injuries among women. Females with menstrual irregularities are at a higher risk for certain injuries, especially stress fractures.[11,13,14] Women have less muscle mass per body weight (23 percent) than do equally trained men (40 percent).[14] Women also have a lower bone mass than men. During running activities, the repetitive loads of the activity will be forced on the weaker musculoskeletal system in women (as compared with a man of equal body weight), thus predisposing to injury of the lower extremity.

A significant association has been reported between the blood group O and chronic Achilles peritendinitis and tendon rupture.[1] This suggests a genetic linkage between ABO blood groups and tendon structure.

CLINICAL EVALUATION

The presentation of overuse injuries is usually of an insidious nature because they arise from repetitive activity. Occasionally, there may have been an acute injury or strain, but this will be the exception rather than the norm. Overuse injuries as a group have similar clinical features in that they often present with a history of nonspecific pain that can be temporally experienced either before, during, or after sport and exercise. Often there is not a lot of swelling except if the joint itself has experienced overload. Nonlocalized tenderness and heat are apparent, whereas thickening or crepitus may be palpable in the patient with tenosynovitis. The diagnosis is based to a great degree on the clinical experience of the treating physician, although a sound and complete history followed by an accurate, thorough physical examination should offer at least a short list of differential diagnoses.

History

One cannot understate the importance of obtaining a detailed history from the athlete regarding these injuries because the diagnosis and treatment will be based to a great extent on the functional inquiry. The history essentially becomes the way for the clinician to delineate the extrinsic risk factors for injury that exist with the particular athlete in question. The clinician must first ascertain the nature of the presenting problem with a specific time frame as to the onset of symptoms, their duration and intensity, and associated symptoms. It may be helpful to categorize the pain in a functional way[5] as it relates to the aggravating or inciting activity (Table 12-3). Pain that is chronic and unremitting is typically found with chronic tendinitis associated with fibrosis and degeneration. It is important to determine if the pain is associated with any swelling, clicking, grating, popping, or locking. Identify any specific relieving factors for the pain aside from rest or medication. The athlete's training program needs to be explored for recent changes in intensity of training, distance, hill work, cross-training, and number of workouts, for example. The types of stretching, strength training, and endurance training need to be identified, plus the location of the activity and the type of playing surface and equipment used, including footwear. Does the athlete usually wear out his or her footwear in a peculiar pattern? The clinician should explore the

TABLE 12-3 Functional Class of Pain Relating to Activity

Level	Description of Pain	Level of Sports Performance
1	No pain	Normal
2	Pain only with extreme exertion	Normal
3	Pain with extreme exertion and 1 to 2 hours afterward	Normal or slightly decreased
4	Pain during and after any vigorous activities	Somewhat decreased
5	Pain during activity and forcing termination	Markedly decreased
6	Pain during daily activities	Unable to perform

Source: From Curwin S, Stanish WD: *Tendinitis: Its Etiology and Treatment.* Lexington, MA, DC Heath & Co, 1984, p 64, with permission.

general health and nutrition of the athlete and identify if he or she has been fatigued more than usual. Perhaps the patient uses an orthotic, a brace, or taping. It is important to discover how the athlete achieves a warm-up and for how long, especially in cold weather.

It is important for the physician treating overuse injuries to be aware of the biomechanics of the particular activity in question to be able to analyze the demands placed on the individual and determine whether excess stress is being placed on the tissues from poor technique or equipment.

Physical Examination

The physical examination likewise requires thoroughness because the objective is not only the diagnosis of the involved tissues(s) but also identification of the physical etiologic risk factors and biomechanical imbalances that hopefully can be modified effectively in the treatment plan. A basic understanding of the biomechanics of the extremities including stresses and joint reactive forces that occur during sport can greatly aid in proper diagnosis and management. There are major textbooks devoted solely to aspects of physical examination of the musculoskeletal system, and it is entirely beyond the scope of this chapter to present any more than limited aspects of the examination of a patient with an overuse injury. First, remember that the human body is a masterfully orchestrated machine with a motor system designed to resist gravity and provide purposeful movement via complex neuromuscular mechanisms. Normal learned movements, and gaits in particular, are highly efficient, with considerable preservation of energy, work, and effort. Second, injuries that are a source of pain induce change in muscle function through reflex inhibition via neural feedback loops. This will be manifest clinically by subtle changes from the normal efficient gait movements. These reflex changes may go unrecognized, however, because of the body's ability to substitute alternative muscles for those inhibited. Thus in upper extremity problems the clinician needs to specifically look for weakness of the scapular stabilizers and rotator cuff muscle. Dysfunction of these muscles, coupled with loss of glenohumeral rhythm, is the functional basis for the extremely common anterior shoulder impingement syndrome. After lower extremity injuries, weakness of the primary hip stabilizers ensues, which will manifest as subtle changes in gait. This is not to say that the athlete is not capable of excellent performance but that inevitably secondary injuries will occur because of loss of efficiency.

It has been stated that the five components of good physical performance are strength, endurance, speed, coordination, and flexibility.[15] Poor flexibility, or the inability of a joint to move through a normal range of motion, is a major factor in the development of overuse injuries. Any time a motion segment in the body is restricted, the adjacent motion segments must increase their relative motion, which increases stress in the associated supporting structures. Tight muscles can cause significant postural adaptations that detract from efficiency of movement. The testing of passive muscle length therefore becomes very useful in examination for flexibility. Imbalance of quadriceps and hamstring strength and flexibility is believed by many to be the fundamental cause of knee dysfunction during running; thus the clinician should examine both passively. Other musculotendinous units that are important to examine are the iliopsoas (Thomas's test) and the iliotibial band (Ober's test) (see Chap. 33).

Analyzing coordination of movement, such as observing walking and running, is subjective but should be performed as part of the routine assessment of the athlete. Gait laboratories (or a gait belt) are not at the disposal of most clinicians examining athletes, but a trained eye and clinical examination of isolated postural muscles can enable one to recognize abnormalities. In performing screening examinations of postural muscles, iliopsoas (hip flexor test), gluteus medius (hip abduction test), vastus medialis obliquus (tested at terminal knee extension), and tibialis posterior (ankle inversion test), it is not the overall strength of the maneuver that is important but ascertaining whether the normally triggered muscle is doing the work or is a substituting muscle. This is exemplified in testing terminal extension of the knee and has long been a pearl of knowledge passed on to junior colleagues by the senior author (WDS). In a healthy patient, there will be a good balance of size of the vastus medialis obliquus (VMO) compared with the rest of the quadriceps. In an injured patient, the strength of terminal extension may not be affected, but often there will be a discernible lack of bulk in the VMO because atrophy occurs more rapidly than in the rest of the quadriceps.

The clinician, aware that poor postural alignment will bring abnormal stresses on joints and muscles and recruit secondary muscles into counteracting the effects of gravity, should include a quick screen for posture in the examination of athletes. This can be done by observing standing posture in the frontal and sagittal planes, posture during gait, and sitting posture. Proper standing posture in the frontal plane is judged by a plumb line drawn from the center of the occiput following equally between the scapulae and through the anal crease. In the sagittal plane the line should pass through the ear, the center of the shoulder, the center of the hips, and slightly anterior to the center of the knee and ankle.

While standing, the back and overall alignment of the lower extremities should be examined. When sitting, in addition to noting the posture, the patient's knee alignment, ankle motion and stability, and foot alignment can be examined. While in the prone position, the sole of the patient's foot can be examined for anatomic abnormalities and callus pattern, the Achilles can be palpated, and the foot-thigh-leg alignment can be viewed. With the patient supine, range of motion of the hip, knee, ankle, and subtalar joints should be examined.

Imaging and Arthroscopy

An x-ray examination often is indicated in the investigation of soft tissue overuse injuries because x-rays can detect or rule out numerous skeletal problems such as fractures, subluxations, diastasis, epiphyseal damage, apophyseal irregularities, spondylolisthesis, and dysplasia. Using a 36-in cassette, one can determine the anatomic and mechanical axes of the lower extremities or postural abnormalities of the spine. Plain radiographs are less helpful for soft tissue pathology but can be used successfully in detecting intratendinous calcific deposits (rotator cuff tendinitis), calcified ligament (Pellegrini-Stieda disease), joint effusions, and some soft tissue swellings. Localized edema and thickening on a soft tissue x-ray strongly suggest a partial tendon rupture.

Computed tomography (CT) provides excellent bony visualization, and when used with contrast material, the CT-arthrogram can offer an improved view of articular cartilage, muscle, and soft tissues in the hips, shoulders, knees, and spine. CT is also valuable in detecting soft tissue calcification, including myositis ossificans.

Technetium bone scanning can be very useful in detecting an occult stress fracture when plain films or CT is normal. It can help in the diagnosis of shin splints (periostitis) where it may be positive in the subacute stage. In soft tissue lesions such as tendinitis and bursitis, the uptake is positive during the early period and is normal in the late period.[16] Bone scanning has been used successfully in identifying insertional iliotibial band injury in an endurance athlete.

Ultrasound examination is a useful and reliable diagnostic tool that provides an inexpensive method to examine muscles and tendons in athletes. It can be used to detect intrinsic muscular defects such as a partial tear, areas of calcification, and fibrous and cystic degeneration. Ultrasound also has been used to detect muscular herniation, but some muscles, such as the biceps femoris, are difficult to examine. High-resolution sonography provides valuable diagnostic information about tendons including rotator cuff rupture, lateral epicondylitis, and tenosynovitis (or nodular tendinitis) of the fingers and wrist. Ultrasound is useful in differentiating tendinitis from partial rupture in achillodynia, and iliopsoas tendinitis, and it also assists in guided local injection of steroids.

Magnetic resonance imaging (MRI) has established itself as an extremely valuable diagnostic modality in evaluating soft tissue overuse injuries. It achieves excellent resolution of soft tissue structures and is sensitive in detecting edema and hemorrhage. In conditions such as tennis elbow (especially if refractory to treatment), not only can MRI evaluate tendon pathology, but it also can determine whether other disorders are present that could give rise to symptoms that are similar to lateral epicondylitis. Examples include entrapment of the posterior interosseous nerve at the arcade of Frohse, synovitis, anconeus or extensor muscle compartment syndrome, lateral ligament incompetence, and degenerative arthritis. With MRI it is possible to delineate the extent of tendon degeneration that must be surgically corrected. In the investigation of other ligament and tendon pathology, MRI has proved extremely valuable.

MRI is currently the optimal noninvasive diagnostic tool to accurately evaluate the status of muscle strains in athletes. It can accurately identify the location and extent of injury to the musculotendinous unit and help identify whether the injury requires surgical intervention to repair a fascial herniation, anastomose a complete muscle tear, or evacuate a hematoma.

MRI is also proving to have an important role in nerve injuries. In cubital tunnel syndrome, for example, repetitive valgus stress may cause inflammation of the ulnar nerve as it passes through an anatomic tunnel posterior to the medial humeral epicondyle. With MRI images, inflammation of the nerve can be seen as areas of thickening and high signal intensity. MRI can delineate the exact position of the ulnar nerve and evaluate the morphology of the perineural soft tissue, osseous structures, and space-occupying lesions such as a ganglion cyst.

Electromyography also has a role in the diagnosis of soft tissue overuse injuries. Decreased activity will be evident in muscles innervated distal to the level of nerve entrapment, whereas increased activity is seen on the injured side of an athlete with an Achilles tendon injury.

Arthroscopy is used both in diagnosis and in treatment. Operative arthroscopy will be discussed later in this chapter. For soft tissue overuse injuries, arthroscopy is used mainly in evaluation of the shoulder for signs of internal impingement, instability, rotator cuff damage, and labral tears. It has a similar role in other joints, including elbow, ankle, knee, and wrist, in the assessment of joint overload and synovitis. The condition of the tissues found at the time of arthroscopy helps dictate the therapeutic course for the athlete in question.

GENERAL CLASSIFICATION OF SOFT TISSUE OVERUSE INJURIES

All major tissues in the musculoskeletal system are subject to overuse injuries. Most commonly overuse problems develop in the muscles and tendons. Although it is convenient to divide these muscles and tendons for ease of presentation, it is important to realize that they function together as a unit—the musculotendinous unit. Other soft tissues, including the bursa, fascia, synovium, and nerves, are also affected by overuse.

Muscle Overuse Injuries

Muscle Strains

The majority of musculotendinous injuries are acute muscle strains, or "pulls." A muscle strain occurs when there is disruption of muscle fibers, either partial or complete. It has been demonstrated that rapid, repetitive cyclic exercise above a rate of 1.0 cycle per second constitutes a high-risk condition. At this frequency of movement, the regulating and stabilizing effects of proprioception and joint antagonist muscle are grossly compromised. Muscle strains occur near the muscle-tendon junction regardless of the amount or rate of deformation of the muscle and regardless of the muscle shape or structure. Partial injuries heal with significant fibrosis, as do intramuscular hematomas. The fibrotic tissue is unyielding and may give rise to a significant inelastic region lying adjacent to normal tissue. This heterogeneity in the muscle may predispose to chronic overuse injuries unless prevented through the use of regular strengthening and stretching.

Muscle Soreness

Three types of muscle soreness are known to be associated with prolonged periods of sustained or intermittent forceful contraction. The first type, and most common, is *delayed soreness*, which is experienced 12 to 48 h after exercise by the athlete as diffuse muscle tenderness, stiffness, and soreness. This discomfort has been experienced by many athletes returning to exercising after a period of inactivity or after a very rigorous workout. It is often experienced in the beginner athlete as well. The phenomenon has been reported in the literature since 1902, when the theory of microrupture was proposed. Initially supported, this hypothesis gave way to the idea that soreness is due to muscle spasms elicited by the *P-substance*: noxious elements that are produced after strenuous exercise. The constituents of this substance, directly or indirectly (via osmotic induced changes), result in edema and produce the soreness. Regardless of the mechanism, there is little doubt that muscle damage is incurred, as evidenced by increased levels of urinary myoglobin and hydroxyproline. This type of soreness seems related to eccentric work.

The second type of muscle soreness is *acute soreness*. This is experienced only during the exercise period and disappears after exercise because it is a reflection of circulation. It can be experienced both by the beginner and by the experienced athlete. It is related to isometric contractions that induce ischemia and lead to anaerobic metabolism with lactic acid production.

The third type is *injury-related pain*, which is experienced during high-speed repetitive exercise and is analogous to a pulled muscle.

Chronic Compartment Syndrome

All muscles are contained within a fascial sheath that acts as a constraint to exercise-induced muscle hypertrophy or increased intramuscular pressure from strong contractions. Either blood inflow or the exit of metabolites becomes impeded, leading to fluid accumulation within the interstitial space, increasing intracompartmental pressures. These syndromes occur most commonly in the anterior or peroneal compartments of the leg, and a diagnosis is suspected with a history of exercise-induced leg pain and associated tightness of the compartment that is palpable. Diagnosis is confirmed with documented intramuscular pressure criteria of one or more of the following: (1) preexercise pressure greater than 15 mmHg; (2) a 1-min postexercise pressure greater than 30 mmHg, and (3) a 5-min postexercise pressure of greater than 20 mmHg. Initial treatment includes a modification of training (including limitation of running), a modification of athletic footwear or orthotic use, and NSAIDs. Surgical decompression by way of fasciotomy is often required to achieve permanent improvement, especially in the anterior compartment (see Chap. 14).

Tendon Overuse Injuries

Painful areas of tendon traditionally have been diagnosed by physicians as tendinitis, implying an inflammatory nature of the lesion. It is not clear whether inflammation is truly present in all forms of the pathology, especially in more chronic situations, where the histologic picture is more in keeping with a degenerative condition.[17] These states, from a pathologic point of view, are probably best designated as *tendinosis*. The problem with the orthopaedic literature is that there has been a lack of agreement on the use of these terms. Some authors question whether tendinitis is appropriate to use at all and have designated conditions wholly as tendinosis.[18] Other authors have given tendinitis an all-inclusive definition of being a syndrome of pain and tenderness including inflammation of sheath and tendon and associated with degenerative changes in structure.[7]

In keeping with anatomic pathology, four conditions of the tendon have been described: paratenonitis, paratenonitis with tendinosis, tendinosis, and tendinitis.[19] For many clinicians it may be easier and more practical to classify the injury based on the clinical entity observed: paratenonitis, tendinitis, tendinosis, or tenoperiostitis (Table 12-4), including whether there is clinically a partial or complete rupture.

Since clinically it is often impossible to determine the exact source of pain around a tendon (i.e., palpation, as well as contraction, involves both tendon and sheath), I wish to reiterate the usefulness of the functional classification presented earlier (see Table 12-3).

Joint Overuse Involving Soft Tissues

Any joint that is subjected to abnormal loads, ranges of motion, or activity is prone to develop a reactive synovitis. This reaction does not necessarily have to be associated with articular surface damage and does not preclude developing arthritis but involves reactive effusion and thickening of the synovial membrane. Most commonly this occurs in the knee, where anterior knee pain is derived from periarticular tendinitis, bursitis, fat pad impingement, plica syndrome, and chondromalacia patellae. Other joints can be affected, including the facet joints in the lumbar and cervical spine.

TABLE 12-4 Classification of Tendon Overuse Injuries

	Definition	Clinical Findings	Clinical Example
Paratenonitis	Inflammation of paratenon sheath	Swelling, heat, tenderness, crepitation	de Quervain's tenosynovitis
Tendinitis	Inflammation of tendon	Swelling, heat, tenderness, redness	Rotator cuff tendinitis
Acute	Symptoms less than 2 weeks		
Subacute	Symptoms present 2 to 6 weeks		
Chronic/refractory	Symptoms present 6 weeks or longer		
With partial rupture		Dramatic limitation in active motion	Partial tear rotator cuff
With complete rupture		Inability to perform active motion	Drummer boy's palsy
Tendinosis	Tendon degeneration, no inflammation	Tender, palpable deformity	Achilles tendinosis
Assoc. with paratenonitis			
Assoc. with partial rupture		Distinct palpable tenderness, swelling	Partial Achilles tear
Assoc. with complete rupture		Palpable defect in continuity	Achilles rupture
Tenoperiostitis	Inflammation of insertion/origin of tendon or muscle into bone	Point tenderness over insertion, pain against resistance during active motion	
Skeletally mature			Adductor longus tenoperiostitis
Skeletally immature			Osgood-Schlatter disease

Overuse Injuries of Nerves

Nerve Entrapment Syndromes

These maladies may develop as a consequence of reactive swelling in the surrounding soft tissues secondary to overuse. The median nerve can be entrapped (carpal tunnel syndrome) under the flexor retinaculum; also, the ulnar nerve in Guyon's canal is sometimes symptomatic for cyclists; tennis players may experience posterior interosseous nerve entrapment; and any running athlete may get entrapment of the medial and lateral plantar nerves. Soccer players may experience nerve entrapments in the groin area.

Neuritis and Neuromas

A nerve may be injured by stretching, friction, compression, or intermittent entrapment. This can lead to an inflammatory state, as in ulnar neuritis secondary to valgus overload of the elbow in pitchers, or to a neuroma, as can be located interdigitally in Morton's neuroma, which is bothersome for some runners.

Overuse Injuries of the Bursa

The bursa can be injured by direct trauma or repeated trauma, leading to the development of an adventitious bursa or hemobursa. This often occurs in bursae overlying the elbow or knee. Such a hemobursa can lead to a chronic bursitis with calcification and loose bodies that are bothersome to athletes. Bursae can be injured by friction, as in the subacromial bursa on the shoulder, the bursa around the Achilles tendon (retrocalcaneal or superficial), the pes anserine bursa of the knee, and the trochanteric bursa of the hip. Trochanteric bursitis often occurs after prolonged running on a banked surface and can be very difficult to treat. Treatment includes rest, compression, protection, NSAIDs, and occasional corticosteroid injections. Surgery is reserved for chronic symptomatic bursitis.

TREATMENT PHILOSOPHY OF OVERUSE INJURIES

From the outset it should be stated that overuse injuries and chronic tendon problems can be very difficult to treat. The impact on an athlete's career can be profound because such injuries have forced many athletes to change their conditioning/training programs, prevented many from returning to competition at an elite level, and have forced some to give up athletic competition completely.[4,20] The following are 12 fundamental principles that guide management of these injuries.

Principle 1: Initiate Treatment Early with Focus on Both Symptoms and Etiology(s)

The treatment of soft tissue overuse injuries should be started as early as possible. If seen early and treated appropriately, injuries such as tendinitis respond quickly. When injuries become chronic, they are more difficult to treat both from a physical and a psychological point of view. The athlete who is suffering from a chronic injury that prevents active participation is often frustrated and looking for a "quick fix" to get back to competition. Once this stage is reached, the athlete requires even more counseling to remain patient with what will no doubt be a lengthy course of treatment.

Appropriate management entails treatment directed toward both cause (intrinsic and extrinsic factors) and effect (the symptoms). The initial treatment of pain, swelling, and inflammation is of paramount importance, and therefore, initial management should include the components of rest, protection, ice, compression, and elevation. The injury should be protected and rehabilitated in parallel with the healing process.[1] The injured tissue needs to be stressed in order to activate collagen remodeling and alignment but also protected from overstress, which will cause reinjury and incite a further inflammatory response. Taping and bracing both can be helpful in providing protection.[21] Ice is useful for treating pain, hemorrhage, and edema. It induces vasoconstriction, which results in a decrease in local blood flow. Ice acts as a topical anesthetic agent to control pain and decrease reflex muscle spasms by reducing the conduction velocity in peripheral nerves. Ice bags compared with cold gel packs elicit the greatest decrease in tissue temperature over the longest period of time, and application for 15 to 20 min is recommended. Treatment may be repeated every 1 to 2 h in acute cases. In lowering the temperature, ice decreases metabolism and enzymatic function; furthermore, it slows down the inflammatory process. It is useful during the first 48 h in acute cases and in chronic cases can be applied postactivity for 30 to 50 min.

Compression in concert with cold therapy helps to reduce the swelling. When properly applied, an elastic wrap provides effective compression without causing a tourniquet effect. Elevation decreases edema by aiding lymphatic and venous return. In acute ankle sprains elevation has been shown to be the most effective method of reducing swelling.

Without treating the cause of the injury, relapse and recurrence are not only possible but predictable. Once the overuse injury occurs, activity must be modified. Training routines and conditioning programs need to be analyzed and changed, if necessary, since continuation of the provocative activity will cause further aggravation of the injured tissue. Participation in sport is allowed within the limits of pain. Often the only modification necessary may be a decrease in duration, frequency, or intensity of participation to achieve effective control of symptoms. For some athletes, the particular provocative activity will have to be eliminated all together. A swimmer, for example, who specializes in the butterfly and is suffering from shoulder impingement may have to switch to the breast stroke for a brief period.

Malalignment needs to be corrected if possible. Foot orthotics are helpful in treating some malalignment conditions (i.e., excessive pronation) that, when combined with overtraining, create excessive or unusual stress on various tissues. The purpose of the molded orthotic is to adjust the subtalar joint in its neutral position during the midstance phase of running. It also provides support for the medial longitudinal arch of the foot. Pronation occurs when the plane of the forefoot shifts so that the medial side drops below the neutral plane. It is the physiologic result of weight on the foot. Orthotics function to shorten the duration of pronation during the stance phase of running. It is important not to overcorrect, and it is always safest to aim for a slight undercorrection. Pronation can be made worse. Overcorrection can cause lateral ligament pain of the ankle and result in peroneal tendinitis. There are advocates for and against the use of orthotics. Most athletic orthotics prescribed are of the semirigid variety and have been shown to reduce loads and balance forces that are creating strain on the musculoskeletal system,[22] although in a competing study in U.S. Marines no beneficial effect was found (see Chap. 41).

A good athletic shoe can provide support and shock absorption, both of which are important for the athlete. The shoes should be flexible in the forefoot, provide support to the medial longitudinal arch, and have a well-fitted heel counter. Modern athletic shoes are marketed as being well designed to provide this cushion and support but have not been shown scientifically to be better than the shoes of yesteryear.

Other intrinsic risk factors such as leg-length discrepancy, poor flexibility, and muscle weakness also need to be addressed in treating the causes of these injuries.

Principle 2: Treatment Depends on the Stage of Healing

The treatment of a particular overuse injury should be chosen based on the stage of healing of the damaged tissue of the musculoskeletal system.[10] There are essentially three phases of healing: (1) inflammation, (2) proliferation of new collagen and ground substance, and (3) scar remodeling and maturation.

In stage 1, the objective is to treat the initial symptoms with the techniques discussed earlier in order to prevent prolonged inflammation and avoid new tissue disruption. In addition, measures of relative rest are used to protect the tissues from further injury. In stage 2, the objective is to gradually introduce stress and apply modalities to increase collagen production, size, cross-linking, and alignment. The rate of collagen fiber formation is directly related to the functional state of the affected area.[5] The collagen fibers reorientate themselves in line with the tensile force applied to the tissue. In stage 3, the objective is to make the collagen as elastic as possible and decrease the formation of scar tissue. Progressive stress is placed on tissue to promote an increase in collagen fibril size and to increase cross-linking in tissues. Flexibility training is needed to decrease cross-linking in the joint capsule.

Principle 3: Specific Treatment Requires an Exact Diagnosis

It is of paramount importance that the clinician make an exact diagnosis before specific treatment is started. An aggressive exercise program, for example, will not be the most appropriate initial treatment for a compartment syndrome, complete tendon rupture, or nerve entrapment.

Principle 4: Active Rest Is Better than Immobilization

Immobilization is not innocuous. Prolonged immobilization of joints may result in loss of collagen ground substance and elastin. Immobilization of newly formed collagen results in a decrease in the number, size, and proper orientation of the fibers (see Table 12-1). It takes 15 to 18 weeks for ligaments and tendons to regain strength after immobilization has ended. Absolute rest should only be used for 1 to 2 days until the inflammation response has settled or in the most severe, chronic cases of tendinitis after active rest has failed.

Active rest means that the injured area can be used, but it should be protected from significant stress, which may cause further damage.[4] Active rest can be accomplished by decreasing the frequency or intensity of the activity, cross-training (i.e., biking instead of running), altering the biomechanics of the activity by decreasing body reactive forces (i.e., pool running), increasing mechanical advantage (i.e., larger grip size or racket head), or changing the athletic techniques (i.e., change in delivery of pitching). It is important as well to maintain cardiorespiratory fitness through nonaggravating exercise.

Principle 5: Physical Therapy Is the Cornerstone of Treatment; Other Modalities Are Adjunctive

Exercise and physical therapy are the keys to a successful rehabilitation program if they are timely and properly applied. Injured joints need to be fully mobilized, and tissues acting around those joints need to be conditioned to optimal levels. It is important to begin an exercise program carefully, gradually increasing the intensity and load within the limits of pain. A properly devised physical conditioning program that emphasizes flexiblity and strength is most appropriate for eliminating the cause of an overuse injury. The use of medication and physical modalities is excellent for relieving symptoms and may greatly facilitate a conditioning program.

Nonsteroidal anti-inflammatory drugs (NSAIDs) are useful in the treatment of acute overuse injuries, especially if used early, when they can decrease the production of arachidonic acid derivatives in the inflammatory pathway. They are probably best prescribed at maximum dose for 10 to 14 days, and if no benefit is noted in the first 3 days, then likely there will be little benefit in continuing their use.[20] They probably do not have a major anti-inflammatory role in the treatment of chronic injuries because there is scant histologic evidence of a true inflammatory reaction.[18,19] They are widely prescribed but have not been shown conclusively to shorten recovery time. NSAIDs used here may still be of benefit, however, for their analgesic effects in allowing patients to comply with physical therapy.

Corticosteroids are very potent anti-inflammatory drugs, and they are occasionally indicated in a few chronic overuse syndromes. Injections should never be given into the tendon because they can lead to tissue breakdown and degeneration, which can predispose the tendon to rupture. Because these injections result in decreased tensile strength, decreased production of collagen and ground substances, and may lead to circulatory stasis, the patient needs to decrease his or her physical activity for 5 to 10 days after injection.[1,4] Tendon sheath injections, in contrast, are quite effective in treating tenosynovitis of the ankle or wrist. Intrabursal injections, e.g., in impingement syndrome, can be effective when care is taken to remain in the bursal space and not to enter tendon or muscle. Local steroid side effects include depigmentation of the skin (particularly in black athletes) and subcutaneous fat dissolution. Steroid injections also can be given intraarticularly when there is significant reactive synovitis with an effusion. Corticosteroids may be administered topically and driven through the skin by the use of ultrasound (phonophoresis) or electricity (iontophoresis).

Ice as a modality in the treatment of acute symptoms has been mentioned, and it also may play an important role once exercise programs have begun. Ice should then be used at the end of each exercise session to help prevent recurrence of inflammation and swelling.

Heat is effective 48 h after the acute phase and in the chronic phase. It is not used acutely in the first stage of healing because the aim is to minimize the inflammatory process. Later in the healing process heat is used to improve blood flow, relieve muscle spasm, and decrease tissue stiffness, allowing greater ease of deformation. Heat can be applied in different ways. Neoprene sleeves help to retain heat during exercise, whereas superficial heat modalities, such as infrared lamps, heating pads, and chemical heat bags, increase heat to a depth of 1 cm.[4] The most beneficial form of deep heat is ultrasound, because the high-frequency waves render the tissues less stiff and more susceptible to remodeling by applied tensile forces.[5] Ultrasound also increases local circulation and has been shown to speed wound healing. Lasers are another modality that has positive effects on wound healing, but unlike ultrasound, they also decrease inflammation.

Two types of electrical stimulation are used in treatment. Transcutaneous nerve stimulation (TENS) is used for pain relief and can be a useful adjunctive modality.[23] High-voltage galvanic stimulation (HVGS) not only produces heat in the tissues but also has been reported to be effective in retarding the formation of edema (see Chap. 33).

Lastly, deep friction massage is a modality used by physiotherapists to prevent the formation of adherent scars early in healing and later break down scar tissue. It should be avoided in the first couple of days after injury because it can produce microtrauma, induce inflammation, and have a deleterious effect on healing.

Principle 6: Develop Tissue Strength (Incorporating Eccentric Contractions)

A strength training program should start as early as possible while being very careful to use incremental increases in load below the threshold of pain. Initially, isometric exercises are recommended and should be performed without a load. Gradually increasing loads can then be applied, but contractions should be done at levels below the "70 percent maximum voluntary contraction level" and should be held for less than 1 min because they do induce ischemia. Isometric contractions can be augmented with the use of electrical muscle stimulation. When isometric exercise can be performed without pain, then active motion (isotonic or dynamic) exercises are initiated. Dynamic exercise correlates better with improved functional performance.[1] These dynamic exercises include both concentric (muscle-shortening) and eccentric (muscle-lengthening) contractions. Concentric exercises, such as flexing the elbow while holding a weight, may begin relatively early in the rehabilitation program as soon as they can be performed without pain. Eccentric contractions attain significantly greater tension in the muscle-tendon unit. This increased tension and force production are the result of the noncontractile connective tissues working together with the contractile tissues. This is to say, concentric contractions stress only muscle tissue, whereas eccentric contractions stress both muscle and connective tissues.[20] Eccentric exercises should be avoided early when there is an increased risk of overloading the newly formed collagen. When they are started, they should be carried out initially without pain or discomfort.

It is vital that eccentric exercises be included in the physical conditioning program because the tissues need to be strengthened to withstand the greatest stress they will endure—eccentric loading. Overuse injuries are commonly the result of cumulative trauma from repetitive eccentric loading.[19]

A proven effective eccentric exercise program (Fig. 12-1) has been devised.[5]

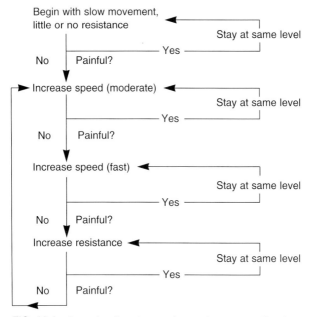

FIG. 12-1 General outline of eccentric exercise program. (Reprinted with permission from Curwin S, Stanish WD: *Tendinitis: Its Etiology and Treatment.* Lexington, MA, DC Heath & Co, 1984, p. 65.)

1. *Stretch*: Hold a static stretch for 15 to 30 s, and repeat three to five times.
2. *Eccentric exercise*: Progress from slow on days 1 and 2, moderate on days 3 to 5, and fast on days 6 and 7. Then increase the external resistance and repeat the cycle. Three sets of repetitions should be performed.
3. *Stretch*: As in 1.
4. Ice for 5 to 10 min.

If one is doing the program correctly, pain should be experienced only in the last set of 10 repetitions. The pain indicates that slight overloading of the tissues is occurring, which will increase its strength. If pain is felt during all sets, then it is a sign that too much force is being applied, which in fact may worsen the injury. If there is no pain, then this indicates insufficient loading, and the patient is not working hard enough to effect benefit or improvement in symptoms. A key factor in this program is not only the progressive use of resistance load but also progressive increase in the speed of the contraction (velocity of the exercise).

Isokinetic exercise is another type of dynamic exercise in which mechanical exercise equipment provides resistance at a controlled velocity. Resistance is increased, but no acceleration is allowed. Isokinetics can be initiated early, within the limit of pain, and like any exercise should be preceded by the application of heat and then stretching and followed by stretching and ice application.

Principle 7: Flexibility Training Must Accompany Strength Training

Strength training alone decreases joint flexibility but is counteracted when combined with flexibility training.[4] The flexibility of a joint is limited primarily by tightness of the bridging connective tissues. Flexible tissue is better able to adapt to the load placed on it without suffering structural damage, and therefore, a flexibility program is essential. Flexibility can enhance athletic performance and aid in preventing or treating injury. There are different methods of flexibility training, including ballistic stretching (utilizes quick movement characterized by bobbing or rebound motions), slow static stretching (involves slowly stretching the muscle as far as possible and then holding the position for 20 to 60 s), contract-relax stretching (includes principles of proprioceptive neuromuscular facilitation in which slow stretch is followed by a maximum isometric contraction and then relaxation and another stretch), and the 3S, or scientific stretching for sport, technique (muscle is passively stretched and then exposed to an isometric contraction while another person maintains the stretch).

In general, slow static stretching is the most widely used method of overuse injuries. Contract-relax stretching is popular as well. Stretching should precede and follow training or competitive athletics and is best done after a brief warm-up. Stretching should last 5 to 10 min and be repeated prior to vigorous activity. The most effective permanent change in connective tissue deformation has been accomplished with increased tissue temperature and slow static stretching.

Principle 8: Sport-Specific Training Needed Prior to Full Return to Sport

Sport-specific training involves training of the muscles and tendons involved in the athlete's specific sport. This is important and should be carried out before a full return to the particular sport, since this is essentially another phase of eccentric conditioning because it is in sporting activities that the trauma is sustained. Whether deceleration is occurring on an upper extremity while pitching or a lower extremity while stopping from a run, significant and specific eccentric loads are placed on the musculotendinous tissues.

Functional activities bridge the gap between rehabilitation of the physical components and full return to sport.[20] While conditioning programs offer a controlled method of loading soft tissue, the joint movement is restricted to a single axis of rotation. When a person participates in athletic endeavors, however, well-coordinated and purposeful movement occurs about multiple axes of rotation. Therefore, even in gifted natural athletes, sport-specific training is mandatory to enable the muscle strength and endurance gains to be integrated in a functional manner. Functional training in a basketball player after knee injury, for example, might involve jogging at first, then running straight, then figure-of-eight drills, and then jumping and pivots. This would be followed by a brief time on the floor playing ball and gradually increasing the length and intensity of participation.

Additionally, it is important to incorporate proprioceptive training into the program by using exercises that require balance, weight shift, and maintenance of center of gravity. This type of training is more important for injuries such as chronic ankle pain and instability.

Principle 9: Treatment Best Involves a Team Approach

To be assured of the best chance of success, a multidisciplinary approach to the injury should be adopted. The need for the physician and therapist to work as a team is obvious, but equally important are the coach, the athletic trainer, and perhaps the family, since they can be instrumental in ensuring compliance with the directed treatment and rehabilitation. In addition, the more active the individual is in the treatment plan, the more informed and educated he or she will become with regard to preventative measures.

Principle 10: Treatment Must Be Individualized

This point cannot be overemphasized. No two athletes are exactly alike, nor will their bodies respond in the exact same fashion to an identically prescribed treatment program. One structured program is not the cure-all for all overuse injuries, and the clinician and therapist must tailor the program to the individual needs of the athlete. The only true guide that the clinician can follow is the patient's subjective complaint of pain. Respect for the individual athlete's report of pain should be a prevailing factor when designing and redesigning the treatment program.

Principle 11: Avoid Surgery until Nonoperative Treatment Fails

With proper diagnosis and recognition of contributing risk factors, most cases of overuse injury can be treated successfully using the nonoperative methods discussed. Only after conservative methods have failed should surgery be employed (unless there is frank rupture), and only then in a limited yet well-defined role.

For conditions such as lateral epicondylitis or chronic partial tears of the Achilles, adductor longus, or rotator cuff tendons, excision of scar and degenerative tissues can give good results. Release of a tight fascial compartment may be required in conditions such as de Quervain's tenosynovitis and similar involvement of the peroneal tendons. Myofascial release may be required to decompress a tense compartment in the lower extremity, as with anterior exertional compartment syndrome. Carpal tunnel or Guyon's canal nerve compression injuries respond well to surgical release.

Arthroscopic surgery of the knee joint in joint overload conditions to lightly debride irritated synovium and a redundant fat pad often allows an early return to sport. Arthroscopic subacromial decompression for impingement problems of the shoulder and use in repairing or debriding lesions of the labrum and rotator cuff are performed capably. Arthroscopy is also used in ankle and elbow pathology in treating synovitis or retrieving loose bodies.

Of all surgery on the body for overuse injuries, the most common is for chronic Achilles tendon pathology, accounting for almost 25 percent of all surgeries in one study.[24] Surgery on tendons and tendon sheaths accounted for over 30 percent of operations, with over 90 percent of operations performed on the lower extremity.

Principle 12: Prevention Is Easier than Treatment

Many factors, both intrinsic and extrinsic, contribute to the production of an overuse injury. The time invested by the athlete in recognizing, minimizing, or eliminating these contributing factors will be rewarded in helping to prevent initial injury and will decrease the risk of recurrence. Physicians and therapists need to stress preventive techniques to the athlete and caution against training sessions that cause fatigue. Fatigue causes imbalances and increased strain on structures less well protected than they would normally be.[20] It is essential for the athlete to preserve a high level of cardiorespiratory fitness, strength, and flexibility.

COMMON SITE-SPECIFIC OVERUSE INJURIES

This section outlines, by region of the body, some of the more common overuse injuries. Along with each body region heading is listed the common names applied to the condition referred to in the text.

Shoulder *(Impingement Syndrome, Swimmer's Shoulder, Rotator Cuff Tendinitis, Dead Arm Syndrome)*

Disorders of the rotator cuff are extremely common. The *impingement syndrome*, manifesting as anterior shoulder pain, is a somewhat ill-defined term for a variety of disorders of the shoulder that can include rotator cuff tendinitis, subacromial bursitis, bicipital tenosynovitis, and rotator cuff tear. Sports requiring repetitive overhead motions, such as baseball, tennis, and swimming, may be important in the genesis of these injuries because microtrauma may lead to instability, subluxation, and secondary impingement resulting in cuff tears. Fifteen percent of all injuries sustained in elite volleyball players have been reported to be overuse injuries of the shoulder. While it has been suggested by some that problems with the rotator cuff are secondary to subacromial impingement, others mandate degeneration as a primary event, since deep intratendinous tears are seen more often than tears on the bursal side. In the throwing athlete, the tremendous forces (up to 80 percent of body weight) required to decelerate the arm after the pitch are absorbed by the posterosuperior cuff muscles (supraspinatus, infraspinatus, and teres minor), thus predisposing to an overuse injury. The history can help in the diagnosis in these athletes. Pain that is associated with a specific phase of the throwing motion, such as late cocking or acceleration, is likely due to mild anterior instability. Pain that is aggravated by progressive activity suggests inflammatory cuff tendinitis or subacromial bursitis. Pain at rest or during the night is suggestive of a cuff tear. To differentiate primary impingement from primary instability with secondary impingement, the relocation test (posteriorly directed force on proximal humerus with shoulder externally rotated and abducted 90 degrees) is performed. Patients with no change in their pain have primary impingement, whereas those with primary anterior instability feel a reduction in pain as the humeral head is reduced posteriorly, relieving impingement on the posterosuperior glenoid rim.

Patients who have shoulder laxity or multidirectional instability have relatively incompetent static stabilizers, since the rotator cuff and other shoulder girdle muscles must work harder to limit glenohumeral translation.[18] This leads to overuse. This relationship between overuse injury and laxity has been documented in competitive swimmers (see Chap. 25). Likely a combination of hypovascularity, fatigue, poor stroke mechanics, and progressive instability in a hypermobile joint results in impingement, and this entity is called *swimmer's shoulder*. Arthroscopy is the most accurate diagnostic tool for shoulder instability. The patient with anterior shoulder instability often describes weakness or giving way in the shoulder with overhead activities such as throwing or serving in tennis. Often the patient describes a complete lack of strength—the *dead arm syndrome*. Despite the argument regarding the primary etiology of shoulder overuse injury, the most important concepts in nonoperative rehabilitation are the same. The first phase of the rehabilitation process is pain control; second is restoration of range of motion; and the third phase is muscle strengthening. Any muscle imbalance must be corrected, especially imbalance in strength between the internal and external rotators. Glenohumeral instability is addressed by strengthening the dynamic stabilizers of the shoulder, including the latissimus dorsi. Operative intervention to achieve stability is required if conservative treatment fails.

Elbow *(Tennis Elbow, Golfer's Elbow, Climber's Elbow, Snapping Elbow)*

The majority of athletic elbow maladies are chronic overuse injuries occurring most commonly in sports requiring throwing and overhead activities and frequently are the result of valgus stress.[25] In pitchers this valgus overload leads to microtrauma, healing of the ulnar collateral ligament in an attenuated state, increased forearm valgus, and an elbow flexion contraction of up to 20 degrees secondary to attempts at repair and stabilization.[25]

Tennis Elbow

Tennis elbow, or lateral epicondylitis, was first described over 100 years ago[18] in a tennis player but is now known to occur also in golfers (hooker's elbow), carpenters, and others nonengaging in sporting activities.[17] It is arguably the most common source of elbow pain in the general population and occurs 7 to 10 times more frequently than medial epicondylitis.[26] The primary pathology involves the extensor carpi radialis brevis tendon, although the origins of extensor digitorum communis, extensor carpi radialis longus, and the supinator also can be involved.[18] It remains very common in tennis players, and half of 30-year-old club players in one study experienced its characteristic aching lateral pain. In treating the pain, phonophoresis with 10% hydrocortisone cream has been found to be useful. Corticosteroid injections can be used in resistant cases, but the number of repeat injections that is acceptable is a matter of debate. Some authors set a limit of three injections in 1 year,[18] whereas others believe that multiple injections are fine because the consequences of tendon degeneration and rupture are, at least in part, the goal of surgery. Once has to balance the loss of surgical risks with local complications from the steroid.

Counterforce braces have been shown to be effective in treatment as well, but if symptoms are aggravated with their use, then entrapment of the posterior interosseous nerve in the forearm should be considered because it is associated with lateral epicondylitis in approximately 5 percent of cases.[25] As with all overuse injuries, an exercise program focusing on eccentric strengthening is of paramount importance.[27] If nonoperative treatment for 1 year has failed, surgical treatment should be considered, but the athlete needs to know that this can result in a lengthy time to return to sports (approximately 4 to 6 months or when strength and endurance are about 80 percent of normal.)[18]

Golfer's Elbow

Medial epicondylitis, or golfer's elbow, results from overuse of the forearm flexor muscles, with the tendons of pronator teres, flexor carpi radialis, and occasionally, flexor carpi ulnaris primarily affected. This condition is seen in throwing athletes, tennis players, golfers, and javelin throwers.[2] Acute disruption of the medial supporting structures of the elbow can present with similar medial pain and needs to be ruled out because this condition is better treated surgically. Nonoperative treatment is the mainstay for medial epicondylitis, but if surgery is required, then care should be taken not to detach the common flexor origin because this can lead to posteromedial instability of the elbow.

Climber's Elbow

Climber's elbow is essentially a strain of the brachialis tendon. In rock climbers this musculotendinous unit is overloaded because the forearms are used in a pronated, semiflexed position. Biceps brachii tendinitis and medial epicondylitis are also common in climbers.

Snapping Elbow and Ulnar Neuritis

Ulnar neuritis is a common cause of medial elbow pain in athletes and can develop secondary to compression, traction, or friction. In the athlete, the earliest symptoms include medial joint line pain and clumsiness or heaviness of the hand and fingers. This neuritis can be secondary to the ulnar nerve subluxing out of the cubital tunnel or to compression by the medial head of triceps snapping over the medial epicondyle. Both are causes of snapping elbow syndrome.[25]

Hand/Wrist (de Quervain's Tenosynovitis, Intersection Syndrome, Drummer Boy's Palsy, Carpal Tunnel Syndrome)

Overuse injuries of this area are seen most frequently in activities that require the hand and wrist to grip a tool or club (racquet sports, golf, rowing), to act as a tool (volleyball, handball), or to support the body's weight (gymnastics, rock climbing). They also occur in activities requiring repeated finger movements to communicate nonverbally (musicians and singers).

de Quervain's Tenosynovitis

Stenosing tenosynovitis of the abductor pollicis longus (APL) and extensor pollicis brevis (EPB) was described by de Quervain in 1895. It is seen with sports that require repetitive wrist radial and ulnar deviations such as golf, racquet sports, fly fishing, and javelin and discus throwing. Pain is usually the first presenting symptom, which can be accentuated by Finkelstein's test. As in all overuse injuries, treatment is dictated by the stage of healing. When seen early, rest and immobilization are effective in 25 to 72 percent of patients, and injection of corticosteroid into the first dorsal compartment achieves cure in 62 to 100 percent of patients. Initial management often includes a thermoplastic thumb spica splint. If no improvement is seen with conservative measures, then surgery is considered to decompress the first dorsal compartment. In doing so, the surgeon needs to be careful in identifying and decompressing all slips of the APL and the two separate compartments for EPB and APL that are present in 20 to 30 percent of people.

Drummer Boy's Palsy

Tenosynovitis of the digital extensors is not common but is seen occasionally in athletes. Likewise, tenosynovitis of the extensor pollicis longus (EPL), or drummer boy's palsy, occurs infrequently in squash players. It is unique because of the potential for rupture, and thus early diagnosis is important. Findings of tenderness, swelling, and crepitus are well localized to the third dorsal compartment. Initial treatment includes splinting, NSAIDs, and activity modification, but early surgery is recommended in the nonresponsive patient to avoid tendon rupture. Steroid injections, which likewise can lead to rupture, are not recommended. Surgical decompression of the third dorsal compartment, subcutaneous transposition of the EPL radial to Lister's tubercle, and closure of the retinaculum to prevent spontaneous relocation are usually curative.[28]

Intersection Syndrome

Intersection syndrome is an inflammatory condition seen in athletes using repetitive wrist extension such as weight lifters, rowers, and canoeists.[28] Pain, tenderness, swelling, and crepitus occur in the area of the crossing point of the first dorsal compartment muscles (APL and EPB) and the radial wrist extensors (extensor carpi radialis longus and brevis). Nonoperative treatment includes splinting, NSAIDs, and steroid injection. Most patients will be cured with this treatment, and at least 6 weeks of conservative treatment is recommended prior to considering surgical exploration and decompression.

Carpal Tunnel Syndrome

Repetitive digital flexion in an individual unaccustomed to such activity can induce tenosynovitis of the digital flexors. This swelling can compress the median nerve under the transverse carpal ligament and lead to symptoms of carpal tunnel syndrome. An excellent example of this occurring in individuals unaccustomed to a specific task is seen in nondeaf signers, who experience symptoms of carpal tunnel syndrome (EMG consistent) significantly more frequently than in native signers (deaf), whose signing is no doubt less stressful and/or learned at an earlier age.

Foot and Ankle *(Achilles Tendinitis, Plantar Fasciitis, Pump Bumps)*

Achilles Tendon Overuse Injuries

The etiology of Achilles tendon overuse injuries is multifactorial, including the anatomic twisting as it passes to its insertion[18] and its somewhat tenuous blood supply proximal to its insertion. Different malalignments and biomechanical faults (including forefoot varus, foot hyperpronation, and decreased calf muscle strength and flexibility) seem to play a role in 60 to 70 percent of athletes with Achilles tendon overuse. Functional hyperpronation produces a whipping action in the Achilles tendon as the heel goes from varus on heel strike to valgus in midstance, thus accounting for the increased risk of injury. Other factors known to predispose to injury include inadequate stretching, training errors, rigid surfaces, and occasionally, systemic disease. Achilles tendon injuries are seen commonly in recreational runners (approximately 11 percent) who train on banked or hard surfaces or who do a lot of hill work. Achilles tendon injury is common (9 percent incidence) among ballet and theatrical dancers. The positions of en pointe and revel demand extreme plantarflexion, whereas the demipile and grand pile positions require ankle dorsiflexion, thus predisposing to injury by eccentric contraction.[29] Achilles tendon pathology can be divided into insertional and noninsertional categories. Noninsertional Achilles tendon injuries occur proximal to the retrocalcaneal bursa and exist as a spectrum of disease ranging from paratenonitis to tendinosis to rupture. Paratenonitis may exist as a separate entity or in association with tendinitis. Insertional injuries include tendinitis and tendinosis, either of which can be associated with a Haglund deformity (a prominence of the posterosuperior aspect of the calcaneus). Retrocalcaneal bursitis often coexists with Achilles tendinitis. Two-thirds of Achilles tendon injuries in competitive athletes are paratenonitis, and one-fifth are either insertional bursitis or tendinitis. The remaining afflictions consist of pain syndromes of the myotendinous junction and tendinopathies. Achilles tendon overuse injuries occur at a higher rate in older athletes than most other typical overuse injuries. Tendon rupture is the most serious Achilles tendon overuse injury and is usually observed with an eccentric contraction. The rupture typically occurs 6 cm proximal to the insertion site.

Most patients with Achilles tendon overuse injuries, particularly noninsertional, respond to a conservative program that emphasizes control of inflammation, correction of limb malalignments, strengthening, and stretching. Stretching is probably the most important component of the treatment and must be performed slowly without bounce. Since these injuries are thought to occur largely as the result of eccentric muscle contraction, it is of paramount importance to strengthen the Achilles tendon in this mode. A proven eccentric program for Achilles tendon pathology has been documented.[5] Steroid injections generally are to be avoided but can be used relatively safely and with good effectiveness in patients with retrocalcaneal bursitis. The injection should enter the bursa alone. If the symptoms fail to respond to these measures, then cast immobilization can be tried for a short period. If nonoperative treatment fails, then surgery can be contemplated. Surgery is required in about 25 percent of athletes with Achilles tendon pathology. The frequency of surgery increases with the older patient, duration of symptoms, and presence of degenerative change (tendinosis). Surgery may be the best treatment for a chronic partial rupture, which is characterized by sudden onset of pain associated with a distinct palpable defect. MRI and ultrasound can help in the diagnosis. In a long-term follow-up study, the patients undergoing surgery for paratenonitis were the most satisfied, whereas those with tendinosis were the least satisfied. Despite this, surgery for chronic partial ruptures gives good results in about 80 percent of patients.[1] For complete rupture, the treatment is surgical, since this is shown to have a lower rerupture rate than if treated nonoperatively.

Clinicians can expect patients with Achilles tendinitis to return to full activities within 3 to 4 months of starting treatment. Following Achilles tendon debridement, patients usually return to running within 6 months.

Plantar Fasciitis

Plantar fasciitis is an overuse injury commonly seen in runners and athletes participating on a hard surface. It is characterized by low-grade pain, insidious in onset, that is located along the plantar fascia at its origin on the medial tubercle of the calcaneus. The pain is accentuated by dorsiflexion of the ankle, which stretches the fascia. The pain is often at its worst during the first few steps taken in the morning or after prolonged sitting. Conservative treatment is successful in over 90 percent of patients. Treatment initially consists of NSAIDs, heel-cord stretching, and an orthotic. The orthotic should support the arch and have a suctioned heel lift and often a cutout over the tender area. Ice massage, phonophoresis, and deep friction massage are also reported to be effective. Manual stretching of the first metatarsophalangeal joint emphasizing dorsiflexion may be necessary. Exercise to strengthen the intrinsic muscles of the foot, such as picking up small objects with the toes, is advisable. Patients often note a significant decrease in pain within 2 weeks and should become essentially asymptomatic within 6 weeks. Steroid injections are sometimes used for resistant cases. Complications including plantar fascia rupture (which is more difficult to treat) and fat pad atrophy limit its indications. Surgical release of the plantar fascia is indicated in less than 5 percent of patients and only after failure of nonoperative treatment.[30]

Pump Bumps

Pump bumps were described originally in 1928 by Patrick Haglund in association with posterior heel pain, a prominence of the calcaneus, and the wearing of rigid, low-back shoes. As we have seen in the preceding discussion, the Haglund deformity is associated with insertional Achilles tendinitis and can be a cause for failure of nonoperative treatment. It is now recognized that the clinically evident calcaneal bump is not diagnostic of Haglund's syndrome but is secondary to a superficial Achilles tendon bursitis. The most common cause is likely from athletic shoe irritation. Other causes of this swelling and/or heel pain aside from Haglund's syndrome are an isolated inflammation of the superficial Achilles tendon bursa, posterior displacement of normal soft tissues because of a significant calcaneal prominence, or systemic articular disorders such as Reiter's syndrome. An x-ray is needed to rule out Haglund's syndrome. Conservative treatment of the pump bump including shoe modification, heel lift, and Achilles stretching is usually curative. Occasionally, a steroid injection into the bursa is required. If associated with a Haglund deformity, surgical excursion of the prominence is considered.

Leg *(Shin Splints, Medial Tibial Stress Syndrome)*

The term *shin splints* has been applied to a symptom complex characterized by exercise-induced pain in the midleg. It has caused confusion because of its name and also because of arguments over its etiology. The use of the word *shin* confuses the issue because this implies pathology in the anterior portion of the leg, but it is commonly agreed that the pain and tenderness experienced refers to the posteromedial border of the tibia in middle to distal third regions. The term used synonymously, *medial tibial stress syndrome*, is therefore probably more appropriate.

The accepted definition states that the diagnosis should be limited to musculotendinous inflammations excluding fractures and ischemic disorders. Therefore, despite stress fractures being identified frequently as a cause of pain in the distal third of the posteromedial tibia, they should be viewed as a separate entity from medial tibial stress syndrome. Intramuscular pressures have been measured in the deep posterior compartment of the leg during exercise. Some authors have found an increase in pressure, but subsequent review of the results by others found that the study was flawed and not convincing. There have been numerous studies showing no increase in pressure. Most authors currently feel that medial tibial stress syndrome is pain secondary to subclinical periosteal inflammation or microtrauma to the muscular insertion of the medial soleus or tibialis posterior.[31]

Contributing factors to this injury include varus hindfoot, excessive forefoot pronation, genu valgum, and other malalignments.[2] In fact, it has been shown that the subtalar joint ratio (the ratio of the transverse plane to the frontal plane components of subtalar joint motion) is related to an athlete suffering an overuse injury in either the leg or the foot.

The medial tibial stress syndrome is typically a problem for long-distance and middle-distance runners, cross-country skiers, and orienteers. It is felt to be secondary to repetitive running on hard surfaces or forcible, excessive use of the foot dorsiflexors. Radiographs are usually normal, and the bone scan is in keeping with periostitis—a linear streaking over the posteromedial aspect of the tibia.

This overuse injury is usually treated successfully with rest and activity modification followed by an exercise program. Surgery should be considered in resistant cases, in which release of the soleus bridge from the posterior tibial border is performed.[31]

Knee (*Runner's Knee, Jumper's Knee, Pes Anserine Bursitis, Popliteus Tendinitis*)

Runner's Knee

Runner's knee is a pain syndrome experienced on the lateral aspect of the knee. Its more anatomically correct name is *iliotibial band friction syndrome* (IBFS). It is very common in runners, especially those who have been running for less than 4 years and regularly run more than 14 km per week.[1] The incidence in running athletes in published series has ranged from as low as 6 percent to over 50 percent. The biomechanics of the iliotibial band (ITB) play an integral role in IBFS. In knee flexion greater than 30 degrees, the ITB lies on or behind the lateral femoral epicondyle, whereas the knee in an extended position places the ITB in front. Thus flexion and extension of the knee under stress can produce irritation and subsequent inflammatory reactions within the ITB, the underlying bursa, and the periosteum of the lateral femoral epicondyle. The pain is often initiated or worsened by running downhill or on banked surfaces and is felt 2 cm above the joint line.

Predisposing factors include training errors (uneven banked running or running downhill), a prominent lateral epicondyle, forefoot pronation, tight ITB, or excessive genu varum. ITB tightness is demonstrated by a positive Ober's test.[18]

Treatment includes relative rest (often reducing mileage and avoiding hills is sufficient), NSAIDs, orthotics, and good shoes. Occasionally, a steroid injection into the inflamed area will help. Stretching of a tight ITB is important. The athlete should be aware that symptoms often will settle with conservative care in less than 1 week, but mild cases may take as long as 6 weeks to resolve. If conservative treatment fails, a 2-cm incision across the posterior iliotibial band proximal to the epicondyle, creating a V-shaped defect, is effective.

Jumper's Knee

Patellar tendinitis, or jumper's knee, is classically characterized by tenderness at the distal patellar pole. The definition today has been broadened to include tendinitis anywhere along the knee extensor mechanism from the quadriceps tendon to the patellar tendon insertion on the tibial tubercle. It is seen commonly in athletes involved in running, jumping, and kicking sports.[18] Volleyball and soccer are sports with a prevalence of this condition. Pain is insidious and is usually localized to the inferior pole of the patella. Radiographs are usually normal but may reveal traction spurs or calcification in the patellar ligament. MRI may reveal degeneration in chronic cases. Ultrasonography is an alternative imaging modality. Four stages of jumper's knee have been described that range from pain only after activity to rupture of the tendon. The key to successful management is prevention using proper training via strengthening and stretching exercises and incorporating sport-specific drills such as jumping.

Patients should be treated a minimum of 6 months nonoperatively before surgery is considered. Local steroid injections are contraindicated because they can predispose to frank rupture; however, phonophoresis or iontophoresis can more safely deliver cortisone to inflamed tissues if the injury is recalcitrant to other modalities. Quadriceps and hamstring tightness is frequently observed and should be treated appropriately with stretching and flexibility exercises. For patients resistant to nonoperative treatment, many surgical procedures have been suggested, including incision and resection of degenerative tendon lesions and resection or drilling of the inferior pole of the patella. In patients with frank disruption, acute repair of the patella tendon is indicated.

Pes Anserine Bursitis

Pes anserine bursitis is characterized by pain, swelling, and tenderness located approximately 6 cm distal to the medial joint line in the region of the pes insertion. The athlete at risk is one with excessive lower extremity malalignment and tight hamstrings. The bursitis usually responds to conservative treatment including rest, ice, NSAIDs, ultrasound, and stretching modalities. When conservative treatment fails (including steroid injections), MRI may be helpful to confirm the diagnosis. Surgical excision of the bursa, if necessary, can be accomplished easily through a posteromedial incision with the patient supine.

Popliteus Tendinitis

The popliteus muscle and tendon resist internal rotation of the tibia during gait. Tendinitis occurs mainly as a result of either hyperpronation or excessive downhill running and is experienced as lateral knee pain that can be confused with IBFS. On physical examination, popliteus tendinitis is most easily detected in a figure-of-four position, where tenderness is detected along the course of the tendon and beneath the fibular collateral ligament.[33]

Conservative treatment is usually effective, and occasionally, a steroid injection is used in refractory cases.

Hip *(Snapping Hip, Trochanteric Bursitis)*

Snapping Hip

The *snapping hip* refers to an audible and palpable snapping with motion of the hip, of which there are two main types: internal and external.[18] Internal snapping hip is usually secondary to the iliopsoas tendon snapping over (1) the femoral head, (2) the lesser trochanter, or (3) the iliopectineal eminence. It commonly occurs in dance and the martial arts. The diagnosis can be confirmed by iliopsoas bursography.[34] Treatment includes avoidance of provocative activities, NSAIDs, and stretching and strengthening of the iliopsoas. A step-cut lengthening of the iliopsoas tendon through a transverse inguinal incision has been recommended if conservative treatment has been exhausted.[34]

The external snapping hip is caused by the iliotibial band or the anterior portion of the gluteus maximus snapping over the greater trochanter. It is most common in cyclists and runners. It is associated with genu varum, leg-length discrepancy, and running downhill or on banked surfaces. Patients presenting to the physician report pain and a high-pitched snapping over the greater trochanter. Many cases are painless. It is difficult to distinguish from trochanteric bursitis, but initial treatment of both conditions is identical, including NSAIDs, activity modification, and physical therapy. Resisted abduction is painful when iliotibial tendinosis is present but not when the patient has bursitis alone.[18] Ober's test can detect ITB tightness. An injection of steroid is often effective for bursitis alone but not for that with associated tendinosis. Stretching is important, and it may aggravate the bursitis initially. Surgery is rarely indicated, but for resistant cases of external snapping hip, a lengthening of the ITB can be considered. Bursitis, on the other hand, has a tendency to become chronic, and surgical excision frequently gives excellent results.

Lumbar Spine, Sacrum, and Pelvis *(Osteitis Pubis, Spondylolysis, Groin Pulls)*

Osteitis Pubis

Osteitis pubis in athletes is a painful condition of the pubic symphysis and surrounding muscular insertions. Although the pathogenesis is unclear, periosteal trauma seems to be an important initiating event. Sports frequently involved are running, soccer, ice hockey, and tennis. Pain is the primary symptom associated typically with difficulty in ambulation, and the patient has a characteristic "waddling gait."[35] The diagnosis is made on the basis of typical findings of pubic tenderness and pain on hip rotation, tenderness of the adductor longus origin, and sacroiliac discomfort. Radiographic changes (which include reactive sclerosis and osteolytic changes) lag behind the symptoms by about 4 weeks.

Treatment is directed at the associated inflammation, and most patients respond to NSAIDs and rest. Refractory cases may require injection with corticosteroids. Full recovery that is documented has been reported to take up to 9.5 months in males and 7 months in females. If there is no improvement in symptoms after 6 months of nonoperative treatment, wedge resection of the symphysis pubis can be considered. Such surgery is rarely necessary.

Groin Pulls

Groin pain is common in athletes. It is most often called a *pulled groin*. Indeed, it is caused most commonly by an overuse tensile force resulting in tendoperiostitis of the adductor muscle/tendon units, especially the adductor longus.[36] Groin pain accounts for around 4 percent of all injuries in soccer.[1] The rectus femoris, rectus abdominis, and iliopsoas muscles and tendons are also commonly affected.[36] Inflammation at the pubic insertion of the inguinal ligament also has been cited as a cause of chronic groin pain. Ultrasound, CT, and MRI are useful in imaging the groin area because the diagnosis may be difficult. Treatment is aimed at the relief of symptoms and a well-directed rehabilitation program. Surgery for acute injuries is rarely indicated; however, tenotomy of the adductor longus has given satisfactory results in athletes after failure of nonsurgical treatment.[36]

Overuse of the Back

Lower back pain is a common problem for many athletes. Running tends to tighten the posterior low back muscles, which leads to increased lordosis of the lumbar spine.[4] This change in structural alignment leads to altered mechanics and predisposes the facets to an overload syndrome. This joint overload can lead to reactive synovitis and accompanying soft tissue inflammation, muscle spasm, and pain. The increased lordosis also predisposes to other posterior elements overloading and possibly leads to spondylolysis. Gymnasts, rowers, and wrestlers are especially at risk.[1] Competitive swimmers are also at risk for back overuse injuries. The etiology of their problems is probably related to a combination of repetitive overuse of the back muscles, imbalance of the back muscles in relation to other muscle groups, and increased lordosis. The back injuries seen most commonly in swimmers include disk degeneration and strain. Since running, cycling, and swimming are sporting activities that individually place the athlete's back at risk for injury, it only stands to reason that back problems would be quite prevalent in a sport combining these disciplines—the triathlon. In a group of triathletes, back pain was experienced by 35 percent over a 1-year period. Most of the pain lasted less than 7 days, suggesting mainly soft tissue involvement, but almost 20 percent lasted over 3 months, suggesting involvement of the intervertebral disks. The amount of time spent training trunk flexors was significantly associated with back pain. Cycling was identified as a major risk.

As is the case with other overuse injuries, prevention is the key to success. In no other body region is it as vital to maintain a general, well-balanced exercise (with flexibility conditioning) program. Based on findings relating duration of back pain to pathology, athletes who have been out of competition for more than 7 to 10 days should undergo a full and comprehensive evaluation.

SOFT TISSUE OVERUSE INJURIES IN CHILDREN AND ADOLESCENTS

The child subjected to repetitive training is susceptible to many of the same overuse injuries as adults: tendinitis, bursitis, nerve entrapment syndromes, joint overload syndromes, and muscle strains. There are, however, several overuse injuries unique to the growing body.

Children must not be thought of as being small adults. Sports programs that match children according to age alone do not understand the difference between age and maturity in adolescence that allows 200 pounds of muscle and moustache to compete against 100 pounds of peach fuzz and baby fat. The growing skeleton is perhaps more at risk for injury than a mature skeleton. Two factors account for this possibility. First is the presence of growth cartilage, and second is the growth process itself.[12] Growth cartilage is located at three locations: the epiphyseal plate, the joint surface, and the apophysis. Each of these sites may be injured, but overuse at the physis is quite rare because most commonly this area is injured by an acute traumatic event. The traction apophyses are sites of active growth in the child, since here columns of growth cartilage unite tendon with bone. These sites are commonly involved in overuse injuries because they are more susceptible to injury than the closed apophyses of adults. Additionally, during periods of rapid growth, there is a measurable increase in tightness in the musculotendinous unit across the joint. This leads to loss of flexibility, which is a known risk factor for overuse.[37] As this tightened unit is stressed, there is an increased risk for repetitive tiny avulsion fractures at the weakest site in the musculotendinous unit: the apophyseal growth cartilage.

Osgood-Schlatter's Disease

This is the most common apophyseal overuse injury. The onset is characterized by an adolescent complaining of low-grade aching pain brought on by activity, developing insidiously, and localized to the area of the tibial tubercle. Both athletically active males and females are at risk for this injury, with males experiencing it between 14 and 15 years of age and girls between 13 and 14 years of age.[37] Physical examination reveals localized tenderness with or without palpable swelling or deformity over the tibial tubercle. Resisted extension of the knee from a flexed position of 90 degrees reproduces the pain. Decreased quadriceps flexibility and patellar maltracking also may be noted. Radiography in the lateral plane may show prominence of the tubercle, fragmentation of the ossific nucleus, or a free bony fragment proximal to the tubercle. Management is individualized and depends on the severity of symptoms. The disorder is almost always self-limiting, with symptoms abating at skeletal maturation of the tibial tubercle apophysis. Treatment includes initial pain control with ice and NSAIDs and is followed by exercise to increase the flexibility and strength of the lower extremity musculature, with particular emphasis on the quadriceps. Quadriceps strengthening is achieved with straight leg raising exercise. Patients are encouraged to achieve normal athletic participation, but activity limitation is necessary in some patients. Rarely, a child who remains symptomatic can be placed on crutches or in a cylinder cast for immobilization for a 3-week maximum. Steroid injection is contraindicated because it may lead to rupture. Occasionally a patient will remain symptomatic after skeletal maturation, and such patients may require excision of free ossific nuclei for symptom relief.

Sever's Disease

Sever's disease, or calcaneal apophysitis, is the preadolescent equivalent of Osgood-Schlatter's disease. It is characterized by heel pain and tenderness localized to the os calcis apophysis. Pain usually follows athletic activities and is bilateral in two-thirds of patients. It usually presents in the 10- to 12-year age group. Children are usually in their growth spurt, and associated malalignment of the feet often is present.[37] Significant dorsiflexion loss is noted in these patients. Treatment consists of orthotics, relative rest, and supervised physical therapy with exercises focused on gastrocnemius-soleus stretching. Foot dorsiflexion strengthening is also included in the program.

An important etiologic factor is inappropriate footwear with hard soles and cleats that have little padding and poor flexibility. Sever's disease resolves naturally in 12 to 18 months, and the patient can participate in athletic activities as symptoms allow. There are no long-term sequelae.

Little Leaguer's Elbow

This is the classic childhood athletic injury. During the acceleration phase of throwing, a valgus moment is generated at the elbow causing radiocapitellar compression, tension on the medial side, and extension overload. The muscles in the vicinity do not protect against valgus overloading, and so the only protection is static: composed of the radiocapitellar joint, the medial ligament, and the olecranon/olecranon fossa articulation. Similar forces can occur following excessive severe or overhead stroking in tennis.

The spectrum of physical and radiographic findings noted depends on the severity and duration of the injury. Medial tension causes an apophysitis at the medial epicondyle resulting in Little Leaguer's elbow. The medial epicondyle becomes prominent and painful. Accelerated growth and widening of the medial epicondylar apophysis are noted frequently. Fragmentation of the medial epiphysis is occasionally noted. Associated pathology includes Panner's disease, osteochondrosis of the capitulum, osteochondral lesions of the radial head, and medial epicondylar fracture.

Initial management consists of relative rest, review of pitching mechanics, and flexibility/strengthening exercises. A triceps-strengthening program of progressive resisted extension exercises and a forearm flexor/extensor-strengthening program using the French curl technique have been found to be particularly helpful. Enforcement of relative rest can be difficult, and a short period of casting may be used to ensure compliance. Gradual return to throwing is allowed when the patient is pain free with a full range of motion. As a general rule, the young athlete should not progress more than 10 percent per week in the amount and frequency of training.[38] Of paramount importance is the enforcement to limit the number of pitches thrown. In some cases, disability may continue for an extended period of time. In these patients, elbow pain may recur when throwing even if the child has been asymptomatic for 4 to 6 months.

Lumbar Scheuermann's Apophysitis and Back Pain

As noted in the adult section on back overuse injuries, increased lumbar lordosis predisposes the back to posterior element injuries including facet joint overload and spondylolysis. Evidence has accumulated that in the pediatric population these injuries and spondylolisthesis are associated with chronic repetitive hyperextension activities such as in gymnastics. Most cases of spondylolysis and mild spondylolisthesis respond to an antilordotic exercise program and bracing. Surgical fusion is rarely needed.

Another cause of back pain in the pediatric population is atypical Scheuermann's disease or lumbar Scheuermann's apophysitis. This is a separate entity from the kyphotic deformity of classic Scheuermann's disease in that it produces pain but not deformity. Lateral radiographs reveal defects in the secondary ossification centers of the lumbar vertebrae. This is a self-limiting condition with no evidence of any long-term complications or predisposition to chronic back syndromes.[1] Although the pain usually abates with reduced activity, occasionally bracing may be necessary. Typically the symptoms are in keeping with a chronic activity-related back pain without radicular features. Athletes at risk include weight lifters, gymnasts, and football players. With maturation, the symptoms and radiographic changes disappear.

SUMMARY

Overuse injuries are the result of repetitive microtrauma to the musculoskeletal system. They are common in recreational and elite athletes. Treatment protocols are based on the stage of the healing process that is active at the time of diagnosis. Most overuse injuries resolve quickly after activity modification. However, they are not always so innocuous, and some leave prolonged symptoms. With the modern-day focus on prevention with identification of risk factors and pathomechanics of injury, many of the overuse injuries can be avoided with scientific coaching and contemporary sports medicine.

REFERENCES

1. Renstrom P: An introduction to chronic overuse injuries, in Haries M, Williams C, Stanish WD, Micheli LJ (eds): *Oxford Textbook of Sports Medicine.* New York, Oxford University Press, 1994, p 531.
2. Herring SA, Nilson KL: Introduction to overuse injuries. *Clin Sports Med* 6:225, 1987.
3. Slocum DB, James SL: Biomechanics of running. *JAMA* 205:720, 1968.
4. Renstrom P: Diagnosis and management of overuse injuries, in Dirix A, Knuttgen HG, Tittel K (eds): *The Olympic Book of Sports Medicine.* Oxford, England, Blackwell Scientific Publications, 1988, p 446.
5. Curwin SL, Stanish WD: *Tendinitis: Its Etiology and Treatment.* Lexington, MA, Collamore Press, DC Heath, 1984.
6. Nirschl RP: Shoulder tendinitis, in Pettrore FA (ed): *Symposium on Upper Extremity Injuries in Athletics.* St. Louis, Mosby, 1986, p 322.
7. Curwin SL: The aetiology and treatment of tendinitis, in Narries M, Williams C, Stanish WD, Micheli LJ (eds): *Oxford Textbook of Sports Medicine.* New York, Oxford University Press, 1994, p 512.

8. Archambault JM, Wiley JP, Bray RC: Exercise loading of tendons and the development of overuse injuries: A review of current literature. *Sports Med* 20(2):77, 1995.

9. Akeson WH, Amiel D, Abel ME, et al: Effects of immobilization on joints. *Clin Orthop* 219:28, 1980.

10. Renstrom AF: Mechanism, diagnosis, and treatment of running injuries, in *Instructional Course Lectures*, vol 42. American Academy of Orthopaedic Surgeons, 1993, p 225.

11. Bennell KL, Crossley K: Musculoskeletal injuries in track and field: Incidence, distribution and risk factors. *Aust J Sci Med Sports* 28(3):69, 1996.

12. Dalton SE: Overuse injuries in adolescent athletes. *Sports Med* 13(1):58, 1992.

13. Rubin CJ: Sports injuries in the female athlete. *N Engl J Med* 88(9):643, 1991.

14. Drinkwater BL: *Female Endurance Athletes.* Champaign, IL, Human Kinetics Publishers, 1986.

15. Cooper DL, Fair J: Developing and testing flexibility. *Phys Sports Med* 6:137, 1978.

16. Byers GE, Berquist TH: Radiology of sports-related injuries. *Curr Probl Diagn Radiol* 25(1):1, 1996.

17. Patten RM: Overuse syndromes and injuries involving the elbow: MR imaging findings. *AJR* 164:1205, 1995.

18. Teitz CC, Garrett WE Jr, Miniaci A, et al: Tendon problems in athletic individuals. *J Bone Joint Surg* 79A:138, 1997.

19. Puddu G, Ippolito E, Postacchini F: A classification of Achilles tendon disease. *Am J Sports Med* 4:145, 1976.

20. Welsh RP, Woodhouse LJ: Overuse syndromes, in Shephard RJ, Astrand PO (eds): *Endurance in Sport.* Oxford, England, Blackwell Scientific Publications, 1992, p 505.

21. Perrin DH: *Athletic Taping and Bracing.* Champaign, IL, Human Kinetics Publishers, 1995.

22. Bull RC: Orthotic devices: Indications, in Torg J, Welsh P, Shephard RD (eds): *Current Therapy in Sports Medicine*, vol 2. Philadelphia, BC Decker, 1989, p 214.

23. Gleck JH, Saliba EN: Application of modalities in overuse syndromes. *Clin Sports Med* 6(2):427, 1987.

24. Orava S, Leppilahti J, Karpakka J: Operative treatment of typical overuse injuries in sport. *Ann Chir Gynaecol* 80(2):208, 1991.

25. Safran MR: Elbow injuries in athletes: A review. *Clin Orthop* 310:257, 1995.

26. Coonrad RW: Tendonopathies at the elbow, in Tullos HS (ed): *Instructional Course Lectures*, vol XL. Park Ridge, IL, American Academy of Orthopaedic Surgeons, 1991, p 25.

27. Thomas DR, Plancher KD, Hawkins RJ: Prevention and rehabilitation of overuse injuries of the elbow. *Clin Sports Med* 14(2):459, 1995.

28. Pyne JIB, Adams BD: Hand tendon injuries in athletics. *Clin Sports Med* 1(4):833, 1992.

29. Fernandez PF, Rivas S, Mujica P: Achilles tendinitis in ballet dancers. *Clin Orthop* 257:257, 1990.

30. Anderson RB: Ankle and foot: Reconstruction, in Kasser JR (ed): *OKU5 Home Study Syllabus*. Rosemont, IL, American Academy of Orthopaedic Surgeons, 1996, p 532.
31. Michael RH, Holder LE: The soleus syndrome. *Am J Sports Med* 13(2):87, 1985.
32. Blazina ME, Kerlan RK, Jobe FW, et al: Jumper's knee. *Orthop Clin North Am* 4:665, 1973.
33. Mayfield GW: Popliteus tendon tenosynovitis. *Am J Sports Med* 5:31, 1977.
34. Schaberg JE, Harper MC, Allen WC: The snapping hip syndrome. *Am J Sports Med* 12:361, 1984.
35. Lentz SS: Osteitis pubis: A review. *Obstet Gynecol Surv* 50(4):310, 1995.
36. Kavlsson J, Sward L, Kalebo P, Thomee R: Chronic groin injuries in athletes: Recommendations for treatment and rehabilitation. *Sports Med* 17(2):141, 1994.
37. Micheli LJ, Fehlandt AF: Overuse injuries to tendons and apophyses in children and adolescents. *Clin Sports Med* 11(4):713, 1992.
38. Gill TJ 4th, Micheli LJ: The immature athlete: Common injuries and overuse syndromes of the elbow. *Clin Sports Med* 15(2):401, 1996.

13 | Dermatology

Thomas N. Helm   Wilma F. Bergfeld

Athletes place extreme stress on their bodies and develop a variety of dermatoses. Skin problems may be more severe or have a different presentation when compared with the population at large. There is a need for rapid resolution so as not to interfere with further physical activity. Mechanical problems from friction or direct injury are most commonly encountered, but physical exposure to cold or sun can lead to skin problems, as can infections, infestations, and miscellaneous other skin disorders. This chapter reviews the most common problems encountered in clinical sports dermatology.

MECHANICAL PROBLEMS OF THE SKIN

Blisters

Strenuous activity in the unaccustomed individual may lead to a variety of changes in the skin. *Blisters* are commonly encountered when individuals run long distances or train or play for long periods of time. Frictional forces cause a dissolution of keratinocytes in the epidermis and the loss of adhesion of keratinocytes. Vesicle and then later blister formation occur. Blisters themselves do not need to be opened or drained unless they impede further activity. If blisters are located in such a place where they interfere with mobility, the overlying skin can be prepped with alcohol or Betadine pads and incised with a number 11 blade or other sharp instrument. The blister fluid is evacuated by gentle pressure on the blister, and the surrounding necrotic epidermis can be left in place. Occlusive ointment such as white petrolatum speeds reepithelialization. Alternative treatments include the use of bacitracin ointment or a triple-antibiotic ointment containing polymyxin and bacitracin. A nonadherent absorbent dressing such as telfa pads can be secured over the area. If expense is not a consideration, hydrocolloid dressings (e.g., DuoDerm, Actiderm, Cutinova) can be used as well and are easier to work with, although much more expensive.

Corns

Corns represent thickening of the stratum corneum seen in areas of increased pressure. They are due to mechanical forces and protect underlying structures. We often use hydrocolloid dressings (e.g., DuoDerm) in our patients. Other products such as Second Skin and Allevyn pads also may be of benefit. The hydrocolloid pads are especially helpful in preventing pain from skates, rollerblades, or ski boots in areas of pressure. Pads may be left on for several days and often stay on despite showering. Cotton socks are worn over the pads. Lamb's wool and moleskin also may be used. Some athletes have irregularities in the shape of their feet. In these instances, padding can be glued into footwear to prevent sliding of the feet.

Subcorneal Hemorrhage

With very vigorous exertion, capillaries in the superficial papillary dermis may rupture, and this leads to a *hemorrhagic bulla*. At times, small hemorrhagic blisters form. They may not be noticed, and as they resorb, they may leave pigmentation within the stratum corneum. This may lead to fear of a pigmented neoplasm such as melanoma. A black discoloration due to blood in the stratum corneum is known as a *calcaneal petechiae* or *talon noir*. A diagnosis can be established by paring the skin. The stratum corneum that houses the hemoglobin pigment can be removed easily and painlessly by paring the talon noir. If paring does not remove the pigment, a biopsy should be entertained to exclude the possibility of a melanocytic neoplasm.

Splinter Hemorrhage

Splinter hemorrhages may occur in an analogous fashion. Sports that involve rapid starts and stops such as tennis, squash, racquetball, and basketball are all associated with the development of splinter or subungual hemorrhages. Worry about an underlying pigmented neoplasm may arise. Subungual melanoma is often preceded by an erroneous history of prior trauma, therefore, clinicians must be wary of this pitfall. If the possibility of a melanocytic neoplasm of the nail bed exists, the pigment should be evaluated closely. A punch biopsy can be obtained through the nail plate. If hemorrhage is suspected, the area of hemorrhage underneath the nail will grow out in an orderly fashion, and the rate of outgrowth can be measured and monitored. It takes approximately 18 months for a new toenail to grow on the hallux. Therefore, the nail would be expected to grow out at approximately 2 mm a month. If the pigment does not grow out or spreads out laterally, further evaluation is indicated.

Ingrown Toenails

Because of trauma to the nails and splitting of the distal edge of the nail, athletes often trim their nails short. If the nails are rounded instead of squared off, an ingrown nail may result. The nail plate stabilizes the distal digit and on the hands allows for precise gripping. If a nail is lost, it becomes harder to pick up small objects with the hands. Loss of toenails may lead to pain with running. Ingrown nails are characterized by erythema, induration, and swelling at the lateral nail fold. Ingrown nails are one of the most common nail complaints of athletes. Improperly fitting shoes or improper cutting of the nails leads to growth of the lateral nail into the nail fold. Trimming the nail shorter often serves only as a temporary solution; when the nail regrows, the problem returns. In many cases the affected areas can be anesthetized and a cotton wedge placed underneath the nail plate. Tannic acid solution (e.g., Outgrow) is applied three times daily. In early and mild cases, this treatment suffices. In refractory cases, we prefer the Jansey technique, in which a wedge of tissue is removed. An incision is made perpendicular to the nail plate at the base of the toe. Another incision is then made parallel to the nail plate, and the involved tissue is removed. Sutures are used to approximate the lateral flap of tissue. Alternatively, phenolic ablation of the nail matrix can be done at the site of involvement after a longitudinal section of nail has been removed. The nail remains permanently narrowed, and mechanical difficulties may result. Therefore, this approach is least favored by us. Topical tannic acid preparations as well as soaks in Epsom salts may help soothe and settle down inflamed tissues. In severe cases, the lateral nail fold may be anesthetized with 1% plain lidocaine, and a cotton pledget can be inserted underneath the nail plate to elevate the nail plate above the surrounding tissue. It is tempting to trim the nail plate back further to alleviate immediate discomfort, but this does not solve the long-term problem. Proper nail trimming is most important in avoiding ingrown nails.

PHYSICAL FACTORS

Sunburn

Athletes train in a broad range of climates. *Sunburn* is commonly encountered in athletes with a fair complexion, especially in individuals with blond or red hair (Fig. 13-1). The sun's rays are most likely to cause sunburn in midday. Depending on latitude, ultraviolet exposure can be maximal at different times. In our area, burning is most likely to occur around 2 P.M. Many athletes do not receive optimal benefit from traditional sunscreens because they lack substantivity and are removed by sweating. Broad-spectrum sunscreens are most advisable, and various sunscreens come in gel or spray formulations that may be preferred by athletes. These formulations do not leave a greasy feel to the skin, nor do they block eccrine coils. Sunscreens should be applied a half hour prior to activity so as to allow the active ingredients to combine with the stratum corneum. Ultraviolet B–blocking sunscreens have been the traditional agent of choice, but it is now known that ultraviolet A

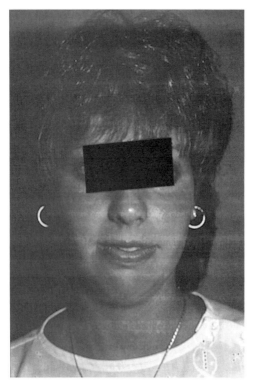

FIG. 13-1   Sunburn is most likely to occur between 10 A.M. and 2 P.M. because of the intensity of ultraviolet B rays. Regular use of sunscreens that include ultraviolet A and ultraviolet B blockers (e.g., oxybenzone and methoxycinnamates) is advisable.

also can hasten photodamage of the skin and photoaging and is associated with the development of skin cancer. For these reasons, a broad-spectrum agent is preferred.

When sunburn does result because of prolonged exposure or exposure to ultraviolet light at high altitudes or from activities in which there is a lot of reflection (such as skiing), treatment with cool compresses and mild topical steroids is beneficial. We typically prescribe nonsteroidal anti-inflammatory agents (e.g., aspirin, ibuprofen) to interfere with the prostaglandin mediators thought to initiate some of the cutaneous damage. Lubrication is especially important because dehydration of the epidermis results after extensive ultraviolet exposure. Some recent research suggests that pretreatment of the skin with vitamin C can inhibit a certain degree of photodamage in laboratory animals. Whether this will be very helpful in humans remains to be determined.

Cold Injury

Cold injury is also commonly encountered. Interestingly, in very cold climates such as northern Canada or Alaska, individuals training outside are well versed in proper skin protection methods and know how to recognize cold injury. They are therefore not at as great a risk as novices. Individuals training in more temperate areas where a sudden change in temperature may not be anticipated are the ones at greatest risk. Prolonged exposure to the cold from running in shoes that are not properly insulated may give rise to pernio or chilblains. Chilblains is characterized by erythematous papules and nodules that occur on the acral toes or on the dorsal toes. These painful lesions persist. Affected athletes may have exposures on the hands, feet, ears, and face. Dampness favors the development of chilblains. Burning, itching, and redness call the lesions to attention. Treatment with vasodilators such as dipyridamole (25 mg) three times daily or nicotinamide (100 mg) three times daily may be of benefit. Calcium channel blockers such as nifedipine have been tried as well.

Prolonged immersion even in warm water may cause difficulties. So-called tropical immersion foot can give rise to itching, burning, and redness as well as a wrinkling of the skin. Proper lubrication and use of thick cotton socks within boots will help prevent this.

So-called trench foot will develop from prolonged exposure to cold. Even if the cold is not below freezing, impeded circulation leads to paresthesias and vascular damage and possibly even gangrene. Removal from the offending environment and keeping the area warm and dry are important in resolution for this problem.

Cold Panniculitis

Some athletes, especially young women, may develop panniculitis on the lateral thighs. This has been noted most in equestrian sports. The cold may lead to a solidification of the panniculus, which in turn leads to painful erythematous nodules. Identifying the cause and wearing proper clothing prevent recurrence.

INFECTIONS

Viral infections are extremely common in athletes as well as in the population at large. Common warts due to human papillomavirus are encountered primarily on the hands and feet and may interfere with sports. A number of treatment options exist for human papillomavirus infection. The standard treatment is that of liquid nitrogen cryotherapy, which if used by an experienced practitioner usually leads to resolution without scarring. Topical cantharone has been a mainstay of therapy in the past but is no longer approved by the Food and Drug Administration (FDA) in the United States. It is available in Canada and all other Western nations. Carbon dioxide laser ablation, electrosurgical removal, and chemical destruction with topical acids such as nitric acid are all of benefit as well.

In our practice, the use of paring and chemical destruction with nitric acid is preferred. Nitric acid must be used with great caution because it can cause severe burns to the skin, but if it is used correctly, it leads to marked desquamation with less pain than liquid nitrogen or other therapies. Topical salicylic acid preparations can be of benefit. The greater the concentration of salicylic acid, the more quickly results are noted. We favor the use of 40% salicylic acid plasters (Mediplast) cut to the size of the wart and applied each night at bedtime. Additionally, other agents such as topical tretinoin (Retin-A) have been used.

Molluscum Contagiosum

Molluscum contagiosum is a poxvirus infection that can affect the skin. Young children and athletes are most commonly affected. There are reports of individuals spreading molluscum contagiosum on cross-country teams or through swimming pools (Fig. 13-2). Molluscum contagiosum is characterized by flesh-colored or white papules that have a central umbilication when lesions are fully mature (Fig. 13-3). Intertriginous folds, the face, and periorbital areas are commonly involved. Favored treatments include liquid nitrogen cryotherapy or curettage. Liquid nitrogen cryotherapy must be used with caution in individuals with dark complexions because of the risk of hypopigmentation. Curettage with or without anesthesia is helpful. In children or sensitive adults, use of a topical anesthetic cream (e.g., EMLA) 1.5 h prior to the procedure will lead to painless removal. Additionally, topical cantharone or a topical irritant such as salicylic acid can be used.

Herpes

Herpetic infections present as painful blisters on erythematous skin. Exposure to cold, biting winds or sunburn on the lip may lead to recurrence of herpes labialis. If an individual with an underlying dermatosis such as severe atopic dermatitis is exposed to herpes, a specific manifestation known as *herpes gladiatorium* may result

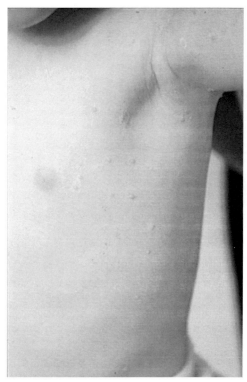

FIG. 13-2 Molluscum contagiosum is common in swimmers, but outbreaks have been noted on cross-country teams as well. Umbilicated papules that are mildly pruritic develop especially in intertriginous areas.

(Fig. 13-4). Herpes gladiatorium is a widespread herpetic infection that is serious and needs to be treated with oral antiviral medications. In the past, acyclovir has been the mainstay of therapy. Now acyclovir is available for use for herpes zoster and genital herpes. In our hands, it is extremely efficacious for herpes gladiatorium when given in a dosage of 500 mg twice daily for 10 days. Other treatment options include famciclovir (e.g., Famvir) given at a dosage of 125 mg twice daily for 5 days.

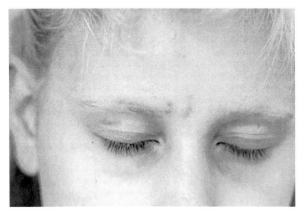

FIG. 13-3 Umbilicated papules of molluscum contagiosum may at times become inflamed.

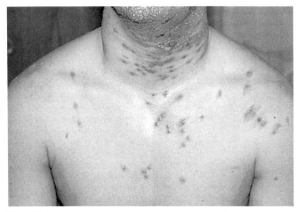

FIG. 13-4 Herpes simplex infection may spread to involve wide areas of skin in individuals with underlying skin disease such as atopic dermatitis or Darier's disease. Wrestlers are particularly prone to this widespread form of herpes simplex known as *herpes gladiatorum*.

Herpes zoster also may be seen in the athlete (Fig. 13-5). Herpes zoster in a young individual should raise the possibility of concomitant human immunodeficiency virus (HIV) infection. Herpes zoster may be a presenting sign of HIV infection, and therefore, risk factors should be explored in individuals affected by herpes zoster. In younger individuals, it may not be necessary to treat, but in individuals older than age 60, the risk of postherpetic neuralgia becomes so prominent as to warrant treatment with antiviral agents. Treatments include valacyclovir at a dose of 1 g three times daily for 7 days, famciclovir at a dosage of 500 mg three times daily for 7 days, or acyclovir given at a dosage of 800 mg five times daily for 7 days. The newer agents valacyclovir and famciclovir are favored because of their increased ability to minimize postherpetic neuralgia.

HIV Infection

HIV infection has continued to increase in our society and now is rising especially in young women. HIV infection may manifest as herpes zoster, candidiasis, or extensive and refractory molluscum contagiosum. Current information suggests that there is no risk of acquiring HIV through sports activity, but it is important for sports

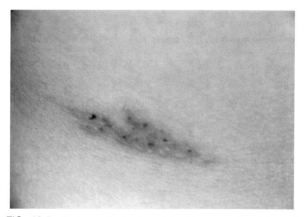

FIG. 13-5 Herpes zoster is characterized by grouped vesicles and pustules occurring on an erythematous base in a dermatomal region. With the increased incidence of HIV infection, young adults with herpes zoster should be questioned for risk factors for underlying immunosuppression.

physicians to practice universal precautions in all treated individuals.

Bacterial Infections

Bacterial infections are extremely common in athletes. *Folliculitis* is perhaps the most commonly encountered bacterial infection and is seen especially in individuals with profuse body hair who participate in sports that involve a great deal of sweating and exertion. Pustules are centered around hair follicles and often have a hair emanating from the center. Treatments include antibacterial soaps (e.g., Lever 2000, Dial antibacterial soap, benzoyl peroxide, or benzoyl peroxide wash) and topical antibiotics (e.g., clindamycin gel, erythromycin gel). In widespread or refractory cases, oral therapy with a penicillinase-resistant penicillin (e.g., dicloxacillin) is extremely efficacious. Erythromycin is also helpful for community-acquired folliculitis and is sometimes preferred because of its excellent safety profile.

Impetigo is characterized by honey-colored crusts that may expand in an annular fashion. Impetigo can be treated with wet compresses of either tap water or aluminum acetate solution (diluted at a ratio of 1:40) and subsequent application of a topical antibiotic such as mupirocin (e.g., Bactroban). Mupirocin in many cases is as efficacious as oral antibiotics. We use oral dicloxacillin or erythromycin and topical mupirocin in severe or extensive cases of impetigo.

Erythrasma is an infection of the intertriginous areas by the organism *Corynebacterium minutissimum*. Dull red plaques are seen in body folds. These lesions are usually asymptomatic. Soap and water cleansing many times will control the problem entirely in most cases. Otherwise, topical erythromycin medications (e.g., Akne-mycin cream) will be of benefit. Oral erythromycin also can be given but is rarely needed. The alcohol-based erythromycin products should be avoided because of the irritation they create in the body folds.

Fungal and Yeast Infections

Fungal and yeast infections are seen most often during warm weather. *Pityriasis versicolor* is a lipophilic yeast infection caused by an organism that is found as a commensal on normal skin. In some individuals, the *Pityrosporon* organism grows to great quantities. On skin scraping, small spores, as well as short hyphae, are identified. The *Pityrosporon* organisms produce azeleic acid, which interferes with normal melanization. Areas are hypopigmented and scaly and are disturbing because of their cosmetic appearance (Fig. 13-6). Treatment includes the use of selenium sulfide topical lotion. The 2.5% lotion is applied for 10 min to the affected areas each day and then rinsed off in the shower (Fig. 13-7). This procedure is continued for 1 week and then once a month thereafter as needed. Athletes must be cautioned that pigmentation will not normalize immediately but may take several weeks to months. If affected areas are showing on the neck or in other places, topical imidazole creams can be used as well (e.g., Spectazole cream). This approach is more expensive and not generally needed.

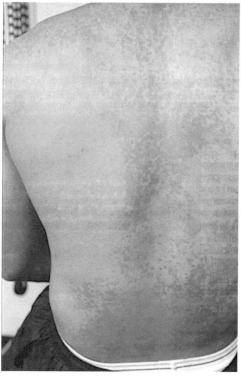

FIG. 13-6   Tinea versicolor may present as tan, scaling macules on the skin. The *Pityrosporon orbiculare* organism produces azeleic acid, which may cause hypopigmentation in individuals with darker skin color.

Tinea cruris and *tinea corporis* are very common in athletes. Affected individuals develop redness in the groin folds. There is often an advancing serpiginous or annular scaling border (Fig. 13-8). Tinea cruris is especially common in individuals with onychomycosis. Heat and moisture in the groin folds will allow tinea to develop, and athletes complain of a burning or stinging sensation. Topical imidazole creams lead to prompt resolution in most cases. Alkylamines (e.g., Lamisil) are helpful also. Tinea cruris does not typically involve the scrotum but is most pronounced in the groin folds and often has a serpiginous or annular edge. Perianal involvement may occur. Aluminum acetate (1/40) compresses applied for 10 min three times daily can help cleanse the affected areas and are soothing. Widespread tinea infections may be encountered in wrestlers and in participants in other contact sports. Our current therapeutic armamentarium has widened substantially with the use of oral azole antifungal agents. Itraconazole, fluconazole, and ketaconazole are all very helpful in leading to prompt eradication of tinea infection.

Tinea capitis is best treated with oral antifungal agents. At the present time, terbinafine (e.g., Lamisil) and itraconazole (e.g., Sporonox) are favored. In the past, griseofulvin was used widely as oral therapy, but the newer agents are effective against a greater range of dermatophytes and have a more rapid onset.

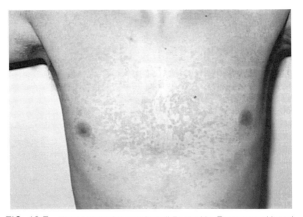

FIG. 13-7 Tinea versicolor may be mildly pruritic. Treatment with topical selenium sulfide 2-1/2% lotion applied for 10 min each day for 1 week is usually very successful in eradicating this common infection. Repeat treatments may be necessary.

If scrotal erythema is present, the possibility of candidiasis should be considered. Candidiasis of the genital region is accompanied by pustules around the areas of involvement known as *satellite pustules*, whereas dermatophyte infections are not. A potassium hydroxide examination of scale will reveal branching hyphae in dermatophytosis and pseudohyphae in candidiasis.

Loose, cool clothing and thorough drying of the affected areas facilitate healing.

Intertrigo and Pruritus Ani

Intertrigo and "skin fold rashes" are common in heavy set or overweight athletes. Friction, moisture, and heat lead to maceration. Secondary infection with dermatophytes, *candida*, and even bacteria (e.g., *Corynebacterium*, streptococci, staphylococci, and *Pseudomonas*) is commonplace. Treatment includes thorough drying of

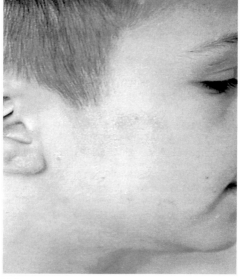

FIG. 13-8 Tinea may have an annular appearance but in some instances may have an acneiform appearance, especially if topical corticosteroids were used previously, as in this case. Scraping the skin and viewing the skin scrapings after digestion with potassium hydroxide solution allow for accurate diagnosis.

the affected areas and the use of protective ointments. We have found the use of aluminum acetate (Burow's solution) 1:40 compresses three times daily for 5 min followed by zinc oxide protective ointment (USP 10%) helpful. Athletes are then advised to apply an imidazole-containing antifungal agent at bedtime (e.g., Spectazole or Exelderm). In acute situations, we favor the immediate application of Castellani's paint.

INFESTATIONS

Scabies

Scabies infestation is very common in young athletes and easily spread with close contact to affected individuals. Scabies is characterized by an intensely pruritic eruption that may involve the flexural surfaces of the wrists, around the ankles, the genitalia, and the feet and arms. The head and neck area is usually spared. Burrows may be seen. In fastidious individuals, the clinical findings may be very subtle. A skin scraping examined under oil emersion may demonstrate the mite, ova, or fecal pellets known as *scybala*. Treatment includes the use of topical permethrin 5% cream (e.g., Elimite) or the use of topical lindane lotion. Although the permethrin product is more expensive, it has an excellent safety profile and is extremely efficacious and is used to treat all individuals in a household unit. If only one individual is treated, one can count on recurrences and longer-lasting difficulties.

Lice

Lice infection (*Phthirius corporis* and *pubis*) may be spread through close contact between individuals. Lice may remain in seams of clothing or bedding and infection is often acquired during travel if accomodations are not properly cleaned or sanitized. Many shampoos help for scalp involvement, and these include permethrin products (e.g., Pronto and Nix) as well as topical lindane (Kwell) products. Nits may be removed by using a formic acid rinse (step 2). Bedding should be washed, and all individuals on a team must be examined to prevent further spread.

MISCELLANEOUS DERMATOSES

Many dermatoses may be exacerbated by athletic activities. Psoriasis will spread to involve areas of injury (the so-called isomorphic or Koebner affect). Discoid lupus erythematosus and lichen planus similarly may show an isomorphic response. Sweating may exacerbate atopic dermatitis by causing increased itching and subsequent scratching of affected areas.

Acne

Acne is characterized by papules and pustules on the face, chest, and back. Blackheads and whiteheads are noted first and then erythematous macules and papules develop (Figs. 13-9 and 13-10). If acne is not treated, pustules and cysts may heal with scarring. Triggering factors should be eliminated where possible. Helmet straps and shoulder pads may exacerbate acne because of direct occlusion of pilosebaceous units. Treatment of mild acne usually consists of an aqueous benzoyl peroxide gel applied in the morning and tretinoin (Retin-A) applied at bedtime. A topical antibiotic (e.g., erythromycin gel) may also be added if pustules are present. When pustules predominate, oral antibiotics such as tetracycline or erythromycin are preferred.

Contact Dermatitis

Contact dermatitis describes an eczematous dermatitis developing from exposure to an allergen. Only sensitized individuals will develop rash, unlike the setting or irritant dermatitis where all exposed individuals would develop an eruption given the same degree of provocation. Nickel in metal snaps, rubber in pads and equipment, and exposure to plants in the outdoor setting (e.g., poison ivy) are common culprits. Potassium dichromate used in the

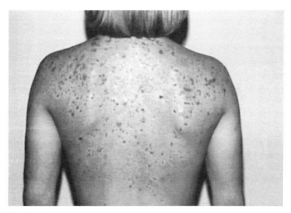

FIG. 13-9   Acne may cause pain and discomfort on the back, especially in individuals who have padding or other protective gear on affected areas.

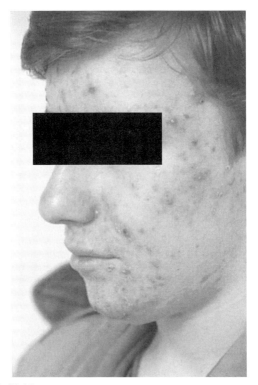

FIG. 13-10 Erythematous papules and pustules may be exacerbated in areas where chin straps or helmets contact the skin.

tanning of leather products and adhesives are other common sensitizers. Allergic contact dermatitis to shoe components often presents on the dorsum of the foot (Fig. 13-11). Avoiding the offending allergen is the most important aspect of treatment. Topical corticosteroids and, occasionally, oral corticosteroids are helpful for symptomatic relief.

In athletes, underlying skin diseases must be controlled with judicious use of topical products. For psoriasis, we favor the use of corticosteroids for mild involvement as well as topical calcipotriene cream or ointment (Dovonex). Approximately 70 per-

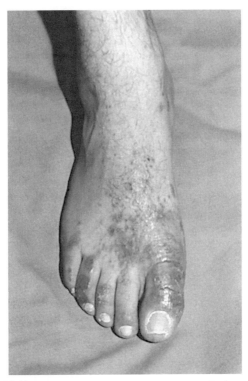

FIG. 13-11 Allergic contact dermatitis to components in shoes is becoming increasingly common. Common shoe allergens include epoxy resins and rubber components.

cent of individuals using calcipotriene show improvement, and for 15 percent of individuals, the improvement is marked. For atopic dermatitis, we recommend the use of bland emollients (e.g., cetaphil moisturizing lotion, Moisturel lotion, or Lubriderm lotion). Atopic individuals may be especially prone to what has been referred to as "joggers' nipples." Joggers' nipples are caused by friction between the nipples and clothing. Lubrication and use of occlusive ointments such as Aquaphor or Vaseline will lead to improvement. Some athletes may need to have cotton patches sewn into jerseys if the problem persists.

The Gunk

Some hockey players are plagued with pruritus from fiberglass. Many hockey sticks have fiberglass components, and the fibers may become loose and come into contact with skin surfaces. Severe pruritus is seen in the absence of objective findings. Biopsy sometimes reveals filamentous material, but a small amount of fiberglass can cause severe pruritus and not be evident on skin inspection or biopsy evaluation. Clinical suspicion is most important, and the dermatitis will resolve within 2 to 3 weeks after exposure to the offending substances has stopped. Many hockey players are themselves familiar with this problem and do not seek or request medical attention.

CONCLUSION

Athletes present with many skin findings and require rapid diagnosis and treatment so as not to interfere with training. Becoming familiar with the various presentations of common dermatoses is especially important in proper management of the athlete.

REFERENCES

1. Bergfeld WF, Helm TN: Skin disorders in athletes, in Grana WA, Kalenak A (eds): *Clinical Sports Medicine.* Philadelphia, Saunders, 1991, pp 110–118.
2. Bergfeld WF, Helm TN: The skin, in Strauss RH (ed): *Sports Medicine* 2d ed. Philadelphia, Saunders, 1991, Chap 6, pp 117–131.
3. Bergfeld WF, Elston D: Skin problems of athletes, in Fu Fit, Stone D (eds): *Sports Injuries.* Baltimore, Williams & Wilkins, 1994, pp 781–795.
4. Sedar JI: Treatment of blisters in the running athlete. *Arch Podiatr Med Foot Surg* (suppl 1):290–340, 1978.
5. Bergfeld WF, Taylor JS: Trauma, sports, and the skin. *Am J Ind Med* 8:403–413, 1985.
6. Levine N: Dermatologic aspects of sports medicine. *J Am Acad Dermatol* 3:415–424, 1980.

| **Stress Fractures and Exertional Compartment Syndrome**

Ned Amendola   David Bell

STRESS FRACTURES

Several terms have been used to describe bone subjected to repetitive forces beyond its ability to repair: *stress fracture*, *fatigue fracture*, *march fracture*, and *pseudofracture*. *Stress fracture* remains the most commonly used term, although *fatigue fracture* may more accurately describe the gradual bone injury from repeated loads. Stress fractures are commonly seen in athletes as a result of overuse in training and competition. They differ from pathologic fractures seen in conditions such as tumors, infection, and postmenopausal osteoporosis, which result from normal stresses to abnormal bone. One exception to this distinction is the amenorrheic female athlete with abnormal estrogen levels and decreased bone density, who is at higher risk for stress fractures.

Pathophysiology

On a cellular level, healthy bone is in a state of simultaneous breakdown and repair. This allows bone to remodel to applied stresses and to adapt according to functional demands. Thus bone, a living tissue, carries a large advantage over nonliving materials that cannot adapt or self-repair. The balance of resorption and formation is influenced by the magnitude and frequency of external forces, piezoelectric effects, circulating hormones, and the availability of substrates such as protein and calcium.

In the case of stress fractures, repetitive forces to bone shift the balance in favor of breakdown. Resorption that outstrips repair leads to miniature cortical defects and subsequent microfractures.[1] If the offending stress is removed, osteoblastic bone formation can be restored, and the bone can heal by callus formation. If the insult persists, further bone resorption occurs. Structurally, this can lead to a painful, weak bone in continuity or eventually to a displaced fracture.[1] Histologic studies have confirmed this sequence of events.[2,3] Johnson and coworkers[2] observed an active osteoclastic resorption with no fracture or callus formation during the first week in biopsies of 30 stress fractures of the proximal tibia. Periosteal callus became evident during the second week, and if the insult continued, a cortical crack was identified with resorption that was completed at the end of 3 weeks.

245

From a biomechanical standpoint, bone is a heterologous, anisotropic material that requires stress for remodeling. Stress fractures occur when forces exceed the ability to remodel. Four mechanisms of excessive bony stresses have been delineated.[4,5] First, repetitive muscle contraction may lead to bony overload, as seen in fibular and calcaneal stress fractures. Second, muscle fatigue may expose bony structures to increased forces, especially in muscles that serve a decelerating function via eccentric contraction. Third, increased ground reaction forces, such as in training on hard surfaces, may lead to stress fractures. This is accentuated in running, with 1000 to 1200 foot strikes per mile at 1.5 to 3 times body weight. A fourth mechanism is high frequency of low-impact repetitive stress seen with activities such as aerobic dancing.

Epidemiology and Risk Factors

Stress fractures are common in young athletes, and 80 to 90 percent have been reported to occur below age 29.[6,7] Stress fractures comprised 10 percent of all injuries in a certain sport medicine clinic population[8] and were seen at a rate of 4.7 and 15.6 percent in groups of distance runners.[9,10] Reports of stress fractures in military recruits have noted an incidence of 2 percent with symptoms and 31 percent with increased uptake on bone scintigraphy.[11–13] Based on bone scans, the incidence of asymptomatic stress fractures has been noted in 9 to 35 percent of predisposed subjects, with the femur being the most common asymptomatic site.[6,12]

Lower extremity stress fractures are located most commonly in the tibia, followed by the foot and ankle and occasionally the femur.[8,14] The metatarsal and tarsal bones are the most common sites in the foot.[7,8] Bilaterality has been noted in 7 to 16 percent of cases[6,8] and in multiple sites in 5 to 12 percent.[6,7,15] Running is the sport most commonly cited as a cause, especially in the tibia, fibula, and metatarsals.[8,15,16] Sudden increases in mileage or intensity, training on hard or cambered surfaces or uneven terrain, and failure to interpose less intense workouts have been noted as possible potentiating factors.[5,13] Basketball players commonly sustain tarsal navicular stress fractures.[17] Football players have a high incidence of fifth metatarsal stress fractures,[18] as do competitive figure skaters.[19] Volleyball has been noted as the most common offending sport in countries where it is immensely popular, such as Korea.[6] Ballet dancers commonly suffer stress fractures of the tarsal navicular, sesamoids, and proximal shafts of the second and third metatarsals.[20] Marching on hard surfaces in combat boots with a heel snap on initial contact was associated with a high incidence of calcaneal stress fractures in military recruits.[14]

Certain characteristics have been identified as risk factors for stress fractures. Caucasians are at a twofold higher risk than other races,[11,21] and females are at higher risk than males.[6,11,12,21] The "female triad" has been described as amenorrhea, eating disorders, and osteoporosis and has been associated with a higher incidence of stress fractures. One study noted that exercise-induced amenorrhea doubled the risk of stress fractures in female distance runners.[22] A lower body weight of less than 75 percent of ideal and eating disorders such as anorexia and bulimia were associated with a higher rate of stress fractures in a group of ballet dancers.[23] In a group of Finnish military conscripts, tall stature and previous inactivity were associated with stress fractures.[24] Varus alignment of the lower extremity and foot has been implicated in lower extremity stress fractures,[1,5,8] whereas other studies found association only with external rotation of the hip.[25] Other studies found no correlation with height, weight, or tibial torsion, alignment, or width.[26] Excessive foot pronation is associated with a higher incidence of tibia and fibula stress fractures.[1] A low longitudinal arch has been associated with metatarsal stress fractures, whereas a normal arch may be associated with a lower incidence of metatarsal stress fractures yet a higher rate of femur and tibia fractures.[27] Rigid pes cavus with a high longitudinal arch has been associated with a higher incidence of stress fractures in the metatarsals and femur, presumably due to reduced shock absorption capability.[8,28]

Footwear has been implicated in the development of stress fractures. The switch from combat boots on hard surfaces to athletic shoes on soft surfaces did decrease the incidence of stress fractures in military recruits. Gradual deterioration of running shoes, especially in the shock-absorbing midsole, has been implicated in stress fractures in runners.[29] Inadequate heel wedging, loose-fitting heel counters, excessive heel wear, and narrow toe boxes also have been implicated.[28] As an attempt at prevention, viscoelastic shoe inserts have been shown to decrease neither loads transmitted to the lower extremity nor the incidence of stress fractures.[30,31] Semirigid arch-supporting insoles added to combat boots decreased the incidence of stress fractures but not significantly.[13]

Clinical Presentation

The patient commonly presents with exertional pain localized to the affected area, which usually worsens after exercise.[6,32] Some consider exertional pain the sine qua non for stress fracture even in the face of a negative bone scan.[12] If the pain of early stress fracture is ignored and training continues, it may progress to a constant ache and may limit training. A traumatic event may bring about an abrupt increase in pain, noted to occur in 10 percent of cases.[8] Asymptomatic stress fractures, however, have been noted with positive bone scans in 9 to 35 percent of predisposed subjects.[6,12] With sudden starts at training, such as in military boot camps, pain usually commences within the first 2 to 4 weeks.[12,14] In recreational athletes, a prolonged onset and a delay to diagnosis are common, and one study found an average delay of 12 to 16 weeks before a diagnosis of stress fracture of the foot and ankle was made.[8] Rarely, displacement occurs, noted in 8 percent of cases.[7] Displacement can have serious consequences in the femoral neck[32] and tarsal navicular.[33]

On physical examination, stress fractures frequently present a paucity of signs. Point tenderness and swelling at the affected site are usually but not always present.[32] Adjunctive physical tests include the hop test, which produces pain at the presumed site with a one-legged hop,[8] percussion tenderness when the bone is tapped at a distant site,[32,34] and the tuning fork test.[6]

Diagnosis and Imaging

A high index of suspicion and a detailed history will lead to an accurate diagnosis of stress fracture in most cases. Training errors often can be identified, such as training on hard surfaces, footwear changes, or a recent transition to more intense or frequent training.[8,32] In addition to eliciting a history of overuse, other disorders predisposing to stress fractures must be suspected. These include amenorrhea, eating disorders, and osteopenia seen in the female athlete triad; metabolic bone disease; neuropathic arthropathy; malnutrition and gastrointestinal malabsorption; and mild variants of osteogenesis imperfecta. The differential diagnosis of exercise-induced leg pain includes exertional compartment syndrome, tendinopathies, and medial tibial stress syndrome. The history must include questions about night pain, fevers, and constitutional symptoms even in the presence of overuse, to avoid missing diagnoses such as infection or malignancy. Other sources of leg pain include lumbar radiculopathy, spinal stenosis, peripheral neuropathy, and peripheral vascular disease.

For the diagnosis of stress fractures, plain radiographs have been found to be a very insensitive tool.[8] Studies have shown only 14 to 28 percent of patients presenting with stress fractures to have plain radiograph abnormalities.[12,14] Several patients in one study required up to 12 weeks to show radiographic findings, and 6 percent failed to ever demonstrate radiographic changes despite having a positive bone scan.[15] Nonetheless, certain findings on plain radiographs have been noted with stress fractures.[35] One pattern is periosteal new bone formation or cortical breaks, commonly seen in diaphyseal or cortical bone, 2 to 3 weeks after the onset of symptoms. A second pattern is focal sclerosis in cancellous bone, such as the metaphyseal sections of long bones or short bones such as the calcaneus or the tarsal navicular.[16,35,36] This second pattern may be difficult to identify and may not be seen for up to 24 weeks after the onset of symptoms. An anteroposterior view with the foot inverted allows better visualization of any abnormalities in the navicular.[36]

Three-phase bone scintigraphy is highly sensitive in identifying stress fractures, although it is nonspecific.[14,31,35,37] Thus careful correlation of clinical and radiographic findings is required to rule out other possible disorders such as infection or tumors. Bone scanning can be considered the "gold standard" of stress fracture diagnosis, especially in combination with a suggestive clinical presentation and positive focal uptake in the symptomatic region.[14,37] Three-phase bone scanning of stress fractures also provides valuable information regarding bone vascularity as well as bone turnover. In addition, an old stress fracture can be differentiated from a new one and a partial fracture from a complete one.[8]

Magnetic resonance imaging (MRI) is emerging as a sensitive and specific tool in diagnosing stress fractures.[35,38] Characteristic MRI findings are bandlike areas of very low signal intensity seen in the intramedullary space and continuous at some point with the cortex. Computed tomography (CT) scanning has some utility in diagnosing difficult stress fractures such as those in the tarsal navicular and calcaneus.[17] Other imaging modalities such as ultrasonography have been used to image stress fractures yet were found inferior to the combination of plain radiographs and bone scans.

Management and Prevention

Prevention is the first line of treatment for stress fractures, accomplished simply by avoiding the risk factors mentioned earlier. Training regimens must be planned to avoid abrupt increases in intensity or duration. Quality footwear, soft training surfaces, and regular rest days should be encouraged, as well as a healthy lifestyle with adequate rest and balanced nutrition. Female athletes, especially those in endurance sports, should receive instruction regarding menstrual irregularities and eating habits and should be referred to a physician for treatment if needed.

The cornerstone of treatment of stress fractures is rest. Training must be modified to rest the affected area to allow healing and repair. The inciting activity should be avoided, and weight bearing is restricted if necessary based on the specific site or level of discomfort.[32] The duration of rest is usually 2 weeks to several months, and a delay in diagnosis or treatment may require longer rest periods. Cast immobilization is not always required[6,7,14,15,39,40] but may be required based on the severity of symptoms, extent of the lesion, and risk of completion of the fracture.[17] We recommend casting for ankle and foot fractures in which a limp is present during walking. The cast can be discontinued when the patient is able to walk normally, usually a period of 3 to 4 weeks. Analgesics, ice, and massage may help bring pain relief. Some studies have shown 83 percent of patients to be free of symptoms by the second month.[6] The patient should be encouraged to maintain aerobic fitness through non-weight-bearing activities such as swimming, cycling, or running in water. Some protocols have allowed resumption of weight bearing after 2 consecutive weeks without pain.[8] Gradually, weight-bearing exercise is increased on soft surfaces and advanced incrementally a few minutes per day, alternating days with non-weight-bearing conditioning. This second phase usually lasts 6 weeks.

Operative treatment is rarely required, except in fractures of the femoral shaft.[7] Fixation and bone grafting of the tarsal navicular or fifth metatarsal base may be required, where displacement and nonunion are more likely.[17,41] In addition, when stress fractures at the fifth metatarsal metaphyseal-diaphyseal junction are diagnosed in competitive athletes, operative fixation is recommended to minimize time lost from competition.

Specific Stress Fractures

Femur

Femoral stress fractures are noted occasionally in athletes, especially runners, and military recruits.[42–46] Training errors and coxa vara may predispose to femoral neck stress fracture, as well as muscle fatigue.[47] Pain is the most common presenting symptom, which may be in the groin, thigh, or knee. It usually worsens with exertion and resolves with rest. Physical signs include an antalgic gait and limitation of hip motion. Bilaterality is common.[48]

Plain radiographs may fail to show findings for 2 to 4 weeks after the injury.[42] Bone scintigraphy is a sensitive tool, and images of both hips are recommended. Two main fracture patterns have been noted in the femoral neck.[48] The transverse pattern shows a crack in the superior cortex, which is seen in older patients and carries a high risk of displacement. The compression pattern shows a haze of internal callus along the inferior femoral neck, which is seen in younger patients with low risk of displacement. Fractures also have been classified as with callus without a fracture line (type I), definite fracture line but nondisplaced (type II), and displaced (type III).[47]

A high index of suspicion must be maintained to avoid the devastating complication of displacement and subsequent nonunion, varus deformity, or osteonecrosis. If plain radiographs are initially negative, weight bearing is restricted with crutches, and a bone scan and repeat radiographs are obtained. If both are negative, they are repeated in 1 week. Alternative diagnoses are investigated if a second bone scan is also negative. Positive scans with negative x-rays and nondisplaced documented compression-type fractures are treated with rest and restriction of weight bearing until pain subsides and studies show healing; then a slow and gradual return to weight bearing and training is allowed. Frequent repeat x-rays are taken to ensure healing and lack of displacement.

Aggressive treatment with internal fixation is recommended for tension-type fractures, even if nondisplaced, to avoid the severe complications of displacement. Weight bearing and activities can be progressed as healing is demonstrated. Similarly, displaced fractures should be reduced anatomically and fixed internally as quickly as possible with protected weight bearing until healing.

Tibia

As noted earlier, the tibia is the most common site of stress fractures in competitive athletes.[8] Some studies have implicated narrow tibial width,[26] whereas others have found no correlation with anatomic findings. Some studies noted that proximal or distal locations are more common than a central location,[7,49] and others noted the opposite.[12,15,50] When found on the proximal or distal sections, stress fractures are usually noted on the posteromedial compression side of the bone and tend to heal well with hypertrophy. When found in the diaphysis, stress fractures are typically on the anterior tension side and tend to heal poorly. In some cases these fractures can be visualized on plain radiographs as the "dreaded black line."

The treatment for stress fractures in the proximal and distal tibia is rest, activity modification, and a gradual return to sports. For the diaphyseal stress fracture, some authors have suggested initial treatment of cast immobilization and no weight bearing for 6 to 8 weeks, followed by additional rest and activity modification until healing.[51] One report noted that athletes with a central shaft stress fracture lost an average of 12 months from competition.[52] In long delays in healing despite rest or in recurrent stress fractures, more aggressive treatment may be required such as electrical stimulation, drilling, bone grafting, or intramedullary fixation.

Ankle

Medial malleolar stress fractures are uncommon but have been noted in basketball players.[16] An antalgic gait and ankle effusion were noted. Ankle instability, hindfoot valgus, and excessive foot pronation have been implicated as predisposing factors.[1] Plain radiographs are usually normal, except for an occasional lucent line extending superiorly and medially from the junction of the medial malleolus and the tibial plateau. Bone scans show uptake in this region.

Soft tissue injury must be ruled out, such as recurrent sprains or instability, which would show no increased uptake on bone scan. Treatment involves a walking aircast for patients without x-ray findings, and internal fixation for patients with findings on x-rays has been advocated.[16]

Lateral malleolar stress fractures have not been reported. A certain pattern of distal third fibular shaft fractures in runners has been reported 4 to 7 cm proximal to the joint line.[15,32] Treatment is activity modification and rest until symptoms subside. If a limp or constant pain is present, casting is recommended for an initial trial of 3 weeks; then a gradual rehabilitation program can be started.

Talus

Talar stress fractures are not uncommon and have been reported to progress to complete fracture. They are associated with repeated ankle inversion in pronated feet.[41] Patients typically complain of chronic discomfort of the midfoot and ankle that is exercise related. Physical findings include tenderness and swelling over the neck of the talus with occasional discoloration. Plain radiographs are often normal. Bone scan commonly shows fractures in the talar neck paralleling the talonavicular joint. The differential diagnosis includes osteochondral lesions of the talus, anterior ankle impingement syndrome, and osteoid osteoma. The treatment is nonoperative, with both non-weight-bearing and weight-bearing regimens advocated.[1,41] Average recovery time has been noted to be 17 weeks.[8]

Calcaneus

Calcaneal stress fractures are common in military recruits who make a sudden transition to intense and frequent marching.[12,14,53] Some military studies have found the calcaneus to be the most common site in recruits,[14] and 52 percent were associated with a medial tibial condyle stress fracture. The calcaneus was second only to tibial stress fractures in one study in runners.[15] No correlation was found with height, weight, or foot architecture in one study in female recruits.[54]

The patient usually presents with heel pain classically within 2 weeks of beginning training. It is usually confined to the posterior half of the calcaneus and is bilateral in up to 37 percent.[1,32,35,39,53] On physical examination, there may be swelling that masks the malleolar contours and tenderness over the posterior and inferior half of the calcaneus. A squeeze test from medial to lateral on the body of the calcaneus will elicit pain, which it will not in heel pain syndrome and Achilles tendinitis.

Plain radiographs show a bandlike sclerosis in the posterior portion of the body of the calcaneus parallel to the posterior contour. This appears only 6 to 10 weeks after the onset of symptoms. The differential diagnosis includes retrocalcaneal bursitis, Achilles tendinitis, plantar fasciitis, plantar nerve entrapment, and subtalar arthritis.

Treatment is nonoperative, and rapid healing occurs in 3 weeks due to the cancellous bone in the body of the calcaneus.[32,53] Rest and avoidance of impact activities should be recommended. Cast immobilization may be required if the patient has a limp. Heel pads, heel lifts, and shoe modification did not alter the course.[55] Healing may require a longer time, especially if a delay in diagnosis and treatment occurred, which is common. Gradual return to sport is allowed after a pain-free interval.

Navicular

Stress fractures of the tarsal navicular are seen in runners and basketball players and can be difficult to diagnose.[17,55,56] This can lead to completion and displacement unless the diagnosis is made early. Forefoot pronation and a wide heel counter in the shoe have been implicated as causative factors.[56] The symptoms on presentation are commonly vague and often are not localized to the navicular. There may be insidious medial longitudinal arch pain that is aggravated by activity, whereas other tendinopathies of the foot and ankle may improve during activity and worsen following the activity. Plain radiographs are commonly underexposed and without abnormal findings. A coned down anteroposterior view of the navicular with the foot inverted allows the entire width of the navicular to be visualized. About 50 percent of fractures involve only the dorsal cortex.[17] The fracture line is usually in the midportion of the navicular with a sagittal split.[55,56] Bone scan, MRI, or CT scan may aid in identifying the fracture.

When the fracture line is incomplete and nondisplaced, nonweight-bearing cast immobilization for 6 to 8 weeks is recommended.[17,57] Failure to use a cast or to limit weight bearing is associated with delayed union or nonunion. The cast is continued until there is radiographic and clinical evidence of union, seen with bony bridging and cystic changes around the fracture site on plain radiographs. Displaced complete fractures are not as common. Open reduction and internal fixation and bone grafting may be required, especially when sclerosis at the fracture site is present.

Metatarsals

Metatarsal stress fractures are a common cause of forefoot pain in the athlete. The differential diagnosis includes metatarsalgia, interdigital neuroma, metatarsophalangeal joint synovitis, flexor tenosynovitis, and peripheral neuropathy. The patient with a metatarsal stress fracture commonly complains of insidious onset of forefoot pain that initially is diffuse and occurs with activity. The pain increases with activity and may become more localized to the area of the stress fracture. Physical examination often shows some forefoot swelling, and metatarsophalangeal joint swelling may be present. The affected metatarsal is tender at the neck as it is palpated dorsally.

Early on, plain radiographs may be normal. Once fracturing occurs with an acute episode, subsequent radiographs will show the fracture with callus formation. Bone scan can be used in the early phases. Second, third, and fourth metatarsal fractures occur most commonly in the neck, and fifth metatarsal fractures usually occur just distal to the metaphysis.

For the early fracture with no limp or healing fracture on x-ray, the treatment is activity modification until pain and tenderness have subsided, with a gradual return to training. For the patient with a limp and pain, cast immobilization for 3 to 4 weeks with a gradual return to sports is recommended. For fractures of the fifth metatarsal base, there is a higher risk of delayed union or nonunion. Treatment with a weight-bearing cast has been associated with a risk of nonunion and refracture.[58,59] Six weeks of no weight bearing in a short leg cast may avoid the risk of nonunion, yet the delay may be untenable for the athlete. Intramedullary screw fixation may allow earlier rehabilitation and return to activity. Bone grafting may be required in chronic stress fractures with sclerosis.

Conclusion

Stress fractures are a common source of pain in the face of overuse, whether the patient is an athlete or a laborer. An accurate diagnosis must be made to administer proper treatment and allow a smooth return to activity. A high index of suspicion is required because physical signs and plain x-ray findings may be sparse. Bone scanning is an important adjunct to help in diagnosis. Correction of training errors and investigation for predisposing factors must be instituted.

EXERTIONAL COMPARTMENT SYNDROME

Exertional compartment syndrome (ECS) is becoming increasingly recognized as a cause of exercise-induced leg pain in athletes. It has been referred to previously as the *anterior tibial syndrome* or *chronic compartment syndrome.* It belongs in the differential diagnosis of shin splints and leg pain in athletes, which includes stress fracture, compartment syndrome, and medial tibial stress syndrome. This section discusses the pathophysiology, diagnosis, and treatment of ECS and also discusses the related medial tibial stress syndrome.

Pathophysiology

The pathophysiology of acute compartment syndrome is well understood.[60–63] An increase in muscle tissue pressure can occur due to blunt or crush injury, hemorrhage, ischemia, or revascularization after arterial injury. Swelling and increased pressure within a noncompliant fascial compartment limit arterial perfusion to the muscle, which in turn leads to the release of inflammatory mediators and increased swelling. The downward spiral results in further ischemia, and muscle necrosis and neurovascular injury can result.

This acute pathophysiologic process, however, cannot necessarily be extrapolated to explain ECS, which is chronic and generally less severe in nature. Many etiologies of ECS have been proposed.[60,64–68] One widely accepted theory is pain due to ischemia from increased compartment pressure. It is known that muscle responds to exertion with increased blood volume, increased intramuscular pressure, muscular edema, and hypertrophy. Expansion may be limited by abnormal unyielding fascia, and arterial pressure may become insufficient to transport oxygen and nutrients to the muscle capillary beds. Pain and diminished performance result. No experimental model, however, has demonstrated this sequence of events. Furthermore, recent MRI and nuclear medicine blood flow studies have not been able to clearly show postexercise ischemia in patients with documented ECS, as evidenced by elevated compartment pressure measurements.[69–71] Using nuclear magnetic resonance (NMR) spectroscopy to reliably evaluate muscle metabolism, ischemia has not been shown to be a significant component of ECS.[72–74] The pathophysiology of ECS is, needless to say, complex, and future research at the cellular level may help elucidate its cause.

Diagnosis

Exertional leg pain is a common complaint in athletes and may afflict up to 15 percent of runners.[75] The clinician must have a practical and sound approach to determine the etiology. Compartment syndrome must be differentiated from other disorders, which include stress fracture, medial tibial stress syndrome, tendinopathy, and superficial peroneal nerve compression. All these disorders are complex in their presentation and must be ruled out before a diagnosis of ECS can be made. Certain predictors for ECS in a group of 74 patients with exertional leg pain were exercise-induced reproducible pain, bilateral symptoms, and no abnormal findings on physical examination. Young age (<30 years) and running or other repetitive stress sports also were associated with ECS.[69] In this group, previous treatments with physiotherapy, orthotics, and nonsteroidal anti-inflammatory medications were ineffective. If the patient has rest pain, unilateral symptoms, or physical findings or is posttraumatic, an alternative diagnosis should be considered and investigated. Plain radiographs, technetium bone scanning, ultrasonography, and nerve conduction tests may help in the investigation for other etiologies. If the patient has bilateral reproducible pain, no rest pain, and no abnormal physical findings, the primary diagnosis is ECS, and exertional compartment pressure measurement is indicated.

Intracompartmental Pressure Measurements

Although it may cause local discomfort in some patients, intracompartmental pressure measurement is considered the "gold standard" for diagnosis of ECS. Measurement techniques include the slit catheter, the wick catheter, the needle manometer, and microcapillary infusion. We use the indwelling slit catheter because of the reproducibility of its results and its relative ease of use. Patients with ECS may have anterior compartment symptoms, posterior symptoms, or both. The measurement is made on the most symptomatic leg and compartments. An indwelling slit catheter is inserted into the compartment and secured to the leg by an occlusive noncircumferential dressing and tape. Pressures are recorded supine, and then the patient is exercised on a treadmill up to the point where his or her symptoms are reproduced or he or she is unable to exercise any further. Immediate postexercise pressures are then studied supine and recorded continuously for 30 min thereafter.

The most important pressure measurement criterion for ECS is prolonged return to resting pressure after exercising.[76] Actual values vary, particularly across differing measurement techniques.[62,67,71,76,77] We use a value greater than or equal to 15 mmHg at 15 min after exercise as the main criterion of ECS. Also, insertional pressure greater than or equal to 15 mmHg and an immediate postexercise pressure greater than or equal to 30 mmHg are consistent with ECS.

Imaging

MRI has a role in the diagnosis of exertional leg pain and related disorders because of its detailed anatomic visualization, especially of the muscle belly itself. Characteristic MRI changes have been described,[78] and these are prolonged in patients with positive-pressure studies. MRI is most useful in patients with unusual presentations of ECS, in whom posttraumatic changes or intracompartmental abnormalities are suspected. Phosphorous spectroscopy (^{31}P-NMR) has provided information in the research of ECS pathophysiology and in the future may assist in diagnosis.[71–75]

Management

Nonoperative treatments such as physiotherapy, anti-inflammatory medication, and foot orthoses are usually not effective in ECS. Fasciotomy has been shown to be very effective by many investigators[61,70,71,76,79] and is recommended if the patient is not interested in ceasing the offending sport activity. When fasciotomy is done properly in the presence of an accurate diagnosis, excellent results can be achieved.

Anterior symptoms are most common and have been noted to comprise 70 percent of ECS patients.[69] Patients with anterior symptoms undergo a release of the anterior and lateral compartments, and those with posterior symptoms have a release of the tibialis posterior and the remainder of the deep posterior compartment. The superficial posterior compartment is not released routinely because of its thin and compliant fascia that is not likely responsible for symptoms.

Surgical Techniques

We perform anterior and lateral compartment releases via a two-incision technique.[80] The anterior intermuscular septum (IMS) is identified superficially between the lateral border of the tibia and medial border of the fibula. Two longitudinal 2- to 3-cm incisions are centered on the IMS in the proximal and distal halves of the leg. The septum and superficial peroneal nerve are identified, and the nerve is released if its exit from the fascia is felt to be tight. Using subcutaneous finger dissection, the entire fascia adjacent to the IMS can be palpated from the knee to the ankle. At both incisions, small longitudinal fascial incisions are made into the anterior and lateral compartments 1 cm on either side of the IMS. Using 8- and 12-in. Metzenbaum scissors, the fasciotomies are completed subcutaneously from distal to proximal. Through the distal incision, the fascia is released distally to the superior edge of the extensor retinaculum of the ankle, with the tips of the scissors pointing away from the nerve. Proximal extension toward the knee is made through the proximal incision. Complete release of both compartments is confirmed by palpation.

A one-incision technique is used for release of the deep posterior and tibialis posterior compartments. The incision is located 1 cm posterior to the posteromedial subcutaneous border of the tibia. It is centered at the level of the distal gastrocnemius curve and is 8 to 10 cm long. The greater saphenous nerve and vein are easily identified and protected. Dissection down to fascia will identify the medial IMS and the periosteal-fascial junction of the tibia. This plane is then carefully developed proximal and distal to the incision. In the distal aspect of the incision, the tibialis posterior muscle and tendon are identified on the posteromedial border of the tibia. Proximally, the flexor digitorum longus occupies this position. A small vertical incision is made at the osseofascial junction. Then, using Metzenbaum scissors and staying directly on the posterior border of the tibia, the fascia is released to the level of the tibialis posterior tendon. Finger dissection is used to ensure a complete release distally. The release is then extended proximally. The soleus will then be encountered in the proximal third of the tibia at the soleus bridge. Release of this stout structure must be complete because it also represents the proximal confluence of the flexor hallucis longus and flexor digitorum longus fascia. This completes the release of the deep posterior compartment. A blunt periosteal elevator such as a Bristow elevator is then used to release the tibialis posterior muscle off the tibia, completing the release of the tibialis posterior compartment. Remaining on the posterior aspect of the tibia ensures avoidance of the posterior tibial neurovascular bundle. The posterior release also must be confirmed by digital palpation.

Compartment releases are performed under tourniquet, which is deflated intraoperatively to obtain hemostasis. A 1/8-in. Hemovac drain is placed within the released compartment. The subcutaneous tissues are closed, and the skin is closed with a subcuticular suture. A sterile dressing and compression bandage are applied.

The surgery is done on an outpatient basis. The drain remains for several hours in the postanesthetic care room and is removed prior to discharge. Training on crutch ambulation and the postoperative therapy protocol are given by the physiotherapist. The first 2 days consist of rest, ice, compression and elevation, and ankle stretching 3 to 5 times per day. On the third day, the patient commences progressive dorsiflexion and plantarflexion stretches 3 times a day and progresses to walking and cycling once weaned off crutches. At 2 weeks, the wounds are checked, and formal physiotherapy for stretching and functional return to sport-specific activity is begun. A gradual return to running and impact activities is stressed, with appropriate warm-up and stretching.

Medial Tibial Stress Syndrome

Medial tibial stress syndrome (MTSS) is commonly noted as a cause of exercised-induced leg pain.[7,81] The syndrome of posteromedial tibial pain has been referred to as *tibial periostitis*, *soleus syndrome*, and *tibial stress reaction*. The patient commonly presents with pain and tenderness of the posteromedial tibia in its distal half along the periosteal-fascial junction. The pain and tenderness are usually more diffuse than tibial stress fracture, which is more localized to the area of the fracture. In MTSS, plain radiographs may show periosteal calcification, but not in all cases.

MTSS has been categorized into four types: IA with discrete stress fracture, IB with diffuse medial tibial stress reaction, II with periosteal injury, and III with deep posterior compartment ECS.[82] Types I and II usually present with exertional pain relieved by rest but may last several days. This differs from ECS, in which pain subsides quickly with rest. Type II involves a more severe form of type I in which pain is constant even with walking or daily activities. Intracompartmental pressure measurements may be required to rule out the presence of ECS in the type III category.

Several factors have been implicated in MTSS, including training errors such as overuse, poor footwear, hard surfaces, and excessive weight. Specifically, MTSS may be associated with malalignment such as pes planus or excessive pronation with increased eccentric stresses to the tibialis posterior muscle.[62,83]

Treatment of MTSS

Prevention is the first step, which includes following wise training principles. Treatment of established MTSS also requires correction of training errors and contributing factors. Pain control may require rest or activity modification, anti-inflammatory medications, and modalities such as ice and ultrasound. If pain occurs during activities of daily living, crutches and short leg casting may be required. Shoe inserts and a straight-shaped, full- or combination-lasted shoe with good hindfoot control may help pes planus or excessive pronation.

For resistant symptoms, surgical release of the posterior muscles off the tibia may be required. Tibialis posterior and deep posterior compartment fasciotomies can be used in the treatment of type III MTSS with ECS present. Even with fasciotomies, stripping of the muscles off the tibia must be included, especially the tibialis posterior and soleus attachment proximally.

Conclusion

Exertional compartment syndrome and medial tibial stress syndrome are commonly encountered as causes of exercise-induced leg pain. The understanding of their complex pathophysiology is improving through recent clinical and basic research. Accurate diagnosis and proper treatment are required to achieve successful results and to allow the patient to return to the demanding levels of sports activities.

REFERENCES

1. Clement DB: Stress fractures of the foot and ankle. *Med Sports Sci* 23:56–70, 1987.
2. Johnson LC, Stradford HT, Geis RW, et al: Histogenesis of stress fractures. *J Bone Joint Surg* 45A:1542, 1963.
3. Li G, et al: Radiographic and histologic analysis of stress fractures in rabbit tibias. *Am J Sports Med* 13:285–294, 1985.
4. Frankel VH: Editorial comments: Stress fractures. *Am J Sports Med* 6:396, 1978.
5. Taunton JE, McKenzie DC, Clement DB: The role of biomechanics in epidemiology of injuries. *Sports Med* 6:107–120, 1988.
6. Ha KI, Hahn SH, Chung MY, et al: A clinical study of stress fractures in sports activities. *Orthopedics* 14:1089–1095, 1991.
7. Orava S: Stress fractures. *Br J Sports Med* 14:40–44, 1980.
8. Matheson GO, Clement DB, McKenzie DC: Stress fractures in athletes: A study of 320 cases. *Am J Sports Med* 15:46–58, 1987.
9. Brubaker CE, James SL: Injuries to runners. *Am J Sports Med* 2:189–198, 1974.
10. Clement DB, Taunton JE, Smart GW, McNicol KL: A survey of overuse running injuries. *Phys Sports Med* 9:47–58, 1981.
11. Brudvig TJ, Gudger TD, Obermeyer L: Stress fractures in 295 trainees: A one-year study of the incidence as related to age, sex and race. *Milit Med* 118:666–667, 1983.
12. Milgrom C, Chisin R, Giladi M: Negative bone scans in impending tibial stress fracture. *Am J Sports Med* 12:488–491, 1984.
13. Schwellnus MP, Jordaan G, Noakes TD: Prevention of common overuse injuries by use of shock absorbing insoles: A prospective study. *Am J Sports Med* 18:636–641, 1990.
14. Greaney, Gerber FH, Laughlin RL, et al: Distribution and natural history of stress fractures in U.S. Marine recruits. *Radiology* 146:339–346, 1983.
15. Sullivan D, Warren RF, Pavlov H, et al: Stress fractures in 51 runners. *Clin Orthop* 187:188–192, 1992.
16. Shelbourne KD, Fisher DA, Rettig AC, et al: Stress fractures of the medial malleolus. *Am J Sports Med* 16:60–63, 1988.
17. Torg JS, Baldwin FC, Zelko RR, et al: Fractures of the base of the fifth metatarsal distal to the tuberosity. *J Bone Joint Surg* 66A:209–214, 1984.
18. Nicholas JA: Injuries in Football, in *Lower Extremity and Spine in Sports Medicine*. 1986.
19. Pecina M, Bojanic I, Dubravcic S: Stress fractures in figure skaters. *Am J Sports Med* 18:277–279, 1990.
20. Hardaker WT: Foot and ankle injuries in classical ballet dancers. *Orthop Clin North Am* 20:621–627, 1989.
21. Protzman RR, Griffis CC: Stress fracture in men versus women undergoing military training. *J Bone Joint Surg* 59A:825, 1977.
22. Barrow GW, Saha S: Menstrual irregularity and stress fractures in collegiate female distance runners. *Am J Sports Med* 16:209–216, 1988.

23. Frusztajer N, Dhuper S, Warren MP: Nutrition and the incidence of stress fractures in ballet dancers. *Am J Clin Nutr* 51:779–783, 1990.
24. Taimela S, Kujala UM, Osterman K: Stress injury proneness: A prospective study during a physical training program. *Int J Sports Med* 11:162–165, 1990.
25. Surissn A, et al: The effect of pretraining sports activity on incidence of stress fractures among military recruits. *Clin Orthop* 245:256–260, 1989.
26. Giladi M, Ahronson Z, Stein M, et al: Stress fractures and tibial bone width: A risk factor. *J Bone Joint Surg* 69B:326–329, 1987.
27. Simkin A, et al: Combined effect of foot arch structure and an orthotic device on stress fractures. *Foot Ankle* 10:25–29, 1992.
28. Cornwell G: Sports medicine and the pes cavus foot. *Br Columbia Med J* 26:573–574, 1984.
29. Cook SD, Kester MA, Brunet ME, et al: Biomechanics of running shoe performance. *Clin Sports Med* 4:619–626, 1985.
30. Nigg BM, Herzog W, Read LJ: Effect of viscoelastic shoe insoles on vertical impact forces in heel-toe running. *Am J Sports Med* 16:70–76, 1988.
31. Gardner LI, Dziados JE, Jones BH, et al: Prevention of lower extremity stress fractures: A controlled trial of a shock absorbent insole. *Am J Public Health* 78:1563–1567, 1988.
32. Hershman EB, Railly T: Stress fractures. *Clin Sports Med* 9:183–214, 1990.
33. Goergren TG, Venn-Watson EA, Rossman DJ, et al: Tarsal navicular stress fractures in runners. *AJR* 136:201–203, 1981.
34. Stechow AW: Fussoedan und Rseutgenstrahleu. *Dtsch Mil Aerztl Z* 26:465, 1987.
35. Sanit M, Sartoris DJ: Diagnostic imaging approach to stress fractures of the foot. *J Foot Surg* 30:85–97, 1991.
36. Pavlov H, Torg JS, Freiberger RM: Tarsal navicular stress fractures: Radiographic evaluation. *Radiology* 148:641–645, 1983.
37. Prather JL, Nusynowitz ML, Snowdy HA, et al: Scintigraphic findings in stress fractures. *J Bone Joint Surg* 58A:869–874, 1977.
38. Lee JK, Yao L: Stress fractures. *Magn Reson Imaging Radiol* 169:217–220, 1988.
39. Anderson EG: Fatigue fractures of the foot injury: *J Bone Joint Surg* 21:275–279, 1990.
40. Markey KL: Stress fractures. *Clin Sports Med* 6:405–425, 1987.
41. Montos MJ, Madad RJ: Conditions of the talus in the runner. *Am J Sports Med* 14:486–490, 1986.
42. Fullerton LR, Snowdy HA: Femoral neck stress fractures. *Am J Sports Med* 16:365, 1988.
43. Hajek MR, Noble HB: Stress fractures of the femoral neck in runners. *Am J Sports Med* 10:112, 1982.
44. Lombardo SJ, Benson DW: Stress fractures of the femur in runners. *Am J Sports Med* 10:219, 1982.
45. McBryde AM: Stress fractures in athletes. *Am J Sports Med* 3:212, 1976.
46. Skinner HB, Cook SD: Fatigue failure stress of the femoral neck. *Am J Sports Med* 10:245, 1982.

47. Blickenstaff LP, Morris JM: Fatigue fracture of the femoral neck. *J Bone Joint Surg* 48A:1031, 1966.

48. Devas MB: Stress fractures of the femoral neck. *J Bone Joint Surg* 47B:728, 1965.

49. Rupani H, Holder L, Espinola D, Engin S: Three-phase radionuclide imaging in sports medicine. *Radiology* 156:187–196, 1985.

50. Roub L, Gumerman L, Hanley E: A radionuclide imaging perspective. *Radiology* 132:431–438, 1979.

51. Andrish JT: The leg, in *Orthopaedic Sports Medicine: Principles and Practice*. Philadelphia, Saunders, 1994, pp 1603–1631.

52. Rettig AC, Shelbourne D, McCarroll J, et al: The natural history and treatment of delayed union stress fractures of the anterior cortex of the tibia. *Am J Sports Med* 16:250–255, 1988.

53. Darby REC: Stress fractures of os calcis. *JAMA* 200:131–132, 1967.

54. Hopson CN, Perry DR: Stress fractures of the calcaneus in women marine recruits. *Clin Orthop* 128:159–162, 1977.

55. Towne LC, Blazina ME, Cozen LN: Fatigue fractures of the tarsal navicular. *J Bone Joint Surg* 52A:376–378, 1970.

56. Ting A, King W, Yocum L, et al: Stress fractures of the tarsal navicular in long-distance runners. *Clin Sports Med* 7:89–101, 1988.

57. Hulkko A, et al: Stress fracture of the navicular bone. *Acta Orthop Scand* 56:503, 1985.

58. Delee JC, et al: Stress fracture of fifth metatarsal. *Am J Sports Med* 11:349, 1983.

59. Zelko RR, Torg JS, Rachum A: Proximal diaphyseal fractures of the fifth metatarsal: Treatment of the fractures and their complications in athletes. *Am J Sports Med* 7:95, 1979.

60. Hoffmeyer P, Cox JN, Fritschy D: Ultrastructural modifications of muscle in three types of compartment syndrome. *Int Orthop* 11:53–59, 1987.

61. Matsen FA, Rorabeck CH: Compartment syndromes, in *Instructional Course Lectures*, vol 38. Park Ridge, IL, American Academy of Orthopaedic Surgeons, 1989, pp 463–472.

62. Mubarak SJ, Gould RN, Lee YF, et al: The medial tibial stress syndrome: A cause of shin splints. *Am J Sports Med* 10:201–205, 1982.

63. Sheridan GW, Matsen FA: An animal model of the compartmental syndrome. *Clin Orthop* 113:36–42, 1975.

64. Fleckenstein JL, Conby RC, Parkey RW, et al: Acute effects of exercise on MR imaging of skeletal muscle in normal volunteers. *Am J Res* 151:231–237, 1988.

65. Hill AV: The pressure developed in muscle during contraction. *J Physiol (Lond)* 107:518–526, 1948.

66. Hoing CR: *Modern Cardiovascular Physiology*. Boston, Little, Brown, 1981, pp 225–262.

67. Jacobsson S, Kjellmer I: Accumulation of fluid in exercising skeletal muscle. *Acta Physiol Scand* 60:286, 1964.

68. Sejersted OM, Hargens AR: Regional pressure and nutrition of skeletal muscle during isometric contraction, in Hargen AR (ed): *Tissue Nutrition and Viability*. New York, Springer-Verlag, 1986, pp 263–283.

69. Amendola A, Rorabeck CH: Chronic exertional compartment syndrome. *Curr Ther Sports Med* 2:250–253, 1990.

70. Qvarforft P, Christenson J, Eklof B, et al: Intramuscular pressure, muscle blood flow and skeletal muscle metabolism in chronic anterior tibial compartment syndrome. *Clin Orthop* 179:284–290, 1983.

71. Styf J, Korner LM: Microcapillary infusion technique for measurement of intramuscular pressure during exercise. *Clin Orthop* 207:253–262, 1986.

72. Inch WR, Serebrin B, Taylor AW, et al: Exercise muscle metabolism measured by magnetic resonance spectroscopy. *Can J Appl Sports Sci* 11:60–65, 1986.

73. Chenton DW, Heppenstall RB, Chance B, et al: Electrical stimulation of human muscle studied using 31P-NMR spectroscopy. *J Orthop Res* 4:204–211, 1986.

74. Balduini FC, Shenton DW, O'Connor KH, et al: Chronic exertional compartment syndrome: Correlation of compartment pressure and muscle ischemia utilizing 31P-NMR spectroscopy. *Clin Sports Med* 12: 151–165, 1993.

75. Bates P: Shin splints: A literature review. *Br J Sports Med* 19:132–137, 1985.

76. Rorabeck CH, Bourne RB, Fowler PJ: The surgical treatment of exertional compartment syndrome in athletes. *J Bone Joint Surg* 65A: 1245–1251, 1983.

77. Pedowitz RA, Hagens AR, Mubarak SJ, Gershrine DH: Modified criteria for the objective diagnosis of chronic compartment syndrome of the leg. *Am J Sports Med* 18:35–40, 1990.

78. Amendola A, Rorabeck CH: The use of magnetic resonance imaging in exertional compartment syndromes. *Am J Sports Med* 18:29–34, 1990.

79. Almdahl SM, Samdal F: Fasciotomy for chronic compartment syndrome. *Acta Orthop Scand* 60:210–211, 1989.

80. Rorabeck CH, Bourne RB, Fowler PJ, et al: The role of tissue pressure measurement in diagnosing chronic anterior compartment syndrome. *Am J Sports Med* 16:146, 1988.

81. Styf J: Chronic exercise-induced pain in the anterior aspect of the lower leg. *J Sports Med* 7:331–337, 1989.

82. Detmer DE: Classification and management of medial tibial stress syndrome. *Sports Med* 3:436–446, 1986.

83. Wallensten R, Eriksson E: Intramuscular pressure in exercise-induced lower leg pain. *Int J Sports Med* 5:31–35, 1984.

II | SPECIFIC SPORTS

15 | Ice Hockey

Shauna Martiniuk   R. Charles Bull
Chris Broadhurst

Ice hockey is theoretically Canada's national sport, with an average annual participation rate of over 500,000 registered amateur players. Although Canada is considered to be the birthplace of ice hockey, the sport is extremely popular in the United States and in Europe. The McGill report states that the first match took place in March of 1875 in Montreal, although a more nostalgic account records the first game as having occurred on Christmas day in either 1855 or 1866 in Halifax. There were reports of 20 men on each side. The game lasted for 6 h and 20 min. The match was between two garrison teams from the Canadian Royal Rifles, one from Halifax and one from Kingston. No victor was recorded.[1] The number of individuals playing hockey has increased during this century, and the inclusion of the best professional players in the world and women's hockey at the 1998 Winter Olympics may provide a tremendous boost to the sport.

Ice hockey is an intensely physical sport that demands both aerobic and anaerobic fitness in combination with great skill execution due to the speed at which it is played. It is a fast and rough game, with varying degrees of aggressive and contact play. In a professional game of three 20-min periods, a player generally plays for 45 to 60 s at one time.[1a] The intense play periods add up to 16 min of playing time on average.[1a] Physiologically, both anaerobic and aerobic energy pathways are used in the game of hockey for both the intense bursts of activity and endurance and power. Overall, 80 percent of injuries are due to trauma and 20 percent from overuse.[2] Most injuries are in the third period, with fewest in the first.

The mechanisms of injury in hockey are several. They involve high skating speeds up to 48 km/h in senior amateur players,[2] high sliding speeds of 24 km/h,[3] plus sticks, pucks, blades, quick changes in direction without stopping, boards, goalposts, and other players. A hockey puck's maximal impact force has been measured at 567.5 kg.[4] The hockey stick has been measured at angular velocities of 100 to 200 km/h, and the puck's speed has been measured at up to 192 km/h in professional hockey.

Several studies have been performed to elicit the type and number of injuries. Variable reports exist because of different reporting characteristics and protective equipment such as visors. A study in 1988 of elite international Swedish hockey players found an incidence of 79.2 injuries resulting in player absence per 1000 player-hours and 70.8 per 1000 for facial lacerations. All injuries were traumatic in nature. Stick injuries accounted for 82.3 percent of the facial lacerations, and many would have been prevented by wearing a visor. Only approximately 40 percent of players were wearing a visor.[5] Another study of elite Swedish hockey players found that contusions made up 33 percent of traumatic injuries, with strains (17 percent), sprains (16 percent), and fractures (13 percent) being next common.[6] The lower limb was most affected (54 percent), with the upper limb (24 percent), back (16 percent), and head (6 percent) following. The most common mechanisms of injury for traumatic injuries were checking (33 percent), player contact (25 percent), puck (14 percent), and stick (12 percent). Cutting and skate contact accounted for less than 10 percent of injuries. Overuse injuries only made up 20 percent of the study, most commonly adductor and patellar tendonitis. Eight major injuries occurred in their study, with five of these being total tears of the medial collateral ligament, working out to between one and four ligamentous tears in each elite hockey team per season.

A 1995 study of injuries in Junior A hockey found an incidence of 96.1 injuries per 1000 player-hours in games.[4] Of all injuries, 51 percent were caused by collision, with the most commonly injured area the face and then the shoulder. A study of intercollegiate ice hockey injuries reported knee injuries to be most common (19 percent) and then the face (18 percent).[7] A full 45 percent of the injuries were caused by legal body checks. Not surprisingly, in ice hockey for youths under 11 years of age, where body checking is illegal, many fewer injuries occur.[8] One concern in youth hockey is the size difference between players of similar ages. One study showed a 357 percent difference in force of impact during simulated body checking between the weakest and strongest players.

In addition to the more common injury patterns mentioned earlier, occasionally, more sinister events occur. According to Dr. Robert Cantu, ice hockey is "the most dangerous sport in the United States for nonfatal catastrophic injury." However, fatalities do occur. One paper published in 1995 outlined case reports of sudden cardiac arrest from blunt chest injury.[9] In these case reports, four sudden deaths occurred in hockey players, two from puck injuries, one from a body collision with another player, and one by the heel of a hockey stock during slashing. The cause of death in most blunt chest injuries such as these is likely ventricular dysrythmia.

The body sites most frequently injured in ice hockey are as follows:

Head and neck	20–30 percent
Upper body	15–20 percent

Trunk	15–25 percent
Arm	8–20 percent
Leg	20–30 percent

These percentages are based on a composite of studies.

The injury rates by player position in ice hockey are as follows:

Forward	49–60 percent
Defense	35–48 percent
Goalie	3–8 percent

HEAD AND NECK INJURIES (Fig. 15-1)

Head

In a study of elite players, 5.3 percent of all traumatic injuries in hockey were head concussions.[6] Death from head injury also has occurred in hockey.[10] One can expect a range of head injuries to occur in hockey, from superficial hematomas to epidural hematomas requiring surgical treatment.

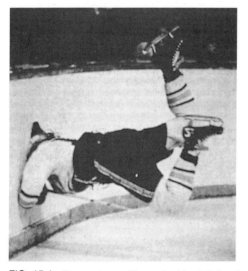

FIG. 15-1 The sports practitioner should watch the play at all times. This is a true emergency, and you must be prepared. Your team should be ready to manage this serious concussion and cervical spine injury.

Concussions

Concussions are the most common head injury in sports, and concussion occurs most commonly in ice hockey when a player strikes the boards head first. A concussion may be a consequence of a direct blow to the head but also may occur when the neck suffers a whiplash injury with enough force being applied to the brain.[11] In ice hockey, approximately 0.27 concussions occur for every 1000 athlete exposures,[12] a number larger than that found for football (0.25 per 1000) and for sports without helmets such as soccer (0.25 per 1000).[12]

A summary statement published in 1997 on the management of concussions in sports was written by the Quality Standards Subcommittee of the American Academy of Neurology.[13] This subcommittee defined *concussion* as a "trauma-induced alteration in mental status that may or may not involve loss of consciousness." A concussion is no longer the diagnosis when loss of consciousness (LOC) lasts longer than 30 min, if the first Glasgow Coma Scale (GCS) score is less than 13, or if posttraumatic amnesia lasts longer than 24 h.[16]

In the minutes to hours following a concussion, patients may complain of headache, vertigo, nausea or vomiting, and lack of awareness of surroundings. In the days to weeks following a concussion, patients may have a persistent low-grade headache, be lightheaded, have poor attention and concentration, evidence memory dysfunction, have disturbed sleep, or be fatigued, irritable, photophobic, phonophobic, anxious, or depressed. On examination, such patients may have a vacant stare, slow verbal and motor responses, confusion, disorientation, slurred or incoherent speech, poor coordination, memory deficits, and a period of LOC. Mental status testing should be done to include orientation, concentration, and memory, and the patient should be asked to perform basic athletic maneuvers to assess appearance of symptoms. The neurologic examination needs to be performed in grade II and III concussions.

Concussion grades are as follows[13]:

Grade I
   Transiently confused, no LOC, symptoms resolve in less than 15 min.
   May return to competition that day if assessment is normal.
   If a second grade I concussion occurs on the same day, the player may only return to play in 1 week if asymptomatic.

Grade II
   Transiently confused, no LOC, symptoms last longer than 15 min.
   No return to competition that day.

Frequent examinations that day, and reexamine the next day.

Neurologic examination after 1 week to clear athlete for return to play.

CT scan or MRI if symptoms worsen or last longer than 1 week.

A second grade II concussion sidelines the player for 2 weeks.

Grade III

Any LOC (seconds and longer).

Transport to emergency room.

Full neurologic examination and possible neuroimaging.

Admit to hospital if there are any signs of pathology or if mental status is abnormal.

May be sent home if all findings are normal.

After seconds of unconsciousness, patient may play after being asymptomatic for 1 week.

After a longer period of LOC, patient may play if he or she is asymptomatic for 2 weeks.

After a second grade III concussion, no playing for at least 1 asymptomatic month.

Neuroimaging if headache or symptoms worsen or last longer than 1 week.

Any intracranial pathology on imagining should sideline the player for the season, and return to play should be discouraged in the future.

The physician also must be aware of an even more dangerous scenario called the *second impact syndrome*. In this situation, a second concussion occurs while the player is still symptomatic from the first. Consequently, the brain loses cerebrovascular autoregulation, leading to brain swelling and increases in intracranial pressure.[11] Articles have been written about hockey players dying from second impact syndrome.[15,16] In addition, the effects of concussion may be cumulative, and chances of getting a second concussion may be four times higher than in athletes without a previous concussion.[17] The number of concussions a player has accumulated in his or her career must be taken into consideration when discussing future play. Unfortunately, we are still without standards for how many concussions are too many and when an athlete should retire. When considering the diagnosis of concussion, always include in the differential diagnosis the following: epidural hematoma, subdural hematoma, intracerebral hematoma, intracerebral contusion, subarachnoid hemorrhage (SAH), cerebral concussion, malignant brain edema syndrome, second impact syndrome, and cervical spine injury. Epidural hematomas occur most commonly with a tear to the middle meningeal artery. This may be the result of a high-velocity impact, such as from a hockey stock or a puck, especially to the temporoparietal region.

On-ice treatment of a suspected head or neck injury begins with not attempting to move the player from the ice. Maintain an airway using jaw-thrust maneuvers, with proper cervical spine precautions. The helmet may be removed only if adequate protection of the cervical spine is maintained. A neurologic examination may then be done, including assessment of consciousness, pupils, arm and leg movements, and strength.

Sideline or off-ice testing mental status should include the following:

Area	What To Do
Orientation	Check for orientation to person, place, and time
Attention	Repetition of digits or months of the year, in backward order
Retrograde amnesia	Memory of previous plays, what player was doing at the time of injury and just before
Anterograde amnesia	Memory of three objects immediately and after 5 min
General appearance	Dazed look, incoherent speech, any changed behavior

Barriers to the evaluation of neuropsychological testing include

- Lack of understanding of the evaluation process
- Apprehension about test results by both athletes and medical staff
- Time constraints placed on the athlete
- Financial considerations
- High rewards compared with low perceived risk
- English as a second language, long road trips, trained physicians not traveling with teams
- Difficulty in evaluating patients rinkside

Vital Cranial Triad

An area of controversy is the jaw disorder as it relates to the vital cranial triad (VCT). The VCT is a complex of bones consisting of the temporomandibular joint (TMJ), the tympanic temporal bone, and the inferior surface of the petrous temporal bone. Clinical examination reveals headaches, earache, nausea, vomiting, vertigo, impaired hearing and balance, muscle weakness, occlusal disturbances, TMJ pain, and other symptoms associated with neurologic and circulatory deficits secondary to trauma. Radiologic findings include compression fractures, condylar neck fractures, degenerative condylar remodeling, obliteration of the articular eminence, atresia of the ear canal, and other damage to the VCT.

Structural damage to the VCT always results in loss of physical strength and endurance. Without corrective measures in athletes with VCT injuries, the athlete will never attain his or her full potential. Thus proper protection and treatment of the VCT are critical.

Facial and Eye Injuries

To adequately protect the face and eyes from injury in this high-risk sport, certified protective visors should be worn at all times, including games, practices, and shinny. One prospective study of injuries in adult recreational leagues revealed that only 35 percent of players wore some form of face shield.[18] It is likely that the role models in professional leagues who do not wear face masks are a negative influence on recreational players.

Prior to the use of face masks, lacerations were the major injury. Facial fractures also occur, but with the use of face masks, the incidence is likely much lower. Helmets with face masks have reduced the number of facial injuries by 70 percent.[19] Minor hockey associations in Canada have required that players wear approved face masks and helmets since 1978. A prospective study of a National Collegiate Athletic Association (NCAA) Division I team with mandatory use of face masks found an incidence of 14.9 facial lacerations per 1000 player-hours.[20] This incidence was lower than that found in other studies not requiring the use of face masks.

Pashby, a Toronto ophthalmologist, researched eye injuries in hockey, and it was his work that brought in a rule requiring face masks in 1976. This rule has reduced the number of injuries substantially.[21] The most common eye injuries prior to face mask use were periorbital soft tissue trauma, followed by hyphema and iris damage. Injuries were caused mostly by sticks and pucks.

In 1996, a prospective study of head, face, and neck injuries was performed.[22] Of 119 patients, only 1 was female. Once again, this low number may represent a low relative rate of participation of females in ice hockey, or it may reflect the less violent nature of the game when played by females, possibly due to checking rules. More directed studies will have to be pursued to answer this question.

Eye injuries With regard to when a player can return from an eye injury, three steps should be followed:

1. The ocular tissue has healed sufficiently to sustain a blow to the head or body that produces a Valsalva maneuver and thereby increases the pressure inside the eye.
2. The eye is comfortable with adequate return of vision. Appropriate, well-fitting eye protectors must be worn.
3. Immediate return to play after injury during a game depends on the complaint.

Danger signs and symptoms of potentially serious eye injuries include a sudden decrease in or loss of vision, loss of visual field, pain with eye movement, photophobia, diplopia, protrusion of the eye, lightening flashes, floaters, an irregularly shaped pupil, a foreign body sensation, and red eye or blood in the anterior chamber. Always obtain an adequate history and determine the force and direction of the blow. Assess visual acuity, visual fields, pupils, and fundi.

Facial fractures Always observe and palpate for facial asymmetry, point tenderness, bony steps, mobility, ecchymosis, and paresthesia. Occlusal (bite) discrepancy, pain, and limitation of mouth opening suggest a jaw fracture. Fracture of the nasal bone and cartilage is common, and findings include bleeding, nasal airway obstruction, nasal asymmetry, crepitus over the nasal bridge, periorbital and subconjunctival ecchymoses, and septal hematomas. Treatment includes controlling the airway and bleeding, protect from further injury, and transport for definitive diagnosis. Malar fractures are common, with loss of opacity of the maxillary sinus a good clue to this type of fracture. Mandibular fractures are also fairly common in hockey.

Neck (Fig. 15-2)

The most common mechanism responsible for fracture of the cervical spine is axial loading in a slightly flexed position, which flattens the normal cervical lordosis. This occurs most commonly when a helmeted player strikes the boards. When the neck is flexed approximately 30 degrees, the cervical spine becomes straight. From the standpoint of force, energy absorption, and the effect on tissue deformation and failure, the straightened cervical spine in axial loading acts as a segmented column. This injury is seen commonly when a player hits the boards head on. According to Tator,[23] sliding is also a common mechanism of neck injury. This may be attributed to the difficulty of changing position or direction while sliding. Rotational forces also manifest in the upper cervical spine, especially at C1, C2, and C3, and whiplash forces are transmitted to the C5–C6 area of the neck.

The management of any potential cervical spine injury is neck immobilization until full evaluation of the injury is undertaken. The helmet of the player should not be removed, but the face mask may be cut off to enable access to the airway if needed. The player should not be moved from his or her position, including turning the patient over or straightening the head.

Regarding return-to-play advice, a player with permanent neurologic damage should not return to competition.[24] A player with a stable fracture according to flexion-extension views with no spinal

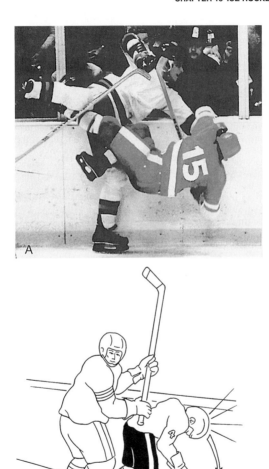

FIG. 15-2   A sudden collision into the boards or a check from behind caused most neck injuries, although the stick is also a major culprit. The mechanism is usually active flexion. The cervical spine is more readily broken in flexion than in hyperextension.

cord injury may return to normal daily activities. A play with any unstable fracture or dislocation, i.e., that requiring a halo brace or surgery, should not return to contact sports because he or she does not have enough spinal strength. Despite healing of the bone, there is loss of normal motion of the segments above and below the injury that predisposes to future injury.[24]

Since the introduction of mandatory helmets, some investigators have reported a possible link between them and increased serious cervical spine injury.[2] This increase may be related to players' perception of invincibility as well as referee leniency with rules if the consequences of actions such as high sticking are less obvious.[25] The incidence of illegal use of the stick has increased.[25] A helmet will decelerate the head, with the neck decelerating the torso. Other factors also have contributed to the increase in neck and spinal injuries, such as increased speed and muscle mass in players and increased play along the boards as skaters use more ice surface with an improved fitness level.[25] The main mechanism of spinal cord injuries is a check from behind, and it is important that players and coaches realize this and take it into consideration when battling for the win.

Laryngeal fractures can be a life-threatening situation. Symptoms include loss of airway, hemoptysis, crepitus, and loss of the "Adam's apple" prominence. The need for a cricothyroidotomy has to be considered. This injury is basically impossible to protect against. Crosschecks over the neck or garroting from behind should be decreased by proper application of the rules (Fig. 15-3). Treatment consists of rest, humidification, and no hockey for 6 to 12 weeks.

Stinger Syndrome

The stinger syndrome is a common injury in hockey that presents as a burning pain down the arm, either acute or chronic. Most commonly this injury has been thought to be caused by traction secondary to lateral flexion of the neck. More recently, a study in football players published in 1993 suggests that a more common mechanism of injury is compression of the brachial plexus between the shoulder pad and the superomedial border of the scapula.[26] This mechanism of injury also may be found in hockey players because shoulder pads are also worn in hockey. It is a brachial plexus injury, most commonly affecting the C5 and C6 roots. The injury is unilateral, typically lasting 1 to 2 min, although prolonged neurologic deficits can occur. In the latter case, imaging and electromyographic (EMG) studies may be done to secure a diagnosis. In the acute scenario, radicular pain is felt and may be accompanied by transient paresis and tenderness at Erb's point, the most superficial

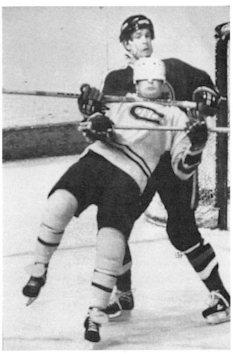

FIG. 15-3 Protection against laryngeal fractures is almost impossible. Symptoms are loss of airway, hemoptysis, crepitus, and loss of the "adam's apple" prominence. The need for cricothrotomy (tracheotomy) has to be considered. *(Canadian Press Photo.)*

site of the brachial plexus. The radicular symptoms resolve in 5 to 10 min, but tenderness persists. With C5 and C6 injury, pain and tingling are felt in the lateral arm, thumb, and index finger, with paresis in the biceps, deltoid, and infraspinatus muscles. If there is any weakness of elbow flexion or shoulder external rotation or abduction, the athlete should not return to competition and should be followed closely.

A player may return to play after symptoms have resolved and with a painless cervical spine range of motion. One needs to ensure that the patient does not have a transient cervical myelopathy. This will involve two extremities, either both arms, both legs, or ipsilateral arm and leg.[27]

The best prevention program for neck injuries is an isometric program or isokinetics using the Nautilus hydragym type of equipment prior to the hockey season. Holding the neck muscles tightly against the points of compass, north, south, east, and west, for periods of 10 s, and repeating for three sets of 30, is a good isometric preventative exercise. Flexibility is also the key to protection against neck and back injuries, and a full preseason flexibility program is mandatory.

SHOULDER INJURIES

Injuries to the shoulder include possible trauma to the neck, shoulder, clavicle, chest, upper ribs, or arm. The greatest proportion of shoulder injuries are classified as minor in nature but can inhibit the ability to play effectively due to the physical nature of the game. The cause of injury is commonly a collision with an opponent or the boards or falling on an outstretched arm. The most common injuries in ice hockey are

Acromioclavicular separation
Glenohumeral joint dislocation subluxation
Sternoclavicular fractures

Acromioclavicular Separation

Acromioclavicular (AC) separation may be caused by a projectile force into the boards, a direct blow onto the AC joint with a stick, a direct fall on the shoulder, and a fall on an outstretched arm or point of the elbow. These mechanisms will temporarily force the tip of the scapula (acromion) away from the collarbone (clavicle).

AC separations can be classified into three main types:

First degree: These represent a complete tear of the joint capsule with no major break in the continuity between the acromion and the clavicle.
Second degree: These involve a complete tear of the joint capsule, but the coracoclavicular ligaments are intact. On visual examination, the distal end of the clavicle appears to ride somewhat higher.
Third degree: These involve a complete disruption of both the joint capsule and the coracoclavicular ligaments. Physical examination reveals an obvious depression of the scapula with what appears to be an elevation of the clavicle.

Often players with a first-degree AC separation never miss a shift in the game and experience point tenderness over the joint.

With a third-degree AC separation, athletes do not need surgical intervention, and immobilization of the joint until the symptoms subside is quite beneficial. Protection over the area is imperative on return to play with well-constructed shoulder pads that emphasize rigid collar protection and possibly a protective doughnut pad over the AC joint. The point tenderness can remain for up to 12 weeks after injury, but if persistent discomfort is felt, suspect a distal clavicular bone irritation, which is positive on bone scan. A few more severe third-degree separations have been documented with complete dislocation of the clavicle at the AC joint, and management of this type of injury is surgical, especially if it occurs on the dominant side. A player also may get posttraumatic osteolysis of the distal end of the clavicle, and this should be considered if pain is persistent. An x-ray will show cyst formation and resorption.

Disability varies with the type of separation, with variable amounts of time off from hockey. Most AC dislocations are treated conservatively because studies comparing nonoperative versus operative treatment have not shown better outcomes with surgery.[28] However, not all patients do well with conservative treatment, and some surgeons recommend surgery for young patients in certain situations.

Glenohumeral Dislocation

This injury is caused most commonly by a direct blow to an arm (humerus) that is extended backward with a violent twisting motion that overcomes the shoulder capsular restraints. The player will note a definite pop and/or sensation that the shoulder is out of place. Shoulder dislocations are often classified in the direction of instability. The most common type of instability in hockey is the traumatic anterior dislocation of the shoulder. Player age appears to be a more important factor than length of immobilization, specific rehabilitation program, or degree of initial trauma. Players who sustain an initial dislocation before the age of 20 years as a result of minimal trauma have the highest risk of recurrent dislocation. There has been a reported 92 percent recurrence rate in individuals aged 20 years or younger at the time of initial dislocation.

The traumatic acute anterior dislocation of the glenohumeral joint should be reduced as quickly as possible. Early relocation eliminates the compression of neurovascular structures and minimizes the amount of muscle spasm that must be overcome to obtain reduction.

With a first-time dislocation, a thorough physical and neurovascular examination should be carried out as well as radiographs if bone injury is suspected. The duration of immobilization is an area of great controversy at this time. Players older than 40 years of age at initial dislocation probably should be immobilized for a briefer period than younger players because the recurrence rate in this age group is low and longer immobilization is more likely to lead to shoulder stiffness. Immobilization in the older player is continued only until pain subsides, which is typically 7 to 10 days. The younger player (<25 years of age) should be immobilized for at least 4 to 6 weeks to allow for healing of the stretched or disrupted anterior shoulder capsule and ligaments.

The treatment concerns with glenohumeral dislocations include the following:

- There may be excessive bleeding internally.
- Weakening of the rotator cuff tendons is more common in patients older than 40 years. This should be suspected especially if persistent pain and weakness do not improve within 2 weeks of reduction. A magnetic resonance image (MRI) should be obtained to rule out a rotator cuff pathologic condition.
- After immobilization is discontinued, the patient should gradually progress through a rehabilitation program that emphasizes strengthening of the rotator cuff and scapular musculature.
- Prerequisites for return to hockey are a full range of motion, return of strength, and absence of pain.
- A harness that limits abduction and outward rotation may be used to avoid recurrent injury.
- Surgical intervention is very successful in hockey players if apprehension compromises the patient's ability to perform despite a conservative trial of treatment.

Clavicular Fractures

Clavicle fractures are usually classified into three groups based on which part of the clavicle is fractured:

Eighty percent of clavicle fractures occur in the middle third.
Fifteen percent of clavicle fractures occur in the lateral third.
Five percent of clavicle fractures occur in the medial third.

Most commonly clavicular fractures are caused by a direct impact to the clavicle. When the middle third of the clavicle is fractured, the shoulder slumps forward and inward as the player attempts to hold the arm against the chest to protect against any shoulder movements. Direct tenderness and palpable deformity are often present at the fracture site. Reduction of a middle-third clavicle fracture is easily accomplished by drawing the shoulders upward and backward as the end fragments are manipulated into alignment. Usually the fragments can be held in place with a figure-of-eight sling or a modified shoulder spica cast. The great majority of clavicle fractures are treated conservatively in this way. Indications for operative treatment are

Neurovascular involvement
Interposition of soft tissue between the fractured segments
Open fractures

Sternoclavicular Dislocations

Sternoclavicular dislocations can occur either anteriorly or posteriorly. A posterior dislocation is usually caused by a direct force and is more significant because of the proximity of important mediastinal structures (e.g., subclavian vein, cardiac vessels, trachea, esophagus, and pleura). Emergency medical treatment of this injury may be required on site. This requires pulling the clavicle anteriorly and away from deeper structures either with a towel clip around the clavicle or even with a towel roll between the scapula. With traction on the shoulder joint in a posterior direction, the joint should reduce. Anterior dislocations are more common and not life-threatening. Surgical repair of the sternoclavicular joint is difficult, but stability is of great importance.

Overuse Injuries

Overuse injuries of the shoulder are fairly common because players shoot repetitively. Players may develop rotator cuff tendonitis and tuberosity impingement. They will exhibit the typical painful arc from 45 to 110 degrees. Rest and strengthening are the first treatments to try, but Cybex testing and arthrograms are useful in extreme cases. Arthroscopy of the shoulder with subsequent Cybex rehabilitation has been quite successful.

UPPER EXTREMITY INJURIES

The most common upper extremity injuries in ice hockey are

Dislocation of the thumb at the metacarpophalangeal joint
Fracture of the wrist at the scaphoid bone
Rupture of the flexor tendon

Dislocation of the First Metacarpophalangeal Joint

Commonly known as *Gameskeeper's thumb* or rupture of the ulnar collateral ligament of the first metacarpophalangeal (MCP) joint, this injury results from a forced lateral stress with the MCP joint in nearly full extension. A player usually falls with the stick in hand and abducts the MCP joint of the thumb.[2] Hockey players are more vulnerable to this injury because of the manner in which the stick is held. It is important to recognize the injury because surgery is often required to reattach the ulnar collateral ligament. Failure to treat this injury adequately will result in a weak pinch and grasp.

A partial tear can be differentiated from a complete tear by obtaining anteroposterior (AP) stress views of the thumb MCP joint. If angulation of the thumb MCP joint is more than 30 degrees with a radially directed stress compared with the uninjured side, the injury is considered a complete tear.

The physical findings with disruption of the ulnar collateral ligament of the thumb is tenderness over the ulnar aspect of the MCP joint and exquisite pain with abduction stress testing. There also will be significant joint laxity when testing the thumb with the MCP and interphalangeal joints both in a flexed position. The Stenner lesion is an interposition of the adductor aponeurosis between the torn ulnar collateral ligament ends. It is a complication that must be recognized and surgically corrected early if treatment is to be successful. Recommended treatment is summarized as follows:

Grades I and II: Incomplete lesions:
Immobilize with thumb spica cast for 3 weeks.
At 3 weeks, reevaluate stability and discomfort and begin active and gentle passive range-of-motion (ROM) exercises.
Removable splint to be worn for protection.
At 8 weeks, patient should be asymptomatic, and the splint can be discontinued except for sports.
Continue strengthening exercises.

Grade III: Complete rupture:
Consider primary surgical repair.
At 3 weeks, remove bulky dressing.
Fit with wrist and thumb static splint.
At 6 weeks, begin dynamic splinting for ROM.
Begin active and gentle passive ROM exercises.
At 8 weeks, begin active strengthening exercises.
At 12 weeks, allow patient to return to activity.
Playing thumb splint should be worn.

Prevention of this type of injury is attempted through "lock thumb" mechanisms within the hockey glove. Protective measures include the leather tab at the end of the glove thumb, which should not be cut.

Fracture of the Scaphoid Bone

This injury is one of the most dreaded injuries by hockey players not only because of the amount of time necessary for proper healing but also because of the complications that can occur in rehabilitation. The classic symptoms are snuff box tenderness, pain over the volar aspect of the scaphoid bone, or pain with forced impaction of the first metacarpal. Any sign of scaphoid fracture, with or without fracture on scaphoid views, requires the player to be treated with a scaphoid cast. It is not unusual for radiographs to first show evidence of fracture at 2 to 5 weeks.

Due to the high nonunion rates for these injuries, early diagnosis and appropriate casting are indicated. The recommended immobilization of this fracture is 8 to 12 weeks with a complete thumb spica cast and incorporating about two-thirds of the forearm. Blood supply is confined to the distal pole in some cases and will increase the healing time and the incidence of nonunion, avascular necrosis of the proximal fragment, and osteoarthritis. During immobilization, the player should not play because of the tremendous amount of motion that the scaphoid has in the cast as a result of gripping the hockey stick. Given the amount of contact in hockey, one has to consider earlier open reduction of a scaphoid nonunion in a professional player. Following cast removal, a player is usually able to regain hand function through activity; thus extensive rehabilitation is not usually warranted.

Jersey Finger

This injury is an avulsion of the flexor digitorum profundus tendon and is a commonly missed injury. The injury occurs when a player grasps an opponent's jersey by flexing the digit, with the distal phalanx forced into hyperextension at the same time. The tendon is avulsed from its insertion and may be associated with an avulsion fracture. The injury commonly involves the fourth or fifth digit. Physical examination reveals swelling and tenderness over the distal interphalangeal (DIP) joint and the distal end of the tendon. The tendon may have retracted to the proximal interphalangeal (PIP) joint level or to the level of the MCP joint. The patient will be unable to flex the DIP joint of the affected finger when testing the tendon in isolation. An x-ray should be taken to rule out a fracture. Treatment must be surgical to reattach the tendon to the distal phalanx. The best prognosis is offered with surgery within 2 to 3 weeks of injury. A missed injury is much more difficult to repair because the tendon has retracted and presents difficulty in being brought back out distally. Unfortunately, this is one of the most commonly overlooked injuries in hockey.

Females

There is no significant difference in frequency or types of injuries in women when compared with men (all sports).[29]

LOWER BACK, THORACIC, AND ABDOMINAL INJURIES

Fortunately, injuries to the spine are not among the most common in ice hockey,[2] but when they do occur, they can be the most devastating and disabling. Back pain is often muscular. After conservative management of back pain, unresolving pain should be evaluated with an x-ray and bone scan to rule out more sinister medical problems, such as disrupted posterior spinal elements in acute spondylolysis.

The most common lumbar region injuries in hockey are as follows:

Lumbar strain: Most common type of back pain and accounts for at least 70 percent of all back pain. Caused by a stretch or microtearing of the muscles of the spine, but it usually responds well to treatment.

Facet joint syndrome: These small joints of the spine can become sprained or inflamed when under extreme force, as with excess twisting or hyperextension of the spine.

Herniated lumbar disk: This is usually the most severe of low back disorders. The motion of skating puts increased pressure on the disk, which can herniate out at a point of weakness or injury. This herniation can place pressure on the spinal nerves, resulting in radiating pain into the buttocks and down the legs.

Degenerative disk disease: Degenerative changes occur after repetitive wear and tear on the spine. As the gelatinous disk becomes thinner, excess pressure is placed on the facet joints and nerves. Eventually, synovitis and osteophyte formation occur.

Although the four conditions just mentioned are the ones found most commonly in active hockey players, there are still many other potential conditions to consider, such as acute spondylolysis. A thorough history and physical examination are required for all back pains, and radiologic imaging will be required for some. The treatment of each individual back problem varies, but the principles remain the same.

1. *Trunk stabilization*. The "rigid cylinder" concept is one in which the muscles of the trunk are fully strengthened to stabilize the vertebral column. This protects the neural elements and the annular portion of the disk by shifting certain force vectors to the stronger muscles without sacrificing flexibility.

2. *Trunk strength*. The quadriceps and gluteal muscles are very important in the skating motion and must be trained to offer both explosive power and endurance. This will improve the resistance to fatigue and protect the spine through improved biomechanical posture.

3. *Trunk flexibility.* Tight hip flexors, hamstrings, and erector spinae muscles increase the compressive forces on the facets and disks when the player assumes the skating position. Therefore, proper stretching of these muscles is imperative.

4. *Overall conditioning.* The player's overall physical conditioning is the single most important factor in the prevention of injuries.

Thoracic and Abdominal

The most common problems are as follows:

Rib Fractures

Rib fractures are commonly caused by forced compression of the rib cage and can result in significant pain. Displaced rib fractures can cause internal trauma with pneumothorax and hemothorax complications. Splenic trauma has been reported in up to 20 percent of left lower rib fractures and liver trauma in up to 10 percent of right lower rib fractures. Never underestimate the severity of rib fractures with regard to medical emergencies. A player may return to play with a minor rib fracture once healing has begun and pain has diminished enough to sustain play in a contact game.

Intraabdominal Blunt Trauma

In contact sports one must consider blunt trauma with all abdominal complaints. Off-ice examination should include vital signs and a full physical examination. Any point or rebound tenderness, guarding, decreased bowel sounds, back pain in the absence of back trauma, shoulder tip pain, hematuria, hypotension, and tachycardia should alert the examiner to the possibility of significant injury. The spleen and liver are the most likely organs to be injured in blunt abdominal trauma. The spleen may sustain a subcapsular rupture with large hematoma formation. This subcapsular structure may rupture at any time in a very lethal fashion (see Chap. 11).

"Slapshot Gut"

This injury is a tear in the external oblique muscle that normally occurs in the external oblique aponeurosis of the lower abdomen. Often conventional investigations including ultrasound, x-rays, CT, and MRI do not show any abnormality because they are performed in a static state and the defect is evident only in a dynamic state. Conservative treatment is usually unsuccessful because the opposing portions of the muscle do not approximate close enough to allow for scar formation. Surgical repair of the tear is relatively simple. Some surgeons perform adductor partial or complete releases to decrease the pelvic tension and increase the blood flow to the groin region.

Females

Breast

The natural support of breasts is minimal, composed mostly of adipose tissue plus skin and some deep fascial structures. Studies of breast motion have been done and have shown considerable breast movement in up-down and spiral motions.[30] In addition, larger breasts exert more force against the chest wall than smaller breasts. A bra is important to reduce movement and should be made of mostly nonelastic material with good absorbing capabilities, restrict movement in all directions and have covered clasps and hooks to limit the amount of abrasion. It is also extremely important to wear proper chest protectors made of an impenetrable material to decrease trauma to the breast.

Nipple abrasions are common if abrasive material is worn next to the skin. A good bra also will help prevent this. Cold injury can occur in female hockey players; perspiration with evaporation and wind chill if in an outdoor arena make the nipple sore and sensitive. This is best avoided by wearing windbreaking material and proper clothing. There is no specific treatment.

Trauma to the breast consists of mild contusions from sticks, pucks, etc. Edema and ecchymosis are the presenting findings and gradually resolve. Treat early with ice. Heavier blows to the breast can cause hematomas. Most resolve spontaneously, but they may need to be evacuated if they are increasing in size or pain or if there is a possible infection. Occasionally, a nodule remains that may need to be excised. There is no evidence that this trauma leads to cancer. Breast augmentation is not recommended in hockey players because trauma can lead to rupture of the prosthesis and bleeding with breast deformity.

LOWER EXTREMITY INJURIES

Groin

The groin is a very common site of muscle strain because skating requires forceful contraction of the hip adductors.[2] Goaltenders are also particularly prone to injure this area. Groin area injuries may include the hip adductor group, the iliopsoas, the rectus femoris, and the internal oblique muscles and peripheral nerve entrapments. Most commonly this injury causes an untimely absence from play with a poor response to treatment using conventional modalities or exercises. The loading of the adductor muscles during high-intensity exercise such as hockey may lead to injury and inflammation along the adductor origin, especially the adductor magnus. Pain may occur along the origin and radiate into the rectus abdominis as well as the symphysis pubis. The differential diagnosis must include inguinal hernia, osteitis pubis, and stress fractures of the hip or pelvis.

Groin Treatment Program

1. Early use of ice packs, compression, and elevation.
2. Second- or third-degree muscle strains require crutches with no weight bearing for 48 to 72 h to allow collagen fibers to scar over the strained area.
3. Soft tissue mobilization is necessary to address the fibrosis and adaptive shortening of the musculature. Fibrosis secondary to injury can predispose the muscle to further injury.
4. Retraining of the injured area once it has healed should progress as follows: Begin with isometrics without external loading, dynamic training without loading (pool workout), isometric training with external loading, dynamic training with loading, stretching, and finally, sport-specific training.

Some athletes with chronic adductor tendonitis will benefit from as much as 6 months away from their sport if they can possibly do it. Players need to be discouraged from repetitively traumatizing the region, leading to chronic tendinitis through reaggravation. Injury can be prevented by stretching prior to every game and practice.

The senior author has operated on several resistant cases of adductor tendinitis or "pulled groin." The adductor tendon is detached from the pectineal and pubic origins. The results are satisfactory in properly selected patients (those with quite localized injury). Cortisone injections three times, each 1 month apart, should be tried first.

Knee

Most knee injuries in hockey are of the collateral ligaments, but the anterior cruciate ligament (ACL) and the menisci are also frequently injured. Most injuries occur from contact, mostly with an opponent's knee, but they also may occur with contact with the boards or posts. Although hockey skates allow the feet to move and the foot is not fixed, there are still very severe injuries.

Medial Collateral Ligament Sprain

The hockey player skates with the knee in an almost constantly flexed position. Injury is caused by an overstretching of the ligament by a valgus and internal torsion strain often when hit by an opposing player on the lateral aspect. This mechanism of injury is also the most common for an ACL injury. In children, it is critical not to miss epiphyseal damage.

Grade I sprains are tearing or stretching of some ligament fibers, with no or minimal loss of function. Grade II sprains consist of rupture of some of the fibers resulting in some loss of function. Grade III sprains are complete ruptures of the ligament from the bone. There is total loss of stability and function.

Surgery is not advantageous in the treatment of this type of injury. Treatment generally is conservative, and return to play should be accompanied by a custom fit or off-the-shelf brace.

Anterior Cruciate Ligament Sprains

Important historical features are the presence of a pop, crack, or noise at the time of injury and immediate swelling suggesting hemarthrosis. The physical examination may be quite difficult to perform initially given the large muscle bulk of many players and the spasm existing after injury. In many players with an increased tolerance to pain, a mere lack of pain does not preclude serious injury.

Treatment concerns include the following:

Reconstructive surgery is a strong possibility.
Joint capsule or cartilage tear increases joint instability, thereby increasing potential complications.
Degenerative changes are seen with an unstable knee joint.
Chronic swelling causes muscular weakness.

Meniscus

Injury it most commonly from a quick rotational, shearing, or squatting force at the knee joint. Physical findings include a positive McMurray's test, joint-line tenderness, and a positive Apley's compression test. Occasionally a player will be unable to extend the knee due to a mechanical block of the meniscus into the intraarticular notch.

Indications for arthroscopy of meniscal tears:

Failure to respond to nonsurgical treatment
Positive physical examination and typical symptoms of joint-line catching and pain, effusions, locking, and giving way

Preventative concepts for knee injuries:

Good quadriceps and hamstring strengthening
Maintenance of good overall body weight and composition
Maintenance of a good overall fitness level
Speed and agility training for the lower extremity

After any injury, strength should be maximized prior to return to play. Players should be able to cut, turn both ways, and pivot with hard forces on their knees without symptoms. A full Cybex examination with 100 percent return to function is an excellent guide for when to return to play.

Chondromalacia and abnormal patellar tracking are common in hockey but less severe than in the jumping sports. The cause in hockey is likely to be drills that involve jumping and squatting and dropping to the knees on the ice.

Females

In the United States, the NCAA records athletic injuries for certain sports, but only for men's ice hockey, not for women's. In the NCAA's comparable sports, i.e., gymnastics, soccer, and basketball, women sustained more knee injuries than men,[31] including between two and four times more ACL injuries in these sports. Other studies also have supported this finding.[11,25,32] Of significance, however, male ice hockey players sustained fewer ACL injuries than men in other sports. Some possible explanations for the increased number of ACL injuries in women include poorer conditioning, increased ligamentous laxity, alignment of the lower extremity (e.g., increased Q angle), and muscle development. The high number of noncontact ACL injuries in women may be related to a smaller ACL and femoral notch space.[31] It is possible that a future study of ACL injuries in ice hockey players will reveal a greater increase in female injuries versus male.

Ankle

Ankle injuries do occur in hockey despite the stiff skate, although the skate does offer some prevention against inversion injury. The force to the knee joint when a player is skating hard can be over 600 lb. The force is less in the ankle joint because it is locked in the skate, but there is still an equivalent force of at least two times the player's body weight.

An important part of prevention in young players is fitting them with the correct skates. Buying oversized skates for a child to grow into is still common but should be discouraged.

Rehabilitation of an ankle injury is most important. Fortunately, hockey players are going back into a skate boot, which also provides additional ankle support after an injury. After an ankle injury, it is possible to have weakness of the hip flexors, quadriceps, hamstrings, and calf musculature. After 8 weeks of inactivity, 40 percent of the strength is lost in the ligaments. Therapy must concentrate on strengthening these groups as well as residual mechanical instability, peroneal weakness, proprioceptive defects, and quick-response fibers of the lower extremity. For the hockey player, therapy should build up to cuts, pivots, tight figure of eights, agility exercises, and jumping.

Foot

Problems with the feet are much less common than one would imagine. Hockey players usually fit their skates very tightly, with a thin cotton sock or none at all. With a tight form-fitting skate there is a tendency to calcaneal bumps, pressure sores on the medial malleolus, or areas of ganglionic type swelling adjacent to the medial malleolus. Tenosynovitis and tendonitis of the anterior tibial tendons and extensor tendons of the feet can occur. Players usually respond by altering the skate. Sorbothane, moleskin, or low-density foam also can be introduced into the skate. For tenosynovitis of the ankle, excision of the synovial material or removal of the tendon sheath may be required. A metatarsal fracture may occur after a direct blow to the foot, and foot x-rays should be performed with management dependent on the degree of injury.

Morton's neuroma may be excruciatingly uncomfortable in a skate. The player may complain of the sensation of a nail sticking up in the skate. Treatment consists of adequate forefoot room in the skate, corticosteriod injections, ultrasound, and padding. Surgery may be required if conservative therapy is not successful.

Females

Bunions, which are an inflammation of the bursa over the medial first metatarsal, are more common in women in general. This may be due to increased pronation as well as inappropriately narrow and high footwear. When looking for footwear, and importantly, an ice skate, one must remember that a women's foot is built differently from a man's. The female foot is wider in the forefoot than in the hindfoot.[33] Since most ice skates are built on a man's last, a women's foot may experience problems. In order to correct movement of the foot in the skate, a tighter fit at the heel may be required, especially since hockey requires many accelerations and decelerations. Surgery eventually can correct the deformity, but the player may be out of play for many months.

Other

Lacerations

Lacerations of the ankle and foot occur, requiring evaluation of underlying tendon function. Boot-top injuries include injury to the anterior tibial tendon, extensor hallucis longus, and extensor communis tendons or the dorsalis pedis artery, vein, or nerve. These injuries are rare in comparison with other injuries in hockey, but several cases have been presented in the literature.[34] One must suspect this injury when injury has occurred to the anterior aspect of the ankle generally by a skate blade. Severe damage can occur with a seemingly small superficial laceration, and missed injuries can be devastating for athletes. A careful physical examination must be performed, and investigations may include an MRI and wound exploration. Surgery is required to correct any obvious deficits. In order to prevent such injuries, all players should wear the skate tongue in the upright position.

Compartment Syndromes

The posterior tibial tendinitis that hockey players develop is treated identically to that of runners. Progression to periostitis and anterior compartment syndrome may occur. The common precipitant in hockey is dry land training such as running and additional exercises in pretraining. In a hockey player who develops shin splints, aerobic training should be conducted in some other sport such as cycling.

Medial Tarsal Tunnel Syndrome

An athlete often will incur entrapment of the posterior tibial nerve as it enters the fiberosseous tarsal tunnel beneath the flexor retinaculum on the medial side of the ankle. At this stage the nerve divides into the medial and lateral calcaneal or plantar nerves, and the player is left with pain, numbness, burning, and a sensation of "impairment" on the sole of the foot. The complaint is accentuated by playing for long periods of time. Occasionally an intrinsic muscle weakness is manifested in the distal lateral surface of the foot and along the medial longitudinal arch. Tinel's sign modified by tapping over the area of entrapment is usually positive. If nerve conduction studies are positive, surgical decompression is indicated.

Females

The female anatomy has a wider pelvis, femoral neck anteversion with varus hip, valgus knees, external tibial tubercle rotation, and pronation of the hindfoot combining to increase the Q angle.[29] There is no proof that these anatomic differences result in any decrease in athletic performance.

Injuries in female athletes of different sports, which are seen more commonly, are as follows:

1. Common around the hip is iliotibial band friction syndrome with pain or snapping over the greater trochanter. Athletes also may suffer lateral knee pain. Treatment is with (ITB) stretches, ice, anti-inflammatories, and vastus medialis strengthening.

2. Greater trochanteric bursitis is common due to anatomic differences of the hip and a tight ITB. Treat with stretching, anti-inflammatories, and conditioning.
3. Retropatellar pain is very common and may be aggravated in hockey conditioning off ice, i.e., with hill running, squats, and knee flexion and extension exercises. The patella comes in contact with the femoral trochlea at 30 degrees of flexion. The differential diagnosis is large, but it is important to look for vastus medialis obliquus (VMO) atrophy. In addition, a triad of fat pad hypertrophy, inflammation of the patellar tendon, and medial plica tenderness may exist. Treatment includes strengthening, anti-inflammatories, Cybex, TENS, and possibly surgery.
4. Lateral knee pain is the second most common problem in the athletic female, either as a result of ITB friction, synovial interposition, or fat pad interposition. Lateral collateral knee sprains, as well as lateral meniscal injury, also must be ruled out.
5. Medial knee pain is often from VMO atrophy; therefore, treatment is strengthening. Treatment of medial collateral ligament sprains in women is slightly different from that in males and may require medial orthotics and increased VMO strengthening.

THE FEMALE HOCKEY PLAYER

Since the 1970s, female participation in sports has increased tremendously. Several factors have played a role: research showing the benefits of exercise; increased media attention to these benefits, the physician's role in encouraging exercise, a change in the societal perception of exercise for women, and new legislation, the largest being Title IX in the United States, providing equal opportunities in physical education and athletics for women in institutions receiving federal funds.[35]

Historians will recall the first time women played hockey back in 1889, when Lord Stanley's daughters played the game in the backyard.[36] Since then, women's hockey has grown substantially and is still doing so, from 6000 participants in the early 1980s to 35,000 in 1997. The first women's world championships took place in 1990, in Ottawa, Canada, with Team Canada taking the gold. Team Canada has since won World Championships in 1992, 1994, and 1996. In Nagano, Japan, in 1998, women's ice hockey will be given full-medal status for the first time. As an Olympic event, women's hockey is expected to grow further and make even more noticeable gains with both the public and the press.

The game is different than men's hockey in that muscle and power are less a component and speed, fast passes, and carrying the puck occur more in the women's game. Body checking was banned in 1990, but contact along the boards is allowed.

Unfortunately, the body of literature on women's hockey is small, with very few statistics and case reports. Two articles reviewing the physiology of ice hockey[1,37] have made no mention of female physiology specifically and no comparisons with male players. This relates primarily to the lack of research on females in general and on ice hockey specifically.

Female injuries are specific with regard to the reproductive organs, but there are many similarities between injuries for both sexes, likely more than there are differences. Studies have indicated that injuries to women are sports related not sex related.[38] However, certain injuries are more common in women than in men: patellofemoral disorders (19.6 percent of all female injuries in sports versus 7.4 percent of males[38]), recurrent patellar dislocations (4.6 percent for females, 0.7 percent for males, in all sports[39]), spondylolysis, stress fractures, shin splints, bunions, and swimmer's shoulder.

After puberty, a major sex difference is in muscle mass, giving men greater power and speed. Women, however, can gain great strength (up to 44 percent) without significant increases in muscle mass.[40] Given the overall increase in muscle mass in males, power is increased, thus subjecting men to increased forces of play. Women, on the other hand, may rely more on speed and agility in their game, in addition to power. If both sexes are subjected to the same coaching, training, and conditioning, the actual injury patterns vary mostly from sport to sport and not between the genders.[29] Differences may well be seen in the same sport depending on how it is played by men versus women. In hockey, for instance, the body checking rules are different, resulting in likely much fewer injuries for women. We see this in many other sports as well, where women bring finesse to the sport and men may be more contact related.

Reproductive System

Despite the concerns early on in female sports about damaging reproductive organs, the female system is well protected within the bony pelvis, with few cases of trauma. One anecdotal case[41] reports an IUD perforating the uterus following a pelvic blow in a field hockey game. It is only during pregnancy, when growth has carried on beyond the pelvis after the fourth month, that protection is decreased. It is best to not participate in contact sports beyond this time. The complaint of pelvic pain in the female athlete may be musculoskeletal, gastrointestinal, or genitourinary.[42] Localizing pain is difficult given the close proximity of the viscera and surrounding musculoskeletal elements. An MRI is very useful in clarifying musculoskeletal injuries of the pelvis.

Female athletes have increased irregularities of the menstrual cycle (28 percent in college varsity athletes).[29] Delayed puberty also occurs with increased frequency in female athletes, and its long-term effects are not clear. During adolescence, normal bone mass gain occurs, but this is lessened in late-maturing females due to the lack of estrogen.[43] In addition, amenorrheic women lose bone mass at the rate of 5 percent per year, similar to the rate seen in menopause. Of greater interest is the bone mass density in female athletes not concerned about thinness, which is often the case in hockey. In a study of female rowers who were oligo/amenorrheic, vertebral bone content was the same as in matched nonathletic women.[43] However, conflicting data are also available that have shown a decrease in bone mass density in athletes with menstrual irregularities.[44] The osteopenia that may result from decreased bone mass density will increase players' risk of injury, including stress fractures. If growth is complete, as measured by closed epiphyseal plates, and menarche has not occurred by age 16, hormonal therapy should be started as prevention.[43]

There are two different types of amenorrhea: one related to low body weight, which is less likely to occur in hockey players, and another hormonal pattern where low weight is not required. The latter pattern may occur in hockey players, since muscle mass is important, and weight and body fat not as much of a concern as in gymnasts, for instance. This "athlete's amenorrhea" has shown increased levels of luteinizing hormone and androgens, but future research is still required.[38] Treatment includes calcium supplement, nutritional counseling, a possible change in training intensity, and hormone replacement.

Recommendations for the evaluation and treatment of amenorrhea in adolescent females from the American Academy of Paediatrics' Committee on Sports Medicine are as follows[45]:

All: Evaluation of menses and diet, counsel on nutrition; monitor menses, diet, growth, weight, and skin fold thickness; calcium supplementation, 1200 to 1500 mg daily.

If amenorrheic: Physical examination, endocrine evaluation, and exclude pregnancy and anorexia.

If less than 3 years after menarche: Decrease exercise intensity, improve nutrition.

If more than 3 years after menarche or after age 16: Start low-dose OCP.

In pregnancy, the American College of Obstetricians and Gynecologists has set out guidelines for exercise[41]: Discourage competitive activities, maternal heart rate not to exceed 140 beats per minute, no longer than 15 min of strenuous activity, and joint instability exists due to connective tissue laxity, and therefore, jarring motions or rapid changes in direction should be avoided. As far as beginning exercise following pregnancy, Shangold states that one should be guided by pain. There will be a difference between the average to top athlete, and cesarean sections also will require more recovery time.

Steroids

In one study, steroid use among older teens was 5 percent in males and 1 percent in females (all sports).[35] Given the nature of hockey and its reliance on speed, power, and strength, it is possible for the percentage of women using steroids to be higher if they are hockey players. In women, side effects include hirsutism, increased muscularity, deeper voice, male-pattern baldness, hypertrophy of the clitoris, acne, menstrual disorders, and increased aggressiveness. Oral steroids may cause elevation of liver enzymes, and long-term use may result in peliosis hepatitis. Other effects include increased low-density lipoproteins, high-density lipoproteins, hypertension, decreased glucose tolerance, decreased thyroid hormones and immunoglobulins, and possibly early growth plate epiphyseal fusion.

HIGH-PERFORMANCE TRAINING IN HOCKEY

Sport-specific training is important to improve performance. Training programs should be task specific to improve fitness and to maximize the energy demands placed on players.[1] Studies have shown that players involved in hockey-related training programs show greater improvement in skating performance than players only training through games.[46] Further studies have suggested that players do not receive enough on-ice game and practice challenge to maintain and increase their level of fitness, leading to detraining. With the average National Hockey League (NHL) on-ice game time being 16 min per player and poor exercise intensities during practices, detraining will occur.[1] Thus proper training programs must be in place for all levels both to improve playing ability and to decrease injury.

Physiologic Characteristics of the Sport

1. Energy requirements of the sport are characterized by fast, explosive skating and quick and sudden changes in direction.
2. Motor development requiring agility for stick handling, passing, shooting, and playmaking with teammates is necessary.
3. Muscular strength and balance are required for on-ice activities including bodychecking, absorbing hits by opponents, and crashing into boards, posts, and ice.

Ice hockey demands a complex interaction of several specific physiologic components, many of which serve to provide a base for advanced high-performance training.

Physiologic components are as follows:

1. Aerobic energy system
2. Anaerobic energy system
3. Muscular strength
4. Power
5. Muscular flexibility
6. Agility

Aerobic Energy System

Aerobic training prepares the on-ice energy supply and recovery process and builds the base needed to handle more intense anaerobic training. The aerobic system is vital to the recovery process between bouts of intense exercise. Adjacent slow oxidative muscle fibers also can contribute by reoxidizing lactic acid if they are well conditioned, even if the slow-twitch fibers have not been recruited for the skating action. Players' heart rates during a single shift could exceed 90 percent of the age-adjusted maximum. During this event, players would have a far greater dependence on the anaerobic energy system.

Anaerobic Energy System

The anaerobic energy system provides the major source of energy for muscle contraction during the exertion phase of hockey. Bursts of maximal effort place explicit demands on the anaerobic system. Fast, explosive movements demand a rapid supply of ATP energy. Anaerobic ATP production peaks at 30 to 45 s and has an upper limit of 120 s depending on the intensity. If the athlete is not trained properly, an inhibitive action on performance will result, providing submaximal efforts.

Muscular Strength

Programs are designed to increase lean body mass, improve absolute strength, and provide a base for power training. Absolute strength is necessary for contact. Sports-specific exercises help to lower the center of gravity and increase inertia. Lower body strength contributes to skating, acceleration, agility, and pelvic stability. Upper body strength improves body checking, shooting, and puck-control skills. Muscle balance is important for injury prevention and sport performance. A joint may be more susceptible to injury when there is a strength imbalance between muscle groups.

Power

Power is a fundamental requirement for on-ice activities, particularly when propulsion of the total body is required. The hockey player often executes sharp changes in direction and accelerates quickly. Explosive power is arguably the most important physical parameter in ice hockey.

Muscular Flexibility

Muscular flexibility is very important when a player must execute powerful, explosive movements. Flexibility decreases injuries and improves execution. Players who fail to extend the rear leg during the skating motion seriously hinder their skating speed and power. Flexibility training should target the lumbar region, hip, groin, quadriceps, and hamstrings.

Agility

Agility becomes vital when the athlete must make quick, sudden changes in direction, such as those during one-on-one situations to maneuver around the opposition. Complex agility skills distinguish the elite player.

In order to make ice hockey safer, the most important change must be that of attitude. Players must be educated about the true protective value of equipment. Coaches need to teach players the correct way to play and not to tolerate or promote intentional violence. Fans and parents must encourage officials to enforce rules and to prevent high-risk behavior.

Females

In strength training, men develop hypertrophy of muscles because they have much higher levels of androgenic hormones. Women may do the same weight training and also become strong, but they do not develop markedly enlarged muscles. In endurance training, women are found to have a lower maximal oxygen consumption compared with men. This difference is due to larger heart size and thus greater stroke volume and more hemoglobin in men. Thus the training target V_{O_2} max in women will be somewhat lower.

The Canadian National Team and university teams in Canada (University of Toronto) have off-season training manuals for female hockey players. For example, the July National training manual includes the following: strength training 3 days a week, plyometric workouts twice a week, pool work twice a week, a long cardiovascular workout once a week, two shorter anaerobic activities each week such as biking or rollerblading (goal is to perform high-intensity exercise for short time period and rest for a short time in between), and an abdominal program, with 1 day of rest each week. By August, the on-ice training begins to increase from twice the first week up to four to five times for the last week. The best training drills are high-intensity scrimmage, which the players are encouraged to do as well as some gamelike drills. The month also continues with pliometrics (such as medicine ball throws, leap frog), anaerobic work, and emphasis on flexibility, especially in the lower back, groin, hamstrings, hip flexors, iliotibial band, quadriceps, and calves. Emphasis is also on abdominals, with a workout 6 days a week.

The University of Toronto training manual for off-season includes a general preparation phase for 2 months, a specific preparation phase for 1 month, and a precompetitive phase for the final month. This off-season training began 2 years ago, and according to coaches, improvement in the players is noticeable. The first 3 months include strength, flexibility, and aerobic activities. The first 2 months build up muscle strength and general physical conditioning, increasing intensity gradually. Coaches and trainers have noticed a lack of strength in the upper body specifically, predisposing players to injury. Thus greater emphasis is placed on these muscles in this training period. The third month aims activity toward sport-specific exercises to achieve greater speed and power. On-ice intensity also increases gradually. In the last month, more speed, power, and specific skills are worked on and include exhibition games prior to the competitive season.

PROPER FITTING OF PROTECTIVE EQUIPMENT

The following will describe what to look for when fitting or buying new equipment. Properly fitted equipment can significantly reduce the chance of injury and improve the athlete's skating performance.

Skates

A hockey skate usually will fit a half size smaller than regular street shoes. Ensure that there are no wrinkles in the sock when tightening the skate up. With foot and toes to the front of the boot, you should be able to place one finger between the boot and the heel of the foot. When lacing up the skate, bang the heel against the floor to ensure support. The first three to four eyelets should be snug, the next three loose, and the final two to four very snug. Do not wrap the lace around the ankle, since this may inhibit circulation and irritate the tendons. The skate tongues should be behind the shin guard to ensure maximum protection for the shins. If the hard shell is cracked, replace immediately because of the increased chance of a serious toe or foot injury. Never buy skates that are too big. This can seriously inhibit skating development.

Shin Guards

The sizes will vary from junior (8 to 13 in) to senior (14 to 16 in). The cup of the shin guard should be centered directly over the kneecap. The top of the skin guard should overlap roughly 2 in with the bottom of the hockey pant. With the skates on, the pads should rest 1 in above the foot when it is fully flexed.

Pants

Hockey pants should be fitted with shin guards in place. The belt should be fitted just above the hip bone and allow for snug adjustment. The pants should have as much padding as possible without restricting movement. The player should be able to fully squat with the pants and shin guards on, with the padding in the pants staying in the same position.

Shoulder Pads

Make sure that the shoulder pads cover the shoulders, upper back, chest, and upper arms to just meet the elbow pads. The protective caps should be placed on top of the shoulders. The back of the shoulder pads should slightly overlap with the pants to ensure maximum protection of the spine. To guarantee full range of motion, the player should be able to lift the arms just above shoulder height without the pads digging into the neck area.

Elbow Pads

Ensure that elbow pads are properly fitted to each arm, since some pads will vary protection depending on left or right elbow. The donut inside the pad should be placed on the point of the elbow. The elbow pad should fit tightly and lock into the elbow. The pads should extend to the bottom of the shoulder pads and down the forearms to where the tops of the gloves start. The player should be able to fully flex the elbow without constriction from the straps. The straps usually will wear out first, so either get new ones or secure them with tape.

Gloves

Hockey gloves should fit like loose winter gloves over the fingers. The top of the glove should extend to the bottom of the elbow pad to ensure full forearm protection. To ensure maximal protection, with your hand in the glove, push the back of the glove with your other fingers. This compression should not be felt inside the glove. Test the glove with a hockey stick and stick handle on the spot for a few minutes to ensure freedom of motion and to locate any spots that might cause blisters.

Helmet

All helmets must be approved by the Canadian Standards Association (CSA) and will have a sticker indicating this. They are generally measured in junior and senior sizes depending on head sizes from $6\frac{1}{2}$ to $7\frac{3}{4}$ in. The helmet should be snug on the head after adjustments are made. Shake the head from side to side, back and forth, ensuring that the helmet does not move and causes no discomfort. The front of the helmet should be just above the eyebrows. The chin strap should be placed securely under the chin for a snug fit. Occasionally check the inside foam of the helmet. Press the thumb against the padding. If the padding returns to the original position, this is a good sign that the foam is still protective. If the padding breaks or cracks, the helmet should be replaced.

Face Protectors/Masks

All masks must be CSA approved and will have a sticker indicating this. Make sure that the cage is compatible with the helmet. The mask should allow for one finger to fit between the bottom of the chin and the chin cup of the protector.

Throat Protectors

The protector should fit snugly, but not too tight. It should completely cover the throat, and, with bib styles, the upper chest area.

Undergarments

Undergarments should be cool and comfortable to avoid irritation of the skin. Always wear a single pair of socks to offer comfort and moisture-absorbing ability. The best combination of material is 50 percent cotton and 50 percent polyester.

Athletic Support

Choose an appropriately sized protective cup and strap that is effective for shock absorption. Females should wear a jill. If the cup is cracked or the strap is frayed, replace it immediately.

Females

Some companies have lines of equipment specifically for females:

- Different sizes.

- Pants: Better fitting waist and thinner kidney pads so they fit better with the shoulder pads.
- Gloves: Smaller fit decreases hand motion inside glove.
- Shoulder pads: Two pieces across the breast area enables better arm movement.
- Neck guards: Normal, although most women do not use the neck flap because it does not fit as well with the shoulder pads.

Goalies

Pads

Always fit the pads with your skates on. Kneel down into each pad and make sure the kneecap is in the middle of the knee roll. The pad should extend from the toe of the skate to 4 in above the knee. The top of the pad should fit approximately 3 in above the bottom of the pants.

Catcher and Blocker

Lower the blocker and glove to the side, and they should not be able to fall off. The blocker should be comfortable, an easy grip, and able to control the stick for a proper fit. The catcher must have a heavily padded cuff that overlaps the arm pads.

Upper Boot Protection

Ensure that all straps are fastened and used properly. The arm padding should extend down past the blocker to the wrist while allowing full range of motion in the wrist and elbow. The body pad should tuck into the pants about 2 in below the navel.

Throat Protectors (Fig. 15-4)

The protector can be either the hanging kind or have a snug fit around the neck. The bib-style protector should be worn beneath the chest protector. *Tip:* Throat protectors will protect against skate lacerations and cuts but *not* against spinal injuries. Make sure that all Velcro straps are in good shape, and replace the protector when it is damaged.

Pants and Athletic Supports

Goaltenders should wear a special athletic support and cup with extra protection. It should be fitted like that for regular players but with this special design. The pants are specifically designed to absorb and disperse the high impact from pucks. Ensure that the pants are loose enough around the waist to allow for the belly pad to tuck into them. *Tip:* Padding is heavier than regular pants and therefore may require the use of suspenders.

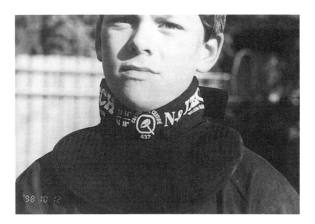

FIG. 15-4   Plastic mesh collar for an 8-year-old goalie. They are larger for older players.

Face Mask Protection

The mask should be CSA approved and specifically designed for goaltenders due to the increased chance of pucks hitting the mask at high speeds.

Sticks

Sticks should be comfortable in the crouch position. The lie of the stick should be flat on the ice when the goaltender is in the crouch position. The length of the paddle also should be comfortable in this position.

HIV IN SPORTS

HIV in athletics has become an issue over the last decade as world-class athletes have publicly announced their infectious state and as HIV has become a more prevalent infection. Athletes such as Earvin "Magic" Johnson have attracted much attention to the issue of HIV in sports. Guidelines have been produced and articles written about how sports should be conducted and how athletes should be educated.

In general, guidelines suggest that bleeding in any game or match be stopped and wounds dressed prior to return to play.[47] Athletes need to be educated about HIV and testing procedures. The largest risk to athletes is off-field activities. These include sexual activities and intravenous drug use. The risk of transmission of HIV is low in athletic competition, but the potential is there. The virus has never been isolated from sweat and rarely and in low concentrations from saliva.[48] The main concern in sporting activities is blood contact. A possible case of transmission has been reported between two soccer players in a 1989 Italian soccer game involving head wounds. One player was known to be HIV-positive prior to play, and the other player converted to HIV positivity after the collision, although no test was performed at the time of injury to state conclusively that conversion occurred as a result of the collision.[49]

Athletes are concerned about both the possibility of contracting HIV from other athletes and the possibility of mandatory testing. The possible consequences of mandatory testing and disclosure include exclusion from sport and discrimination. Athletes who have engaged in high-risk behavior do benefit from testing and should be encouraged to do so. They will then be able to make educated decisions regarding treatment, controlling transmission to sexual partners, and participation in counseling and education programs.[50]

Specific recommendations have been written by the American Academy of Pediatrics in order to facilitate decisions on HIV testing and precautions when faced with these issues in the athletic setting.[51] The recommendations include allowing athletes with HIV infection to participate in all competitive sports unless further evidence is provided regarding HIV transmission in sports, encouraging known HIV-positive individuals to choose sports with less risk of blood exposure, respecting confidentiality of all athletes with regard to HIV status, and not recommending routine HIV testing. Personnel are to use gloves when in contact with body fluids and to follow universal body substance precautions. Wounds are to be well covered and blood washed from body surfaces and from sporting equipment and surfaces.

In a study published in 1993, 548 NCAA schools were surveyed regarding HIV policies and precautions.[52] Interestingly, 2 of 548 schools required mandatory HIV testing of athletes, and 426 schools did not offer HIV testing within the athletic department. Policies on participation of athletes with HIV infection were present in 33 schools; 15 of these restricted participation in some manner. All 15 schools restricted ice hockey and wrestling to non-HIV-positive individuals only. Sixty-two percent of schools had universal precautions education programs for staff, yet adherence to such programs still showed a need for improvement.

In the HIV-infected individual, exercise has been shown to be beneficial and safe.[48] For those not HIV-positive, sports may be carried out in a competitive and enjoyable fashion as long as proper universal precautions are taken, as mentioned previously.

REFERENCES

1. Schlerer KA: The seventy year history of the International Ice Hockey Federation, 1908–1978. Munich, Prospect Presse Service, 1978.

1a. Cox MH, Miles DS, Verde TJ, Rhodes EC: Applied physiology of ice hockey. *Sports Med* 19(3):184–201, 1995.

2. Daly PJ, Sim FH, Simonet WT: Ice hockey injuries: A review. *Sports Med* 10:122–31, 1990.

3. Sim FH, Chao EY: Injury potential in modern ice hockey. *Am J Sports Med* 6:378–384, 1978.

4. Stuart MJ, Smith A: Injuries in Junior A Ice Hockey. A three-year prospective study. *Am J Sports Med* 23(4):458–461, 1995.

5. Lorentzon R, Wedren H, Pietila T, Gustavsson B: Injuries in international ice hockey. A prospective, comparative study of injury incidence and injury types in international and Swedish elite ice hockey. *Am J Sports Med* 16(4):389–391.

6. Lorentzon R, Wedren H, Pietila T: Incidence, nature and causes of ice hockey injuries. A three-year prospective study of a Swedish elite ice hockey team. *Am J Sports Med* 16(4):392–396.

7. Pelletier RL, Montelpare WJ, Stark RM: Intercollegiate ice hockey injuries. A case for uniform definitions and reports. *Am J Sports Med* 21(1):78–81, 1993.

8. Stuart MJ, Smith AM, Nieva JJ: Injuries in youth ice hockey: A pilot surveillance strategy. *Mayo Clin Proc* 70:350–356, 1995.

9. Maron BJ, Poliac LC, Kaplan JA, Mueller FO: Blunt impact to the chest leading to sudden death from cardiac arrest during sports activities. *N Engl J Med* 333:337–42, 1995.

10. Benoit BG, Russell NA, Richard MT, Hugenholtz H, Ventureyra ECG et al: Epidural hematoma: Report of seven cases with delayed evolution of symptoms. *Can J Neurol Sci* 9:321–324, 1982.

11. Kelly JP, Rosenberg JH: Diagnosis and management of concussion in sports. *Neurology* 48:575–580, 1997.

12. Dick RW: A summary of head and neck injuries in collegiate athletics using the NCAA Injury Surveillance System. In: Hoerner EF, ed: *Head and Neck Injuries in Sports*. Philadelphia: American Society for Testing and Materials, 1994.

13. Practice Parameter: The management of concussion in sports (summary statement). *Neurology* 48:581–585, 1997.

14. Report of the Mild Traumatic Brain Injury Committee of the Head Injury Interdisciplinary Special Interest Group of the American Congress of Rehabilitation Medicine: Definition of mild traumatic brain injury. *J Head Trauma Rehabil* 8:86–87, 1993.

15. Fekete JF: Severe brain injury and death following minor hockey accidents: The effectiveness of the "safety helmets" of amateur hockey players. *Can Med Assoc J* 99:1234–1239, 1968.

16. Cantu RC, Voy R: Second impact syndrome: A risk in any sport. *Phys Sports Med* 23, 1995.

17. Leblanc KE: Concussions in Sports: Guidelines for Return to Competition. *Am Family Phys* 50(4):801–806, 1994.

18. Voaklander DC, Saunders LD, Quinnery HA: Correlates of facial protection use by adult recreational ice hockey players. *Can J Public Health* 87(6):381–382, 1996.

19. Pashby TJ: Eye injuries in Canadian amateur hockey, still a concern. *Can J Opthalmol* 22:293–295, 1987.

20. LaPrade RF, Burnett QM, Zarzour R, Moss R: The effect of the mandatory use of face masks on facial lacerations and head and neck injuries in ice hockey. A prospective study. *Am J Sports Med* 23(6):773–775, 1995.

21. Pashby TJ: Eye injuries in Canadian hockey. Phase III: Older players now most at risk. *Can Med Assoc J* 121:643–644, 1979.

22. Deady B, Brison RJ, Chevrier L: Head, face and neck injuries in hockey: A descriptive analysis. *J Emerg Med* 14(5):645–649, 1996.

23. Tator CH. Neck injuries in ice hockey: A recent, unsolved problem with many contributing factors. *Clin Sports Med* 6:101–114, 1987.

24. Maroon JC, Bailes JE: Athletes with cervical spine injury. *Spine* 21: 2294–2299, 1996.

25. Murray, TM, Livingston LA: Hockey helmets, face masks, and injurious behaviour. *Pediatrics* 95:419–421, 1995.

26. Markey KL, Benedetto MD, Curl WW. Upper trunk brachial plexopathy. The stinger syndrome. *Am J Sports Med* 21(5):1993.

27. Akau CK, Press JM, Gooch JL: Sports medicine: 4. Spine and Head Injuries. *Arch Phys Med Rehabil* 74:S443–S446, 1993.

28. Weinstein DW, McCann PD, McIlveen SJ, et al: Surgical treatment of complete acromioclavicular dislocations. *Am J Sports Med* 23(3):1995.

29. AJ Pearl (ed): *The Athletic Female*, American Orthopaedic Society for Sports Medicine, Champaign, IL, Human Kinetics Publishers, 1993.

30. Lorentzen D and Lawson L: Selected sports bras: A biomechanical analysis of breast motion while jogging. *Physician Sportsmed* 15(5): 128–139, 1987.

31. Hutchinson MR, Ireland ML: Knee injuries in female athletes. *Sports Med* 19(4):288–302, 1995.

32. Gray J, Taunton JE, McKenzie DC, et al: A survey of injuries to the anterior cruciate ligament of the knee in female basketball players. *Int J Sports Med* 6:314–316, 1985.

33. Arendt EA: Orthopaedic issues for active and athletic women. *Clin Sports Med* 13(2):483–503, 1994.

34. Simonet WT, Sim L: Boot-top tendon lacerations in ice hockey. *J Trauma* 38(1):30–31, 1995.

35. Warren MP, Shangold MM: *Sports Gynecology: Problems and Care of the Athletic Female.* Cambridge, MA, Blackwell Science, 1997.

36. Webb, M: Hockey Moments with Marg. *Univ Toronto Magazine* XXV (2):10–13, 1997.

37. Montgomery DL: Physiology of ice hockey. *Sports Med* 5:99–126, 1988.

38. Rubin C.J: Sports Injuries in the female athlete. *NJ Med* 88(9):643–645, 1991.

39. DeHaven KE, Lintner DM: Athletic injuries: Comparison by age, sport and gender. *Am J Sports Med* 14(3):218–224.

40. Wilmore J: Alteration in strength, body composition, and anthropometric measurements to a ten week training program. *Med Sci Sports* 6:133, 1979.

41. Mueller FO, Ryan AJ: *Prevention of Athletic Injuries: The Role of the Sports Medicine Team.* Philadelphia, F.A. Davis, 1991.

42. Short JW, Pedowitz, RA, et al: The evaluation of pelvic injury in the female athlete. *Sports Med* 20(6):422–428, 1995.
43. Constantini NW, Warren MP: Special problems of the female athlete. *Bailliere's Clin Rheum* 8(1):199–219, 1994.
44. Fruth SJ, Worrell TW: Factors associated with menstrual irregularities and decreased bone mineral density in female athletes. *JOSPT*, 22(1): 26–38, 1995.
45. American Academy of Paediatrics Committee on Sports Medicine. *Pediatrics*, 84:394–395, 1989.
46. Greer N, Serfass R, Picanatto W: The effects of a hockey-specific training program on performance of bantam players. *Can J Sports Sci*, 17: 65–69, 1992.
47. Drotman DP: Professional boxing, bleeding and HIV testing (Letter) *JAMA*, 276(3):193, 1996.
48. Calabrese LH, LaPerriere: Human immunodeficiency virus infection, exercise and athletics. *Sports Med* 15(1):6–13, 1993.
49. Torre D, Sampietro C, et al: Transmission of HIV-1 infection via sports injury (Letter) *Lancet,* 335:1105, 1990.
50. Seltzer DG: Educating athletes on HIV disease and AIDS. The team physician's role. *Physician Sportsmed* 21(1):109–115, 1993.
51. American Academy of Pediatrics Committee on sports medicine and fitness: Human immunodeficiency virus in the athletic setting. *Pediatrics*, 88(3):640–641, 1991.
52. McGrew CA, Dick RW, Schniedwind K, Gikas P: Survey of NCAA institutions concerning HIV/AIDS policies and universal precautions. *Med Sci Sports Exerc* 25(8):917–921, 1993.

16 | Basketball Injuries

Douglas W. Richards   *Ato Sekyi-Out*
Paul H. Marks

Basketball is a sport that enjoys wide popularity among people of many ages and both sexes in most parts of the world. In this chapter, we examine the epidemiology, prevention, and management of basketball injuries

INCIDENCE OF INJURY IN BASKETBALL

Information about injury rates in basketball may be derived from several different types of studies. Prospective longitudinal examinations of all injuries occurring within a given team or league, provide the best estimates.[1-4] Other studies, based on retrospective questionnaires[5-6] or analysis of emergency room or other medical encounters[7-10] suffer from sample bias and underreporting of injuries but add some additional information. In all of these paradigms, the estimates vary widely, at least in part because of different definitions or detection thresholds for injury (the protocols requiring an athlete to miss time from participation fail to report the mildest injuries). Various authors report injury rates per athlete-year, per athlete-hour, or per athlete-exposure (where an exposure is one game or practice, regardless of actual minutes of participation). Table 16-1 combines and summarizes the range of available estimates of the overall incidence of injury in basketball, expressed as injuries per 1000 athlete-exposures.

Many authors have reported a breakdown of injury incidence by time-course and/or anatomic region of injury.[1-5,7] Not surprisingly, the reported relative incidence of different injuries in basketball varies somewhat among them, likely due to the variation in tracking methods, thresholds of injury detection, and injury definition used in these studies. Nonetheless, certain trends emerge clearly and are approximated in Table 16-2. Acute injuries most commonly affect the ankle, knee, hand, or face, while chronic or overuse syndromes are most common in the knee, low back, foot, and ankle. Our discussion of specific injuries later in this chapter will focus on these problems with significant incidence in basketball.

TABLE 16-1 Incidence of Injury per 1000 Athlete-Exposures

Sex	Level of Play	Incidence of Injury
Female	Elite	4–18 injuries/1000 AE
	Recreational	0.5–4 injuries/1000 AE
Male	Elite	5–12 injuries/1000 AE
	Recreational	0.3–6 injuries/1000 AE

TABLE 16-2 Relative Incidence of Injuries by Anatomic Region

Anatomic Region	Acute Injuries (%)	Chronic/Overuse Injuries (%)
Ankle and foot	30	10
Knee	20	40
Other lower extremity (calf, shin, thigh, groin, hip)	15	15
Hand/wrist	10	5
Face/eyes/mouth	10	—
Low back	5	15
Other	15	15

FACTORS AFFECTING BASKETBALL INJURIES

A number of factors can be seen in the literature to correlate with, perhaps cause, or contribute to the variance in the incidence of basketball injuries. While some of these are obviously predetermined or cannot be regulated, many of them can be affected through timely appropriate intervention by trainers, coaches, officials, and physicians. Such interventions are the cornerstone of injury prevention.

Sex

Some disagreement exists in the literature as to whether overall injury rates differ between participants of the different sexes. Some studies have reported higher rates for female participants,[8,11] but many others have found no difference or even slightly higher rates for males.[3,9,10,12] The highest reported estimate of injury rates in basketball is by the NBA Trainers' Association[1]; this includes only males. Considering all of these data, we can say that overall injury rates reported for women's and men's basketball at comparable levels of play have not consistently been shown to be statistically significantly different.

However, certain specific injuries are more common in females (and presumably others among males, although these have not been focused on in studies). Among acute injuries, disruption of the anterior cruciate ligament (ACL) while playing basketball is more common in females by a ratio of perhaps 4:1.[13–15] Among women, noncontact mechanisms of ACL injury are more common.[14] Speculation on why this may be includes theories of less favorable muscle balance, coordination, or proprioception,[16,17] intercondylar notch width,[18,19] and the effect of female hormones on tissue strength. Further research is required to assert the cause of this problem with any confidence. In the meantime, all players, but especially women, would perhaps be well advised to pay particular attention to muscle balance and neuromuscular coordination during training (see below in "Training and Conditioning").

Playing Surfaces

Basketball is played on a variety of surfaces, from the asphalt and concrete of urban playgrounds to double-sprung maple hardwood gym floors. Personal experience providing medical coverage for three-on-three tournaments on asphalt reveals what would be expected in terms of acute injuries—more abrasions and contusions from falling down than occur on a wooden floor. With respect to overuse syndromes from accumulation of microtrauma, many of us suspect that tendinopathies, enthesopathies, and stress fractures are all more common when the game is played on harder surfaces. One of us (Richards), who has traveled with a Canadian national team to many tournaments, has seen the number of athletes on the team suffering from patellar enthesis (jumper's knee) go from 4 to 12 after 1 week of tournament play on a rubberized concrete floor (the team had practiced only on hardwood before the tournament). Interestingly, the host team (Brazil), which trained regularly on this surface, did not experience a higher incidence of enthesitis than is normal in elite basketball. Perhaps gradual conditioning to playing on harder surfaces may actually strengthen entheses, tendons, or other tissues.

Minkoff and coworkers[20] cite a study performed by an independent research company for a flooring manufacturer,[21] which showed almost twice the incidence of injuries on synthetic surfaces as on maple hardwood floors in high schools. They point out that a lesser difference (10 percent higher incidence on synthetic floors) has been observed in college basketball.[3]

Games versus Practices

The intensity of practices varies with the time of season, level of play, particular team and coach, and other circumstances. Nonetheless, it comes as no surprise that injuries are relatively more frequent in games. The relative incidence of injury in games has been reported[1,4] to be between 2 and 7 times as high in games as in practices[1,4] Most teams need some amount of gamelike drills or intrasquad scrimmaging to be ready for competition, but coaches would be well advised to remember that their athletes' risk of injury is significantly higher in these situations.

Position Played

Insufficient data, and/or insufficient analysis thereof, do not allow any confident assertion about the vulnerability of certain positions to general or particular injuries. No significant positioned trends have been observed in the NBA[1] or other leagues.[2,3,5,7,11]

Shoes and Ankle Stabilizers

Most basketball players wear high-top or medium-cut sneakers designed specifically for basketball. Many also wear ankle stabilizers (braces) or have their ankles strapped with trainer's tape. There are two issues to consider in choosing sneakers and deciding whether or not to use additional ankle support: effects on injury and effects on performance.

In the laboratory, ankle stabilizers, ankle taping, and high-cut shoes have all been shown to reduce the range of motion of rearfoot inversion, with no reliable differences across studies.[22–29] Several of these studies showed that the restricting effect of tape was reduced after exercise,[23,26,30] leading the authors to question whether reusable stabilizers (braces) are not a better choice. However, all of these laboratory studies suffer from questionable extrapolation from restriction of range of motion to prevention of ankle sprains.

More importantly, some clinical studies have analyzed the effect of stabilizers or tape on the actual incidence of ankle sprains. In a retrospective multisport study, it was found that the combination of lace-up braces and low-cut shoes was most effective.[31] The authors suspect the low-cut shoes encouraged brace wearers to retighten their braces during competitions. The only published randomized prospective clinical trial of ankle braces in basketball was associated with a statistically significant reduction in the frequency of ankle sprains.[32] Another prospective, randomized trial examined the effect of high-cut versus low-cut shoes on ankle sprains in basketball and found no significant differences in injury rates.[33]

Braces or tape may reduce ankle injury, but many athletes are concerned or have a perception that they inhibit athletic performance. Several studies have provided some evidence of this.[34–36] However, several others disagree, finding no significant effect on performance.[37–40] These latter studies include several prospective, randomized, longer-term trials, lending more credence to their findings. It may be that wearing braces or taping requires some habituation to negate a temporary inhibition of performance found when they are first used.

In the end, it is (or should be) an athlete's choice whether or not to wear protective stabilizers or tape and what type of shoes to wear. In our opinion, athletes would be well advised to use either professionally applied tape or a reputable ankle stabilizer (brace). Lace-up shoes and/or braces should be retightened during a game if they loosen perceptibly. We feel the evidence warrants assurance to athletes that these preventive measures will not significantly alter their performance but will prevent some ankle sprains.

Training and Conditioning

We believe that proper training and conditioning is the single most important intervention in preventing injuries in basketball or sports in general. There is some literature to bolster that contention[42]; however, that is based to some extent on conventional wisdom and common sense. Aside from injury prevention, physical conditioning also has the important goal of improving athletic performance. Although it is not the focus of this chapter, we will examine several aspects of training and conditioning for basketball from a combined injury preventive and performance-enhancing perspective.

Adaptation to Specific Overload

Commonly accepted wisdom in sports medicine includes the principles of "overload" and "specific adaptation to imposed demand," which collectively assert that gradually progressive training and conditioning prevents injuries through strengthening of tissues in response to overloads which stimulate hypertrophy without significantly exceeding those tissues' envelope of load acceptance. There are many laboratory studies that corroborate that connective tissues respond to physical activity with hypertrophy.[42] In spite of the obvious inference that stronger tissues should lead to less trauma, there are few clinical studies that convincingly demonstrate this. Nonetheless, it remains conventional wisdom. Coupled with the demonstrated improvements in performance flowing from specific overload, it forms the cornerstone of athletic training and conditioning.

Training Variables and Training Errors

Many variables in the design of a training program can affect the desired outcomes. The frequency and duration of training sessions are the two most apparent; taken together, these are sometimes said to represent the "volume" of training. Equally important is the intensity of training in each session, which includes the strength, work, and power involved in executing prescribed movements or activities.

Attempts to increase any of the variables which determine volume or intensity of training by too much in one increment, or too quickly, are commonly called training errors. These errors of commission have been shown to cause injury.[43]

It is common practice in basketball, as in many other sports, to start the preseason training camp with "two per day" workouts. This volume and intensity is often more than the athletes are accustomed to (in spite of being warned to "report to camp in shape"). Our experience at the university, national team, and professional levels in basketball reveals an unfortunately high injury rate during this preseason training camp (unpublished data). Dialogue with coaches and trainers is an important mechanism to induce change in this aspect of the culture of sport, including basketball. Having said that, it is equally or perhaps more important for basketball players in elite leagues to train during their off-season so that "training camp" does not represent a "training error."

Periodization

Training regimens in basketball should be periodized across a 1-year cycle, so that attempts to alter an athlete's anatomic (e.g., hypertrophy) or physiologic (e.g., strength, power, endurance) substrate significantly occur during the competitive off-season. At other times, training can focus on technical skill development, game strategies, and so on, while maintaining adequate anatomic and physiologic substrate.[44]

Flexibility

That flexibility prevents injury and/or improves performance is another item of conventional wisdom with less scientific corroboration than one might expect. There are no studies that specifically show injury reduction through flexibility in basketball. The literature on flexibility and injury prevention in sports in general is controversial[45]; nonetheless, stretching is widely practiced and recommended.

It is increasingly common to avoid static stretching as part of the warm-up routine. Many believe that warming up tissues through gradual active movements is better. Attempts to improve flexibility through static stretching or proprioceptive neuromuscular facilitation may best be reserved for sessions between games or practices.

Strength, Power, and Endurance

Basketball is demanding of most aspects of locomotion. It requires strength, speed, and power over a wide range of time intervals. Hence, the basketball athlete requires truly balanced or broad development of muscular strength, speed, and strength endurance, and well-developed energy provision by all three systems for the production of resynthesis of intramuscular ATP (phosphocreatine, anaerobic glycolysis, and aerobic glycolysis).

Basketball athletes' training programs must, therefore, incorporate regimens of activity of sufficient specificity as to develop all of the necessary physiologic substrates for the game.

Balance, Coordination, Stability, and Proprioception

It is important to balance the strength and flexibility of agonists and antagonists across each motion segment (for example, strengthen flexion and extension of the knee, and stretch both quadriceps and hamstrings). Although this is true in general, it has received most attention with respect to the contribution of muscle imbalance to the rupture of ACLs.[16,17,46-48]

It is also important to strengthen the short, stabilizing muscles across each motion segment as much as the stronger, prime movers of that segment (for example, the rotator cuff muscles must be strengthened as well as pectoralis major).

Accumulated Exposure

Data from the National Basketball Association[1] indicates that more experienced players are injured more frequently. One obvious reason explaining this might be that virtually all "overuse" injuries have some component of accumulated microtrauma in their etiology. Accumulated exposures would be expected to generate such accumulated microtrauma. However, other confounding factors exist (such as more playing time for some more experienced players).

Fatigue

Data from the most detailed prospective observations of basketball injuries reveal that injuries are perhaps twice as common in the second half of games and much less common in the first quarter.[1,3] Whether this is due to fatigue as the game goes on or confounding factors such as increased participation of less experienced or skilled players (nonstarters) or increased intensity of play in the late parts of the game is not clear.

Level of Competition

As seen in Table 16-1, injury rates are higher among elite competitors than their recreational counterparts. No good statistical analyses exist to tell us what amount of this variance is due to the increased intensity or skill level of play per se, but we suspect that some of it is. Confounding variables correlated with elite play which might contribute to the increased injury rate independent of the intensity or skill level of play include length of games, frequency of exposure (less rest time between exposures), accumulated exposures (see above), or different officiating/interpretation of rules (see below).

Rules and Their Interpretation

Basketball is, in the rulebooks, a "noncontact" sport. Given this, one would expect that traumatic injuries due to collisions (other than with the floor) would be minimal. However, all that have played or watched it at a competitive level know that certain amounts of contact are explicitly or implicitly tolerated. At the highest competitive levels, collisions with considerable transfer of momentum occur routinely, and collisions with other players are responsible for a significant percentage of injuries.[1]

It follows that proper enforcement of the rules of the game and some control over the level of collisions tolerated might contribute to the prevention of basketball injuries, as it does in other sports.[49] Certainly, the extent to which elbows to heads, or hands on faces, are tolerated has such an effect.

Preexisting Disease or Injury

As in any sport, a basketball player with a past history of injury or illness may face increased risk of recurrence or other new injuries. Three situations warrant comment.

History of significant musculoskeletal injury or disease may predispose to a higher risk of further injury. Appropriate screening for, and advice about, such predisposing conditions should be provided to participants in organized basketball programs.

Cardiovascular problems may predispose a basketball player to further illness or even sudden death with intense activity. Recommendations for screening and guidelines for participation are discussed in "Sudden Death Syndrome" below.

Past history of concussion has been shown to increase risk of future concussions. Previous loss of consciousness (grade 3 concussion using the AAN classification[50]) increases relative risk of concussion by a factor of four in high school football.[51] Although this may not be exactly the case in basketball, it would seem reasonable to suspect that prior history of significant concussion in a basketball player may have increased risk of a recurrence with further competition. Athletes with prior history of head injury should be advised of these risks before competing.

GENERAL MEDICAL CONSIDERATIONS

Athletes playing basketball are subject to the same wide spectrum of general health disorders as those in most other sports. A physician caring for a basketball team or athlete needs to consider and attempt to prevent or be prepared to deal with all these issues, such as exercise-induced bronchospasm, diabetes, exercise in pregnancy, dermatologic conditions, and respiratory infections. We will not consider these further, as their prevention, diagnosis, and management are not specific to basketball. There is one general medical problem that stands out as having a significant incidence in basketball, which warrants closer consideration.

Sudden Death Syndrome

The American College of Cardiology and the American College of Sports Medicine have sponsored two conferences in Bethesda to formulate recommendations or guidelines for participation in sports for people with known cardiovascular disease or risks.[52,53]

One of the task forces in each of these conferences has classified sports according to their static and dynamic cardiovascular requirements. Basketball is classified as a high-intensity sport with moderate static and high dynamic demands.[54,55]

Approximately 35 percent of the sudden deaths occurring in sports in the United States occur in basketball.[56] However, it is not clear how disproportionate that may or may not be when compared to sports of similar intensity and normalized for participation rates in the United States. Nonetheless, publicity associated with the deaths of several well-known basketball players has generated a perception that playing basketball confers disproportionate risk of sudden death,[57-59] which may or may not be true.

Of sudden deaths among young people playing sports in the United States, 85 percent are of cardiovascular cause. Most of these are due to hypertrophic cardiomyopathies, with fewer due to anomalous or otherwise deficient coronary circulation.[56,60-62] Hypertrophic cardiomyopathy is more common in African-Americans than in Caucasian-Americans. The high participation rate in basketball among African-Americans may explain the apparent high incidence of sudden death in basketball to some extent. Even fewer of these sudden deaths are caused by cardiovascular anomalies such as aortic root dilatation and aortic dissection associated with Marfan's syndrome[63]; however, the high prevalence of Marfan's among tall people and the prevalence of tall people in basketball has led to obvious concern for possible risks to Marfanoid hoopsters.

The two Bethesda conferences[52,53] have generated detailed and specific recommendations for participation among people with identified disease, including coronary artery disease, congenital malformations, acquired valvular disease, cardiomyopathies, systemic hypertension, and arrhythmias. The reader is referred to these sources for details.

These recommendations have led to scrutiny of the efficiency and effectiveness of screening for abnormalities which would predict risk and/or preclude or limit participation based on the Bethesda guidelines. Routine history taking and physical examination appear to be of limited value,[56,64] but 12-lead resting electrocardiography may yield as much as one potentially high risk individual per 255 tests.[64] Stress electrocardiography is even more effective but inefficient such that it is only useful as a routine screening test at the elite levels of the game.

SPECIFIC COMMON INJURIES IN BASKETBALL

Ankle and Foot

As noted in Table 16-2 above, foot and ankle injuries represent the most commonly seen acute and chronic problems arising from basketball.

Ankle Ligament Injuries

By far the most common acute injury in basketball (other than minor contusions, which go unreported) is a sprain of the lateral ankle ligaments, especially the anterior talofibular ligament.[6,12,65] The bony architecture of the ankle is the primary stabilizer of the mortise in the weight-bearing position. The anterior talofibular ligament becomes the significant static stabilizer when the ankle is plantarflexed or rotated. The basketball court provides an ideal situation for the usual mechanism of first-time injury to the lateral ligamentous complex, as the player lands on the plantarflexed foot after a jump. In crowded situations under the "boards," this plantarflexed foot too often has ample opportunity to land on another player's foot.

The calcaneofibular ligament is rarely injured in isolation but is usually injured in association with the anterior talofibular ligament during massive inversion injuries.

The medial deltoid ligament consists of strong superficial and deep fibers that originate from the medial malleolus and fan out to the navicular, sustentaculum, and the talus. The dorsiflexion and eversion or external rotation forces necessary to rupture the deltoid ligament are not commonly seen on the basketball court.

In addition to the mechanism of injury, the physician should determine whether the patient was able to bear weight following the injury, as this is often an indicator of severity of injury. The presence of an audible snap or crack, the degree of swelling, and the presence of bruising following injury should be noted. In adolescent patients, it is important to determine whether the patient is skeletally mature, since physeal injuries to the distal tibia and fibula are more common than ligamentous injuries in children, and these areas should be palpated. The areas of maximum tenderness should be determined by examination. Palpation should also include the proximal fibula and the remainder of the foot to rule out associated injuries. Range of motion should be compared to the uninjured limb and is often limited by both pain and swelling. In the acutely injured ankle, stability testing can be difficult and is best performed early, while swelling is minimal. The anterior drawer test is positive when the talus subluxes forward out of the ankle mortise. A clunk may or may not be heard. The test signifies disruption of the anterior talofibular ligament. Positive inversion stress at neutral dorsiflexion signifies injury to the calcaneofibular ligament.

The need for roentgenographic evaluation of the ankle following injury is now more clearly defined by the "Ottawa Rules" (see Chap. 8).[66–68] When pain and tenderness are more directly over the malleoli (other than their anterior aspects where commonly injured ligaments originate) or when there is an inability to bear weight, anteroposterior, lateral, and mortise views are recommended. Foot x-rays are required if the tenderness is localized on either the base of the metatarsal or the navicular. MRI evaluation of the acutely injured ankle may reveal subchondral bone contusions or other lesions not easily detected by either clinical examination or x-rays (Fig. 16-1).

Management of ankle sprains has been well reviewed elsewhere.[69] Immediate management of the injured ankle includes protection from reinjury through modified activity (non-weight-bearing if this causes significant pain) and taping or bracing, compression and elevation to prevent swelling, ice or other cryotherapy, early mobilization, and perhaps nonsteroidal anti-inflammatory drugs. Immobilization and surgery have not been shown to yield better results and are not indicated except perhaps in the most severe injuries, such as complete dislocations. This is followed by muscle and tendon strengthening and postural stability exercises. Gradually, functional activities that are part of basketball, such as sudden stops and starts, lateral cuts, and landing on toes, are incorporated into the rehabilitation protocol. The ankle should be protected by taping and/or a stabilizer for the return to basketball, if this was not already being done prior to injury.

Tendon Injuries

The Achilles tendon, posterior tibialis, flexor hallucis, and peronei tendons are susceptible to both acute and chronic overuse injuries that can lead to disabling dysfunction. The Achilles tendon must support forces about the ankle during normal gait that are up to five times body mass. The repetitive jumping activity in basketball subjects the tendon to even higher forces. Furthermore, the region of the Achilles tendon 2 to 6 cm proximal to its bony insertion has a precarious blood supply that makes it most prone to injury.[70]

Insertional Achilles tendinitis is seen within the last 2 cm over the distal tendon. Tendinitis in this area can be associated with a calcaneal posterosuperior prominence that contributes to the symptoms of local tenderness and impingement pain. Retrocalcaneal bursitis may be a resulting or exacerbating factor. Intratendonous

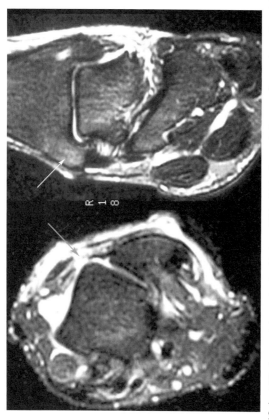

FIG. 16-1 MRI of an acutely sprained ankle in an NBA athlete. Arrows indicate a disrupted anterior talofibular ligament and an area of bone contusion medially.

318

calcification and fibrous degeneration have been observed in surgical specimens.

Noninsertional Achilles tendinitis is classified by stage and histology.[71] Isolated peritendinitis involves acute, chronic, or recurring inflammation of the peritenon with localized symptoms of pain, warmth, swelling, tenderness, and difficulty bearing weight. In stage 2, peritendinitis with tendonosis, there are fibrovascular degenerative changes with the tendon substance. Symptoms are similar to stage 1; however, a mass may be palpated. Pure tendonosis is seen in stage 3 with areas of atrophy, fibrovascular degeneration, or calcification without inflammatory changes. Swelling is minimal in this stage, and the palpable nodule is nontender. The latter stages may lead to rupture in the watershed region.

Initial treatment of Achilles tendinitis is nonsurgical. Basketball activities are modified, or in severe cases discontinued, until sufficient progress allows for nondestructive return to previous levels of functional activity. Gradually progressive strengthening, with careful attention to the magnitude and speed of eccentric loads, is often successful.[72] Adjuvant therapy such as nonsteroidal antiinflammatory drugs (NSAIDs) and ice can be used. A heel wedge of 1 to 2 cm in height can significantly reduce pain.[73] Cortisone injections are not recommended, even for stage 1 disease, as these can weaken the tendon and predispose it to spontaneous rupture. Insertional Achilles tendinitis may be difficult to treat in the basketball player. Modifications of the heel counter in the shoe may be necessary to alleviate direct pressure there.

Only when all conservative therapy fails should debridement of degenerative and calcified tissue and excision of any posterosuperior bony prominence be considered.

Complete ruptures of the Achilles tendon typically occur in the middle-aged males involved in activities that produce eccentric elongation of the tendon. Rupture of the tendon in the young adult or adolescent is unusual. A history of sudden onset of pain and swelling following minor trauma is common. Patients describe a sudden pop or a sensation of being hit from behind. There is a palpable defect in the tendon, although significant swelling and ecchymosis may mask this sign. The patient is unable to perform a single heel rise. The Thompson test is used to confirm the diagnosis. This is performed by having the patient kneel over a chair and squeezing the calf. The absence of a passive plantarflexion of the foot during this maneuver is diagnostic. Ultrasonography and MRI have both been used to evaluate both acute and chronic Achilles tendinopathy. Ultrasound can distinguish inflammation of the peritenon from either complete or partial rupture.[74] MRI also distinguishes rupture from inflammation or degeneration of tendon or peritenon.[75] The optimum treatment for the acute ruptures of the Achilles tendon remains controversial. In a prospective randomized study comparing operative and nonoperative management of acute ruptures of the Achilles tendon, the rate of rerupture was 8 percent in the nonoperative group compared with 4 percent in the surgical group.[76] However, no significant difference in the strength of plantarflexion was demonstrated. In general, the management of an acute Achilles tendon rupture in a basketball player needs to be individualized following a detailed discussion of the risks and benefits with the patient. At the elite level, the normal practice would lean toward surgical repair.

Basketball players can present with dysfunction of the tibialis posterior (TP) tendon. Biomechanical factors expose this tendon to stresses of repeated trauma in the region of the medial malleolus. In this same area, the mesotenon is scarce, and a consistent area of hypovascularity is produced just distal to the medial malleolus.[77] Johnson and Strom[78] have classified this entity into three stages. The young basketball athlete is most likely to present with stage 1 disease characterized by pain, swelling, and mild weakness of the posterior tibial tendon but no secondary foot deformity.[79] The pain may not be confined to the region between the navicular and the medial malleolus but may extend to behind the malleolus proximally for some distance. Local tenderness and swelling are consistent with the tenosynovitis. While the patient is able to perform a single limb stance, the task is often painful. Rupture of the tibialis posterior tendon without foot deformity, stage 2, is even more uncommon in young athletes. The diagnosis of tibialis posterior tendon dysfunction in the basketball player is made clinically. MRI has been found to be useful in evaluating the status of the tendon preoperatively when conservative measures fail.[80] Early diagnosis is crucial to prevent the onset of progressive foot deformity. The basketball player who presents with stage 1 tendinopathy can be managed conservatively with general principles of rehabilitation to resolve the acute symptoms. An orthosis that provides support to the longitudinal arch while limiting heel valgus, such as the UCBL (University of California Biomechanics Laboratory) orthosis, may be helpful. Acute rupture, when seen in the young athlete, may be treated surgically with augmentation with flexor digitorum longus or flexor hallucis longus.[81]

The flexor hallucis longus (FHL) tendon is also prone to repetitive trauma in the basketball player. At the level of the talus, the FHL tendon passes through a restrictive fibro-osseous tunnel. Functionally the long flexor of the great toe is important for push off. This explains why the highest incidence of FHL tendinitis occurs in ballet dancers and jumpers. Overuse activities can lead to a stenosing tenosynovitis and secondary posterior ankle impingement, if the cycle is not halted. In addition to the usual site of impingement at the entrance of the fibro-osseous tunnel, stenosis may occur proximally behind the medial malleolus or distally between the hallux sesamoids. Pain is localized deep to the medial side of the Achilles tendon. This can be exacerbated by resisted plantarflexion or passive dorsiflexion of the great toe with the ankle and first metatarsal supported in a neutral position.[82] MRI is useful when the diagnosis is unclear. Nonsurgical treatment with rest, ice, and nonsteroidal anti-inflammatories is usually successful. In the early phase of treatment, taping the great toe in a position of plantarflexion may also help. When conservative measures fail, tenosynovectomy and debridement are indicated.

The peronei play a role as dynamic lateral stabilizers of the ankle joint. The peroneus longus tendon is necessary for normal lateral push off. Despite its long course from behind the fibular malleolus to its insertion on the first metatarsal, acute rupture and tenosynovitis of peroneus longus are rare. The peroneus brevis is closer to the fibula and the lateral malleolus, and while acute rupture of the peroneus brevis tendon is rare, degenerative tears of this tendon are common.[83] The severity of the pathology can range from mild fraying to extensive longitudinal tears.[84] Pain and swelling are located behind the lateral malleolus and can be exacerbated by passive inversion of the ankle or eversion against resistance. The ankle should also be assessed for associated recurrent instability. MRI can localize abnormal pathology. Temporary modification of activity, orthotic support for the medial longitudinal arch, and strengthening exercises for TP and FHL are cornerstones of treatment. NSAIDs may be adjuvant therapy. Only if nonsurgical measures are unsuccessful may intratendonous debridement be indicated.

Subluxation of the peroneal tendons may occur when the superior peroneal retinaculum avulses from its fibular attachment during acute dorsiflexion of the ankle coupled with a forced contraction of the peronei.[85] These injuries are often mistaken for ligamentous injuries; however, the pain and tenderness of the acute peroneal subluxation is retromalleolor. Radiographs may demonstrate small fragments of bone at the site where the retinaculum avulsed form the distal fibula. Recurrent instability of the peroneal tendons is unusual and presents with a history of recurrent and often painful snapping over the distal fibula. This can sometimes be managed adequately with taping that includes a pad over the peroneal tendons. When symptomatic recurrent subluxation of the peronei is unmanageable and sufficiently bothersome, soft tissue reconstruction may be considered.[86]

Fractures

Anterior avulsion fractures of the calcaneus can occur in basketball players. The bifurcate ligament, originating from the anterior calcaneal process and attaching to both the cuboid and the navicular, avulses off its proximal attachment during an inversion-plantarflexion mechanism. These fractures may initially be diagnosed as severe ligament sprains, and recovery may be prolonged. Pain is localized to the region of the sinus tarsi. The oblique radiograph of the foot may identify an avulsed fragment of bone. Nonoperative treatment with cast immobilization usually yields good results. Surgery is reserved for fractures with large avulsion fragments or for symptomatic nonunions.[87]

Fractures of the navicular tuberosity occur with forced eversion of the foot and subsequent avulsion of the posterior tibial tendon as it forcefully contracts. The fracture is usually held in an undisplaced position by the multiple slips of the tibialis posterior tendon to other bones and the insertion of the deltoid to the navicular. Tenderness is localized, and x-rays are helpful in distinguishing the lesion from an accessory os naviculare. Cast immobilization is usually all that is required of the acute injury. Although they usually heal with fibrous union, this often is asymptomatic. Excision of the avulsed fragment is indicated for symptomatic nonunions. Stress fractures of the navicular can also be seen in basketball players, and the diagnosis should always be considered in any athlete with chronic vague midfoot pain from repeated jumping and running.[88] Undisplaced fractures are treated with non-weight-bearing for 6 to 8 weeks. Displaced fractures require stabilization.

The os trigonum is a posterolateral accessory ossicle seen in only 10 percent of the population. Fractures of the os trigonum are most commonly seen in dancers or soccer players but can be seen in basketball players when the plantarflexed foot takes the weight of another player's body.[89] Stress fractures of the os trigonum can also occur in the absence of any specific history of trauma. Pain is posterior although symptoms may be vague. Swelling and bruising may be present. Because of the proximity to the flexor hallucis longus tendon, motion of the great toe may exacerbate the pain. The lateral x-ray is used to identify the irregular borders suggestive of an acute fracture of the os trigonum. Bone scan is also used to distinguish the normal os trigonum for fracture or fibrous detachment. Early immobilization is usually successful. When pain is persistent in the presence of increased uptake on bone scan, excision is advocated.

The Jones fracture of the proximal diaphysis of the fifth metatarsal and the avulsion fracture of the same bone are two distinct entities with varying locations, injury mechanisms, and prognoses.[90] Either can occur in isolation in the basketball player, and they must be distinguished from each other in order to implement adequate treatment. The region of the proximal diaphysis of the fifth metatarsal is relatively hypovascular, and this contributes to the significant risk of delayed or nonunion of the Jones fracture.[91] Historically, the avulsion fracture is felt to arise from force contraction of the peroneus brevis tendon at the tuberosity. In contrast, the acute Jones fracture occurs when the forefoot is loaded laterally while pivoting. The chronic form is a fatigue fracture typically in the young athlete. Fractures at the base of the fifth metatarsal will present with local tenderness. Radiographs may initially be normal in the fatigue fracture, and bone scan may be needed to confirm the suspicion. The current standard care for the elite basketball athlete with an acute Jones fracture is percutaneous screw fixation (Fig. 16-2); however, the acute Jones fracture and the more benign tuberosity avulsion fracture may be treated in a below-knee non-weight-bearing cast for 6 weeks. Longer periods of casting are needed for delayed unions of Jones fractures, but operative treatment is again advised for the young or high-level athlete with this problem. Established nonunions require internal fixation.

HEEL PAIN AND FASCIITIS

Heel pain is extremely common among all athletes. The differential diagnosis for this complaint is large and includes plantar fasciitis, bursitis, tendinitis, apophysitis, fracture, nerve entrapment, tumor, foreign body, and infection.[92] History and physical examination will usually help to differentiate the pathology. Radiographs, bone scan, MRI, and electrophysiology are ordered as needed when the diagnosis remains unclear. The pain of plantar fasciitis is accentuated by running or jumping activities. Pain can be intense in the morning following a prolonged sleep with the foot in the plantarflexed position. Tenderness is typically plantar and medially where the fascia originates from the medial calcaneal tuberosity. The mainstay of treatment of plantar fasciitis is nonsurgical with a strict regimen of NSAIDs, heel pads, and stretching of the plantar fascia and Achilles tendon. Cortisone injections in the region of pathology may be useful. A night dorsiflexion splint can be used for both acute flare-ups and as a preventive measure. Plantar fascia release should only be performed after a prolonged period of unsuccessful conservative therapy.[93]

ANTERIOR ANKLE IMPINGEMENT

The pathogenesis of anterior ankle impingement in the basketball player probably begins with a traumatic injury to the lateral ankle

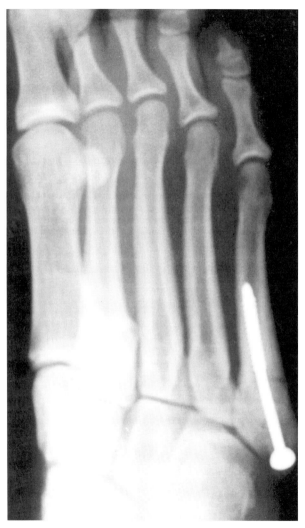

FIG. 16-2 Postoperative x-ray after percutaneous screw fixation of an acute Jones fracture in an NBA athlete.

ligaments. Subsequent laxity and synovial and capsular soft tissue scarring contribute to the pathology. Osteophytes then develop specifically between the distal tibia and the neck of the talus. Pain is with dorsiflexion activities, and as osteophytes enlarge, range of motion can be restricted. Lateral x-rays will reveal the site of disease. Conservative therapy may begin with a heel lift and manual mobilization of the talocrural joint to increase its range of motion. If this fails to alleviate the symptoms, an excision of the osteophyte may be performed either openly or arthroscopically.[94]

OSTEOCHONDRITIS DISSECANS

Osteochondral defects of the talar dome can occur insidiously. Traumatic lesions are more commonly posteromedial, while atraumatic lesions are usually anterolateral. Symptoms are related not only to the size and the location of the lesion, but also to its stability. Pain, locking, or a feeling of giving way can all be presenting symptoms. When pain radiographs do not show the defect, computed tomography or MRI is indicated.[95] In the skeletally immature basketball player, the prognosis with conservative therapy is good, and a brief period in a patella tendon bearing cast will usually suffice. Operative treatment in adults who do not respond to conservative measures depends on the size, location, and stability of the fragment.[96]

KNEE INJURIES

Basketball players are prone to a variety of acute and overuse injuries about the knee. The great majority of these injuries arise from noncontact mechanisms.

Acute Knee Injuries

With frequent episodes of acceleration and deceleration, internal and external tibial rotation, and continuous pivoting, the opportunity to injure the anterior cruciate ligament (ACL) during basketball activity is high. The player with an acutely injured ACL is almost always unable to return to the basketball court following the traumatic event. A pop or tear heard on the court is indicative of an ACL injury. Early swelling is suggestive of an acute hemarthrosis. Weight bearing will be difficult but may not correlate with injury severity. Injury-specific tests such as the Lachman, anterior drawer, and the pivot shift usually confirm the diagnosis but may be difficult to perform in the acutely swollen knee. The Lachman test appears to be the most reliable in the acutely injured knee.[97] MRI will demonstrate the acute or chronic tear as well as associated bone bruises and meniscal injuries (Fig. 16-3).[98] The definitive management of the ACL-deficient knee is individualized to the patient's activities and level of participation. While the initial management involves physical therapy to restore range of motion and muscle strengthening, the young basketball athlete who wishes to continue playing competitively is unlikely to tolerate the cutting and pivoting that the game demands without reconstruction. The role of functional or rehabilitative braces following ACL injuries remains controversial. Braces are generally used to supplement the nonoperative rehabilitation regimen or the surgical ACL reconstruction; the player who returns back to basketball should not be under the impression that the brace will prevent further injury.[99,100]

Meniscal injuries can occur in isolation or in association with ACL or medial cruciate ligament (MCL) tears. Pain is localized over the joint line, and the painful arc of motion depends on the location of the pathology. Mechanical symptoms such as locking, giving way, and swelling may also be evident. McMurray's test is helpful when present but is not specific for meniscal disease. MRI is the investigation of choice when physical examination remains unclear. When symptoms are significantly disabling, therapeutic arthroscopy is required for repair or partial meniscectomy, followed by rehabilitation and gradual return to sports. The reparable meniscus lesion requires protected weight bearing for 4 to 6 weeks. The basketball player with a reparable meniscus tear and a torn ACL warrants more aggressive treatment of the ligament injury to increase the chance of a successful cartilage repair.[46]

Overuse Injuries of the Knee Extensor Mechanism

Derangement of the patellar mechanism is extremely common in basketball players, particularly at the competitive levels.[1,3,101] Microscopic tissue failure and/or inflammation along the patellar or quadriceps tendons or their insertional entheses at the patella or tibia are collectively known as jumper's knee. Eccentric contractions during repeated jumping predisposes the basketball player to this sometimes disabling problem.[72] Patients can present with activity-related anterior knee pain and tenderness over the patellar tendon at its bony insertion. Pathological changes in this area include acute or chronic inflammation and mucoid degeneration. MRI is valuable in demonstrating the extent of disease (Fig. 16-4).[102] A strict training program with eccentric strengthening is critical in avoiding or treating jumper's knee.[72] Early diagnosis is the key to implementing prompt treatment and halting the cycle of inflammation. Nonsteroidal anti-inflammatory drugs, ice, ultrasound therapy, and a period of avoidance of jumping is the initial treat-

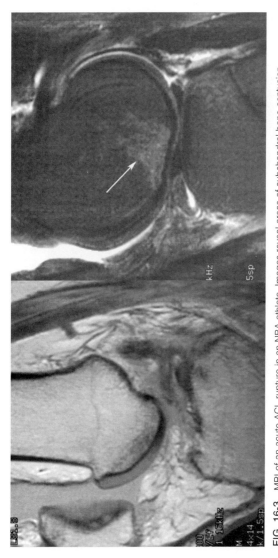

FIG. 16-3 MRI of an acute ACL rupture in an NBA athlete. Images reveal areas of subchondral bone contusion in addition to the disruption of the ligament.

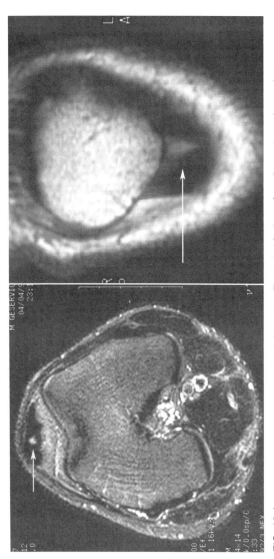

FIG. 16-4 MRI of acute "jumper's knee" in an NBA athlete. The typical findings of patellar tendon enthesopathy are seen as an area of increased signal in the central third of the tendon just distal to the inferior pole of the patella (*arrows*).

ment. Eventually, eccentric contractions can be attempted, but isometric and concentric activity must be mastered first.

The requirement to temporarily curtail jumping is usually the biggest barrier to successful treatment in basketball players. It is often difficult to obtain a suitable interval free of further damaging eccentric exercise (jumping) during which the extensor mechanism can be gradually strengthened. Noncompliance in this regard explains the high prevalence of chronic patellar enthesopathy in basketball.

Cortisone injections in the region of the patellar tendon should be completely avoided; steroids weaken the tendon and may lead to spontaneous rupture.[103] Ruptures of the patella tendon or the quadriceps tendon may also occur after weakening by chronic inflammation or following an acute eccentric contraction. Disruptions of the extensor mechanisms warrant surgical management, and when treated early, good results are achieved.[104] Rarely, a chronic case of jumper's knee is refractory to all nonoperative measures when they are given adequate trials. Only then is surgical debridement indicated.

In the skeletally immature player, jumper's knee presents as a traction apophysitis at the tibial tubercle called Osgood-Schlatter disease. Sinden-Larsen-Johanssen syndrome refers to inflammation of the patellar tendon at the inferior pole of the patella in the adolescent. Signs and symptoms of these entities are similar to the adult forms, and treatment is nonoperative.

Patellofemoral pain and eventually arthrosis often occur with repeated running and jumping. It comes as no surprise that basketball is fertile ground for this problem. Maltracking of the patella caused by dynamic forces (imbalance of quadricep strength between vasti medialis and lateralis, or rotation of the knee with hyperpronation of the foot) or rotational abnormalities of the femur or tibia are often implicated in this syndrome.[105]

Patellofemoral pain is best prevented and treated by proper training, conditioning, and equipment. The basketball player regardless of caliber should avoid open-chain kinetic exercises that tend to place excessive stress on the patellofemoral joint. Increasing endurance and strengthening gradually will avoid sudden stresses of the patellar mechanism. Careful attention to alignment of the foot and knee and awareness of muscle tone in vastus medialis are critical to achieve strengthening of the quadriceps mechanism. Motion control features in the shoe can be helpful in preventing contributory hyperpronation. Unfortunately, basketball shoes do not come with as wide a spectrum of stabilizing features as shoes for running per se. It is, therefore, often necessary to replace or supplement the manufacturers insole with one custom-fitted to the athlete's foot, with built-in corrections or support to prevent hyperpronation.

Conservative therapy is usually successful, and surgery is rarely indicated for the patient with a documented structural abnormality whose symptoms do not resolve with therapy. Such surgery is usually limited to minimal debridement.

UPPER EXTREMITY INJURIES

As noted above, injuries to the hand and wrist are very common in basketball.[1–3,5,7,10,11,106]

Before commenting on specific hand and wrist injuries, we note that the treatment of these injuries in basketball is very aggressive. Early consultation with a hand specialist is critical. Early mobilization and functional splinting often allow a return to activity much quicker than is suggested by the hand surgery literature. Early compression of injured digits, with an elasticized wrap such as Coban, is critical to prevent excessive swelling. Where hand specialists often use volar splints, we will fashion a dorsal splint to allow volar contact with a basketball. Although the ideal angle of flexion for splinting of some injuries may vary, we will usually splint a finger with the hand placed on a basketball, such that the flexion of the digits matches the curve of the ball. This allows as early as possible return to partial basketball activities and minimizes the loss of ball skills during rehabilitation from hand injuries. This is most critical for injuries to the primary shooting hand.

Injuries to the Fingers

Injuries to digits 2 to 5 are most common. Commonly referred to by players as a "jammed finger," there are several variations on this theme. The proximal interphalangeal joints (PIPJs) are most often injured, followed by the distal interphalangeal joints (DIPJs), phalanges, metacarpals, metacarpophalangeal joints (MCPJs), and the carpometacarpal joints (CMCJs).

Injuries to the PIPJs include fractures and dislocations, as well as sprains and ruptures of the collateral ligaments. Collateral sprain or tears occur with hyperabduction or hyperadduction at the PIPJ. Treatment is conservative with buddy taping and early range of motion. Usually the athlete is able to return to basketball quickly with functional splinting or taping.

Volar plate rupture occurs with hyperextension of the PIPJ and leads to dorsal PIP dislocation. Tenderness is over the volar plate of the joint, and lateral x-rays confirm the direction of the distal fragment (Fig. 16-5). These isolated dislocations are usually stable following closed reduction and can be treated with 4 to 5 days of immobilization followed by early range of motion.[107] Dorsal PIPJ fracture-dislocations may be more difficult to treat. The fracture is

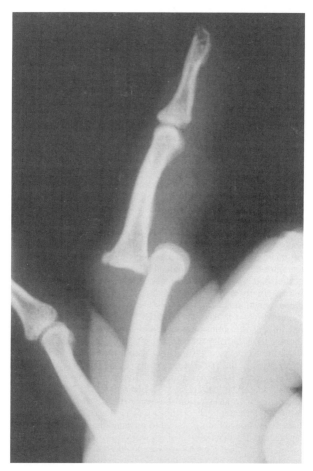

FIG. 16-5   X-ray of a dorsal PIPJ dislocation in an elite female basketball player.

an avulsion of the volar base of the middle phalanx that can vary in size, and when the collateral are attached to this fragment, the fracture is unstable. Stable fracture-dislocations can be treated with early mobilization, similar to the isolated dislocations. Unstable fracture-dislocations require extension block splinting or open reduction with fixation, if the fragment involves more than 50 percent of the articular surface, or excision and volar plate advancement, if the fragment is irreparable. The principle of any treatment option should be to obtain and maintain joint congruity and to initiate early motion and maximize joint function.

Volar dislocations at the PIPJ are less common. They occur after forced varus or valgus load with a volar impact. The pathology includes injury to one of the collaterals, an incomplete volar plate tear, and a disruption of the central slip. The acute finger is swollen at the PIPJ. The injury may be missed because the patient may use the lateral bands to extend the PIPJ. However, weakness is demonstrated with resisted extension, and pain is dorsal. It is the central slip injury, which if left unrecognized, will lead to a posttraumatic boutonniere deformity. For this reason, these injuries are best treated early with extension splinting and close observation.[108]

Soft tissue injuries of the metacarpophalangeal joints are common in basketball players. Dorsal dislocations occur with forced hyperextension of the joint. Simple dislocations are easy to reduce and should temporarily be splinted in 70 degrees of flexion to avoid contracture of the collateral ligaments and subsequent stiffness. Complex dislocations are irreducible due to soft tissue interposition of the volar plate. The metacarpal head is trapped between the lumbrical radially and the flexor digitorum profundus tendon ulnarly. Open reduction is necessary.

Intraarticular fractures at the MCPJ can usually be treated nonoperatively with brief immobilization and buddy taping and early mobilization. Surgery is reserved for fractures with large fragments that can be reduced and surgically stabilized.

Avulsion of the extensor mechanism at the DIPJ may result in a mallet finger if left unrecognized.[109] This injury is common in basketball with axial loading of the finger against the ball. It may be associated with an avulsion fracture of the distal phalanx. In the skeletally immature patient, this is a Salter-Harris type I or III fracture. Extension splinting is used to prevent a late mallet deformity and recurrent subluxation. This is worn full-time for 3 weeks followed by another 3 weeks of wear as the player returns back to activities.[110] Surgery is recommended for joint subluxation associated with large fragments.

Fractures or dislocations of any of the CMCJs other than the thumb (discussed separately below) may occur after direct trauma or crush from the weight of an opponent's body. Dorsal dislocations are more common at this joint, and it is often the lateral or oblique x-rays that demonstrate the pathology. These are usually stable following reduction. Dislocation of multiple CMCJs should be treated surgically. The reverse Bennett's fracture is an intraarticular fracture at the base of the fifth metacarpal that mirrors the thumb fracture. The deforming force is the extensor carpi ulnaris tendon. This fracture must be reduced and held reduced by casting or preferably pin fixation.

Thumb Injuries

The human thumb by nature of its mobility and ability to oppose in space is prone to a number of very common injuries. Bony stability is imperative in controlling and handling the basketball. The thumb is commonly injured in falls on the floor, when "jammed" on the rim during a "dunk," or when struck by an opponent.

Gamekeeper's thumb, or injury to the ulnar collateral ligament (UCL) at the MCPJ of the thumb, is the most common of these injuries and occurs with hyperextension and hyperabduction of the joint. The UCL usually avulses distally, and the adductor pollicis aponeurosis may come to interpose and prevent proper reduction and healing of the ligament to bone, a complication known as the Stener lesion.[111] Acute injuries present with pain and tenderness directly over the site of the ulnar collateral ligament at the thumb MCPJ. Plain radiographs are taken to demonstrate any avulsion fractures from the proximal phalanx. Only after plain radiographs are assessed should stress views be taken. Angulation of greater than 35 degrees, or 15 degrees compared to the uninjured side, confirms a complete tear of the UCL, and surgery is recommended to prevent chronic instability and joint incongruity. Surgery is also indicated if the joint is irreducible or if intraarticular bony fragments are seen on plain radiographs. Incomplete tears can be treated with immobilization in a thumb spica for a period of days to a few weeks (depending on severity) with the MCPJ at 30 degrees of flexion, followed by functional taping or splinting.

Other thumb injuries such as dislocation of the MCPJ, Bennett's fracture, and the Rolando fracture are more rare and are treated in the manner dictated by current practices of consulting hand specialists.

Wrist Injuries

Injuries to the carpus can be bony, ligamentous, or cartilaginous. History usually reveals a fall on the outstretched hand. The exact site of pain and tenderness must be determined on physical examination, and radiographs including anterorposterior, lateral, and oblique should be taken when indicated. Bone scan, CT scan, or MRI may assist in the diagnosis of occult carpal fractures. MRI or ultrasonography may be used to assist diagnosis of triangular fibrocartilage injury.

The management of wrist injuries in basketball does not differ significantly from what is done for athletes in other sports (or nonathletes).

OROFACIAL INJURIES

The aspect of the game of basketball played "in the paint," or in the key under the basket, generates many injuries to the face. Players jostling for position under the net, holding their opponents at bay ("boxing out") with arms and elbows, and fighting for possession of a ball rebounding from a missed shot attempt all make for many elbows and fingers in faces.

Eye Injuries

The frequency and types of eye injuries in elite basketball have been well documented.[112] Corneal abrasions, lid lacerations, orbital blow-out fractures, and scleral lacerations all occur with significant frequency.

Symptoms that contraindicate a return to play without ophthalmologic (slit lamp) examination and/or treatment are significant loss of vision, photophobia, diplopia, or sudden onset of visual flashes or floaters.

Initial examination must include visual acuity, visual fields, close inspection of the eyelid margins and canthi, ophthalmoscopic examination of iris detail and the fundus, extraocular movements, pupil shape and responsiveness, corneal/conjunctival integrity (using fluorescein stain and cobalt blue light), and palpation of the orbital margins and periorbital tissues. Return to play without further examination or treatment is contraindicated by loss of visual acuity (this makes a baseline assessment important); loss of visual fields (suspected detached retina); unclear iris details (suspected hyphema); loss of extraocular movements or diplopia with extremes of range (suspected blow-out fracture); subcutaneous emphysema or palpable tender deformity of orbital margins (suspected blow-out fracture); laceration of lid margins, canthi, cornea or sclera; or swelling that prevents adequate opening of the palpebral fissure.

Many of these injuries, certainly the ones caused by fingers poking eyes, could be prevented by the use of polycarbonate lens protective eyewear. While frames and lenses of sufficient strength to merit CSA approval for racquet sports would probably also help prevent some blow-out fractures, thinner polycarbonate lenses (inadequate for racquet sports), such as Oakley eyeguards, perform admirably in basketball. The ball is large enough that impact with such thinner polycarbonate lenses will not cause them to crack into the eye.[113] An increasing number of players in the NBA are starting to "see the light" and protect their vision.

Oral and Dental Injuries

Injuries to the lips, cheeks, jaw, and teeth are also common in basketball. These are also caused mostly by contact with opponent's elbows. Lip and cheek lacerations, maxillary and mandibular fractures, temperomandibular sprains and contusions, and dental fractures, luxations, and avulsions occur all too frequently.[114] Some tooth avulsions have been reported from entanglement with the net.[115]

Prevention is most desirable. Aside from issues surrounding officiating and interpretation of the rules of the game, the most obvious preventive measure is the use of custom-fitted mouthguards. It is also important to have elective dental work taken care of in a timely fashion, to prevent in-season dental emergencies, as well as to reduce the risk of mandibular fracture after extractions (elective extractions should occur as soon as possible after the end of a season, to allow maximum time for bone healing before the next season).

When covering basketball games without the luxury of an attending dentist, the physician's kit should include a few dental supplies: eugenol (oil of clove) for the relief of dental pain, a stock or "boil and bite" mouthguard for emergency use in the absence of a custom-fitted guard, a container of Hank's balanced salt solution (available from 3M Company as the Save-a-Tooth kit) for the preservation of avulsed teeth, and temporary filling material (such as zinc oxide paste). Luxated teeth should be reduced immediately. Avulsed teeth should be replaced in the socket from whence they came, if that can be identified. If multiple teeth have been avulsed, it may be better to place them in Hank's solution (milk, saline, or water are better than nothing) and let a dentist sort them out. Avulsed teeth should not be debrided of any loose tissue remaining attached to them.

REFERENCES

1. NBTA: Injury Report, 1995-98. National Basketball Trainers Association, 1998.
2. Henry JH, Lareau B, Neigut D: The injury rate in professional basketball. *Am J Sports* 10:16-18, 1982.
3. NCAA: 1989-90, Basketball. National Collegiate Athletics Association injury surveillance statistics. National Collegiate Athletics Association, 1990.
4. Gomez E, DeLee JC, Farney WC: Incidence of injury in Texas girls' high school basketball. *Am J Sports Med* 24:684-687, 1996.

5. Rocca G: Basketball traumatology. Epidemiologic study. *Medicina dello Sport* 50:317-324, 1997.

6. Leanderson J, Nemeth G, Eriksson E: Ankle injuries in basketball players. *Knee Surg Sport Traumatol Arthrosc* 1:200-202, 1993.

7. Hickey GJ, Fricker PA, McDonald WA: Injuries to young elite female basketball players of a six-year period. *Clin J Sport Med* 7:252-256, 1997.

8. Chandy TA, Grana WA: Secondary school athletic injuries in boys and girls. A three year comparison. *Physician Sports Med* 13:106-111, 1985.

9. Brison RJ, Macnab RB, Arthur-Quinney H, Voaklander DC: The epidemiology of contact sport injuries treated in an emergency department. Gloucester, Ontario, Canadian Fitness and Lifestyle Research Institute, 1992.

10. Kujala UM, Taimela S, Antti-Poika I, et al: Acute injuries in soccer, ice hockey, volleyball, basketball, judo, and karate-Analysis of National Registry data. *Br Med J*, 311:1465-1468, 1995.

11. Zelisko JA, Noble HB, Porter M: A comparison of men's and women's professional basketball injuries. *Am J Sports Med* 10:297-299, 1982.

12. DeHaven KE, Lintner DM: Athletic injuries: Comparison by age, sports and gender. *Am J Sports* 14:218, 1986.

13. Ireland ML, Wall C: Epidemiology and comparison of knee injuries in elite male and female United States basketball athletes. *Med Sci Sports Exercise* 22:592, 1990.

14. Arendt EA, Dick R: Knee injury patterns among men and women in collegiate basketball and soccer: NCAA data and review of literature. *Am J Sports Med* 23:694-701, 1995.

15. Arendt EA, Teitz CC: The lower extremities, in Teitz CC (ed): *The Female Athlete*. Rosemont, IL, American Academy of Orthopaedic Surgeons; 1997, pp. 45-62.

16. Huston LJ, Wojtys EM: Neuromuscular performance characteristics in elite female athletes. *Am J Sports Med* 24:427-436, 1996.

17. Hewett TE, Stroupe AL, Nance TA, Noyes FR: Plyometric training in female athletes-Decreased impact forces and increased hamstring torques. *Am J Sports Med* 24:765-773, 1996.

18. Souryal TO, Freeman TR: Intercondylar notch size and anterior cruciate ligament injuries in athletes: A prospective study. *Am J Sports Med* 21: 535-539, 1993.

19. LaPrade RF, Burnett QM, II: Femoral intercondylar notch stenosis and correlation to anterior cruciate ligament injuries: A prospective study. *Am J Sports Med*, 22:198-203, 1994.

20. Minkoff J, Simonson BG, Sherman OH, Cavaliere G: Injuries in basketball in Renström PAFH (ed): *Clinical Practice of Sports Injury Prevention and Care*. Oxford, Blackwell Scientific Publications, 1994, pp. 303-353.

21. MFMA: Incidence of Injury Study: Maple flooring vs. synthetic. Maple Flooring Manufacturers Association, 1988.

22. Garrick JG, Requa RK: Role of external support in the prevention of ankle sprains. *Med Sports Exercise* 5:200-203, 1973.

23. Greene TA, Hillman SK: Comparison of support provided by a semi-rigid orthosis and adhesive ankle taping before, during, and after exercise. *Am J Sports Med* 18:498-506, 1990.

24. Wilkerson GB: Comparative biomechanical effects of the standard method of ankle taping and a taping method designed to enhance subtalar stability. *Am J Sports Med* 19:588-595, 1991.

25. Karlsson J, Sward L, Andreasson GO: The effect of taping on ankle stability: Practical implications. *Sports Med* 16:210-215, 1993.

26. Shapiro MS, Kabo JM, Mitchell PW, et al: Ankle sprain prophylaxis: An analysis of the stabilizing effects of braces and tape. *Am J Sports Med* 22:78-82, 1994.

27. Gross MT, Batten AM, Lamm AL, et al: Comparison of DonJoy ankle ligament protector and subtalar sling ankle taping in restricting foot and ankle motion before, during, and after exercise. *J Orthopaed Sports Physical Ther* 19:33-41, 1994.

28. Ottaviani RA, Ashton-Miller JA, Kothari SU, Wojtys EM: Basketball shoe height and the maximal muscular resistance to applied ankle inversion and eversion moments. *Am J Sports Med* 23:418-423, 1995.

29. Stacoff A, Steger J, Stussi E, Reinschmidt C: Lateral stability in sideward cutting movements. *Med Sci Sports Exercise* 28:350-358, 1996.

30. Furnich RM, Ellison, AE, Guerini GJ: The measured effect of taping on combined foot and ankle motion before and after exercise. *Am J Sports Med* 9:165-170, 1981.

31. Rovere GD, Clarke TJ, Yates SC, Burley K: Retrospective comparison of taping and ankle stabilizers in preventing ankle injuries. *Am J Sports Med* 16:228-233, 1988.

32. Sitler M, Ryan J, Wheeler B, et al: The efficacy of a semirigid ankle stabilizer to reduce acute ankle injuries in basketball-a randomized clinical study at West Point. *Am J Sports Med* 22:454-461, 1994.

33. Barrett JR, Tanji JL, Drake C, et al: High-top versus low-top shoes for the prevention of ankle sprains in basketball players-a prospective randomized study. *Am J Sports Med* 21:582-585, 1993.

34. Burks RT, Bean BG, Marcus R, Barker HB: Analysis of athletic performance with prophylactic ankle devices. *Am J Sports Med* 19: 104-106, 1990.

35. MacKean LC, Bell G, Burnham RS: Prophylactic ankle bracing vs. taping: Effects on functional performance in female basketball players. *J Orthopaed Sports Physical Ther* 22:77-81, 1995.

36. Brizuela G, Llana S, Ferrandis A, Garcia-Belenguer AC: The influence of basketball shoes with increased ankle support on shock attenuation and performance in running and jumping. *J Sports Sci* 15:505-515, 1997.

37. Robinson JR, Frederick EC, Cooper LB: Systematic ankle stabilization and the effect on performance. *Med Sci Sports Exercise* 18:625-628, 1986.

38. Gross MT, Everts JR, Robertson SJ, et al: Effect of DonJoy ankle ligament protector and Aircast sport-stirrup orthoses on functional performance. *J Orthopaed Sports Physical Ther* 22:77-81, 1994.

39. Pienkowski D, McMorrow M, Shapiro R, et al: The effect of ankle stablizers on athletic performance-a randomized prospective study. *Am J Sports Med* 23:757-762, 1995.

40. Locke A, Sitler M, Aland C, Kimura I: Long-term use of a softshell prophylactic ankle stabilizer on speed, agility, and vertical jump performance. *J Sport Rehab* 6:235-245, 1997.

41. Renström PAH (ed): *Sports Injuries: Basic Principles of Prevention and Care.* Oxford: Blackwell Scientific Publications, 1993.

42. Chandler TJ, Kibler WB: Muscle training in injury prevention, in Renström PAFH (ed): *Sports Injuries: Basic Principles of Prevention and Care.* Oxford, Blackwell Scientific Publications, 1993, pp. 252-261.

43. Taunton JE: Training erros, in Renström PAFH (ed): *Sports Injuries: Basic Principles of Prevention and Care.* Oxford, Blackwell Scientific Publications, 1993, pp. 205-212.

44. Stone WJ, Steingard PM: Year-round conditioning for basketball, in Steingard PM (ed): *Basketball Injuries.* Philadelphia, W. B. Saunders Company, 1993, pp. 173-191.

45. Stanish WD, McVicar SF: Flexibility in injury prevention, in Renström PAFH (ed): *Sports Injuries: Basic Principles of Prevention and Care.* Oxford, Blackwell Scientific Publications, 1993, pp. 262-276.

46. Johnson RJ, Beynnon BD, Nichols CE, et al: Current concepts review: The treatment of injuries of the anterior cruciate ligament. *J Bone Joint Surg* 74A:140-151, 1992.

47. Ball, KA, Evans RE, Marks PH, Richards DW: *The Effect of Hip and Knee Angle on Force Generation in Quadriceps/Hamstring Knee Strength: Implications for ACL Injury.* Québec, Canadian Orthopaedic Association.

48. Marks PH, Ball KA, Evans RE, et al: *Effect of Hip and Knee Angle on Hamstring/Quadriceps Knee Strength: Implications for ACL Injury.* Beaver Creek, Colorado, ACL Study Group, 1998.

49. Jørgenson U: Regulations and officiating in injury prevention in Renström PAFH (ed): *Sports Injuries: Basic Principles of Prevention and Care.* Oxford Blackwell Scientific Publications, 1993, pp. 213-219.

50. Kelly JP, Rosenburg JH: Diagnosis and management of concussion in sports. *Neurology* 48:575-580, 1997.

51. Gerberich S, Priest JD, Boen JR, et al: Concussion incidences and severity in secondary school varsity football players. *Am J Public Health* 73:1370-1375, 1983.

52. Mitchell JH, Maron BJ, Epstein SE: 16th Bethesda Conference-Cardiovascular abnormalities in the athlete. Recommendations regarding eligibility for competition. *J Am Coll Cardiol* 6:1185-1232, 1985.

53. Maron BJ, Mitchell JH: 26th Bethesda Conference: Recommendations for determining eligibility for competition in athletes with cardiovascular abnormalities. *J Am Coll Cardiol* 24:845-899, 1994.

54. Mitchell JH, Blomqvist CG, Haskell WL, et al: Classification of sports. *J Am Coll Cardiol* 6:1198-1199, 1985.

55. Mitchell JH, Haskell WL, Raven PB: Classification of sports. *J Am Coll Cardiol* 24:864-866, 1994.

56. Maron BJ, Shirani J, Poliac LC, et al: Sudden death in young competitive athletes—Clinical, demographic, and pathological profiles. *J Am Med Assoc* 276:199-204, 1996.

57. Thomas RJ, Cantwell JD: Sudden death during basketball games. *Physician Sports Med* 18:75-78, 1990.

58. Maron BJ: Sudden death in young athletes-lessons from the Hank Gathers affair. *N Engl J Med* 329:55-57, 1993.
59. Van Camp SP: What can we learn from Reggie Lewis' death? *Physician Sports Med* 21:73-74, 1993.
60. Maron BJ, Gaffney FA, Jeresaty RM, et al: Task Force III: Hypertrophic cardiomyopathy, other myopericardial diseases and mitral valve prolapse. *J Am Coll Cardiol* 6:1215-1217, 1985.
61. Epstein SE, Blomqvist CG, Buja LM, et al: Task Force V: Ischemic heart disease. *J Am Coll Cardiol* 6:1222-1224, 1985.
62. Thompson PD, Klocke FJ, Levine BD, Van Camp SP: Task Force 5: Coronary artery disease. *J Am Coll Cardiol* 24:888-892, 1994.
63. Lazar JM: Marfan syndrome: Cardiovascular manifestations and exercise implications. *Physician Sports Med* 25:34-39, 1997.
64. Fuller CM, McNulty CM, Springer DA, et al: Prospective screening of 5,615 high school athletes for risk of sudden cardiac death. *Med Sci Sports Exercise* 29:1131-1138, 1997.
65. Garrick JG: Epidemiology of foot and ankle injuries. *Med Sport Sci* 23:991-997, 1987.
66. Steill IG, Greenberg GH, McKnight RD, et al: A study to develop clinical decision rules for the use of radiography in acute ankle injuries. *Ann Emerg Med* 21:384-390, 1992.
67. Steill IG, Greenberg GH, McKnight RD, et al: Decision rules for the use of radiography in acute ankle injuries: Refinement and prospective validation. *JAMA* 269:1127-1132, 1993.
68. Leddy JJ, Smolinski RJ, Lawrence J, et al: Prospective evaluation of the Ottawa Ankle Rules in a university sports medicine center, with a modification to increase specificity for identifying malleolar fractures. *Am J Sports Med* 26:158-165, 1998.
69. Shrier I: Treatment of lateral collateral ligament sprains of the ankle: A critical appraisal of the literature. *Clin J Sport Med* 5:187-195, 1995.
70. Carr AJ, Norris SH: The blood supply of the calcaneal tendon. *J Bone Joint Surg* 71B:100-101, 1989.
71. Puddu G, Ippolito E, Postacchini F: A classification of Achilles tendon disease. *Am J Sports Med* 6:731-734, 1976.
72. Curwin S, Stanish W: *Tendinitis: Its Etilogy and Treatment*. Churchill, Livingstone; 1985.
73. Lowdon A, Bader DL, Mowet AG: The effect of heel pads on the treatment of Achilles tendinitis: A double blind trial. *Am J Sports Med* 12:431, 1984.
74. Kainberger FM, Engel A, Barton P, et al: Injury of the Achilles tendon: Diagnosis with sonography. *Am J Roentgenol* 155:1031-1036, 1990.
75. Quinn SF, Murray WT, Clark RA, et al: Achilles tendon: MR imaging at 1.5 T. *Radiology* 164:767-770, 1987.
76. Nistor L: Surgical and non-surgical treatment of Achilles tendon rupture: A prospective randomized study. *J Bone Joint Surg* 63A:394-399, 1981.
77. Frey C, Shereff M, Greenidge N: Vascularity of the posterior tibial tendon. *J Bone Joint Surg* 72A:884-888, 1980.
78. Johnson KA, Strom DE: Tibialis posterior tendon dysfunction. *Clin Orthop* 239:196, 1989.

79. Woods W, Leach R: Posterior tibial tendon in athletic people. *Am J Sports Med* 19:495, 1991.

80. Conti S, Michelson J, Jahss MM: Clinical significance of magnetic resonance imaging in preoperative planning for reconstruction of posterior tibial tendon ruptures. *Foot Ankle* 13:208-214, 1992.

81. Mann RA, Thompson FM: Rupture of the posterior tibial tendon causing flat foot: Surgical treatment. *J Bone Joint Surg* 67A:556-561, 1985.

82. Gould N: Stenosing tenosynovitis of the flexor hallucis longus tendon at the great toe. *Foot Ankle* 2:46-48, 1981.

83. Sammarco GJ, DiRaimondo CV: Chronic peroneus brevis tendon lesion. *Foot Ankle* 9:163-170, 1989.

84. Sobel M, DiCarlo E, et al: Longitudinal splitting of the peroneus brevis tendon: An anatomical and histological study of cadaveric material. *Foot Ankle* 12:165, 1991.

85. Eckert WR, Lakes M, Davis E: Acute rupture of the peroneal retinaculum. *J Bone Joint Surg* 58A:670, 1976.

86. Zoellner G, Clancy W Jr: Recurrent dislocation of the peroneal tendon. *J Bone Joint Surg* 61A:292-294, 1979.

87. Degan T, Morrey B, Braun D: Surgical excision for anterior process fracture of the calcaneus. *J Bone Joint Surg* 64A:519, 1982.

88. Torg JS, Pavlov H, Cooley LH, et al: Stress fractures of the tarsal navicular. A retrospective review of twenty-one cases. *J Bone Joint Surg* 64A:700- 712, 1982.

89. Ihle CI, Cochran RM: Fracture of the fused os trigonum. *Am J Sports Med* 10:47-50, 1982.

90. DeLee JC, Evans JP, Julian J: Stress fracture of the fifth metatarsal. *Am J Sports Med* 11:349-353, 1983.

91. Smith JW, Arnoczky SP, Hersh A: The intraosseous blood supply of the fifth metatarsal: Implications for proximal fracture healing. *Foot Ankle* 13:143-152, 1998.

92. Graham CE: Painful heel syndrome: Rationale of diagnosis and treatment. *Foot Ankle* 3:261-267, 1983.

93. Leach RE, Seavey MS, Salter DK: Results of surgery in athletes with plantar fasciitis. *Foot Ankle* 7:156-161, 1986.

94. Ferkel R, Karsel R, Del Pizzo W, et al: Arthroscopic treatment of anterolateral impingement of the ankle. *Am J Sports Med* 19:440, 1991.

95. DeSmet AA, Fisher R, Burnstein MI, et al: Value of MR imaging in staging osteochondral lesions of the talus (osteochondritis dissecans): Results in 14 patients. *Am J Roentgenol* 154:555-558, 1990.

96. Alexander AH, Lichtman DM: Surgical treatment of transchondral talardome fractures (osteochondritis dissecans); Long term follow up. *J Bone Joint Surg* 62A:646-652, 1980.

97. Torg JS, Conrad W, Kalen V: Clinical diagnosis of anterior cruciate ligament instability in the athlete. *Am J Sports Med* 4:84, 1976.

98. Marks PH, Fowler PJ: Imaging modalities for assessing the anterior cruciate ligament deficient knee. *Orthopaedics* 16:417-424, 1993.

99. Ott JW, Clancy WG: Functional knee braces: Review. *Orthopaedics* 16:171- 176, 1993.

100. Mishra DK, Daniel DM, Stone ML: The use of functional knee braces in the control of pathological anterior knee laxity. *Clin Orthop* 241:213-220, 1989.

101. King JB, Perry DJ, Mourad K, et al: Lesions of the patellar ligament. *J Bone Joint Surg* 72B:46-48, 1990.

102. El-Khoury GY, Wira RL, Berbaum KS, et al: MR imaging of patellar tendonitis. *Radiology* 184:849-854, 1992.

103. Kennedy JC, Willes RB: The effects of local steroid injections on tendons. *Am J Sports Med* 4:11, 1991.

104. Kelly DW, Carter VS, Jobe FW, et al: Patellar and quadriceps tendon ruptures-jumper's knee. *Am Sports Med* 12:375, 1984.

105. van Kampen A, Huiskes R: The three-dimensional tracking pattern of the human patella. *J Orthop Res* 372-382, 1990.

106. Choyce MQ, Potts M, Maitra AK: A profile of sports hand injuries in an accident and emergency department. *J Accident Emerg Med* 15:35-38, 1998.

107. Kahler DM, McCue FC, III: Metacarpophalangeal and proximal interphalangeal joint injuries of the hand, including the thumb. *Clin Sports Med* 11:57-76, 1992.

108. Incavo SJ, Morgan, JV, Hilfrank BC: Extension splinting of palmar plate avulsion injuries of the proximal interphalangeal joint. *J Hand Surg* 14A:659-661, 1989.

109. Culver JE: Sport-related fractures of the hand and wrist. *Clin Sports Med* 9:85-109, 1990.

110. Crawford GP: The moulded polythene splint for mallet finger deformities. *J Hand Surg* 9A:231-237, 1984.

111. Abrahamsson SO, Solerman C, Lundborg G, et al: Diagnosis of displaced ulnar collateral ligament of the metacarpophalangeal joint of the thumb. *J Hand Surg* 15A:457-460, 1990.

112. Zagelbaum BM, Starkey C, Hersh PS, et al: The National Basketball Association Eye Injury Study. *Arch Ophthalmol* 113:749-752, 1995.

113. Easterbrook M: Eye protection for basketball. Personal communication, 1998.

114. Flanders RA, Bhat M: The incidence of orofacial injuries in sports: A study in Illinois. *J Am Dent Assoc* 126:491-496, 1995.

115. Kumamoto DP, Winters J, Novickas D, Mesa K: Tooth avulsions resulting from basketball net entanglement. *J Am Dent Assoc* 128: 1273-1275, 1997.

17 | **Football**

Don Johnson

Football is a collision, contact sport and injuries are an integral part of the game. It is the responsibility of the team doctor and trainer to provide a high standard of urgent care to the athlete. This immediate attention to proper assessment and treatment may prevent long-term disability from the injury. In this section the common athletic injuries are discussed.

PREVENTION

We all would like to find cause of the current epidemic of anterior cruciate ligament injuries. However, in the meantime we can advise the athlete that the best prevention is proper conditioning.

Cardiovascular Conditioning

This means elevating the heart rate into the target zone for 20 to 30 min. The target zone is between 70 and 85 percent of the maximum rate, which is 220 − age. For the 20-year-old, this is about 160 bpm. There is a wide variation of normal maximum heart rate, and most trainers will design an individual program that includes both endurance and interval training. The most efficient exercise is running. For the lineperson, the exercise bike or stairmaster will work better. "Big people" do not like to run. The program should be specific to their position.

Strength

Most football players are advocates of lifting. The key is emphasizing their weaknesses. When they are tested in training camp, the weak muscle parts should be specifically trained. The hamstrings are one of the common injuries for receivers and deep backs. If there is a detectable weakness, then this should be addressed. Not only are free weight exercises important, but also strengthening with sport-specific plyometric exercises should be instituted.

Flexibility

The other key area to emphasize is the flexibility of muscles groups that are commonly injured. The wide receivers and deep backs, who are sprinters, should emphasize strength and stretching of the hamstrings to prevent tearing. Most of the anterior cruciate ligament injuries occur with a noncontact twisting injury. This is often

343

a maneuver that the athlete has done many times. It is hard to believe that some specific exercise can prevent this injury. The best prevention is to run the pattern many times to condition the muscles by specificity of the sport.

COMMON INJURIES

Shoulder

Most upper extremity injuries are owing to a fall on the out-stretched arm (Fig. 17-1).

Anterior Shoulder Dislocations

The mechanism of injury is by abduction and external rotation of the shoulder. The pathology is tearing of the capsulolabral complex from the anterior glenoid rim. The symptoms of pain, limited motion, and a square deformity of the shoulder make the diagnosis. The treatment of the dislocation should be early reduction. I do not think that it is appropriate to reduce the dislocation on the field. On occasion, it is possible to reduce it on the bench with the athlete in the prone position and the arm hanging over the side of the bench.

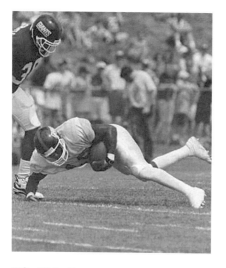

FIG. 17-1 Most upper extremity falls are due to a fall on the out-stretched arm.

I think that it is more prudent to take the athlete into the dressing room to do the reduction.

The easiest method is to lie prone on the bench, letting the arm hang over the edge of the bench. Many times, with gentle traction downward on the elbow, the shoulder will reduce. If it does not reduce easily, the tip of the scapula may be rotated medially with the other hand. If the shoulder still does not reduce, the athlete should be transported to the hospital.

The question of whether or not to attempt a reduction without an x-ray is a difficult one. If you are experienced at the diagnosis and manipulation of the dislocated shoulder, and do not believe that this is a fracture of the surgical neck of the humerus, then an attempt at reduction is indicated.

Acromioclavicular Joint Sprains

Injuries to the acromioclavicular (AC) joint still occur in spite of shoulder pads (Fig. 17-2). The diagnosis is made by pain, tenderness, and deformity at the AC joint. The injuries are classified into three grades.

1. Grade 1: pain, tenderness, with no deformity.
2. Grade 2: pain, tenderness, and slight separation with a prominent end of the clavicle.
3. Grade 3: pain, tenderness, and marked separation of the joint with a prominent end of the clavicle.

There are three other grades, but they are very rare. Treatment is based on the grading of the injury.

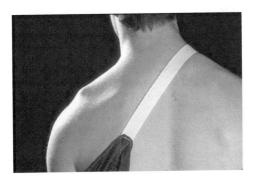

FIG. 17-2 A second-degree AC separation responds to a sling, analgesics, and intensive physiotherapy.

1. Grade 1: needs symptomatic treatment only and may return to play the next game.
2. Grade 2: needs sling, analgesics, physiotherapy, and may be out of play for 2 to 4 weeks, depending on the severity of the symptoms.
3. Grade 3: needs to have protection and reduction in a varney brace. In some instances, an open reduction and internal fixation is the best treatment. This will depend on the athlete's position. For example, a quarterback with a grade 3 AC joint should have an operative reduction. He or she will be out for 6 to 8 weeks and will need to have the hardware removed.

Clavicle Fractures

The cause of the fracture is a fall on the outstretched arm. The diagnosis can be made on the sidelines, by palpating the clavicle. This injury should be confirmed by an x-ray and immobilized in a figure eight bandage if displaced and a sling if undisplaced.

This fracture will take 6 to 8 weeks to heal. There is very little physiotherapy that can be done in the early fracture healing stages. Riding an exercise bike will maintain some cardiovascular fitness during the healing stages.

Most clavicle fractures will heal with conservative treatment. The only indication for operative fixation is if there is marked displacement of the fragments or neurovascular compromise.

Tendon Ruptures

Tendon ruptures of the upper extremity are common but sometimes overlooked. The rupture of the long head of the biceps is caused by a violent flexion of the elbow and shoulder. Pain, swelling, and deformity of the biceps are quite evident and make the diagnosis easy. When the biceps is flexed it looks like a "Popeye" muscle. The treatment is generally conservative.

The distal rupture of the biceps at the elbow is more difficult to diagnose and is always treated surgically.

Tendon ruptures also occur in the hand. The long flexor of the finger may be ruptured distally when the player grabs another player's shirt. The violent flexion ruptures the tendon from the distal phalanx. The diagnosis is made by examining for lack of flexion of the distal phalanx.

Wrist and Hand

Scaphoid Fracture

The scaphoid can be injured by a fall on the outstretched arm. Pain, swelling, and tenderness in the anatomic snuff box of the wrist make the diagnosis of a scaphoid fracture. The fracture may be confirmed by an x-ray. It is common that the fracture does not initially show up on plain x-rays. The wrist should be immobilized, and a bone scan performed. If the plain x-rays and bone scan are negative, then the possibility of a scaphoid fracture is remote. A clenched fist view of the wrist may reveal a scapholunate instability that may mimic a scaphoid fracture. The treatment of a scaphoid fracture is cast immobilization for 6 to 12 weeks until healed.

Phalangeal Dislocation

Dislocations of the fingers are extremely common and used to be called "coach's finger," since they used to reduce them in the past (Fig. 17-3). Pain, swelling, and deformity make the diagnosis of a joint dislocation. The management is gentle longitudinal traction to reduce the joint. The association of a fracture is fairly common, and an x-ray is mandatory. It is acceptable to attempt a gentle closed reduction without an x-ray. To confirm the reduction, and to rule out a fracture, an x-ray after the reduction is important.

Metacarpal and Phalangeal Fracture

Fractures are produced by direct blows or crush injury. The diagnosis is by pain, swelling, and local bony tenderness. X-ray is essential to confirm any suspicious injury. Treatment of undis-

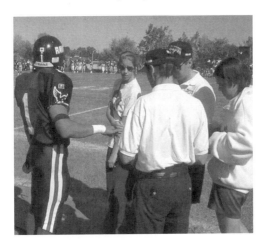

FIG. 17-3 The medical team providing sideline care for a finger dislocation.

placed fractures is cast immobilization. Displaced fractures may require closed reduction and some surgical reduction and fixation.

Bennett's Fracture

The Bennett's fracture is a displaced fracture at the base of the thumb. The mechanism is by jamming the thumb. Pain, swelling, and tenderness at the base of the thumb make the diagnosis. The fracture is confirmed by x-ray. Closed reduction of the fracture may be adequate, but usually an open surgical reduction is necessary.

Closed Head Injuries: Concussion

In recent years there has been much greater emphasis on a more conservative approach to the cerebral concussion. The evaluation of the athlete on the bench must be thorough and accurate. The brief examination should test for orientation (where are you), immediate memory (score in the game), concentration (adding numbers), and delayed recall (phone numbers).

The severity of the injury should be categorized. There are three grades of concussion:

1. Grade 1: Conscious, transient confusion for less than 15 min; the player returns to play after 15 min. If there are several concussions, he or she should sit out for a week.
2. Grade 2: Conscious, transient confusion for more than 15 min; the player returns to play after 1 week, or 2 weeks if multiple concussions.
3. Grade 3: Loss of consciousness and need of emergency care; the player returns to play after 1 week if the loss lasted seconds, 2 weeks if it lasted minutes, and 1 month or longer if multiple concussions.

If an athlete has three concussions in a session, then he or she should not continue to play that year.

Spine

Burners and Stingers

These are traction injuries to the brachial plexus. When the athlete falls on his head and the neck is flexed to the side, traction on the nerves will produce a sensation like hitting your "funny bone" in the elbow. These may be a mild nuisance or quite severe and prevent the athlete from playing for most of the season. Many times the first one is mild, and the reinjury is what causes the prolonged disability.

The diagnosis of stingers is made by the history of injury and by the examination of flexing the neck to the side of the injury and reproducing the symptoms.

Treatment is to protect the neck with a "horse" collar attached to the shoulder pads to prevent excessive lateral flexing. If the symptoms persist, then the athlete must be taken out of play until the symptoms subside. Gentle range of motion mobilization exercises and heat applications give symptomatic relief.

Musculoligamentous Sprain of the Spine

There are many injuries that occur to the spine in football that we categorize as back sprain. The diagnosis is by the history of back pain, local spinal tenderness, with restricted range of motion but a normal neurologic examination. These are usually minor, and the athlete may miss a few practices but is ready to play the next game. If the symptoms persist or worsen, then further examination and investigation is indicated.

Disk Injury

Many of the so-called "back sprains" are injuries to the disk, but it is difficult to diagnose. However, if the sprain does not improve quickly, then more investigation is necessary. If the athlete has radiating pain with or without neurologic symptoms, then an MRI should be ordered to assess the disk protrusion. Most disk injuries may be treated conservatively without surgery. The exception is the neurologic deficit that should have early surgical intervention. Conservative treatment may keep the athlete out for 6 to 12 weeks.

Fracture and Stress Fracture of the Pars Intraarticularis

Persistent back pain that does not settle in the lineperson is often a pars intraarticularis fracture. This is produced by repeated extension of the spine. Routine x-rays of the spine will reveal fractures or spondylolysis. A bone scan may also help to determine if this is of recent origin. The CT scan is the best method to evaluate this injury. The initial treatment is conservative with rest and back exercises.

Fracture Dislocation of the Cervical Spine

Although this is rare, it is the one most feared injury of any sports physician or trainer who has spent much time on the sidelines. Every time an athlete goes down and does not move for a few minutes you always say to yourself, "Please move your legs."

Since this scenario is uncommon, it helps to review the sequence of events to evacuate the player from the field with a serious neck injury. In the CFL we always have an ambulance on the sidelines. If this is a serious neck injury, I will call for the ambulance and the stretcher. The neck is immobilized in a collar with the helmet left on, and the athlete is transferred to the hospital for x-ray and evaluation. The helmet is then removed at the hospital, without moving the neck, and suitable x-rays are done. If there is suspicion that this is a fracture, it is more prudent to move the athlete to the hospital than to try to evaluate this in the training room.

Pelvis

Contusion to Anterior Superior Spine: "Hip Pointer"

This common injury is owing to a direct blow by a helmet to the anterior crest of the pelvis. There is bleeding on the bone and exquisite tenderness. The treatment is by padding to prevent a further blow on the area. Sometimes some local anesthetic may be used to allow the athlete to run pain free. Local infiltration can be safely used in this situation where no long-term harm will ensue from the injection.

Thigh

Contusion to Quads: "Charley Horse"

A "charley horse" is a bruise to the quadriceps muscle owing to a direct blow. Pain, swelling, local tenderness, and limited range of motion of the knee make the diagnosis of a quads contusion.

The treatment is with ice, compression, and elevation. The injury may be evaluated by the degree of loss of knee flexion. If there is only 45 degrees of knee flexion, this injury will take several weeks to improve. Physiomodalities, such as ultrasound, contrast baths, and local stretching of the muscle, will also speed healing.

Adductor Sprain

A strain of the adductors may be diagnosed by pain, swelling, local tenderness in the muscle or at the tendon-bone junction, and by limited abduction range of motion at the hip.

The treatment should be initially ice, compression, and anti-inflammatory medication. Ultrasound and stretching will also help heal the injury. In some chronic tendon-bone junction pain syndromes, an injection of cortisone may be indicated.

Knee

Medial Ligament Sprain

The medial collateral ligament is injured by a valgus or lateral force against the knee. The diagnosis is made by pain, swelling, local tenderness over the ligament on the medial side, and limited range of motion of the knee. The injury is separated into three grades to aid in planning treatment.

1. Grade 1: local pain and tenderness, no instability on examination.

2. Grade 2: local pain, swelling, tenderness, and laxity of the ligament on valgus stress, but an endpoint can be felt on stressing the ligament.
3. Grade 3: often very little pain, moderate swelling, and marked instability on valgus stress with no endpoint to the examination (Fig. 17-4).

Management depends on the grade.

1. Grade 1: ice, compression, and protection only, return to sport in 2 to 3 weeks.
2. Grade 2: ice, compression, and protection for 4 to 6 weeks in a double upright brace with full range of motion. Strengthening exercises using the bike and Stairmaster may be instituted early.
3. Grade 3: ice, compression, and protection with a knee brace for 4 to 6 weeks. Strengthening exercises may be started when comfort allows. It will usually take 10 to 12 weeks to return to sports. This is the injury to be very certain that an associated anterior cruciate ligament is not present. It is extremely rare to have an isolated grade 3 medial ligament sprain. It has also been shown that conservative treatment of this injury gives the best results.

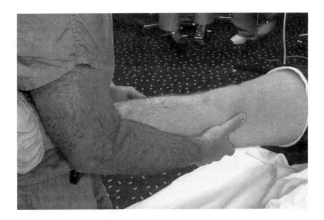

FIG. 17-4 The early and accurate clinical examination of the knee is important to avoid missing an injury that may require surgical intervention. The exam within the first 30 min is always easier than the exam the next day when there is more pain and swelling.

Anterior Cruciate Ligament Tear

The commonest mechanism of injury of the ACL is a noncontact pivot injury. The athlete hears a "pop" and experiences immediate pain and swelling. The examination on the sidelines reveals a positive Lachman test. The athlete will often walk around and feel better in 10 to 15 min and want to go back in the game. It is important that the seriousness of the injury is impressed on the athlete. It is at this stage that he or she can sustain more injury to the meniscus and have a poor outcome.

Approximately half the cruciate ligament injuries are isolated and have no meniscal injury associated with them. With proper management these have a good long-term outlook.

The diagnosis of an anterior cruciate ligament injury is made by pain, swelling, limited range of motion, and a positive Lachman test.

The Lachman test This is the most important test to learn how to perform well. The main feel that you are looking for is the endpoint. This should be compared to the opposite side. This should also be well documented in the preseason physical examination. This can be referred to later in the season when the athlete has an injury to his or her knee. It is unusual to be able to do a pivot shift test on the acute knee, so you have to rely on the Lachman test. Since many of the football players have large legs, and are difficult to get to relax, the drop leg Lachman test is much easier to perform (Fig. 17-5).

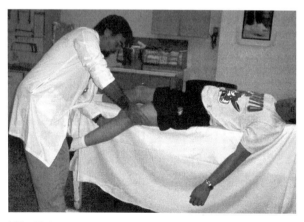

FIG. 17-5   Drop leg Lachman test.

Drop leg Lachman test If the Lachman test is positive, and the athlete is going to have surgery, you do not have to order an MRI to confirm the ACL tear. The only indication for an MRI is to rule out a meniscal injury in someone who you are considering delaying surgery until the end of the season. If the MRI was positive, then surgery would be scheduled during the season. In this situation the MRI would change the course of treatment. A routine preoperative MRI does not change the treatment plan. The treatment for a tear of the anterior cruciate ligament is surgery. The timing of the surgery may be controversial. If a lineperson has an isolated ACL tear, he or she may be rehabilitated and return to play in 1 month in a brace. Surgery may be done at the end of the season. The risk to reinjure is low. The presence of a meniscal tear will not allow the athlete to return to play in a brace. If the MRI is negative for meniscal injury, then you can feel safe in allowing the athlete to return to play.

The criteria to return to play are: no pain, full range of motion, no effusion, and equal strength measured on the cybex.

This program will usually not be successful in a running back or receiver. Such athletes should have surgery when the swelling subsides and the range of motion is nearly normal.

Meniscal Tear (Fig. 17-6)

Compression and rotation tear the meniscus. The duck walk (or baseball catcher's squat position) is a good way to tear the posterior horn of the medial meniscus. It is also a good provocative test for the chronic meniscal tear. The history of flexion and rotation of the knee followed later by pain and swelling make the diagnosis of meniscal injury. The swelling often does not occur until the next

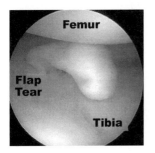

FIG. 17-6 The arthroscopic view of the flap tear of the meniscus. This flap gets caught between the tibia and femur, producing pain, swelling, catching, and giving out symptoms.

day. The clinical signs of a meniscal tear are: effusion, tenderness, and pain with flexion and rotation (the McMurray test) (Fig. 17-7).

The Apley compression test is useful. It is performed by flexing the knee to 90 degrees in the prone position and compressing the tibia against the femur. A positive test is pain and snapping of the meniscus between the femur and the tibia.

If the knee has full extension (that is not "locked") then conservative treatment should be instituted; that is, ice, compression, and elevation. Contrast baths in the whirlpool and gentle range of motion exercises should be started early.

If the knee lacks full extension, x-rays should be done to rule out avulsion fractures and loose bodies. The MRI will confirm the bucket handle tear of the meniscus. This should be surgically dealt with as quickly as possible.

Posterior Cruciate Ligament Injury

The mechanism of injury to the posterior cruciate ligament (PCL) is a direct blow to the anterior aspect of the tibia. This may occur by falling on the front of the knee with the foot plantar flexed. The blow occurs directly to the tibial tubercle and drives the tibia backward to tear the posterior cruciate ligament.

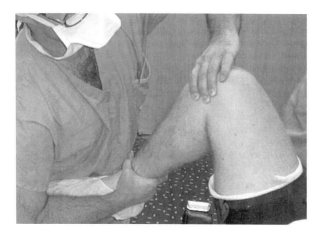

FIG. 17-7   The McMurray test. The flexion and rotation of the knee catch the flap tear between the femur and tibia. This produces a clunk, or snap, and the athlete experiences pain.

Pain, swelling, limited motion, and a positive posterior drawer test make the diagnosis (Fig. 17-8).

Once you determine the neutral tibial step off, by comparing the tibial plateau on both knees, you can grade the posterior drawer test. The quadriceps neutral position may also be determined by having the patient contract his or her quadriceps with the knee at 70 to 90 degrees. This pulls the tibia forward to the neutral position.

1. Grade 1: tibial plateau palpated and forward of the femur, 0- to 5-mm posterior displacement.
2. Grade 2: tibial plateau slightly palpable or equal with the femur, 5 to 10 mm of posterior displacement.
3. Grade 3: tibial plateau posterior to the femur, 10 to 15 mm of posterior displacement.

Most of the isolated PCL injuries are grade 1 or 2. The grade 3 injuries are usually associated with other ligament injuries such as the posterolateral corner.

It is important to determine if there is any associated injury. The isolated injury may be treated conservatively, but the combined in-

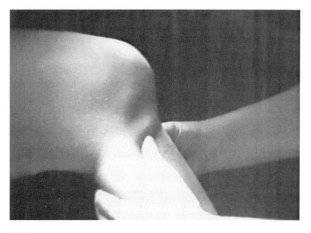

FIG. 17-8 The posterior drawer test is performed with the knee at 90 degrees and pushing the tibial backward. You must make sure that you start at the neutral point. You can do this by pulling the tibia forward to match the opposite side.

juries usually require surgery. The common posterolateral corner injury may be detected by examining for external rotation of the tibia at 30 and 90 degrees.

Tendon Rupture

The patellar tendon and quadriceps both can be ruptured by sudden quick stops while running. These injuries are massive and require urgent surgical treatment. Pain, swelling, local tenderness, and lack of active knee extension make the diagnosis. The defect in the tendon is palpable. The treatment is surgical repair and may require 6 months to recover.

Lower Leg

Stress Fracture

Stress fractures are less common in football than other sports. The mechanism is overuse in an unconditioned player. They are more likely to occur at the end of training after twice-a-day workouts. The common sites are the proximal tibia, the distal fibula, and the metatarsal shafts. Uncommon sites are the tarsal navicular and the calcaneus. Pain, swelling, and local bony tenderness make the diagnosis. The stress fracture may not show clinical signs on the x-ray for 3 to 4 weeks. The bone scan will be positive within a few days of injury.

The treatment is rest. No immobilization is required.

Shin Splints and Compartment Syndrome

"Shin splints" are a pain syndrome along the front of the tibia caused by running in the unconditioned state. The shin splint is a stress syndrome of the muscle attachment to bone. It is important to differentiate shin splints from compartment syndrome. The latter is pain and swelling in the anterior or lateral muscle compartments of the lower leg. The muscle will swell up to 30 percent with exercise. If there has been a bruise to the compartment or the fascia sheath is tight, the muscle may swell enough to obstruct the venous outflow, increasing the volume in the compartment. This may eventually obstruct the arterial inflow. This may become a surgical emergency if the swelling is sufficient to cut off the arterial blood supply. The severity of the pain will alert the medical staff to the more important compartment syndrome. The diagnosis of compartment syndrome is pain, pallor, pulselessness, and peripheral neuropathy. The treatment for a compartment syndrome is to release the fascia around the involved muscle.

Pain, swelling, and local tenderness along the posterior medial border or the anterolateral border of the tibia make the diagnosis of shin splints. The treatment is ice, compression, elevation, stretching, and rest.

Calf Muscle Pull: Strains and Tears

Muscle pulls and tears are extremely common in football owing to the explosive nature of the activity. Muscle tears are graded into three levels, mild strain, partial tear, and complete tears. Pain, swelling, local muscle tenderness, and deformity make the diagnosis. The treatment is ice, compression, and elevation. Ultrasound and interferential current treatments help reduce the pain and swelling. The degree of tear will be an estimate for the length of time to return to sport. The criteria for return to sport are: no pain, no swelling, full range of joint motion, and equal strength on cybex muscle testing.

Ankle

Lateral Ligament Sprain

Rolling over on the ankle or an inversion sprain injures the lateral ligament. Pain, swelling, local tenderness, and instability of the ankle joint make the diagnosis. The anterior drawer test of the ankle and the inversion test determine the instability. The degree of instability can be measured by performing the preceding tests and taking an x-ray at the maximum degree of laxity. Ankle sprains are graded like all ligament sprains into three levels. However, all grades are treated conservatively. The grade 3 sprain may be treated in an aircast that is removable for physiotherapy exercises. The grade 3 sprain also may benefit by a protective ankle brace for the first 3 months after injury.

Chronic persistent ankle pain 3 months after injury may prevent the player from returning to sport. The ankle joint may have to be injected with steroids to reduce the synovitis. If pain persists in spite of the injection, then arthroscopy of the ankle may be necessary to alleviate the pain.

Deltoid Ligament Injury

The medial deltoid injury is less common. The mechanism is by eversion injury of the ankle. Pain, swelling, and local tenderness make the diagnosis. The initial treatment is ice, compression, and elevation. Ultrasound and range of motion exercises are necessary to regain full function.

Osteochondral Fracture of the Talus

The inversion injury may be severe enough to produce a shear to the dome of the talus and detach a fragment of bone and articular surface. This osteochondral fracture may heal if undisplaced. If displaced, arthroscopy and removal of the loose fragment may be required.

Pain, swelling, and loss of range of motion are the clinical signs that make the diagnosis. Plain x-rays will show the lesion. Occasionally a CT scan of the talus may be required to evaluate the osteochondral lesion.

Achilles Tendon Sprains and Tears

The Achilles tendon is torn by a violent contraction of the gastrocnemius muscle in sprinting. A loud pop, followed by pain and swelling make the diagnosis. A palpable defect in the tendon and a positive Thompson test are the clinical signs of a complete rupture of the tendon. Squeezing the gastroc muscle when the patient is supine comprises the Thompson test (calf compression test). A positive test is the failure of the ankle to plantarflex when the muscle is squeezed. The opposite side is used for comparison. The treatment of most athlete Achilles tendon tears is by surgically suturing the torn ends of the tendon. The athlete usually is out for the season.

Posterior Tibial Tendon Rupture

This is an uncommon tendon rupture. It produces a flat foot appearance. The athlete is unable to toe raise without the foot remaining in a pronated position. The treatment is to surgically suture the tendon or to augment the repair with another tendon.

Foot

Plantar Fascial Injury

The plantar fascia may be injured with a sprinting action or a forced dorsiflexion of the foot. Pain, swelling, and local tenderness of the fascial insertion on the os calcis make the diagnosis. The treatment is ice, compression, and taping of the arch to protect it while the soft tissues heal.

Metatarsal Fracture

Fractures are caused by direct blow by someone stepping on the foot. Pain, swelling, and local bony tenderness make the diagnosis. The x-ray confirms the fracture. The treatment is by cast immobilization for 4 to 6 weeks. Physiotherapy after the cast removal regains the range of motion and strength of the foot.

Jones Fracture versus Avulsion Fracture of the Base of the Fifth Metatarsal

The Jones fracture is a fracture of the base of the fifth metatarsal caused by an inversion sprain of the ankle. Pain, swelling, and local bony tenderness of the fifth metatarsal base makes the diagnosis.

The x-ray confirms that the fracture is through the metaphyseal region of the bone. The avulsion fracture of the base of the fifth metatarsal has a different outcome. The avulsion can be treated by cast immobilization. The Jones fracture should be treated with surgical reduction and pinning to return the athlete to sport.

Metatarsophalangeal Joint Injury: "Turf Toe"

The turf toe is caused by hyperextension of the great toe. Pain, swelling, and limited motion of the metatarsophalangeal joint make the diagnosis of turf toe. The x-ray is negative for fracture. The treatment is conservative with ice, compression, and elevation. Anti-inflammatory medications help to reduce the swelling. Other physiotherapy modalities such as interferential current will also help to reduce the pain and swelling. This injury may persist most of the season and only gets better when the athlete has time to rest in the off-season.

RETURN TO SPORT: DIFFICULT DECISIONS ON THE SIDELINES

Knee Ligament Sprain

A careful sideline examination must determine if there is any laxity of the joint. If laxity is detected, then the athlete must be sidelined. Type 1 injuries, or those with no laxity, may return to play, based on degree of pain.

The anterior cruciate ligament assessment is the most difficult, due to muscle contraction to protect the joint. You may have to do the Lachman test several times to catch the athlete relaxed. The drop leg Lachman test is the best test to relax the hamstrings after acute injury.

AC Joint Injury

If there is no significant prominence of the outer end of the clavicle, the athlete may return to play. Make sure that you stress the joint by adduction of the shoulder.

Shoulder Dislocation

If this is a first-time dislocation that reduces, the athlete should be protected and kept out of play. If this is a recurrent dislocation that reduces easily, and the athlete has minimal pain and a good range of motion, he or she may return to play.

Hamstring Injury

Return to play after a hamstring injury is a difficult assessment. After a period of rest and icing, I usually have the athlete run on the sidelines to assess the degree of functional impairment. If the strain is grade 1, and he or she is able to run, cut, and stop, then he or she may return. Often this is a call by the athlete, who feels that he or she is not able to perform satisfactorily.

Quads Contusion

Quadriceps contusions are like the hamstring strain. The minor injuries may be iced, wrapped, and the athlete returned to play. An athlete with a serious quads hematoma with less than 90 degrees of knee flexion may take up to 6 to 8 weeks to return to play.

SPECIFIC INJURIES NOT TO MISS

Be overcautious and have a high index of suspicion for these injuries. Always think the worst-case scenario. If you always have these injuries in mind, you will not overlook them.

- Anterior cruciate ligament injuries
- Cervical spine injuries
- Occult fractures—scaphoid

18 | Baseball Injuries

Richard G. Clarnette   *Anthony Miniaci*

Baseball is one of the most popular sports in North America. In 1981 there were estimated to be approximately 13,000,000 children playing baseball. Approximately half of the amateur players are aged between 6 and 12. A survey of over 2800 Little League baseball players in 1994 concluded that baseball was a safe activity with a low rate of injury.[1]

Severe injuries occurred in only 11 cases, giving a rate of only 0.008 severe injuries per 100 player-hours. Impacts by the ball caused more than half of the severe injuries and were usually facial. Overuse injuries were generally not severe but accounted for 19 percent of the injuries incurred.

In the assessment of an injured baseball player of any age and any grade, the physician must have a thorough and systematic approach in order to arrive at the correct diagnosis. In the acute setting one must rule out fractures, dislocations, ligament injuries, and musculotendinous injuries.

In those with chronic symptoms the differential diagnosis may include the following: stress fractures, osteochondral lesions, arthritic conditions, joint instability and subluxation, neuropathies, and tendinitis or tendinopathy.

This chapter does not discuss acute injuries, as the diagnosis and treatment of these are well detailed in standard texts. Instead, we have focused on the chronic and overuse injuries that are specifically related to baseball, with particular emphasis on those areas where diagnosis and treatment may be difficult. The mechanics of throwing is discussed in detail, as this helps in our understanding of how most of these injuries occur. This is followed by a review of specific injuries of the shoulder and elbow in adults and in the skeletally immature.

THROWING

Throwing is a very important aspect of baseball for all players involved, not exclusively for the pitcher. Most chronic and overuse injuries in baseball are caused by throwing; it is an activity that has been extensively researched by many authors using electromyographic (EMG) analysis.[2–4] Studies have been performed on both professional and amateur pitchers, allowing interesting comparisons between the two groups. The pitch motion is a continuous flowing motion, but for the purpose of description and analysis it can be divided into five stages (Figs. 18-1, 18-2, and 18-3).[2]

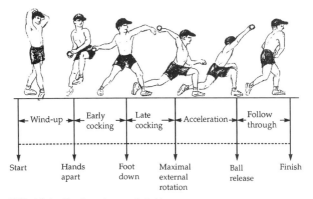

FIG. 18-1   The five phases of pitching.

Stage 1: Windup

The windup occurs from the initial movement until the ball leaves the gloved hand. This is a very important phase whereby the leading leg is lifted and the pitcher's center of gravity is placed over the pitching rubber. From here the pitcher is well balanced to move into the cocking phase. There is little strain on any particular muscle group during this phase.

Stage 2: Early Cocking

This phase begins when the ball leaves the gloved hand and ends as the front foot strikes the ground. During this phase the arm is elevated and abducted to 90 degrees together with early external rotation of the shoulder. EMG studies show the deltoid is the dominant upper limb muscle during this phase and mainly acts to hold the shoulder in abduction.[5] During this phase there is also a lot of lower limb and trunk activity. The pelvis rotates toward the target, causing a coiling effect on the trunk. The leading leg is powerfully extended toward the home plate, which increases the coiling effect.

Stage 3: Late Cocking

This phase begins as the front foot contacts the ground and ends with the first forward motion of the ball. During this phase the enormous amount of energy that has been built up in coiling of the trunk is now transferred to the arm. As the trunk and lower body unwind and begin to translate toward the home plate the hand and

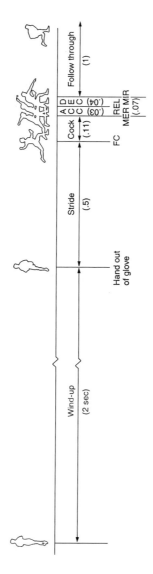

FIG. 18-2 Approximate time lengths for pitching phases.

363

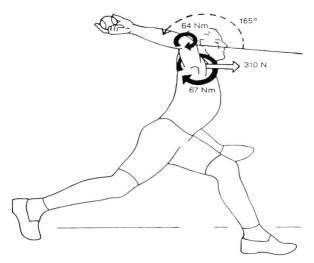

FIG. 18-3 Rotation of shoulder in throwing motion.

ball remain relatively motionless. To allow this to occur, the shoulder moves into a position of extreme external rotation. At the beginning of this phase the shoulder is usually in a position of approximately 90 degrees of abduction and 90 to 120 degrees of external rotation and by the end of the late cocking maximal external rotation will be reached that may be up to 180 degrees. In nonathletes, 90 degrees of shoulder external rotation is considered "normal"; therefore, we can begin to appreciate the enormous stress being placed on the pitcher's shoulder as it is rotated externally to almost 180 degrees.

It is during this phase, as the shoulder and trunk move ahead of the hand and forearm, that the elbow, which is flexed to approximately 90 degrees, is put under an extreme valgus load that stretches the medial structures and compresses the lateral structures. EMG studies show an enormous amount of rotator cuff activity during this phase. Infraspinatus and teres minor work concentrically during stage 2, acting as external rotators of the shoulder. During late cocking their activity peaks as these muscles function to stabilize the humeral head and draw it posteriorly, thus protecting against anterior subluxation. Supraspinatus contracts isometrically to help with humeral head stabilization. Subscapularis is inactive initially but then undergoes its peak activity late in stage 3 as it contracts eccentrically to decelerate the external rotation and protect the anterior of the joint from ligament damage and subluxation. Latissimus dorsi and pectoralis major also act eccentrically during late cocking to decelerate the external rotation of the humerus.[4]

Stage 4: Acceleration

This phase begins with the first forward motion of the ball, which corresponds to the beginning of internal rotation of the humerus. The angular velocity achieved here is up to 7000 degrees per second, and the ball velocity goes from 0 to 90 miles per hour in about 50 ms. The large amount of energy stored in the previous stages is transferred to the ball during this phase with surprisingly little muscle activity required.

Strong contraction of triceps muscle forces the elbow into rapid extension, at velocities averaging over 4000 degrees per second. During this phase the triceps muscle, its tendon, and the olecranon are all exposed to injury.

EMG studies show that the rotator cuff muscles of professional pitchers are relatively inactive during this phase, although in injured and amateur pitchers this is often not the case. It has been shown that amateurs have high levels of activity in both the rotator cuff and the biceps during the acceleration phase, and this may predispose them to an increased likelihood of overuse injuries and possibly to superior labral injuries.[6]

The major activity in professional athletes is in the pectoralis major and latissimus dorsi, which act concentrically to accelerate the humerus into internal rotation. Triceps activity is also maximal during this phase, acting to extend the elbow, but it begins to fire in late cocking and may have some role in helping to stabilize the shoulder by its long head attachment.[4]

Stage 5: Follow-Through

This phase begins with ball release and ends when motion ceases. It is a very violent phase as the muscles of the upper limb attempt to resist the 200-lb outward force on the arm, mostly by the use of powerful eccentric contraction. Despite the strong contraction of the biceps, the elbow still reaches full extension, and at this point the olecranon strikes the olecranon fossa of the humerus.

EMG studies show activity particularly in the rotator cuff muscles, which act to stabilize and decelerate the glenohumeral joint, and also in the trapezius, serratus anterior, and the rhomboid muscles, which control and decelerate the scapular. Teres minor is particularly active in this phase as it contracts eccentrically to decelerate the humerus, which is forcefully rotating internally at this point.[2]

Biceps and brachialis have been shown to fire synchronously through this stage and are thought to act mainly to decelerate the elbow, which is undergoing quite violent extension.[5,7] The strong pull of the biceps may be important in the development of labral and SLAP (superior labrum from anterior to posterior) lesions in the shoulder.[6,8]

Understanding the mechanics of throwing helps the clinician to appreciate the extreme forces placed on the bones, ligaments, and muscles of the body. We know that eccentric loading of muscles places them at most risk of injury and that is partly why the act of throwing is so stressful, particularly on the rotator cuff. If the rotator cuff is weakened or injured, then more stress will be placed on the static stabilizers, especially the glenoid labrum and the anterior glenohumeral ligaments.[6] The untrained or injured athlete will often place even more stress on the rotator cuff and biceps as they attempt to compensate for a deficiency in technique or shield an injury.[9] This may lead to an overuse injury and tendinitis of the rotator cuff that will weaken the rotator cuff and thereby predispose the individual to further damage to the ligaments of the shoulder. Instability, through physiological laxity or pathological ligament damage, can then allow secondary rotator cuff damage owing to impingement, and thus a vicious cycle is entered.[10]

In the elbow, pathology occurs owing to tension on the medial side of the joint, compression on the lateral side of the joint, and implication posteriorly. The region of the joint most affected is partly determined by the age of the individual and their skeletal maturity, as this determines which anatomical structures are most vulnerable.

THE SHOULDER IN ADULTS

Throwing places very high demands on the shoulder, and in the pursuit of speed the anatomical structures of the shoulder are put under loads that may be greater than can be tolerated. The shoulder enjoys the greatest freedom of motion of any joint, and this is owing largely to the lack of bony congruity between the humeral head and glenoid. The shoulder is mainly reliant on the ligaments and muscles to give it stability, and in particular the superior, middle, and inferior glenohumeral ligament and the rotator cuff muscles play a key role. Athletes and especially throwing athletes tend to have relatively lax ligaments, allowing them the advantage of an increased range of motion but putting them at increased risk of instability. Throwing injuries in skeletally mature athletes can be grouped into two main categories, macrotrauma and microtrauma.[11]

Macrotraumatic injuries, such as acute rotator cuff tears, acute shoulder dislocations, and fractures, are generally specific events that are relatively simple to diagnose. A large rotator cuff tear in a throwing athlete is likely to require investigation and surgical repair to optimize the final result. Dislocations require reduction and a short period of immobilization, but the risk of subsequent instability in young athletes is very high and surgical intervention will probably be required.

Microtraumatic or overuse injuries are more common and tend to be insidious in their onset and may be difficult to diagnose. In understanding the biomechanics of throwing, one can appreciate those structures most at risk of failure. The rotator cuff is placed under extreme loads and often contracts eccentrically, which puts it under even greater stress. Subscapularis is loaded maximally in late cocking and teres minor in the follow-through stage. Tendinitis, fatigue, or failure of the rotator cuff leads to further stress on the glenohumeral ligaments, particularly anteriorly. Excessive external rotation with reduced internal rotation of the shoulder is a common finding in pitchers and is presumably an adaptive phenomenon that allows greater velocity to be achieved. This, however, results in posterior capsular tightness that forces the center of rotation anteriorly, and this places further stress on the anterior ligaments and also predisposes to impingement.

IMPINGEMENT AND INSTABILITY

These entities are discussed together, as they are interrelated and interdependent. Subacromial impingement was described by Neer in 1972 and refers to the impingement of the superior portion of the rotator cuff against the anterior acromion and coracoacromial ligament.[12,13] Bigliani's work showed that hooked acromions were more commonly associated with rotator cuff tears, and this added support to the concept of a mechanical injury occurring as the rotator cuff was impinging against the anterior acromion.[14]

Associated with the mechanical impingement are subacromial and acromioclavicular spurs, subacromial adhesions, fibrosis, and bursal-sided partial-thickness tears. This type of impingement syndrome is usually seen in patients over the age of 40 unless there is an anatomical variant, such as an os acromiale. Based on this, Neer described the anterior acromioplasty, and given the appropriate pathology good results have been achieved with this operative technique.[12,13]

Unfortunately, shoulder pain became synonymous with the term "impingement" and this led to some patients being treated inappropriately. Young overhead athletes treated with anterior acromioplasty, whether open or arthroscopic, were achieving good results and returning to their sports in less than 50 percent of cases, and it was realized that the pathology was different in this group of patients.[9,15]

It is now becoming clear that there are different types of impingement requiring different treatment regimes.[10]

Classic Anterior Impingement

This is impingement syndrome as described by Neer.[12] It is rare under the age of 40 years and in throwing athletes, and therefore the clinician should consider other types of impingement syndrome. Anatomical variations, such as an unstable os acromiale or a type III (hooked) acromion, need to be excluded, as they will predispose an individual to this type of impingement.

Anterior Impingement Secondary to Tight Posterior Capsule or Instability

Posterior capsular tightness is a common finding in throwing athletes and can be recognized by an excess range of external rotation with a limited range of internal rotation. Its effect is to shift the center of rotation anteriorly and predispose the individual to anterior impingement. Ligamentous laxity particularly in an anterior direction can also result in secondary anterior impingement. Acromioplasty and coracoacromial ligament resection are contraindicated in these instances, as it will further destabilize the shoulder.

Internal Impingement (Superior Glenoid Impingement)

More recently the concept of internal impingement has been recognized, and this is especially important in throwing athletes.[16–18] Arthroscopic examination in many of these individuals did not show subacromial bursitis or bursal-sided rotator cuff pathology, but instead revealed incomplete articular-sided tears of the posterosuperior cuff, injury, and reaction of the posterosuperior labrum. This is owing to internal impingement of the cuff against the glenoid and occurs with the arm in abduction and external rotation. (This can be visualized arthroscopically.) Bony changes on the greater tuberosity and posterosuperior glenoid were also occasionally seen.

The relationship that this type of impingement has with instability is not yet fully established. Jobe believes weakness of subscapular or incompetence of the inferior glenohumeral ligament results in hyperangulation and inferior subluxation of the shoulder during abduction and external rotation and that this allows impingement of the rotator cuff against the glenoid.[10]

Instability can also occur without impingement and can be classified according to direction (anterior, posterior, inferior, or multidirectional), etiology (traumatic or atraumatic), frequency (acute, recurrent, or chronic), degree (subluxation or dislocation), and volition.[19] Typically, the throwing athlete has anteroinferior or multidirectional instability that is atraumatic (owing to overuse).

Having recognized that there is a spectrum of pathology from pure impingement to pure instability, Jobe and colleagues have classified throwing athletes with shoulder pain into four groups.[9,20]

1. Group 1: pain secondary to pure impingement
2. Group 2: pain secondary to instability owing to anterior ligament and labral injury with secondary impingement
3. Group 3: pain secondary to instability owing to hyperelastic capsular ligaments with secondary impingement
4. Group 4: pain secondary to pure instability without secondary impingement.

Clinical Features

Anterior impingement with rotator cuff tendinitis is suggested by shoulder pain related to overhead activities and often by night pain. There is tenderness along the subacromial bursa, a painful abduction arc, and positive impingement tests as described by Neer and Hawkins.[12,21,22]

Superior glenoid impingement gives a slightly different clinical picture with chronic dorsal shoulder pain that is characteristically worse in the acceleration phase of the pitch when the impingement is maximal.[10] Examination reveals tenderness along the posterior joint line with impingement in a position of 90 degrees of abduction together with full external rotation and horizontal extension. This is the same arm position used to test for anterior instability in the apprehension test, although with superior impingement the athlete experiences pain rather than apprehension. Applying a posterior force to the proximal humerus while repeating the test will often reduce the pain in much the same way as the apprehension can be reduced using the relocation test in a patient with anterior instability.[23]

Rotator cuff tears are unusual in young athletes, but can occur and are suggested by atrophy and weakness of the rotator cuff. Subscapularis is best assessed using the liftoff test (see Fig. 6-4) as described by Gerber and Krushell.[24] This is performed with the arm internally rotated so that the dorsal surface of the hand rests on the lower back. Actively lifting the hand away from the back and resisting force suggests integrity of the subscapularis. The external rotators, teres minor, and infraspinatus can be tested with the arm by the side and elbow flexed to 90 degrees. In this position impingement should not be present so that painful inhibition of muscle activity is eliminated. Supraspinatus can be most effectively isolated and tested with the arms in 90 degrees of scapular elevation and full internal rotation.

Instability usually takes the form of repeated transient subluxations that may be symptomatic to the athlete as a feeling of instability with the shoulder feeling "loose," or it may cause pain that is usually felt over the posterior aspect of the shoulder in the late cocking or early acceleration phase. Occasionally, the subluxation may cause momentary traction on the brachial plexus giving rise to the "dead arm syndrome."[25]

On examination, shoulder instability may be anterior, posterior, or inferior. It may be very obvious and easy to demonstrate, or it may be very subtle and difficult to diagnose. In all cases you need a relaxed cooperative patient and a gentle technique.

In the shoulder it is difficult to know if the translation felt is subluxation to an abnormal position or relocation to a normal position. It is also important to remember that a normal shoulder has a degree of physiological laxity and can translate significantly, and this can be particularly evident under anesthesia.[26] Comparison to the opposite side is vital, as is very careful palpation to feel when the joint is properly located.[27] Subluxation, apprehension, and the reproduction of the patient's pain may all be positive examination findings.

The following examination tests are used to determine the degree and direction of instability.

Load-and-Shift Test

With the patient comfortably seated and with hands in the lap, one can perform the anteroposterior translation or load-and-shift test. To perform this test the right humeral head is grasped with the right hand while the left hand is positioned over the top of the shoulder girdle so that the scapular can be stabilized. Simultaneously, the posterior joint line is palpated with the thumb while the anterior shoulder is palpated with the index and middle fingers. The right hand then loads the joint to ensure concentric reduction and then applies anterior and posterior shearing forces. The direction and translation can then be determined and graded using a scale of 0 to 3 (grade 0 for no instability; grade 1 for mild translation of less than 1 cm; grade 2 for moderate translation of 1 to 2 cm or to the glenoid rim; and grade 3 for severe translation of greater than 2 cm or over the glenoid rim). The fingers of the left hand should be positioned with the middle finger on the coracoid and index finger on the humeral head. In this way abnormal anterior translation can be appreciated, as the index finger moves forward of the middle finger. To perform the apprehension test, move the right hand to the patient's right wrist and keep the left hand on the shoulder. With the arm in adduction and internal rotation the shoulder will not be anteriorly subluxated. From this position bring the arm into abduction and external rotation while using the left hand to palpate any anterior subluxation.[25] Using the left thumb to push the humeral head forward can augment the test.

Apprehension (Crank) Test and Relocation Test (see Fig. 6-1)

The remaining tests are best performed with the patient supine with the shoulder brought just beyond the edge of the examination table beginning with the apprehension or crank test. The test is performed by external rotation of the abducted arm. Classically, it is performed with the arm at 90 degrees of abduction, but this can be varied in order to stress different portions of the glenohumeral ligament complex. While one hand rotates and abducts the arm the other should be used to palpate the anterior and posterior shoulder in order to reference the direction of any movement. The test can be augmented by pushing the humeral head anteriorly from behind. Finally, the relocation test can be performed by pushing posteriorly on the upper part of the humerus. This part of the test is positive if the apprehension or pain is relieved, thereby allowing further external rotation before reemergence of the patient's symptoms. Patients with classical anterior impingement often experience pain on apprehension testing, but it is unrelieved by performing the relocation test.[23] Patients with internal impingement will often experience pain without apprehension during the apprehension test, with the pain being relieved by the relocation maneuver.[10]

Sulcus Sign

Inferior instability is assessed by applying inferior traction to the arm. Gross instability is demonstrated by visible widening of the subacromial space with a sulcus appearing in the adjacent area just distal to the lateral acromion ("sulcus sign"). It is important to remember that normal shoulders can translate significantly.[26] It is important to appreciate the significance of generalized ligamentous laxity particularly in those patients with multidirectional instability, and the examiner should test for this by looking for elbow, finger, and thumb hyperextension together with knee recurvatum and increased ankle dorsiflexion.

Posterior Apprehension

Posterior apprehension is elicited by maximally internally rotating the humerus with the shoulder in 90 degrees of abduction and then applying a posteriorly directed force on the humeral head. In a positive test the patient feels as if the shoulder is about to dislocate. O'Driscoll has found this test to be highly sensitive and specific for posterior shoulder instability.[28] It can be differentiated from impingement by the absence of relief after injecting local anesthetic into the glenohumeral space. Often, however, posterior instability is not associated with pain or apprehension, and so most clinical tests rely on the detection of the subluxation that occurs in certain arm positions.

Posterior Subluxation Testing

Posterior subluxation usually occurs with the arm in adduction and internal rotation combined with some degree of flexion. Abduction and external rotation will relocate the subluxated shoulder. This test, devised by the senior author, utilizes these observations in a clinical test similar to Ortalani's test for hip subluxation. To assess the right shoulder the examiner stands in the axillary region of the patient who is supine with the right shoulder off the edge of the bed. The examiner's left hand takes the elbow and positions the arm in a position of adduction, internal rotation, and 70 to 90 degrees of flexion. The examiner's right hand is positioned over the top of the shoulder with the thumb on the anterior shoulder and fingers on the posterior joint line. With the arm in this position the thumb of the right hand is used to apply a posterior force on the humeral head to achieve posterior subluxation. With the shoulder subluxated the humeral head fills the normal hollow that is present below the acromion. From this position the arm is brought out slowly into abduction and external rotation and will, at some point, relocate with a clunk, which is palpable with the right hand.

Investigation

Routine radiographic evaluations are an essential component of the assessment and should include an anteroposterior, axillary, and lateral view of the shoulder in the plane of the scapula. These can be supplemented with the caudal/tilt view (a 10-degree tilt of the x-ray beam) for assessing the supraspinatus outlet.[29] Pathological findings predisposing to impingement include subacromial spurs, acromioclavicular spurs, a hooked acromion, or an os acromiale. Evidence of instability may include a bony Bankart lesion, glenoid erosion, a Hill-Sachs lesion, or subluxation of the glenohumeral joint. Supplementary radiological tests such as arthrography, CT, and MRI are usually not necessary. CT is the best modality to assess any bony defects if required. MRI is very sensitive and will show signal changes in the rotator cuff in asymptomatic individuals. It is, however, the modality of choice in the evaluation of rotator cuff tears if suspected.

Treatment

Group 1: Pain Secondary to Pure Impingement

This is an uncommon group of athletes, usually over the age of 35, with impingement and no instability. Treatment is initially conservative with avoidance of throwing, stretching, and rotator cuff strengthening. Only after 6 to 12 months of conservative treatment should surgical treatment be considered. Arthroscopic acromioplasty may then be indicated if there are acromial spurs or an acromial hook together with bursal inflammation or bursal-sided rotator cuff pathology.

If the athlete has a rotator cuff tear and no instability then operative repair may be indicated if conservative measures fail or if the tear is large. The prognosis for return to the athlete's former level of performance is, however, very poor.[30]

Group 2: Pain Secondary to Instability Owing to Anterior Ligament and Labral Injury with Secondary Impingement

This group has superior or anterior impingement owing to a definite anteroinferior ligamentous or labral injury. They do not have multidirectional laxity and therefore will not have posterior subluxation. Initial treatment is conservative with rest from throwing activities and anti-inflammatory medication to resolve the rotator cuff tendinitis. This is followed by therapy with particular emphasis on rotator cuff strengthening, scapular stabilization, and posterior stretching. This leads to an improvement in some; however, others will fail, especially if they have significant structural pathology, such as a large Bankart or Hill-Sachs lesion. Surgery may then be indicated in the form of a capsulolabral repair (unless there are very large bony defects requiring more complex reconstructive surgery).

Group 3: Pain Secondary to Instability Owing to Hyperelastic Capsular Ligaments with Secondary Impingement

This group is similar to group 2 except they tend to have multidirectional laxity that affects both shoulders and often have generalized ligamentous laxity. They also have features of rotator cuff tendinitis and impingement. For this group nonoperative treatment is the mainstay of therapy with emphasis on rotator cuff strengthening and scapular stabilization. Surgery may be indicated if there is failure of nonoperative management, but without a discrete pathological entity and laxity in all the ligaments success cannot be guaranteed. Surgery usually takes the form of a capsulolabral reconstruction together with a capsular shift to effectively tighten the ligaments. In this case the balance between obtaining stability and not overtightening the shoulder is difficult to achieve.

The other concern is that tightening the anterior structures alone may accentuate a previous subtle posterior instability. It is partly owing to these technical difficulties that nonoperative treatment is pursued so vigorously in these cases.

Group 4: Pain Secondary to Pure Instability without Secondary Impingement

These athletes have instability without impingement. If the instability is multidirectional and associated with generalized ligamentous laxity as in group 3, then they are managed along similar guidelines with emphasis on nonoperative management. If they have a more discrete pathological lesion such as a Bankart lesion they are more likely to fail nonoperative management and have a better prognosis with surgery.

SUPERIOR LABRAL AND BICEPS LESIONS

The long head of biceps tendon runs up the bicipital groove under the transverse ligament and then runs through the shoulder joint to attach to the superior glenoid via the superior labrum. The biceps tendon and superior labrum can be involved in various pathological processes, including bicipital tendinitis, biceps rupture, biceps tendon subluxation or dislocation, and tears of the superior labrum. Since the advent of arthroscopy, lesions of the superior labrum and biceps anchor have been more clearly defined and classified.[8] Throwing is associated with high activity in the biceps, and this is thought to predispose the athlete to superior labral tears, including SLAP lesions (superior labral tears from anterior to posterior) (Fig. 18-4).

Clinical Features

Superior labral lesions are often associated with instability, and the symptoms may be nonspecific. Anterior shoulder pain, clicking, and popping may, however, be due to labral or biceps lesion.[8] The following tests may help to isolate a biceps or labral pathology.

Yergason's Test

In Yergason's test the elbow is flexed to 90 degrees and the forearm is pronated.[31] At this point the examiner holds the patient's wrist to resist active supination by the patient. Pain in the bicipital groove is a positive test and indicates possible wear or tendinitis of the biceps tendon.

Speed's Test

Speed's test involves having the patient forward flex the shoulder against resistance while maintaining the elbow in extension and the

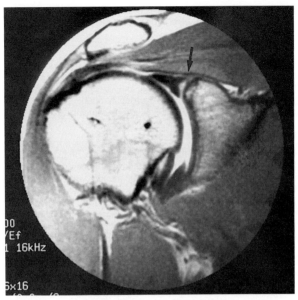

FIG. 18-4   Slap lesion (superior labral tears from anterior to posterior).

forearm in supination. Pain or tenderness in the bicipital groove indicates bicipital tendinitis. Field and Savoie found this test to cause nonspecific shoulder pain in all of their series of patients with superior labral lesions, suggesting that it does test for the competence of the biceps anchor.[32]

Clunk Test

The "clunk" test has been described, whereby the arm is rotated and loaded from a position of extension to one of forward flexion. A clunklike sensation may be felt if a free labral fragment is caught in the joint. This test is similar to the McMurray's test of the knee. Studies have shown that a click on manipulation of the glenohumeral joint was a common finding in patients with labral tears even in the absence of joint instability.[33,34]

Investigation

These lesions are difficult to diagnose and certain investigations may be very valuable. Usually contrast is required to show the pathology with any degree of sensitivity. CT arthrography and MR arthrography have both been shown to be effective.

Treatment

Treatment is dependent on the degree of damage to the labrum and the stability of the biceps. In many cases involving young athletes there will be superior labral damage and associated mechanical instability of the biceps anchor requiring fixation.[35] In most cases repairs of this type can be achieved arthroscopically.

BENNETT LESION (FIG. 18-5)

Posterior ossification of the shoulder is a lesion first described by Bennett in 1947.[36] He described a deposit of bone on the posterior inferior border of glenoid fossa that he thought was owing to traction by the origin of the long head of triceps and was an exostosis. He believed the lesion caused symptoms by local irritation of the capsule, synovium, and axillary nerve. Further studies since then using arthrography, computerized tomography, MRI, arthroscopy, and histological evidence have provided further knowledge. The lesion is extraarticular, in the region of the posterior band of the inferior glenohumeral ligament complex (IGHLC) and is not re-

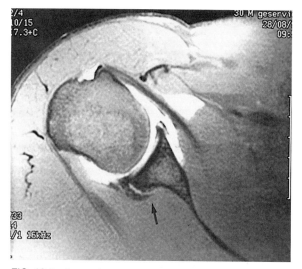

FIG. 18-5   Bennett lesion.

lated to the long head of the biceps.[37,38] The lesion is commonly associated with intraarticular pathology, most commonly tears of the posterosuperior labrum, but also posteroinferior labral tears, posterior instability, and posterior undersurface rotator cuff tears.[38] Histological and MRI studies have not demonstrated any cancellous bone or bone marrow and this suggests that the lesion is not either an exostosis or an osteophyte. It has been shown to be reactive new bone formation at capsular insertion to the posterior glenoid. The cause of the lesion remains unclear, but it seems most likely to be owing to traction on the posterior band of the IGHLC, either during late cocking when subscapularis contraction may cause posterior subluxation of the glenohumeral joint, or during follow-through when there are large distractive forces on these ligaments.

Clinical Features

Symptoms may be gradual in onset or develop suddenly.[36] Pain is felt posteriorly with occasional radiation to the deltoid region. Pitchers can throw hard only for a limited time, and as the pain increases the performance declines. Often the shoulder will be asymptomatic and function normally unless the athlete attempts to throw hard. In a series of seven pitchers with Bennett lesions, all had posterior shoulder pain, mostly in the follow-through phase of the pitch but some experienced it only during cocking. All had posterior glenoid tenderness, two had evidence of posterior instability, and none exhibited any anterior instability.[38]

Investigation

The lesion cannot usually be seen on standard shoulder radiographs. A modified anteroposterior radiograph with the arm in 90 degrees of abduction and in maximal external rotation and the beam tilted 5 degrees cephalad will bring the abnormal area of the glenoid into relief.[36] Computerized tomography is the investigation of choice to demonstrate the bony abnormality and shows extraarticular curvilinear calcification originating from the posterior inferior glenoid extending toward the humeral head. MRI will show the lesion, although it is not as good as CT in demonstrating cortical bone. It is, however, more sensitive in defining the commonly associated intraarticular pathology, particularly if combined with arthrographic techniques.

Treatment

Bennett described how the lesion could be approached and removed using a posterior approach to the shoulder but stated that operative treatment was not advisable.[39] There is no agreement as to the cause or treatment of the lesion. Most agree that a trial of nonoperative management involving rest, nonsteroidal anti-inflammatory drugs (NSAIDs), and rehabilitation should be untaken before anything more aggressive is considered. Lombardo et al.[40] had a series of four pitchers who failed nonoperative treatment and underwent open posterior excision of the lesion with "encouraging" results. It is not clearly stated if they returned to their formal level of competition. In Ferrari et al.'s series of seven pitchers (six professional) all but one returned to their former level of performance after surgery, which involved arthroscopy and treatment of the intraarticular pathology without visualization or treatment of the lesion itself.[38]

THE SHOULDER IN CHILDREN

Even though the elbow is more commonly affected in skeletally immature baseball players than the shoulder, significant lesions can occur at this site owing to the unique stresses encountered as a result of pitching. The pathology seen in children is different from adults owing to the presence of growth plates, which are weaker than the surrounding ligaments and joint capsule. The proximal humerus has three centers of ossification involving the head and the greater and lesser tuberosities, which coalesce at age 7 and fuse to the shaft at approximately 20 years. Acute injuries to the shoulder girdle can occur in baseball owing to falls and collisions, and these may result in variety of fractures and growth plate injuries.

The chronic overuse injury that occurs due to repetitive trauma associated with pitching is termed "Little Leaguer's shoulder." This was first described by Dotter in 1953, who believed that the injury was owing to fracture through the proximal physeal plate.[41] Adams reported a similar injury in 1966 in five adolescent pitchers.[42] He believed the injury was owing to a repetitive traction injury of the proximal humeral physis. All boys in his series were between 13 and 15 years of age and presented vague shoulder pain at the end of a hard throwing motion. All had overdevelopment of the affected shoulder but there was little else to find on examination, except for occasional local tenderness and pain on jerking the outstretched arm. Comparative x-ray studies are the key to making the correct diagnosis, revealing widening of the proximal humeral epiphysis and demineralization of the proximal epiphysis, without evidence of avascular necrosis.

The condition usually responds rapidly to rest, and there is unlikely to be any long-term sequelae. Some authors have recommended that pitching be ceased until the physis has closed, although others suggest that one season of rest is usually adequate.[42,43]

THE ELBOW IN ADULTS

Acute and chronic valgus and hyperextension stress produce a different set of pathological entities in the adult than in the child. The weakest link in the growing immature elbow is the growing epiphysis and the intervening physeal plates. In the young adult it is the ligaments that tend to fail initially.[44] The medial collateral ligament complex consists of three parts: an anterior oblique bundle, a posterior oblique bundle, and a transverse band, which is of little functional significance. The anterior oblique band arises from the medial epicondyle and inserts into the medial border of the coronoid process, and it is the primary stabilizer against valgus stress with the elbow in extension. The posterior bundle is a fan-shaped ligament, which arises from the medial epicondyle and inserts into the olecranon and is taut with the elbow in flexion.[45,46]

Repetitive forceful valgus stress is associated with the development of the medial stress syndrome that can involve a number of different pathological entities, including the valgus-extension overload syndrome, medial collateral ligament injuries, and ulnar neuritis.

Andrews and Timmerman found that in professional baseball pitchers undergoing surgery for elbow injuries the most common types of pathology were posteromedial olecranon osteophyte, ulnar collateral ligament injury, and ulnar neuritis.[47]

VALGUS-EXTENSION OVERLOAD

Pitching results in very high valgus and extension forces on the elbow, and this can lead to a specific impingement syndrome in the posterior compartment of the elbow. Wilson et al. drew attention to this syndrome and the importance of recognizing the medial as well as posterior osteophyte formation that occurs on the olecranon owing to attenuation of the medial ligament.[48] Hypertrophy of the distal humerus adds to the impingement by narrowing the olecranon fossa.

Clinical Features

Pain is felt posteromedially and often increases during the game. Pain is often associated with poor pitching control that the pitcher may attempt to compensate for by "snapping" the elbow, which may further reduce control. Localized tenderness with pain or valgus stressing in extension is the classic examination findings. There may be an associated ulnar neuritis owing to impingement of the ulnar nerve on the osteophyte.

Investigation

Plain x-rays with axial images will usually demonstrate the posteromedial osteophyte formation on olecranon. Occasionally the lesion is cartilaginous and recognized only at arthroscopy.[48]

Treatment

Rest and anti-inflammatory medicines should be used initially to reduce any associated synovitis. An attempt should be made to improve the range of motion without producing pain using a careful stretching program. If this fails to resolve the symptoms, surgical excision carries a high chance of success.

MEDIAL COLLATERAL LIGAMENT INJURIES

The anterior bundle is the most important stabilizer against valgus stress. Injury is usually a chronic overuse syndrome but may be an acute event.

Clinical Features

Often there is a history of chronic medial-sided elbow pain related to throwing. In the acute situation there will be tenderness and swelling that is maximal toward the ulnar attachment of the ligament, as this is where the ligament avulsion occurs. Stability testing of the medial collateral can be performed by applying a valgus stress to the elbow held in approximately 25 degrees of flexion, which unlocks the olecranon from its fossa. The clinician must look carefully for evidence of ulnar neuritis, which is often associated.

Investigation

Stress views comparing both elbows will often aid in confirmation of the diagnosis. X-rays may show spur formation in the region of the coronoid process of the ulna and calcification in the region of the medial ligament. A quite distinctive change seen in baseball pitchers is single or multiple ossicles of bone seen along the course of the medial ligament.[39]

Treatment

Most athletes are managed conservatively with a period of rest, ice, and anti-inflammatory medication followed by therapy to regain motion and strength. Chronic instability with pain and inability to throw after 6 months of conservative therapy may be an indication for ligament repair or reconstruction. Jobe et al. reported that 10 out of 16 throwing athletes returned to their former level of sport after a ligament reconstruction using autologous tendon grafts.[49]

ULNAR NEURITIS

This is common in throwing and pitching athletes and is usually owing to mechanical irritation, which can be from repetitive tension, compression, or friction. In the arm the nerve passes from the extensor compartment to the flexor compartment about 8 to 10 cm above the elbow joint. Here it passes through the fibrous arcade of Struthers where it may be compressed. It passes distally to course posterior to the medial epicondyle and enters the cubital tunnel. Within this tunnel the nerve lies adjacent to the medial epicondyle and medial edge of trochlea and is roofed by the triangular arcuate ligament, which extends from the medial border of the olecranon to the medial epicondyle. After exiting the tunnel the nerve then passes between the two heads of flexor carpi ulnaris.

Compression of the nerve can occur at any point along its course but in the case of throwing athletes one of several pathological entities tends to occur.

1. Traction neuritis may exist due to valgus deformity or valgus instability.
2. Compression of the nerve against posteromedial osteophytes that is seen as part of the valgus extension overload.[50]
3. Subluxation of the nerve with friction of the ulnar nerve.[50]

Clinical Features

Usually there is insidious onset of ulnar-sided elbow pain with associated paresthesia in the ulnar nerve distribution. Examination may reveal tenderness or instability of the nerve at the elbow together with a positive Tinel's sign. Neurological abnormalities may be present but are often subtle or absent.

Investigation

Radiographs of the elbow may reveal spur formation or calcification in the region of the ulnar nerve or medial collateral ligament. EMG studies should be done but may be negative in up to half of the cases.

Treatment

Initial treatment involves rest, activity modification, and anti-inflammatory medication followed by therapy, particularly aimed at strengthening of the flexor and pronator groups. The likelihood of resolution if symptoms are chronic is relatively poor, and surgery may be indicated. This usually involves anterior transposition of the nerve.

THE ELBOW IN CHILDREN AND ADOLESCENTS

Chronic conditions affecting the elbow are rare in the general population but are relatively common in baseball owing to the stress of throwing. The elbow is the most frequent area of complaint in children and adolescent baseball players.[51] As previously outlined, the main forces are tensile on the medial side of the elbow and compressive on the lateral and posterior aspects of the elbow.

Little Leaguer's elbow is the term given to the abnormal changes that occur in the pitching elbows of the skeletally immature. It may refer to medial epicondylar abnormalities (accelerated growth and separation or fragmentation of the epiphysis), osteochondritis of the capitellum, or osteochondritis of the radial head in any combination.[52]

It is important to have some understanding of the way the elbow ossifies and the order in which the epiphyses appear and fuse. At birth the entire elbow is a radiolucent cartilaginous anlage. During childhood the different regions of the elbow undergo ossification in a predictable sequence starting with the capitellum, which begins to ossify at approximately 2 years of age. This is followed by ossification in the radial head epiphysis at about 4 to 5 years, the medial epicondylar epiphysis at about 5 to 7 years, the trochlear epiphysis at 8 to 9 years, and the lateral epicondyle and olecranon that appear between 9 and 11 years of age. There is quite a significant amount of variation depending on the physiological maturity of the individual, and for this reason the epiphyses tend to appear earlier in girls. Fusion of the ossified epiphyses to the shaft of the bone occurs at between the ages of 13 and 16 in boys and 11 and 14 in girls, with the trochlea being the first to fuse.[53] Pappas uses skeletal maturity to define three stages of development that render the elbow susceptible to different pathological processes.[53]

Childhood

This includes children up to the age of about 11 to 12 when the secondary ossification centers are appearing but have not yet fused to the shaft. During this time the cartilage anlage is being vascularized and ossified and is highly vulnerable to excess physical forces. Injury at this time is likely to cause degeneration and necrosis of the epiphysis followed later by regeneration. This is an osteochondrosis and it may affect the medial epicondyle, olecranon, trochlea, or capitellum. Osteochondrosis of the capitellum is known as Panner's disease.

Adolescence

This is the period that begins when all secondary centers have appeared and ends when all long bones physes have fused (up to the age of approximately 14 in females and 17 in males). In this time period, the secondary center has been formed and is now most vulnerable at its periphery, which is at its junction with the physis (growth plate) and at its articular surface. Injury at this time results in subchondral avascular necrosis (osteochondritis dissecans), which usually affects the capitellum and physeal separations and nonunions, which usually affect the medial epicondyle or olecranon.

Young Adult

This period encompasses the first 3 to 5 years after closure of the physes. During this period we begin to see the emergence of adult types of pathology, but one can still see late presentations and sequelae of the adolescent problems.

OSTEOCHONDRITIS DISSECANS OF THE CAPITELLUM

In this condition there is fragmentation and possible separation of a portion of the articular surface.[53] Repetitive compressive and shearing forces are thought to be important etiological factors.[53,54] In adolescents it is commonly seen in conjunction with abnormalities of the medial epicondyle together with enlargement and deformity of the radial head, and it is then often called Little Leaguer's elbow.[52]

Clinical Features

The first symptom may be pain after a season of pitching, which later becomes more severe and activity-related and may be associated with intermittent swelling. As the disease progresses there is often a loss of full extension followed by the loss of pronation and supination. Catching, locking, and intermittent severe pain suggest the presence of loose intraarticular fragments.

Examination may reveal a joint effusion, local tenderness over the capitellum, loss of range particularly in extension, and crepitus on movement.

Investigation

Sequential changes can be seen on plain x-ray, although tomograms or CT scanning may be more sensitive in evaluating the more subtle changes. Evaluation of the overlying articular cartilage requires the use of either arthrography or MR imaging. The earliest changes on plain radiographs are an area of subchondral rarefaction surrounded by a sclerotic rim. Later there is flattening of the capitellum seen particularly on the lateral view, followed by fragmentation and possibly the development of loose body formation.[54]

Treatment

The mainstay of treatment is conservative with rest and avoidance of throwing. This needs to continue until healing of the capitellum, which can be followed by serial x-rays taken at 6-month intervals. Arthroscopic surgery is reserved for those cases where there is evidence of loose or unstable fragments causing mechanical symptoms.[55]

PANNER'S DISEASE: OSTEOCHONDROSIS OF THE CAPITELLUM

This is a disease of the growth or ossification of the capitellar epiphysis and occurs at a younger age than osteochondritis dissecans. It was first described by Panner in 1927 and was likened to Legg-Perthe's disease of the hip.[56]

It is seen most commonly in children between the ages of 5 and 10 and is more common in baseball players and gymnasts than in the general community. It is thought to occur as a result of vascular insufficiency during the critical stages of ossification.

Clinical Features

Pain, local tenderness, and loss of motion are the most common features. The development of unstable or loose osteochondral fragments causing mechanical symptoms such as locking is unusual in this condition.

Investigation

The radiological changes are similar in sequence to those occurring in Perthe's with sclerosis and fragmentation followed by lucency and later by reossification. MR imaging can also be used and shows the typical sequence seen when there is avascular necrosis of bone with loss of the high signal normally seen in healthy bone marrow on T1-weighted images. These changes occur much earlier than radiographic changes.

Treatment

Rest and cessation of throwing activities will usually result in the resolution of symptoms. Radiological follow-up until there is reossification and healing should occur before consideration is given to resumption of activities.

DISORDERS OF THE OLECRANON

Depending on the age and development of the olecranon the following disorders may be seen.

Osteochondritis of the Olecranon

These adolescents present with pain, swelling, and tenderness. Radiological investigation reveals fragmentation and irregularity of the epiphysis, and in these cases comparison to the opposite side is often helpful. Treatment is symptomatic with rest and activity modification until resolution, which may take several months.

Olecranon Epiphyseal Nonunion or Stress Fracture

This is owing to failure of fusion of the olecranon physeal plate, which normally occurs at about 16 years of age in males. It has been reported in baseball players and may be related to the repetitive stress of pitching. Radiographs may show widening of the physeal line or simply failure of the epiphysis to fuse. There is a lot of variation in the appearance and position of the physeal line so comparison with the opposite side is vital. Treatment initially involves a period of immobilization in an attempt to achieve union, but it may require operative fixation if this fails.

DISORDERS OF THE MEDIAL EPICONDYLE

The medial epicondyle is the site of origin of the medial collateral ligament and the powerful forearm flexors. Throwing and in particular pitching places enormous stresses through this region, and in those who are skeletally immature it is the medial epicondylar epiphysis and the intervening growth plate that are most susceptible to injury.

It is also important to consider ulnar nerve pathology, which may be coexistent. The ulnar nerve may be unstable in the ulnar groove, allowing irritation and an ulnar nerve palsy to occur.

Clinical Features

This overuse syndrome is characterized by insidious onset of medial-sided elbow pain with localized tenderness and pain on valgus stressing of the joint. Occasionally, an acute separation of the epiphysis can occur with sudden onset of severe pain.

Investigation

Adams showed radiographic changes in 100 percent of Little League pitchers between the ages of 9 and 14.[52] These changes included accelerated growth, separation, or fragmentation of the epiphysis as compared to the nonthrowing side. At least 45 percent of the pitchers were symptomatic but only on direct questioning, and the study concluded by recommending guidelines for young pitchers that would limit the amount of pitching and abolish the throwing of curve balls, which places even more stress on the elbow.

Treatment

Separation of the epiphysis by 1 cm or more together with valgus instability is an indication for surgery, with open reduction and fixation of the fragment being the goal. Most cases are less severe without instability and can be managed by rest and activity modification.

SUMMARY

Baseball continues to be a popular sport with increasing numbers of participants over a wide age range. Falls, collisions, and direct impact injuries occur, but these are relatively easy to diagnose with appropriate diligence. Injuries that are relatively unique to baseball occur owing to repetitive chronic stress overload, most commonly owing to pitching. An understanding of the mechanics of throwing gives the clinician important insight into how these injuries occur and which anatomical structures are most at risk. The clinician also needs to appreciate how the age of the individual will significantly alter the likely spectrum of pathology that will be encountered in a given joint or region. This is because the anatomical structures that are most susceptible to injury change as the individual matures.

Appropriate injury prevention strategies are also important and can be logically developed with knowledge of the pathology that occurs with overuse, particularly in the skeletally immature, who are most susceptible to long-term complications, especially in the elbow joint.

REFERENCES

1. Pasternack JS, Veenema KR, Callahan CM: Baseball injuries: A Little League survey. *Pediatrics* 98:445–448, 1996.
2. Hancock RE, Hawkins RJ: Applications of electromyography in the throwing shoulder. *Clin Orthop Rel Res* 84–97, 1996.
3. Andrews JR, Timmerman LA, Wilk, KE: Baseball, in Petrone FA (ed): *Athletic Injuries of the Shoulder*. New York, McGraw-Hill, 1995.
4. Jobe FW, Moynes DR, Tibone JE, et al: An EMG analysis of the shoulder in throwing and pitching. A second report. *Am Sports Med* 12:218–220, 1984.
5. Jobe, Tibone, Perry, and Moynes, 1983.
6. Fleisig GS, Andrews JR, Dillman CJ, et al: Kinetics of baseball pitching with implications about injury mechanisms. *Am J Sports Med* 23:233–239, 1995.
7. Basmajian JV, Latif A: Integrated actions and functions of the chief flexors of the elbow: A detailed electromyographic analysis. *J Bone Joint Surg Am* 39:1106–1118, 1957.
8. Snyder SJ, Karzel RP, Del Pizzo W, et al: Slap lesions of the shoulder. *Arthroscopy* 6:274–279, 1990.
9. Glousman RE: Instability versus impingement in the throwing athlete. *Orthop Clin North Am* 24:89–97, 1993.

10. Jobe CM: Superior glenoid impingement. current concepts. *Clin Orthop Rel Res* 330:98–107, 1996.
11. Jobe FW, Kao JT: Throwing sports, in Hawkins RJ, Misamore GW (eds): *Shoulder Injuries in the Athlete.* New York, Churchill Livingstone, 1996, pp. 389–401.
12. Neer CS, 2d: Anterior acromioplasty for the chronic impingement syndrome in the shoulder. *J Bone Joint Surg* 54A:41–50, 1972.
13. Neer CS, 2d: Impingement lesions. *Clin Orthop Rel Res* 173:70–77, 1983.
14. Bigliani LU, Morrison DS, April EW: Morphology of the acromion and its relationship to rotator cuff tears. *Orthop Trans* 10:459–460, 1986.
15. Tibone JE, Jobe FW, Kerlan RK, et al: Shoulder impingement syndrome in athletes treated by anterior acromioplasty. *Clin Orthop Rel Res* 198:134–140, 1985.
16. Jobe CM: Superior glenoid impingement. *Orthop Clin North Am* 28:137–143, 1997.
17. Walch, Boileau, Noel, and Donell, 1992.
18. Jobe and Sidles, 1993.
19. Cofield RH, Irving JF: Evaluation and classification of shoulder instability. With special reference to examination under anesthesia. [Review] [46 refs]. *Clin Orthop Rel Res* 32–43, 1987.
20. Jobe FW, Tibone JE, Jobe CM, et al: The shoulder in sports, in Rockwood CA, Matsen FA (eds): *The Shoulder.* Philadelphia, Saunders, 1990, pp. 961–990.
21. Neer CS 2d, Welsh PR: The shoulder in sports. *Orthop Clin North Am* 8:583–591, 1977.
22. Hawkins RJ, Kennedy JC: Impingement syndrome in athletes. *Am J Sports Med* 8:151–157, 1980.
23. Kvitne RS, Jobe FW: The diagnosis and treatment of anterior instability in the throwing athlete. [Review] [58 refs]. *Clin Orthop Rel Res* 107–123, 1993.
24. Gerber C, Krushell RJ: Isolated rupture of the tendon of the subscapularis muscle: Clinical features in 16 cases. *J Bone Joint Surg* 73B:389–394, 1991.
25. Leffert RD, Gumley G: The relationship between dead arm syndrome and thoracic outlet syndrome. *Clin Orthop Rel Res* 20–31, 1987.
26. Harryman DT 2d, Sidles JA, Clark JM, et al: Translation of the humeral head on the glenoid with passive glenohumeral motion. *J Bone Joint Surg Am Vol* 72:1334–1343, 1990.
27. Miniaci A, Dowdy PA, Fowler PJ: Clinical assessment of shoulder injuries, in Chan KM (ed): *Sports Injuries of the Hand and Upper Limb.* New York, Churchill Livingstone, 1995.
28. O'Driscoll SW: A reliable and simple test for posterior instability of the shoulder. *J Bone Joint Surg* 73B:50, 1991.
29. Neer 2d and Popper, 1977.
30. Tibone JE, Jobe FW, Kerlan RK, et al: Surgical treatment of tears of the rotator cuff in athletes. *J Bone Joint Surg* 68A:887–891, 1986.
31. Yergason RM: Supination sign. *J Bone Joint Surg* 13A:160, 1931.
32. Field LD, Savoie FH: Arthroscopic suture repair of superior labral detachment lesions of the shoulder. *Am J Sports Med* 21:783–791, 1993.
33. Glasgow S, Bruce RA, Yacobucci GN, et al: Arthroscopic resection of glenoid labral tears in the athelete. *Arthroscopy* 8:48–54, 1992.

34. Liu SH, Henry MH, Nuccion S, et al: Diagnosis of glenoid labral tears. A comparison between magnetic resonance imaging and clinical examinations [see comments]. *Am J Sports Med* 24:149–154, 1996.

35. Rames RD, Karzel RP: Injuries to the glenoid labrum, including SLAP lesions. *Orthop Clin North Am* 24:45–53, 1993.

36. Bennett GE: Shoulder and elbow lesions distinctive of baseball players. *Ann Surg* 126:107–110, 1947.

37. O'Brien SJ, Neves MC, Arnoczky SP, et al: The anatomy and histology of the inferior glenohumeral ligament complex of the shoulder. *Am J Sports Med* 18:449–456, 1990.

38. Ferrari JD, Ferrari DA, Coumas J, Pappas AM: Posterior ossification of the shoulder: The Bennett lesion. Etiology, diagnosis, and treatment. *Am J Sports Med* 22:171–175, 1994.

39. Bennett GE: Elbow and shoulder lesions of baseball players. *Am J Surg* 98:484–492, 1959.

40. Lombardo, Jobe, Kerlan, Cartra, and Shields, 1977.

41. Dotter WE: Little Leaguer's shoulder. Fracture of the proximal humeral epiphyseal cartilage due to baseball pitching. *Guthrie Clin Bull* 23:68–72, 1953.

42. Adams JE: Little League shoulder osteochondrosis of the proximal humeral epiphysis in boy baseball pitchers. *Cal Med* 105:22–25, 1966.

43. Tibone JE: Shoulder problems of adolescents. *Clin Sports Med* 2:423–426, 1983.

44. Pincivero DM, Heinrichs K, Perrin DH: Medial elbow stability. Clinical implications. [Review] [25 ref]. *Sports Med* 18:141–148, 1994.

45. Morrey BF, An KN: Functional anatomy to the ligaments of the elbow. *Clin Orthop Rel Res* 201:84–90, 1985.

46. Regan WD, Korinek SL, Morrey BF, et al: Biomechanical study of ligaments around the elbow joint. *Clin Orthop Rel Res* 271:170–179, 1991.

47. Andrews JR, Timmerman LA: Outcome of elbow surgery in professional baseball players. *Am J Sports Med* 23:407–413, 1995.

48. Wilson, Andrews, Blackburn, and McClusky, 1983.

49. Jobe FW, Stark H, Lombardo SJ: Reconstruction of the ulnar collateral ligament in athletes. *J Bone Joint Surg* 68A:1158–1163, 1986.

50. Wadsworth TG: The external compression syndrome of the ulnar nerve at the cubital tunnel. *Clin Orthop Rel Res* 124:189–204, 1977.

51. Guggenheim JJJ, Stanley RF, Woods GW, et al: Little League survey: The Houston study. *Am J Sports Med* 4:189–200, 1976.

52. Adams JE: Injury to the throwing arm: A study of traumatic changes in the elbow joints of boy baseball players. *Cal Med* 102:127–132, 1965.

53. Pappas AM: Elbow problems associated with baseball during childhood and adolescence. *Clin Orthop Rel Res* 164:30–41, 1982.

54. Clanton TO, DeLee JC: Osteochondritis dissecans. History, pathophysiology and current treatment concepts. *Clin Orthop Rel Res* 167:50–64, 1982.

55. Morrey BF: Osteochondritis dissecans, in DeLee JC, Drez D (eds): *Orthopaedic Sports Medicine: Principles and Practice.* Philadelphia, Saunders, 1994, pp. 908–912.

56. Panner HJ: An affection of the capitulum humeri resembling Calve-Perthes' disease of the hip. *Acta Radiologica* 8:617, 1927.

19 | Soccer Injuries

Rejean Grenier

Soccer is a running sport demanding rapid deceleration, pivoting, lateral and backward displacement, jumping combined with the kicking motion, and contact with other players. All that represents factors of vulnerability to injury.

Ankle sprain is the most common joint injury in sports. The knee is the joint most frequently operated on, and injuries to the knee frequently lead to permanent disability. That statement is also true for soccer injuries.

THE IMPORTANCE OF SOCCER IN THE WORLD OF SPORTS

As a team sport, soccer is played most regularly in the greatest number of countries of the world. In most of them, it is known as football, which is quite different from rugby and American football. Furthermore, it has become more popular among women in the past 20 years.[1] In 1989, the number of registered participants was estimated at more than 60 million in about 150 countries, and undoubtedly, more players were not registered.[2] Until recently, soccer was considered a minor sport in North America.[3] Because of the dynamic involvement of national federations and state and regional sport authorities, more and more leagues at the young, high school, college, and professional levels evolved, making soccer the fastest growing team sport in North America.[4] It has even become a popular indoor game.[3]

One possible reason for its popularity is the perception that soccer is a safe sport.[5–7] As a matter of fact, compared with American football, which is a more contact-oriented sport, soccer appears to be relatively safe for younger players who, under 12 years of age (start at age 5 years), sustained twice fewer injuries than their counterparts playing football; whereas in the teenage group, the number of injuries is five times more in American football than in soccer.[3,8] The hazards most likely to cause injuries are related to physical conditioning and training, equipment, playing field, and skills.

FACTORS OF INJURY

Soccer is a hybrid game (played on a field 105 × 70 m) in which players must rapidly run short distances at various speeds and also cover substantial distances over the course of a 90-min game. This is why soccer demands a lot of flexibility to kick, run, and reach.

389

The use of the head to advance the ball is also unique to soccer. The rules of the professional game are felt to contribute to the occurrence of serious injuries in soccer as it is provided for two halves of 45 min (juniors, two 30-min halves), substitutions—three professional, house league unlimited. Thus, exhaustion is a major factor of injury. Offensive forwards, defensive fullbacks, and the goalkeeper suffer the most injuries.

The goalkeeper is the only player on the field who can legally use his or her hands on the ball provided it is done inside the penalty zone. So, even if soccer is not a contact-oriented sport, it is in fact a bodily contact game played with little or no equipment and because it puts great demands on stamina, numerous injuries do occur. According to Ekstrand, factors related to players, such as joint instability, muscle tightness, inadequate rehabilitation after injury, or lack of training, account for 42 percent of injuries.[2] In his report, 24 percent were owing to unsatisfactory playing surfaces, 17 percent to equipment or inadequate shoes or nonuse of shinguards, 12 percent to rule infractions and foul play, and 29 percent to chance. A combination of factors also is fairly common.

EPIDEMIOLOGY

Many injuries occur in soccer players, but this may more reflect the popularity of the game than its dangers. We also must consider the exposure factor, which is the time that a player is at risk. The examination of the distribution and patterns of injury in soccer players reveals that, overall, 35 percent of the injuries may cause absences of more than 1-month duration. The injury incidence during games is highest among players participating at higher levels. Injuries during practice seem to be more common than in the lower series.[9] Injuries during games occur twice as often as during training. More than 80 percent of injuries involve the lower extremities, with ankle sprain being the most common (35 percent). Tackling causes more than 50 percent of the knee injuries. A total of 45 percent of all injuries result from contact, and affect more often the lower and the youth divisions (45 percent), whereas players at the senior level are reported to have only a 30 percent incidence of tackling injuries. On the other hand, overuse syndromes represent about 37 percent of all the injuries.[9]

In indoor soccer, male players aged 25 years old or older have the highest injury rate.[3] The most common cause of injury is collision with another player, which accounts for about 30 percent of all injuries; about 16 percent of all injuries occur when a player is kicked by an opponent. There does not seem to be a significant difference in the rate of ligament injuries for male and female players. (This is similar to basketball, where anterior cruciate ligament

[ACL] injuries are double in females.) However, male players sustain more ankle injuries than female players do; whereas the latter have a higher rate of knee ligament injuries. The injury rates are similar for goalkeepers and the other players. Goalkeepers more often injure fingers, heads, elbows, or hands, whereas the others more commonly incur ankle or thigh injuries.[3] About 75 percent of soccer injuries are considered as minor injuries, such as strains, sprains, and contusions.[7] In the youth, nearly 60 percent of the injuries occur in the lower extremities, about 20 percent involving ankle sprains and strains. Twenty percent are contusions and 6 percent are knee sprains and strains. It is reported that 75 percent of all amateur soccer players are less than 19 years old, suggesting a tremendous potential for future growth of soccer.[10]

Unlike other contact sports, such as American football and rugby, serious injuries in soccer are the exception but not the rule. To understand the nature of soccer injuries as compared with rugby and American football, it is necessary to review some basic movements of the game. In soccer, the goalie is the only one among the 11 team members who can touch the ball with the hands (only within certain areas of the field). The soccer player may kick the ball but also hit with the head or any other part of his or her body except the upper extremities. Pardon cited a Spanish report by Naves of all soccer injuries at various areas of the body (Table 19-1).[11] The lower extremities sustain 70 percent of all injuries.

The youth groups of soccer players who account for about 5 percent of active players are susceptible to sustain soccer injuries. The overall injury rate is 19:1000 player hours.[5] It seems that older girls have the highest injury rate and younger girls have the lowest incidence in this age group. The lower extremities predominate, but more injuries tend to occur in the upper extremities. Contusions occur in one-third of all soccer injuries, and this is less frequent in children than adults. Injuries become more prevalent with advancing age and occur more often in girls. The lower extremities, especially

TABLE 19-1 Injuries in Soccer

Area of Body	(%)	Injuries of Extremities	(%)
Lower extremity	70	Ankle	22
Upper extremity	19	Knee	20
Trunk	6	Thigh	15
Head and neck	5	Elbow	9
		Foot	8
		Wrist	8
		Hand	7
		Shoulder	6
		Others	5

the foot and ankle, again are involved most often. Fractures occur more often in the upper extremities. However, severe injuries fortunately are rare. Injury rates and severity increase with the onset of adolescence. Fields reported an injury rate of 24:1000 h of play among boys and 32:1000 h among girls.[12] Sixty-eight percent of the injuries involve the lower extremities and 10 percent the head and face.

Mortality over a period of 20 years, between 1938 and 1959, was 0.6 to 1.2 per 100,000 players, 33 percent secondary to head injuries.[12] Compared to American football, which is responsible for about 35 fatalities per year, it is estimated that the rate for soccer is lower nowadays because of improved safety measures, such as better conditioning, training, and environment.[13] As far as severity of injuries, about 60 percent of all injuries are considered to be minor, 27 percent moderate, and 11 percent severe.[2]

WOMEN IN SOCCER

The development of girls' and women's soccer has provided an increasing opportunity for women to experience popular team and contact sport activities.[1,14] Soccer has become more and more popular among girls and women, and it is now played in more than 50 countries. Lack of proper conditioning was cited as responsible for many of the injuries in female athletes by early reports that demonstrated that more injuries occur in female athletes than in male.[14,15] Soccer data showed an increase in serious injuries in women and girls during the 1970s. Later studies showed more equal distribution in injury rates, probably owing to the improvement in the level of play.[5,16]

A review of an NCAA Injury Surveillance System (ISS) supports the notion that there are generally similar injury rates in men and women sports with comparable rules. In the same study, female soccer players experienced a higher percentage of severe knee injuries than their counterparts, especially with respect to the ACL.[15] On the other hand, comparing with all injuries for men and women, there was an equal percentage of occurrences but exposure was twice for men. In other words, the distribution of injury is the same but the nature differs and women are more susceptible to injuries. Knee injury rate is similar in men (16 percent) and women (18 percent). Men generally sustain more knee injuries to all structures of the knee except for ACL. Women sustain twice as many ACL injuries as men, and more than half of all ACL injuries are noncontact in nature.[15]

The most common injuries in female soccer players are sprains to the lower extremity, and overuse injuries, which are responsible for more than 40 percent of persistent symptoms, are a consequence of those injuries. Women are more prone to sustain patellar dislocations than men, whereas men incur more dislocations to the upper extremity.[1]

CLASSIFICATION OF INJURIES

1. Trauma: 70 percent
   Direct—Contusion: 20 percent
      Bone
      Soft tissues
   Indirect—Sprain
      Strain
2. Overuse injuries: 30 percent
   Tendinitis
   Shin splint

Injuries are then classified as trauma, which may be caused by the direct blow or an indirect mechanism. Trauma accounts for about 70 percent of injuries. Overuse injuries account for 30 percent. In injuries involved, sprains occur for 29 percent, bursitis or tendinitis for 23 percent, contusions for 20 percent, and strains for 28 percent.[17]

TRAUMATOLOGY

Ankle sprains are much more prevalent in players with previous ankle sprain or clinical instability.

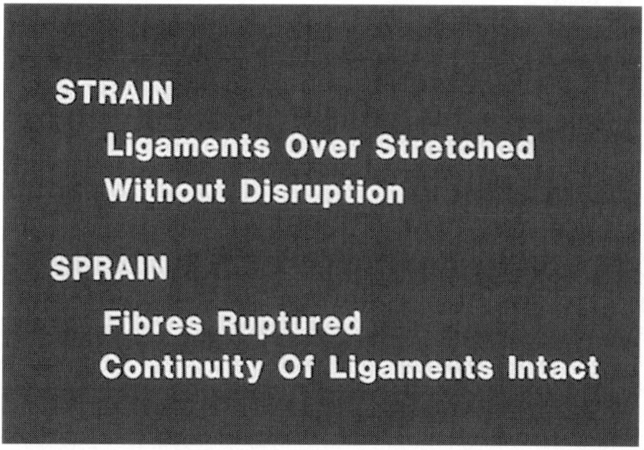

STRAIN

**Ligaments Over Stretched
Without Disruption**

SPRAIN

**Fibres Ruptured
Continuity Of Ligaments Intact**

FIG. 19-1   Strain versus sprain.

THIGH MUSCLE HEMATOMATA "CHARLEY HORSE"

Thigh muscle strains are found in 60 percent of players, and strains commonly affect this particular group.[17] Soft tissue injuries of the thigh can result in an inter- or intramuscular hematoma (charley horse). The very serious ones are intramuscular, where the muscle sheath remains intact. Thus, the hematoma remains intact. Untreated, this can lead to myositis ossificans, which can leave the individual sidelined with a partially mobile knee for as long as 1 year in some cases. Treatment includes hospital admission, ice, elevation, and no massage. Some experts suggest a fully flexed position, if possible, with the knee flexed to 140 degrees and held by a Velcro strap. Monitor the extent of the clot with x-ray and repeated "Doppler" ultrasound studies. Repeated measurement of limb circumference is important. Antibiotics and analgesics should be given. If active bleeding is noted, immobilization of the vessel can be attempted.

Some serious third-degree hematomas should be operated on. If the patient is worse after 72 h with unremitting severe pain and increasing immobility, take the patient to the operating room (OR). Well-trained experts have used the plastic surgical technique of high-vacuum liposuction. Open reduction and direct release of the hematoma, which lies right on top of the bone, is the accepted treatment. Once the clot has been evacuated, treatment is the same as first-degree injuries.

SPECIFIC INJURIES

The Ankle

The ankle is the part most often injured in soccer. The most common injury is sprain produced by a forceful inversion of the plantar-flexed foot. It may happen when a player is running and booting the ground instead of the ball. The severity of the sprain may vary from a single elongation to complete disruption of multiple ligaments, mainly the anterior talofibular, calcaneofibular, or posterior talofibular ligament. The ultimate injury, dislocation of the joint, may be associated with a fracture of one or many components of the ankle and foot (Fig. 19-3). Another mechanism of injury of ankle sprain is forceful eversion of the foot resulting in a deltoid ligament injury that may be associated with a fibular fracture or dislocation and sometimes rupture of the syndesmotic inferior talofibular ligament, which may result in a serious injury requiring a long period of recovery.

Ankle sprains are usually treated conservatively with successive compressive taping protection for a long period of time. It is recommended that a player wear ankle orthosis as a preventive

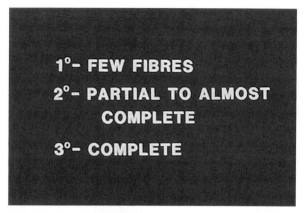

1°- FEW FIBRES

2°- PARTIAL TO ALMOST COMPLETE

3°- COMPLETE

FIG. 19-2 Classification of sprains.

measure to minimize the high risk of recurrence. Definitive treatment of complete dislocation is controversial in the elite athlete, and the orthopaedic surgeon may recommend operative treatment to repair all the ligaments, to promote optimal healing and early rehabilitation, and prevent late sequelae as much as possible.

Time Frame for Return to Sport after an Ankle Sprain (Fig. 19-4)

First-degree No symptoms of instability, lateral or medial or syndesmosis (tib/fib ligament): The athlete should perform single leg hopping, cutting, side step, cross step, forward and backward running comfortably, then tape and/or brace and return with a 3/4-cut or well-padded boot over the ankle.

Second-degree If there is lateral laxity, but a solid endpoint, sports physiotherapy rehabilitation should be initiated for 6 weeks. There should be tightening of the ligament and joint. Examination should not cause pain. The patient should allow taping, bracing, and stage 4 physiotherapy. Return the athlete to competition when he or she is stage 4 pain free and has attained equal agility to the normal leg.

Third-degree In a case of ruptured ligaments with laxity of mortice, after 6 to 8 weeks of full rehabilitation this patient normally needs to be treated surgically; then the patient can return to sports with a brace after 4 more months of rehabilitation; the patient should also get to stage 4 physiotherapy. Even a minimally displaced fracture should be treated operatively after the appropriate radiological as-

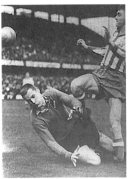

A

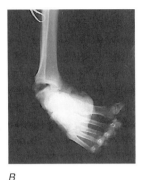

B

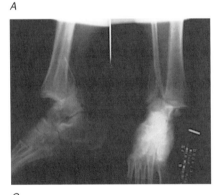

C

FIG. 19-3 Fracture-dislocation of left ankle. This patient required an open reduction. He would be out of action for 6 months or more. Soccer players have to be among the fittest of all athletes to tolerate this demanding sport. Fracture-dislocations of the ankle require immediate relocation if possible and early operation.

sessment to facilitate anatomical restoration and achieve the best functional result.

Contusion of the foot and fracture of the metatarsals, especially the fifth, are common. They are produced by kicking or when a player's foot is stepped on. Fracture of the base of the fifth metatarsal is usually caused by a strong pull on the peroneus brevis tendon. Subtalar joint may also be sprained. The treatment is surgical when there is displacement.

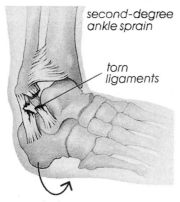

second-degree
ankle sprain

torn
ligaments

FIG. 19-4   The first-degree injury is the most common and most minor if not neglected. It is actually a sprain of the ligaments connecting the bones of the ankle. They are stretched but not torn, with very little swelling and no instability. The person is usually back to sports within a couple of weeks. The second-degree injury is more serious. The ankle ligaments are partially torn. There is some blood in the tissues and there will be bruising of the ankle after a couple of days. This condition requires at least 3 to 6 weeks before returning to full activity. The third-degree injury is the most severe. It is a more serious tear of the ligaments but rarely requires surgery. It takes 8 to 12 months for ligaments to fully heal in third-degree injuries.

Footballer's Ankle

This condition is a chronic periostitis or peritendinitis with calcification, which may occur on the anterior margin of the lower end of the tibia and over the talus. It is owing to the way in which the player ordinarily kicks the ball with the foot in plantarflexion or slight inversion, the ball making contact with the dorsal and medial aspects of the foot.

One complication of ankle sprain in soccer players has been described as a meniscoid lesion of the ankle.[18] This lesion is rare and characterized by pain, persistent swelling, and trapping. If the same complaints persist after a minimum of 6 months of conservative treatment that includes rehabilitation protective devices and anti-inflammatory medication and occasional periods of rest, surgery may be indicated. The pathology of the internal derangement of the ankle is a band of white fibrotic meniscus-like tissue from an old torn ligament lying between the fibula and the talus. The removal of this lesion appears to be an effective treatment and can be done arthroscopically.

The Knee

Injuries to the knee are sprain of the collateral ligament, mainly medial; tear of the meniscus; and damage to the cruciate ligaments, more frequently the ACL. Soccer causes the highest incidence of meniscus injuries, accounting for more than 35 percent of the cases.[1] Since the leg may be fixed in the ground by the cleats of the soccer shoe, sudden uncontrolled rotation and flexion changes of the body position during passing, running, or collision with another player (Fig. 19-5) may produce sudden rotation of the femur relative to the fixed lower leg, causing indirect injuries to the meniscus and knee joint. Even though soccer is a sport with great demands on the knee, the incidence of knee injuries in soccer players is one-fifth of the comparable population of American football players. The distribution of knee injuries in both groups is similar, but not the frequency.[19] Tackling causes more than 50 percent of knee injuries.[9] Ligament sprain often occurs when a player is tackled with the loaded leg fixed on the ground. High friction between the shoe and surface may produce excessive force on the knee or ankle, but too little friction can lead to slipping, which itself can cause injury. Thus, the use of shoes with cleats would lower the risk of such joint injuries.[2]

The incidence of chondral injuries in soccer players has been reported and may result from high velocities and repetitive pivoting, deceleration that the knee experiences, placing extreme stress on the articular cartilage.[20] Chondral injuries are believed to occur through two distinct mechanisms. They may arise through abrasive

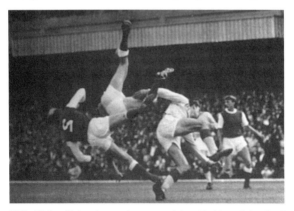

FIG. 19-5 All the players shown were injured in this collision. Dr. Bass calls it his "full house." Evidence of great speed, impact, and agility of play.

wear, which results in superficial fibrillation, and also by disruption of the deep cartilage ultrastructure by large shear forces.

The pathology found at arthroscopy is chondral delamination, which is a full-thickness chondral lesion exposing subchondral bone at the base of the lesion. The lesions are more often seen on the femoral condyle, but the patella facet or the trochlea may also be involved in the knee. It is possible that the same type of lesion occurs in other joints such as the ankle.

Recently, a great deal of attention has been focused on the treatment of chondral lesions. At the present time, debridement to bleeding bone and stimulation of fibrocartilage remains the most common surgical treatment. Partial-thickness lesions may be treated by an open vertical lesion and drilling or microfracturing of the subchondral bone. Autogenous core osteochondral (mosaic) graft has been tried. Allograft is another avenue. Attempts to fill isolated chondral lesions with laboratory-grown cartilage cells and to stimulate chondrogenesis with reversed periosteum have offered new treatment options. Currently, those techniques are experimental, the nature of the cartilage regrowth is controversial, and long-term outcome unknown or unpredictable.[21]

The Groin

Since soccer players manipulate the ball with their legs, groin injuries are fairly common. These are caused by sudden powerful overstretching of the leg and thigh in abduction and external rotation, especially if there is an opposing force such as a wet, heavy ball, an opponent's foot at full speed and in full swing, or the ground. These forces may overstretch the fibers of the muscles or tendons, the bony tissue of the pelvic ring, and the pubic symphysis.

Adolescent soccer players may sustain avulsion fractures of pelvic apophysis, such as the anteroinferior iliac spine where the rectus femoris originates or the anterosuperior iliac spine, where the sartorius is inserted, or even the ischium from a pulled hamstring (Fig. 19-6). The author has personally seen an avulsion of the lesser trochanter site of insertion of the psoas iliac muscle. Those avulsions are treated nonoperatively with excellent functional outcome.

Groin pain also occurs as an overuse syndrome that begins with an adductor strain, leading first to tendinitis followed by chondritis, osteitis, and formation of necrotic foci in the pubis or ossification along the pubis or in the attached muscles appearing as a calcifying tendinitis. This may cause a temporary or even permanent disability. Those, fortunately, are rare. Other pathologies in the regional area should be looked at, such as abdominal wall strain, hernia, hip, sacrum, or lower back afflictions. Groin pain is treated by rest, physical therapy, anti-inflammatory drugs, and rehabilitation. Steroid injection is not generally recommended but if it has to be done, one

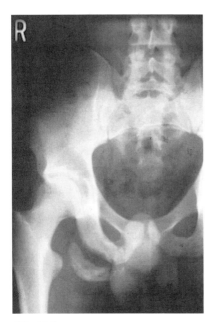

FIG. 19-6 Pictured is a seventeen-year-old male sprinter who lunged at the finish line and sustained avulsion of ischium, hamstring origin. This heals with 2 to 3 months judicious rest.

infiltration of the painful area with a local anesthetic along with a water-soluble corticosteroid solution may be cautiously used.[22] This can be operated on rarely. The adductor origin is partially detached from the pubic tubercle and pectineal line.

Shin Splint and Anterior Tibial Compartment Syndrome

Pain along the medial half distal border of the tibia is sometimes encountered. It usually represents a periostitis (shin splint). A stress fracture of the tibia or the fibula on the lateral side may be suspected. Pain, swelling, and limping are the main symptoms. A radiographic investigation may be normal at the beginning, but a bone scintigraphy confirms the diagnosis.

The treatment is a restriction from sport activities until complete bone healing has occurred.

Anterior tibial compartment syndrome has been reported in soccer players.[23] It may be produced by a kick from another player or result from running. Pain, swelling, and tenderness are the precursors of the onset, followed by weakness of the foot. The patient must be followed up closely and may be monitored for sensation and muscle activity. Development of the acute syndrome occurs in a matter of hours, and unremitting pain and progressive loss of dorsiflexion and motor function of the foot after trauma is a much clearer indication of the compartment syndrome than when overuse is the etiology. Peroneal nerve injury and shin splint must be considered in the differential diagnosis.

In the case of acute compartment syndrome (Fig. 19-7) (see Chap. 14), a surgical fasciotomy must be performed. In chronic cases as in recurrent cases the same treatment may be considered. The compartment syndrome may also be associated with a leg fracture often owing to direct trauma.

The Upper Extremity

Injuries to upper extremities in soccer account for nearly 20 percent of all injuries.[11] Sprain of the shoulder joint, with or without rotator cuff injury, or acromioclavicular or sternoclavicular separation may occur. A forceful backward motion while throwing the ball from the sideline with the arm highly extended or in abduction and external rotation may dislocate the shoulder joint.

The elbow is the most frequently affected joint in the upper extremity, and contusion is the most frequent cause. Radial head

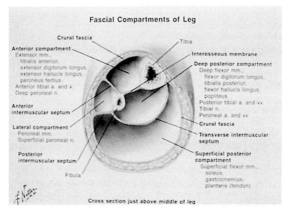

Fascial Compartments of Leg

Crural fascia
Tibia
Anterior compartment
    Extensor mm.
    tibialis anterior,
    extensor digitorum longus,
    extensor hallucis longus,
    peroneus tertius
    Anterior tibial a. and v.
    Deep peroneal n.
Interosseous membrane
Deep posterior compartment
    Deep flexor mm.
    flexor digitorum longus,
    tibialis posterior,
    flexor hallucis longus,
    popliteus
    Posterior tibial a. and vv.
    Tibial n.
    Peroneal a. and vv.
Anterior intermuscular septum
Crural fascia
Lateral compartment
    Peroneal mm.
    Superficial peroneal n.
Transverse intermuscular septum
Posterior intermuscular septum
Superficial posterior compartment
    Superficial flexor mm.,
    soleus,
    gastrocnemius,
    plantaris (tendon)
Fibula
Cross section just above middle of leg

FIG. 19-7   Acute compartment syndrome is a true surgical emergency. Chronic compartment syndrome can be operated on electively. The medial tibia and posterior and lateral (anterior) compartments are released.

fracture with sprain may be seen, but dislocation is rare. Because the goalie is the only player allowed to handle the ball with the hands, he or she sustains the most of the hand injuries. Soft tissue injuries, such as sprain and dislocation of the fingers, are more frequent than fractures.

The Trunk

Injuries to the trunk represent about 6 percent of all injuries.[11] Contusion or bruise, muscle strain, or fracture of the ribs caused by a blow from knees and elbows is common.

The Head and Neck

Injuries to the head and neck represent about 5 percent of all injuries.[11] Injuries ranging from sprain to muscle strain are frequent on all players, especially the goalkeeper. Fatal head injuries may even occur on rare occasion.[12] The mechanism of injury varies. First, when a player heads the ball incorrectly with the neck flexed or extended, he or she may experience increased head motion. A change in momentum of the head is a critical factor producing concussion. Second, a player may also sustain injury when a forcefully kicked ball strikes the head. Goalkeepers most commonly sustain collision injuries when the head strikes a goalpost, the ground, or another player's elbow, foot, or head. A third mechanism of injury may result from head-to-head contact.

Concussions, skull fractures, and epidural or subdural hematomas have all been reported following collision injury.[4] Improvement in the ball construction, particularly the addition of a plastic coating, seems to cause less severe head injuries and is considered the most important change in the prevention of head injuries. In fact, an older leather ball could absorb water, increasing its weight by 20 percent or more. However, we have to remember that even heading the ball correctly requires forcible impact and can cause headaches that may last for several days.

Proper coaching of techniques may help prevent soccer-related head-to-head injuries. Minor head injuries soccer players sustain in collisions are probably underdiagnosed or overlooked. Perhaps use of protective headgear, particularly by goalies, would make soccer an even safer game.

Heading the ball or a blow to the head may also result in neck injuries, and it has been reported that probably soccer players may develop premature degenerative changes in the cervical spine.[23] Understanding the etiology of head and neck injuries can initiate preventive measures.

Controlled head contact with the ball or heading is as valuable a skill as shooting on goal, but it places the player at risk of injury from ball as well as from other players simultaneously trying to head the ball.

The Eye

Blunt trauma to the eye occurs in soccer. Hyphema is the most common disorder and may lead to secondary glaucoma, corneal abrasion, lens trauma, pupillary defects, orbital fracture, and involvement of the retina and the vitreous, including hemorrhage and detachment.[24]

Injuries are unilateral and are caused by a kicked ball striking the eye and periorbita from close range, a kicking foot of another player, or a hit by the skull of an opponent attempting a head butt. Athletes who need to wear glasses should avoid wearing ordinary glasses. Those needing correction for refractive error should wear polycarbonate sport goggles that are lightweight and effective nowadays. It is estimated that serious complications occur in 25 percent of sports-related eye injuries. Protective devices are therefore mandatory in order to minimize any risk of eye injury.[24]

MANAGEMENT OF SOCCER INJURIES

Knowledge of the responsibility of the physician, trainer, coach, and organization authorities as well as certain principles of management and a logical approach to on-the-field diagnosis are essential prerequisites in order to make proper on-the-field decisions and institute necessary first aid measures.

All decisions regarding playability of the injured athlete during a game situation are the sole responsibility of the team physician. In the absence of a physician, the decision becomes the responsibility of the athlete trainer or the coach if a trainer is not available. As a matter of fact, as it is necessary to determine the nature as well as the extent of injury, the physician, trainer, or coach on the field is the privileged individual who can be most helpful in assessing the acute soccer injury. Understanding the mechanisms of injury is usually more informative than any other single piece of information in arriving at the correct diagnosis.

Basic principles of management following an injury must be respected. One must restrict play of the injured athlete and observe, listen, examine, and then initiate treatment when indicated. Before and following return to play, a functional evaluation is necessary. Anytime that it becomes obvious that a player has been injured, the player should be removed from play.

Field Examination

The immediate management of soccer injuries entails an evaluation of the injured athlete at or near the site of injury, the proper determination of his or her playability, and the initiation of treatment when needed.

The best time for accurate assessment of the degree of damage is immediately following injury when muscle spasm is absent, pain is not severe, and swelling has not yet developed. Initial observations and assessment should be made on the spot. The priority is the evaluation of the state of consciousness and the general appearance of the athlete, the color of the skin, the ability to move, the respiratory rate, and the presence of abrasions, lacerations, pain, deformity, or bleeding.

If the athlete is conscious, he or she should relate the experience of injury, indicate the site injured and the mechanism of injury, either by a direct or indirect blow, a fall, or a twist. It is important to know if the athlete felt something popping, breaking, or going out, and if he or she was immediately disabled. Those are expressions of severity. Has there been any previous injury to the same site? If so what was the extent of previous injury? What is the precise location and nature of the pain? Any area of swelling, deformity, or muscle spasm must be noted. One must search for tenderness and crepitus and assess stability, weakness, or dysfunction in the extremities; any sensory defects; and the range of motion.

During the 5 or 10 min after injury, there is usually not much pain. This is especially true with complete ligament disruption. Localizing the point of maximum tenderness with a fingertip is a reliable indicator of the site of injury.

On the field, careful evaluation of the site of injury should precede any movement of an injured player so that appropriate precautions may be taken. In the face of a suspected severe injury, it is important to assist the player off the ground, keeping his or her weight off the injured part. Usually, the athlete can bear partial weight. One should not hesitate to take the injured athlete to a more appropriate area and even use a stretcher if there is any question of aggravating an injury by any other method of removal or to put the player in an ambulance, sending him or her to the hospital when the findings or symptoms indicate that this is necessary. The main thing is to make sure that there is not any obvious instability or deformity, and it is something you can take care of right away.

The next steps would be to put ice on the part until an x-ray can be taken. X-ray examination should always be made as promptly as possible when serious injuries are suspected.

Playability

If after careful examination, the injury appears to be insignificant, then a functional evaluation should be done, and if normal function is present, the athlete can safely be allowed to return to play. If abnormal function is observed, then further participation should be delayed until a more thorough evaluation or definitive treatment can be concluded. If the injury is significant then restriction should be continued and treatment instituted immediately. An on-the-sidelines decision is often required to determine an athlete's ability to return to play. It is the physician's responsibility to make a judgment on the severity of injury sustained as well as the risk of aggravating it with continued play. The decision is usually based on incomplete information. In case of doubt, the athlete should not be returned to play.

There are several findings that suggest significant injury and militate against a return to play.

1. A "pop" at the time of injury
2. Inability to bear full weight on the leg while walking
3. The inability to run or change direction
4. Loss of motion
5. Instability or false motion
6. Pain or immediate swelling

The presence of any of the foregoing findings demands the removal of the athlete from the game and a more thorough evaluation of the injured part.

The importance of making a good diagnosis after the examination on the field can be summarized in two points; first, determine the severity of injury, and second, the playability of the player.

Transportation

Transportation with adequate aids and in proper condition should be assured and provided. The transportation to medical facilities is important in order to have proper radiographic examination, either simple or more elaborate, such as stress films or even tomodensitometry (TACO) or magnetic resonance (MRI).

Initial Treatment

Initial treatment is based on the acronym RICE (rest, ice, compression, evaluation). They are the key steps in the initial management of acute injuries. Application of ice is used for controlling pain and hemorrhage, compression to increase the pressure on the tissue, decreasing the extravasation of fluid and minimizing the hemorrhage and swelling. Elevation increases venous return, helping to prevent swelling, and immobilization helps decrease and minimizing pain and swelling of the injured part. The rapidity of swelling development after injury is an important guide to assess both the severity and the type of injury sustained. Swelling that develops immediately after injury indicates bleeding within the joint, resulting in a hemarthrosis. If the swelling appears the day after injury, usually it is owing to synovial fluid as a result of a reactive synovitis.

Aspiration

Aspiration of a swollen joint may be useful as a diagnostic tool. In case of a hemarthrosis we may be able to distinguish between a ligament disruption and a fracture. In the latter case we will find fat bubbles in the blood. Also aspiration may be used as a therapeutic tool in relieving pain by decompressing a tense swollen joint. However, it has to be followed by a proper compressive immobilization in order to put the joint at rest and minimize the amount of recurrent swelling.

Arthroscopy

Arthroscopy is used not only for diagnostic purpose but also for treatment. The indication for arthroscopy is pain of increasing severity that, in the athlete's opinion, limits the performance on the field; presence of persistent or recurrent effusion; and failure of a proper conservative treatment. Clinical diagnostic accuracy of knee pathology ranges from 70 percent to 75 percent, whereas arthroscopic diagnostic accuracy exceeds 95 percent in the hands of experienced arthroscopists. Synovial lesions can be visualized, biopsied, and evaluated. The mechanics and the tracking of the patella on the femur can be assessed. The function and integrity of the cruciate ligaments can also be tested. One can probe the entire lateral and medial menisci. Arthroscopy may be used to follow up studies on damaged articular cartilage of a joint.

Arthroscopic surgery is a well-accepted technique for several procedures, such as cartilage shaving, drilling, release of tight structures, resection or division of thickened shelf or plica, removal of loose bodies, or fixation of osteochondral lesion such as osteochondritis dissecans. Partial or complete arthroscopic meniscectomy are currently done but we can do more and more repair of meniscal tears. We now use arthroscopy to perform limited meniscectomy and whenever possible to repair or resuture it, to reconstruct unstable joints, and even to reduce articular fractures, thus minimizing the incision and morbidity as well as facilitating rehabilitation.

Safety

It is known that muscle tightness predisposes to strain, and the question has been raised whether soccer training itself can lead to muscle shortness. It has been observed that most ranges of motion would be reduced after training without stretching and that all motion is reduced at 24 h. The situation could be easily corrected if a stretching exercise program is undertaken.[25] Contract-relaxed stretching may prevent certain types of injuries such as muscle strain. A session of stretching exercises seems to be effective in countering the decrease in range of joint motion normally caused by a standard soccer workout. The stretching consists of isometric contractions followed by relaxation and then passive lengthening or elongation of the muscle.

Playing in Hot Weather

Soccer players who are unacclimated to heat and play in hot humid weather risk being incapacitated by heat exhaustion or even killed by heat stroke. When this kind of environment occurs, the trainer, team physician, or sport authorities must promptly initiate modifications in play, including shorter playing periods, more water breaks, and unlimited substitutions that will decrease the number of heat-related injuries despite continued extreme temperature during the rest of the game.

A big part of the coaching plan on a humid day should be regularly scheduling substitutions. At the end of the game, the players will not be exhausted from the heat, and one should remember that the best preventive measure is water, water, and water. Athletes practicing or playing on hot, humid days cannot get too much water before, during, and after the competition.

Players, coaches, officials, and parents need to be made aware of the potential for heat injury. Elias suggested guidelines according to wet bulb globe temperature (WBGT), with quarterly fluid breaks at WBGT over 65°F, shortened game times or unlimited substitution at WBGT over 73°F, and moving midday games to earlier or later times at WBGT over 82°F.[26] An event should not be scheduled at the hottest time of the day or year and the insidious nature of dehydration should be recognized. Presenting symptoms usually include dizziness, light-headedness, weakness, headache, mild disorientation, nausea, and syncope. Players should be allowed to rest in an air-conditioned area with ice packs applied to the groin, neck, and axillae. Oral hydration should be begun. Intravenous hydration is occasionally required.

Another aspect of safety and prevention is the fact that soccer is played either outdoors or indoors, that is, on various surfaces. Soccer is played on grass or Astroturf or on the floor indoors. It is known that Astroturf is not a stable static surface. With use and exposure, irreversible changes occur in its physical makeup. Even if the diminished impact absorption capacity clearly seems detrimental to player safety, players seem to prefer to play on artificial turf instead of grass field because grass surfaces provide a less uniform playing surface in wet and dry conditions than the artificial surface. It seems that the artificial surface is better for the techniques of the game but not for the safety and prevention of injury of the players; as it is known that there are more soccer injuries on artificial surfaces than on grass.

On the other hand, the general use of shin pads by the players and headgear by the goalie is still to be seen. Also, the usefulness of padded goalposts is still to be proven in preventing soccer injuries. Soccer is one of the least expensive sports; approximately $60 outfits a young player and a $40 registration fee allows kids to enjoy the sport all summer long.

CONCLUSION

Soccer is a dynamic ball game and the most popular team sport in the world. It is considered a safe sport for both sexes in youth soccer, even on a highly competitive level. It is a sport with few and generally minor injuries, but unfortunately permanent disability and even fatalities may result from soccer injuries. Relative to safety, according to international rules, there are no game stoppages and few substitutions; thus, fluid replenishment may be a problem that may be minimized and prevented by simple rule modifications and by providing fluid intake with fluid as simple as water.

REFERENCES

1. Brynhildsen J, Ekstrand J, et al: Previous injuries and persisting symptoms in female soccer players. *Int J Sports Med* 11:489–492, 1990.
2. Ekstrand J, Gillquist J: Incidence of soccer injuries and their relation to training and team success. *Am J Sports Med* 11:63–67, 1983.
3. Lindenfeld TN, Schmitt DJ, et al: Incidence of injury in indoor soccer. *Am J Sports Med* 22:364–371, 1994.
4. Darley SW, Barsan WG: Head injuries in soccer. *Phys Sports Med* 20(8):79–85, 1992.
5. Sullivan JA, Gross WA: Evaluation of injuries in youth soccer. *Am J Sports Med* 8:325–327, 1980.
6. Tegner Y, Henriksson A, et al: Avulsion of the anterior-inferior iliac spine in young soccer players. *Clin Sports Med* 2:143–148, 1990.
7. Ward A: Soccer: Safe kicks for kids. *Phys Sports Med* 15(8):151–158, 1987.
8. Schmidt-Olsen S, Bunemann LKH: Soccer injuries in youth. *Br J Sports Med* 19:161–164, 1985.
9. Nielsen AB, Yde J: Epidemiology and traumatology of injuries in soccer. *Am J Sports Med* 17:803–807, 1989.
10. Keller CS: The medical aspects of soccer injuries: Epidemiology. *Am J Sports Med* 15:230–237, 1987.
11. Pardon ET: Lower extremities are site of most soccer injuries. *Phys Sports Med* 43–48, 1977.
12. Fields KB: Head injuries in soccer. *Phys Sports Med* 17(1):69–73, 1989.
13. Smoklaka VN: Death on the soccer field and its prevention. *J Sports Med* 9(8):101–107, 1981.

14. Engstrom B, Johansson C, et al: Soccer injuries among elite female players. *Am J Sports Med* 19:372–375, 1991.

15. Arenth EA: Orthopaedic issues for active and athletic women. *Clin Sport Med* 13(2):483–503, 1994.

16. Nilsson S, Rooas A: Soccer injuries in adolescents. *Am J Sports Med* 6:358–361, 1978.

17. Ekstrand J, Gillquist J: Avoidability of soccer injuries. *Int J Sports Med* 4:124–128, 1983.

18. McCarrol JR, Schrader JW, et al: Meniscoid lesions of the ankle in soccer players. *Am J Sports Med* 15:255–257, 1987.

19. Pritchett JW: Cost of high school soccer injuries. *Am J Sports Med* 9:64–66, 1981.

20. Levy AS, Lohnes J, et al: Chondral delamination of the knee in soccer players. *Am J Sports Med* 24(5):634–639, 1996.

21. Leach R, Corbett M: Anterior tibial compartment syndrome in soccer players. *Am J Sports Med* 24(5):634–639, 1996.

22. Smodlaka VN: Groin pain in soccer players. *Phys Sports Med* 8(8):57–61, 1980.

23. Kurosawa H, Yamanoi T, et al: Radiographic findings of degeneration in cervical spines of middle-aged soccer players. *Skeletal Radiol* 20:437–440, 1991.

24. Orlando RG: Soccer-related eye injuries in children and adolescents. *Phys Sports Med* 18(11):103–106, 1988.

25. Moller MHL: Stretching exercises and soccer: Effect of stretching on range of motion in the lower extremity in connection with soccer training. *Int J Sports Med* 50–52, 1985.

26. Elias SR, Roberts WO, et al: Team sports in hot weather: Guidelines for modifying youth soccer. *Phys Sports Med* 19:67–80, 1991.

SUGGESTED READINGS

Chantrane A: Knee joint in soccer players: Osteoarthritis and axis deviation. *Med Sci Sports Exerc* 17:434–439, 1985.

Ekstrand J, Nigg BM: Surface-related injuries in soccer. *Sports Med* 8:56–62, 1989.

Ekstrand J: Soccer injuries and their mechanism: A prospective study. *Med Sci Sport Exerc* 15:267–270, 1993.

Engstrom B: Does a major knee injury definitely sideline an elite soccer player? *Am J Sports Med* 18:101–105, 1990.

Hanson PG, Angevine M, et al: Osteitis pubis in sports activities. *Phys Sports Med* 111N114, 1978.

Kirkendall DT: The applied sport science of soccer. *Phys Sports Med* 13(4):53–59, 1985.

Maehlum S, Dahl E: Frequency of injuries in a youth soccer tournament. *Phys Sports Med* 14(7):73–79, 1986.

McMaster WC, Maarten W: Injuries in soccer. *Am J Sports Med* 354–357, 1978.

Neyret P, Donedll ST: Partial meniscectomy and anterior cruciate ligament rupture in soccer players: A study with a minimum of 20 years follow-up. *Am J Sports Med* 21:455–460, 1993.

Mark Heard   Carol Gibson-Coyne

Cross country skiing is gaining in popularity as both a recreational and competitive sport. There are over 16 million participants in this highly aerobic and basically safe sport worldwide.[1] Injury in the sport can be either traumatic or, as is more commonly the case, overuse from repetitive trauma through training or racing. Restrom and Johnson quote a study that looked at the Swedish National Team in 1983 to 1984 and found 75 percent of injuries were from overuse and 25 percent were traumatic.[2] Incidence studies put injury rates between 0.049 to 5.63 injuries per thousand skier days, depending on the population studied.[1] Owing to varied terrain, snow conditions, waxing, equipment, and ability, it is difficult to determine the risk of injury of any given participant.

With the advent of skate skiing technique popularized by Bill Koch in the early 1980s, there have been some changes in injury patterns in the sport. Speeds of 60 to 80 km per hour can be reached with the latest equipment and waxing techniques.[2] Considering the noticeable lack of safety features in cross country ski equipment, we may see a change in the incidence of traumatic injury as these speeds are being reached by more participants. The skating technique also has a different pattern of overuse injury than the classic technique, and an attempt is made to identify the etiology of different injuries.

The goal of this chapter is to supply the reader with a means of identifying the common overuse and traumatic injuries in cross country skiing (Diagnosis). An approach is given to the management of these injuries from the perspective of the coach, trainer/therapist, and physician (Treatment). Last, an attempt is made to provide ways to avoid these injuries (Prevention).

UPPER EXTREMITY INJURIES

Shoulder

Impingement syndromes of the shoulder, whether subacromial bursitis, rotator cuff tendinitis, or impingement secondary to instability of the glenohumeral joint, are one of the most common groups of injuries in the sport. Impingement is more common in the skating technique owing to longer pole length and asymmetrical poling.

Diagnosis

Indications include insidious onset of shoulder pain that is aggravated by poling, especially up hill, pain with overhead activities, positive impingement test (grimace with forward elevation of the arm as the greater tuberosity impinges on the acromion), and pain improvement with a subacromial injection of zylocaine.

Differential Diagnosis

If there is a traumatic history of a fall on the shoulder, don't miss a rotator cuff tear. Masters skiers with a long history of impingement may have a cuff tear through attrition with no specific trauma. If there is significant rotator cuff weakness after rest and physical therapy, an arthrogram, MRI, or arthroscopy is indicated. Instability, whether posttraumatic anterior instability or multidirectional, can present in the skier as an impingement syndrome. Osteolysis of the acromial clavicular (AC) joint in the young racer and arthritis in the masters skier are not uncommon. Zylocaine in the AC joint can help sort out this problem.

Management

The initial goal is to decrease inflammation. Rest, ice, anti-inflammatories, and electrical modalities are initiated, usually for a period of 2 to 4 weeks. A rotator cuff and scapular-thoracic assessment and strengthening program commence once the inflammation subsides. The therapist should also assess the cervical spine and ribs for abnormalities.

The coach should review the poling technique with the following concerns. Pole length should be lowered to a maximum of chin height until symptoms resolve. Shrugging of the shoulders on pole plant and positioning of the arms too far away from the shoulders laterally are technical errors that put the skier at risk. The rigidity and weight of the pole should be assessed, as a stiff, heavy pole is more likely to give problems. The skier should alternate classic with skating techniques and, if severe, should perform legs-only workouts to rest the shoulders. The physician can consider an injection of cortisone into the subacromial bursa. This can play a role in the very acute shoulder or when therapy is not effective. The use of the drug is to decrease the amount of inflammation and must be followed by a shoulder and scapulothoracic strengthening program. A maximum of three injections is recommended owing to weakening of the cuff tendon and thus having an increased risk of rotator cuff tear with multiple injections.

For refractory cases, an orthopaedic assessment for an arthroscopic subacromial decompression is indicated. As previously mentioned, occasionally shoulder instability is the primary problem and surgically addressing the instability can alleviate the impingement symptoms.

Prevention

Prevention includes pre- and midseason assessment of rotator cuff and scapulothoracic strength and function; a core strengthening program to improve shoulder girdle stability; and pole length, weight, and stiffness assessment by coach therapist and athlete. The athlete's training program should have a good balance of classic and skating techniques. Poling techniques should be reviewed to prevent shoulder shrugging, lateral pole placement, and excessively high elbow elevation.

Acromial Clavicular Joint

Direct trauma to the shoulder region by a fall, where the arm is kept in and at the skier's side while the athlete lands directly on the shoulder, produces injuries to the AC joint. The most common injury is a separation of the joint, referred to as an AC separation.

Diagnosis

Tenderness when directly palpating the joint is a very accurate method of picking up this injury. There is often swelling and hematoma directly over and around the joint. Deformity is present in severe separations where the distal end of the clavicle protrudes upward.

Differential Diagnosis

Fractures of the clavicle can present clinically, such as an AC separation. An x-ray of the shoulder area should be taken if there is any doubt, as a fracture of the distal clavicle often needs surgical fixation. Injury to the rotator cuff should always be suspected with this type of fall. Repeated exams of rotator cuff strength or an arthrogram, ultrasound, or MRI should be performed if any weakness persists.

Management

Rest, ice, analgesia, anti-inflammatories, and a return to skiing as symptoms permit is the appropriate treatment for the vast majority of AC separations, even with mild deformity. Taping and slings offer symptomatic relief in the acute stages. There are special splint designs that attempt to reduce separations; however, it is questionable as to whether they are successful in preventing residual deformity and discomfort. In cases with major deformity (grade 3) controversy still persists regarding treatment; thus, an orthopaedic referral should be made so that a full discussion of options may ensue.

Prevention

The coach must make the appropriate decision regarding location of training, as well as safe race course design when snow conditions are poor to prevent high-speed falls.

Hand

Ulnar Collateral Ligament of the Thumb

One of the most common traumatic injuries in cross country skiing is spraining of the ulnar collateral ligament of the first metacarpal phalangeal joint of the hand.[3] The injury is caused by the ski pole creating a varus force to the first metacarpal phalangeal joint when the skier falls on an outstretched hand.

Diagnosis

Examine the ligament for laxity in the flexed and extended position. A local anesthetic or median nerve block may be necessary to accurately diagnose a complete tear. It is necessary to compare laxity of the ligament with the uninjured thumb. An x-ray is recommended to avoid missing an avulsion of bone. Complete tears with or without a bony avulsion are at risk of flipping behind the adductor apponeurosis and will not heal. This has been termed the stenner lesion and emphasizes the importance of proper diagnosis of the complete tear.

Management

Acute management includes rest, ice, compression, and elevation (RICE). Partial tears (first- or second-degree) can be managed with the use of a thermal plastic splint that is molded to a ski pole for 4 to 6 weeks. Taping techniques are helpful but tend to stretch out during workouts. Complete tears (third-degree) should be managed surgically. These athletes can return to skiing in 10 days to 2 weeks in a molded fiberglass cast or with a high-temperature thermal plastic splint. Continued splint protection should be maintained for at least 3 months.

Prevention

Preventative splinting for poor or icy ski conditions may be helpful, especially if there has been a history of past or recent injury. Pole design modifications in the future may decrease the incidence of this injury.[3]

LOWER EXTREMITY INJURIES

Overuse injuries in the lower extremity are commonly related to a multitude of factors. Overlay of lumbar spine or pelvic dysfunction can make a lower extremity injury difficult to treat and should be assessed as a factor in this group of injuries.

Hip Strains

Strained muscles around the hip girdle are commonly seen in the skier using the classic skiing technique, from back slipping when the waxing conditions are poor. They can also occur traumatically with a fall. Strains commonly occur to iliopsoas and hip adductors and less often to hamstrings and hip extensors.

Diagnosis

A good history of the pain pattern and the aggravating motions are helpful (i.e., repetitive back slipping). Question radiating pain in the hip region as coming from the back. With strains, direct palpation of the muscle and tendon should elicit the athlete's discomfort. Chronic iliopsoas bursitis or tendinitis shows loss of hip extension.

Differential Diagnosis

Hip strains can be mimicked by lumbar disk or facet irritation of lumbar nerve roots (L1 to L4). Sacral iliac joint dysfunction can be the primary or secondary cause of pain in the hip region.

Treatment

Avoid the offending action, such as steep hills, that can cause back slipping in classic skiing. Use rest, anti-inflammatories, and electrical modalities until the inflammation settles. This can take as long as 6 to 8 weeks in a bad psoas strain. Perform gentle stretching of the hip flexors, hamstrings, and adductors. Avoid overstretching the strained muscle, as this will continue to irritate the injury. Optimizing lumbosacral mechanics and strengthening of the abdominal muscles should be incorporated into the rehabilitation.

Prevention

An appropriate year-round stretching program of the hip girdle muscles, especially hip flexors, and strengthening program for trunk and abdominal stability is encouraged. Try to avoid classic skiing in poor waxing conditions. Incorporate partial or full herringbone techniques for hill work in poor waxing conditions. Regular assessment of lumbosacral function and trunk and abdominal strength is prudent.

Knee Sprains

Injury to the medial collateral ligament (MCL) of the knee can occur from a traumatic event or from repetitive spraining by over-pronating while skate skiing, thus creating a valgus force across the knee with every stride.

Diagnosis

In the case of a traumatic MCL injury, there is usually a history of a fall with a valgus force to the knee often associated with a tearing or "popping" sensation on the medial aspect of the knee. Physical exam reveals swelling and bruising on the medial side, with tenderness along the femoral (most common) or tibial insertion of the ligament. Gapping of the joint in extension suggests a complete or third-degree tear of the ligament. Complaint of pain without instability suggests a first-degree tear. A second-degree tear is typically characterized by instability and gapping while in 30 degrees of flexion but stable while in extension.

The nontraumatic repetitive MCL sprain injury is usually a first-degree tear. The history is usually an insidious onset of medial knee pain that is aching in nature and not mechanical. Observing the overpronation of the foot, internal rotation of the hip, and excessive riding of the inner edge of the ski in the skating technique helps make the diagnosis. A physical exam reveals a stable knee with tenderness along the MCL.

Differential Diagnosis

A torn medial meniscus can mimic a MCL sprain in both the acute-traumatic and repetitive sprain situation. Suspicion of a meniscal injury should occur if the injury is not responding to treatment or if there is a mechanical component to the symptoms (i.e., locking and catching).

In the traumatic MCL injury, care should be made to avoid missing a torn anterior cruciate ligament or a fracture of the tibial plateau.

Treatment

For the acute sprain of the MCL; rest, ice, compression, and anti-inflammatories are initiated as soon as possible. For second- and third-degree sprains, or a first-degree sprain in a valgus knee, the use of a hinged knee brace will prevent permanent ligament laxity. The brace should be worn full time (night included) for a period of 4 to 6 weeks. Early range of motion, particularly extension, is helpful to prevent stiffness. Crutches should be used until good quadriceps control is achieved and a normal gait pattern is demonstrated. Second- and third-degree sprains should be given at least 6 weeks of rest prior to returning to skate skiing, with a return to classic technique possibly 1 to 2 weeks earlier. The use of a hinged knee sport brace may facilitate an earlier return during the competitive season. Some MCL sprains in the older skiing population can take 3 to 6 months to resolve.

For the chronic repetitive first-degree MCL sprain, rest, ice, and anti-inflammatories help to settle symptoms. The coach or therapist should assess the athlete for a valgus thrust in the skating technique. A full assessment of foot mechanics should be made as orthotics, or canting, of the boot binding complex may eliminate the problem. The use of a hinged knee brace or proprioceptive taping of the knee may enable the athlete to continue skating in the competitive season.

Prevention

The coach should watch for excessive valgus in the skating technique. Balance drills during the glide phase can help prevent repetitive trauma. The use of orthotics or canting should be considered early if the athlete demonstrates imbalance. The coach needs to assess foot position in a downhill track before canting for permanent repositioning.

For the prevention of traumatic sprains, the use of quick step turning drills for those fast, icy corners may train the athlete to avoid a fall in this common scenario for an MCL sprain.

Lower Leg Injuries

Exercise-induced anterior compartment syndrome should be suspected in the elite skier with "shin splints."

Diagnosis

Anterior compartment syndrome is characterized by an insidious onset of anterior lower leg pain. The pain usually appears after a fairly predictable length of time (i.e., 15 min of skiing), this time factor decreases in length as the intensity of the training increases or the condition gets worse. The athlete complains of a tightness in the anterior compartment and occasionally of numbness in the distribution of the deep peroneal nerve (between the great and second toe). In its worst form, it can cause a foot drop from compromise of the anterior compartment structures. This condition is most common in the athletes with a mesomorphic build. The diagnosis can be best made in an exercise lab where compartment pressures can be taken during exercises.

Differential Diagnosis

Tendinitis and periostitis can occur from overtraining. A stress fracture should be ruled out, in the atypical picture with a bone scan.

Management

If an early diagnosis is made, this condition can be averted by decreasing the amount and intensity of training until the athlete is asymptotic. This may require a period of complete rest. Ice and anti-inflammatories may also help. Gentle massage followed by ice and elevation may help mobilize the fascia and rid the compartment of fluid from inflamed muscles. Some athletes' symptoms have been made worse by aggressive massage. The coach should make sure the bindings on the ski are mounted properly, because, if the binding is too far back, the athlete has to lift up the front of the ski with every stride, which stresses the anterior compartment muscles. For the more chronic and severe cases, the only solution is a surgical release of the fascia overlying the compartment.

Prevention

Proper mounting of the bindings on skate skis is essential to prevent this problem. The coach and trainer should avoid accelerating the volume and intensity of training too quickly, primarily of the skating technique. Early detection is important to prevent surgical intervention.

Foot and Ankle

Injury around the foot and ankle make up about 15 percent of all cross country skiing injuries.[1] Achilles tendinitis, ankle sprains and fractures, subluxing peroneal tendons, plantar fascitis, and sesmoiditis are prevalent injuries in the cross country skier.

Achilles Tendinitis

This is most common in those performing the classic technique. It can be caused by the mechanical rubbing of the low-cut boot or by the eccentric load in the "preload" just prior to the kick phase. This is amplified when waxing conditions are poor and the athlete back slips, causing increased strain on the Achilles tendon.

Management

Initially rest, ice, anti-inflammatories, and local modalities are used to decrease inflammation. Topical anti-inflammatories are particularly helpful. A gentle stretching program of both gastrox and soleus complexes should be included. A heel raise and boot modifications can decrease the stresses to the tendon. A night dorsiflexion splint can help in the chronic case. In rare cases, surgical debridement can help the refractory case.

Prevention

A proper stretching program is key to preventing this problem. Proper boot fit and orthotics with a heel lift can help. Adjusting technique for hill climbing when waxing conditions are poor is helpful. Treating this condition aggressively at an early onset can prevent the long chronic condition that affects so many athletes (Fig. 20-1).

Ankle Sprains and Fractures

In the traumatic situation, it is important to differentiate the injured lateral ligaments (talo-fibular and calcaneo-fibular) from a fracture of the lateral maleolus. External rotation of the ankle is involved in both of these injuries. An inability to weight bear or any bony tenderness should get an x-ray.

Management

Fractures require casting or surgery. Ankle sprains require all the usual modalities to reduce inflammation. Casting is rarely used; however, function splints are very popular. The function splint can facilitate an earlier return to sport. Proprioception and balance exercises are important to prevent reinjury (Fig. 20-2).

Prevention

Development of higher boots for use while performing skating technique has helped. Further design work in boot and bindings is

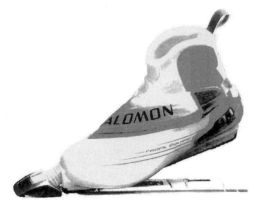

FIG. 20-1   Classic ski boot with binding.

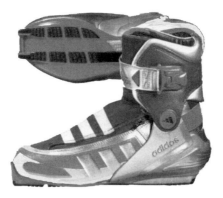

FIG. 20-2   Skate ski boot.

needed to help prevent ankle injury. At present there are no releasable bindings on the market. Preseason plyometric and balance programs help prevent injury.

Sesamoiditis

This injury occurs most commonly in the skating technique, with the pronating foot repetitively inflaming the sesamoids of the great toe flexors.

Diagnosis

The diagnosis is pain directly on the sesamoids of the great toe flexors.

Differential Diagnosis

The differential diagnosis is a stress fracture of a sesamoid and arthritis of the first metatarsal phalangel joint. A bone scan can help differentiate these problems.

Management

Rest, ice, and anti-inflammatories reduce inflammation. The use of orthotics with a medial metatarsal pad to unload the sesamoids is helpful. For the refractory case or the stress fracture, sometimes 4 to 6 weeks in a walking cast is necessary to allow this problem to settle down.

Prevention

Rigid-soled boots with orthotics for the hyperpronating athlete help. The coach should assess the glide phase to make sure the ski is flat on the snow.

Spine and Sacral Iliac Joint

The presence of back pain and sacral iliac joint dysfunction is common in cross country skiers. Eriksson et al. looked at elite Scandinavian skiers and found an incidence of 64 percent who had back pain that affected their skiing ability. This seemed to be associated with the classic diagonal technique.[4] In a Canadian study that look at sacral iliac dysfunction, abnormal function was felt to be found more with the skating technique.[5] Many other injuries seem to be related to dysfunction of the spine and pelvis and it is important to assess them as a key biomechanical link to the extremities.

Diagnosis

These injuries are usually insidious in onset and caused from overuse. Try to determine the offending activity. Common situations include rigid hyperextension of the lumbar spine throughout the classic striding and double poling technique in classic skiing, and pain and malalignment of the sacral iliac joint from excessive pelvic rotation during weight shift in the offset skating technique. The physical exam should include a full assessment of the lumbar spine and sacral iliac joint. This should include muscle length and strength of the major muscle groups around the pelvis, lumbar facet joint movement, pelvic symmetry, and rotation of the sacral iliac joint.

Differential Diagnosis

A neurologic exam in the athlete with radiating pain down into a leg should be performed to avoid missing a herniated vertebral disk. If unsure, a CT scan or MRI should be arranged. In the athlete with very tight hamstrings and lumbar back pain, a plain x-ray of the lumbar spine will pick up a spondylolysis and spondylolysthesis. In the masters skier, stenosis of the lumbar spine should be ruled out by CT or MR scan.

Management

Decreasing training or completely ceasing to ski are often necessary to settle symptoms. Anti-inflammatories can help acute situations. Physiotherapy with stretching and core strengthening are the main features of treatment. Occasional lumbar spine and sacral iliac mobilization by a trained therapist or chiropractor are indicated. Repetitive manipulations can lead to hypermobile joints and result in a worse problem than the athlete started with. The sacral iliac joint once hypermobile is very difficult to treat. Massage therapy can be an excellent adjuvant to treatment.

Prevention

An ongoing core strengthening and stretching program is helpful to prevent injury. Analysis of the athlete's technique may pick up some high-stress components to the spine and pelvis. Avoid overtraining, as lumbosacral problems are often the first signs of the overstressed athlete.

The sport of cross country skiing is becoming an increasingly popular competitive and lifestyle sport. At present its relative safety as a sport is part of its appeal. With some preventative body maintenance and further equipment design this can continue to be a healthy and enjoyable sport.

SUGGESTED READINGS

1. Smith M, Matheson GO, Meeuwisse WH: Injuries in cross-country skiing: A critical appraisal of the literature. [rev] *Sports Med* 21(3):239–250, 1996.
2. Renstrom P, Johnson RJ: Cross-country skiing injuries and biomechanics. [rev] *Sports Med* 8(6):346–370, 1989.
3. Clancy WG Jr: Cross-country ski injuries. *Clin Sports Med* 1(2):333–338, 1982.
4. Eriksson K, Nemeth G, Eriksson E: Low back pain in elite cross-country skiers. A retrospective epidemiological study. *Scand J Med Sci Sports* 6(1):31–35, 1996.
5. Lindsay DM, Meeuwisse WH, Vyse A, et al: Lumbosacral dysfunctions in elite cross-country skiers. *J Orthop Sports Phys Ther* 18(5):580–585, 1993.

| **Lacrosse**

Barry Bartlett   Doreen Cress
R. Charles Bull

Lacrosse is North America's oldest sport. It was first recorded in 1636 by the Jesuit priests. It originated with the Indians as a method of training warriors, and it may have had some religious significance. Games could last for 2 or 3 days and were quite violent. It is officially Canada's national sport.

It is a marvelous sport to play. It really is three-dimensional hockey. Many of the professional hockey players consider it a better sport than hockey. Several noted NHL hockey players who are former lacrosse players are Wayne Gretzky, Joe Newendiuk, Adam Oates, Brendan Shanahan, and John Ferguson.

THE GAME

Box Lacrosse

This is a fast-paced, high-intensity game that is played in indoor hockey arenas or outdoor boxes. Each team is made up of 20 players including two goalkeepers. Five players plus a goalkeeper are on the floor at one time. There is a 10-s limit on moving the ball past center and a 30-s limit on shots on the opposition's goal. Slashing and cross-checking from behind are not permitted, and players are penalized for their actions.

> The sport of Box Lacrosse originated 60 years ago and is played by people of all ages. Competition begins during the spring and ends late summer for both All-Star and house leagues. Boys and girls play this highly exciting arena game with the championships taking place at both the provincial and national level. The major skills performed in Box Lacrosse are passing, catching and shooting. Passing and catching are skills that must be developed early in a player's career. Contrary to hockey, there is no offside in Box Lacrosse; this adds to the speed, scoring and fun of this unique sport. (OLA Promotional Pamphlet for Box Lacrosse.)

The Stick

The player's stick has to be between 42 and 46 inches in overall length. The width of the inside frame is a minimum of $4\frac{1}{2}$ inches and a maximum of 8 inches. The goalkeeper's stick can be of any length suitable to the player, but the maximum width for the inside

423

frame cannot exceed 15 inches. Sticks can be made of wood or plastic.

Shoes

Cross-training or basketball shoes with a sturdy heel counter, medial arch supports, flexible forefoot, and shock-absorbing capabilities work well. High-cut shoes can give good stability to the ankle joint. Goalkeepers should also consider wearing shoes with hard rubber toes for protection against shots.

Padding

The player's padding can include kidney pads, rib pads, spine guards, shoulder pads, elbow pads, and gloves. Equipment must be checked regularly for wear and replaced or repaired to ensure proper protection is given. Many players cut out the palms of their gloves for better contact with the stick, but this drastically reduces the protection offered for their hands and fingers. Players often add padding to the upper arms by taping extra pads over the lateral aspect of the upper arm. This aids in deflecting and absorbing cross-checks and slashes.

Goalkeepers wear leg protectors, padded pants, chestpads, kidney pads, rib pads, shoulder pads, elbow pads, and gloves. The leg guards cannot have any felt or other material extending past the shin protectors. No modifications can be made to a goalkeeper's gloves, so it is important to obtain the correct glove the first time around. It is suggested that goalkeepers wear hockey gloves instead of lacrosse gloves, because they offer better protection. Blocking and trappers are not allowed.

If further padding is required over the rest of the body, it is best to use dense foam for absorption and a plastic piece over the top of the foam for deflection. The most common areas to pad for goalkeepers are between the neck and shoulder cap, over the shoulders and upper arms, and inside of the glove hand. Goalkeeper pads must conform to the player's body and may not exceed 3 inches from any point of the body.

Helmets

All members of a team wear the same colored helmet with an approved wire mask. Cutting bars out of the mask is illegal and can lead to serious injury if the ball penetrates the face mask. Mouthguards are mandatory in some leagues and are highly recommended. To help prevent concussions, helmets must be secured appropriately with straps done up. Throat protectors are mandatory for goalkeepers and are usually suspended about 1 inch below the bottom of the face mask by a string or leather.

Protective Devices

Players on the floor may wear protective devices. Any cast or splintlike material must be appropriately padded.

On-Field Injury Care

Medical help must be called onto the floor by the referee. Any player other than the goalkeeper must leave the playing surface after being tended to. No blood-soaked clothing or open wounds are permitted.

Men's Field Lacrosse

Field Lacrosse is played in a 110 yard by 60 yard field. The field is divided into two zones, offensive and defensive zones, by a center line. The goal is six feet square and is surrounded by a 9-foot radius crease. There are 10 players on the field: 3 attack, 3 mid fielders, 3 defense and a goalkeeper. Substitutions are done on the fly, with some restrictive substitutions rules, and are generally made for mid fielders. Play begins with a face off and the main theme for the game is ball control. Teams try to set up plays and work for the high percentage shot. There is no time requirement to take a shot, so the team can maintain control of the ball. (OLA Promotional Pamphlet on Field Lacrosse)

Stick

The sticks used by field players usually have a plastic head with a wooden shaft. The minimum length for any stick is 40 in. and the maximum is 72 in. Attack and midfielders play with short sticks, and defensive players use long sticks. The minimum width for a stick head is 4 in. Goalkeepers have no limit on the length of stick use.

Shoes

Players may use rubber-soled boots or shoes with cleats or studs. A larger number of cleats shorter in length help decrease the chance of injury found with longer, fewer-cleated shoes. Shoes should include the following: a sturdy heel counter, medial arch supports, a flexible forefoot, and shock-absorbing qualities.

Padding

Players wear gloves, kidney, shoulder, rib, and elbow pads. Goalkeepers wear leg protectors, padded pants, chestpads, kidney pads, rib pads, shoulder pads, elbow pads, and gloves. The leg guards cannot have any felt or other material extending past the shin protectors. No modifications can be made to a goalkeeper's gloves, so it is important to obtain the correct glove the first time around. It is suggested that goalkeepers wear hockey gloves instead of lacrosse gloves because they offer better protection. Blocking and trappers are not allowed.

Helmets

Helmets are specifically designed for field lacrosse. The helmets have a brim to help shield the face from the sun and are tied in the back to ensure a good fit, and a four-point chinstrap keeps the helmet in place. An approved face mask is required for all players, and a throat protector is mandatory for goalkeepers.

Protective Devices

Protective devices are permitted on the field. Casts and splints require the appropriate padding.

On-Field Injury Care

Medical help must be called onto the floor by the referee. If play is stopped for an injured player, they must leave the playing field for the game to resume. No blood-soaked clothing or open wounds are permitted.

Women's Field Lacrosse

This is essentially a noncontact sport. The stick has a shallow pocket (not deeper than the diameter of the ball). Players must stand when the whistle is blown, except following a goal, and play resumes on the whistle.

The goal is 6 ft square, surrounded by a crease of 2.6 m (7-ft). There is also an 11-m (33-ft) working area and 15-m (40-ft) fan area for attacking and defensive players. The officials are two or three umpires, and dangerous stick-checking results in a "free position" for the fouled player. High-sticking around the player's head is a major foul—the only player allowed to wear protective equipment other than a mouthguard is the goaltender. She can wear small tight-fitting gloves and a protective eye- and nose-guard.

Like football, the women's field lacrosse is played outdoors in all kinds of weather and varying field conditions.

Stick

Sticks are made of wood, plastic, fiberglass, nylon, leather, rubber, or gut. Only the handle is allowed to be aluminum or graphite. The length of the stick must be between 0.9 and 1.1 m in length and cannot exceed 567 g in weight. A goalkeeper's stick must measure between 0.9 and 1.22 m in length, and it cannot exceed 733 g in weight. The pockets of the stick cannot be mesh but must be made of four to five vertical thongs supported by cross-lacing. The pocket must be no deeper than the diameter of the ball.

Shoes

Players may use rubber-soled boots or shoes with cleats or studs. A larger number of cleats shorter in length help decrease the chance of injury found with longer fewer-cleated shoes. Shoes should include the following: a sturdy heel counter, medial arch supports, a flexible forefoot, and shock-absorbing qualities.

Padding

The only player to wear any form of protection is the goalkeeper, who is able to wear a chest or body pad, leg pads, arm pads, and gloves. The goalkeeper's gloves are tight-fitting at the wrist without webbing between the fingers. The pads worn cannot exceed 3 cm in thickness at any point. Jewelry cannot be worn by any player unless it is for medical reasons and then it is required to tape the piece down to the skin. Close-fitting gloves are optional for other players.

Helmets

It is mandatory for the goalkeeper to wear a helmet and a throat protector. Other players are *not* permitted to wear headgear or face masks, but nose- and eyeguards are permitted. Mouthguards are mandatory for all players.

Protective Devices

Protective devices must be padded. The umpire has the final ruling if they may be worn during play, with the concern being a hazard to other players.

On-Field Injury Care

An umpire must call medical help onto the field. Incapacitated players have 2 min, whereas goalkeepers have 5 min in which an assessment must be made as to whether they can continue play. After the appropriate time limit, the game will restart without the player. The player may return to play as long as she is able to, no substitutions were made for her, and the umpire agrees. No open wounds or blood on clothing is permitted.

Inter-Lacrosse

This is a coed game played in elementary and secondary schools. There is no stick or body contact permitted, and protective equipment is not required. The stick is made of flexible plastic. This game can be played indoors or outdoors. The number of players on the team can be adapted, but five is recommended for indoor play. Goals can be hockey nets, hoops, pylons, or even a target on the wall. A goalkeeper may or may not by used.

> Because of the simplicity and flexibility of Inter-Lacrosse, it is adaptable to just about any situation. There are four basic rules: possession is limited to five seconds, players must run with the ball, no physical contact is allowed and covering a loose ball with the stick to gain immediate possession is not allowed. (OLA/CLA Promotional Pamphlet Inter-Lacrosse)

Younger Players

Many lacrosse players start at an early age; therefore, it is important not to forget the prepubescent players and their particular circumstances. With younger players there are different rules and contact is limited. Their skill level is lower. Their diminished speed, size, and strength decreases the probability of sustaining some of the more serious injuries. They are, however, more prone to other injuries that need to be kept in mind. As younger bodies develop, their muscles, tendons, and ligaments are stronger than their bones, thus predisposing them to fractures. The most common fractures are Colles fracture of the ulna and radius and the clavicle. Particular attention should be paid to severe sprains that occur where growth plates exist. Growth plate fractures are often misdiagnosed as sprains. This missed diagnosis can lead to the closing of the growth plate prematurely. Osgood-Schlatter's disease and jumper's knee are common in the younger player group. They are three times more common in males, especially between the ages of 10 and 15; although they do occur in females between the ages of 8 and 13 years. The younger players are typically developing their coordination at this age and tend to trip, fall, and run into each other habitually, predisposing them to contusions, lacerations, and fractures.

COMMON LACROSSE INJURIES

Owing to the collision nature of lacrosse, it is important to remember that anything is possible with regard to injury. This section reviews the uniqueness of lacrosse and its most common injuries, their mechanisms, and some suggestions for their prevention and treatment. It is important to remember that other injuries are not foreign to lacrosse; the reader may find them elsewhere in this volume.

Heat Conditions

Cause

- Heat conditions are very common, especially in box lacrosse, as it is played in poorly ventilated and stifling arenas, where the temperatures can rise to dangerous levels, especially to the players. Field lacrosse players are also susceptible to heat conditions during the hot weather and in direct sunlight.
- When the temperature rises to 26°C (79°F), only the sweating mechanism is working.
- Sweating then becomes the only cooling defense; one must therefore ensure that he or she does *not* become dehydrated.
- Goalies are especially vulnerable owing to the excessive amount of protective equipment they wear and their inability to drink during the periods.
- Muscle cramping is also a result of partial dehydration and salt depletion.

Prevention Tips

- Provide buckets of ice water on the bench with towels in it to help the players cool down between shifts and periods.
- Monitor the players closely, to ensure that they do not get heat exhaustion or heat stroke.
- Ensure that there is plenty of water on the bench and allow the players to drink regularly during the practice or game.
- Supply and encourage water consumption up to 1 h prior to activity.
- Suggested water intakes include:
  16 to 20 oz 1 h prior to training or games
  4 to 8 oz every 15 min during a practice or game
  Water at 10°C (50°F) is the ideal temperature
- Electrolyte drinks may be advantageous (see Chaps. 34 and 39).

Treatment Tips

- Showing signs of heat exhaustion or heat stroke warrants immediate removal of the player from the game. Get the player to a cooler area and start immediate treatment with wet towels and cold drinks.
- Monitor the players closely.

HELPFUL HINTS FOR MINOR INJURIES

Blisters

Try to reduce the friction that is the cause of the blister. Hot spots are a sign of impending blister. Using lubrication such as Vaseline or ointment, powders, moleskin, and a pair of thin nylon socks under a pair of thick socks can help to reduce friction. Be sure that the cause of friction is not owing to poor shoe fit. Always tie laces snugly and work in new shoes gradually.

Treatment for blisters involves decreasing the friction by applying a foam or felt donut pad, with the friction area in the center of the donut. Clean the area well. If the blister has broken, apply an antibiotic cream to fill the donut hole. Cover with a clean dressing and stabilize the pad in place using tape.

Lacerations

To stop the bleeding, apply direct pressure until controlled. Clean the cut with an antiseptic agent and sterilized gauze. Apply a dressing strip, taking down one side of the cut and peel over to close the cut. If sutures are required, attempt to bring the skin together temporarily with butterfly closures by applying the closures to the bottom side and pulling up so the lacerated edges are held together.

Nose Bleeds

Have the player sit on the bench with his or her head tilted forward. Apply direct pressure by pinching the lower two-thirds nostrils. Ice can be applied to the bridge of the nose, forehead, or the back of the neck. *Hold* the pressure for a minimum of 5 min to control the bleeding. Never tilt the head back or blow the nose. Tilting the head back may result in the player choking on his or her blood and blowing the nose may restart the bleeding. If it is necessary to play the athlete before the bleeding is controlled, pack the nose with wet sterile gauze folded to fit in the nostril and then remove after the shift. Ensure the gauze is not too small, as it could be sucked back into the throat, causing the athlete to choke. If it is suspected that the nose is broken or dislocated, do not send the player back into the game or practice.

Winded Athletes

This is usually the result of a blow to the solar plexus. Help the player to relax by instructing him or her to pant in and out or hold breath for 10 s. This allows the chest cavity to expand, relieving the spasm so that breathing returns to normal. Always be aware of the possibility of internal bleeding and injury.

MORE SERIOUS INJURIES

Concussion

This can be caused by a direct or indirect blow to the head. Fighting, usually a punch to the head, can cause a rapid head rotation. The force from hitting the floor or ground can be very significant. Fighting is unusual in lacrosse, because the stick is a better weapon than your fists.

An appropriate, well-fitted helmet with straps properly done up and a mouthguard with superior absorption qualities decreases the amount of force transmitted to the brain. However, a lacrosse helmet is quite different from a hockey or football helmet. It is loose-fitted, vented, and much more flexible. It is effective in deflecting blows with the stick, but it is relatively ineffective in high-speed collisions and contact with the floor.

Specific management of head and neck injuries are discussed later in this chapter.

Whiplash

A quick jarring of the cervical or lumber spine from an unexpected cross-check or body check can cause acute and prolonged pain. This involves forced extension and then rapid flexion with a slight rotation, similar to the mechanism in a rear end motor vehicle accident.

Prevention is most important. Lacrosse players must develop strong cervical, abdominal, lumbar erector spinae, and quadratus lumborum muscles. Isometric neck exercises and full neck and back stretching and warm-up exercises should be done for 10 min before every practice and game (see Chap. 34). Look for signs of concussion and neurologic signs and symptoms after a whiplash.

Spinal Loading Problems

These can occur after a cross-check from behind into the boards or a goalpost. This should be prevented by encouraging players to use appropriate checking skills and proper rule enforcement.

Lumbar Back Pain

This can be caused by pounding on the hard, unforgiving floor in box lacrosse or the uneven terrain of the field in field lacrosse. Rapid acceleration and deceleration and rotation with a pivot or fake move can strain the lumbar, psoas, hamstring, or adductor muscles.

Prevention involves intensive conditioning and strengthening with appropriate fast-twitch dexterity drills. Shoes with sufficient shock-absorbing qualities are important.

Back problems are hard to diagnose on the field, and although they are more apt to be associated with muscle spasm, a serious back problem cannot be ruled out. The physician must be aware that an acute disk herniation or facet injury can occur, and a spondylolisthesis is a possibility. The best prevention of neck and back injuries is a strengthening program in the preseason period, using isometric strengthening exercises both in a buddy system and with proper weight training equipment. A full pregame stretching should be done in the neck and back, and for a more serious back problem either a neoprene brace or support or type of power belt can be used. Remember that a player with serious back injury must be removed from the game on the back board and full precautions taken, as with a serious neck injury.

Groin (Adductor and Quadriceps)

Hamstring Strains

These are caused by overstretching or overcontracting the fatigued muscle. This is usually an overtraining, overuse, repetitive strain injury. Moisture on the floor in box lacrosse causes decreased traction and resultant splits and groin pulls. Explosive sprints (acceleration) and sudden stops (deceleration) can cause partial hamstring ruptures and recurrent tendinitis.

Although the player may be well enough to return to play, repeated strains increase the amount of scar tissue and therefore decrease the amount of flexibility of the entire muscle. This increases the severity and frequency of the injury.

Prevention involves proper quad/ham balancing. A ratio of 60 for quads and 40 for hams is acceptable, that is, lift 60 lbs with quads and 40 lbs with hams. However, the quads are usually much stronger than the hams. The abductor/adductor ratio is also important. If the abductors are 1.25 times stronger, the chance of groin injuries increases.

Thus, stretch the quads, hams, and adductors before and after practices and games. A player with a moderately pulled groin should be taken out of the game because the problem will become more severe soon after the game.

Immediate Treatment Tip

Use a hip spica wrap for an adductor or iliopsoas strain, placing a pressure pad over the lesion site. For a quad/hamstring strain, use a herringbone technique, placing a pressure pad under the wrap.

A Hip Pointer

A direct blow to an inadequately protected iliac crest by a helmet, stick, or the floor may cause a contusion along the crest, which is usually associated with a hematoma of the tissue adjacent to and beneath the periosteum covering the crest.

This is a very painful injury. There is immediate muscle spasm and immobility. The patient is unable to rotate the trunk or flex the thigh without pain. Most comfort is obtained by trunk flexion, leaning forward and toward the side of the injury. Rule out a fractured pelvis. This injury can develop into a type of fibrosis and prolonged myositis. The central area in which it occurs can be opened readily in the hospital setting and drained for maximum speed in rehabilitation in the most severe cases. However, the majority of cases respond to the "pier" method (*p*ressure over the area, *i*ce applied, *e*levated above the heart, *r*est—remove from action). This is the principle for immediate care of any acute injury.

The pier method will control the accompanying pain and swelling, which can reduce the amount of time the player is sidelined. The ice should be applied for 15 min every hour and continued for 48 to 72 h until swelling is under control (not to be applied during sleep). The pressure can be applied continuously except when sleeping.

Contusions

Owing to the nature of lacrosse, the ball can travel over 100 miles an hour and the possibility of contusions occurring is enormous anywhere on the body. The lacrosse ball is made of a dense rubber compound that is roughly 170 g. In comparison to baseball, the padding is light. Although the rules discourage slashing on places such as the quads, it is not uncommon to receive blows from the stick on the forearms, deltoids, hands, lower legs, and back.

Bodychecking is encouraged, especially in field lacrosse. If a player continuously gets contusions in the same area, a piece of permanent, custom equipment may be used to protect the injury from recurring. Create your own customized pieces of equipment to best meet the needs of your player and the injury.

Treatment: Ice on Stretch (PIER)

Wrap the contusion to provide compression. Placing a felt donut with the hole over the lesion site and a hard protective plate over the donut would help to deflect and distribute the forces to a larger area. Secure the donut and plate in place with a supportive wrap technique. This would provide the injury with an optimum protection. Watch for the onset of myositis ossificans. Returning a player too soon can expose them to an increased degree of injury and myositis ossificans.

Myositis Ossificans

This is an inflammatory disease of the muscle marked by a bony deposit within a muscle owing to trauma. It is caused by repeated blows. The most common muscles affected in lacrosse are the vastus lateralis of the thigh and the deltoid insertion to the humerus. This causes excessive bleeding in the area which cannot be reabsorbed by the body and over time causes a calcium buildup within or between the muscles.

Prevention Tips

If there are repeated contusions to an area, protect the area with a support wrap that has a donut and a hard plate under it to deflect and distribute the forces to a greater area. Ensure the player rests or decreases the activity level long enough to allow the hematoma to be reabsorbed.

Treatment Tips

Look for a hard lump within a muscle belly that has sustained a contusion or strain that is not healing within normal limits. Attention should be paid especially to a bruise that is not resolving within the normal limits of approximately 7 to 14 days (see Chap. 19).

Blocker's Exostosis

Repeated blows to the deltoid insertion, especially from cross-checking, may result in blocker's exostosis. This can be prevented by using a deltoid cup to protect the deltoid insertion from repeated blows. Increase biceps, triceps, and deltoid development. Reassess regularly for myositis ossificans, especially with players who are offensive specialists. Add an extra pad, taped on, to help disperse the force.

Acromioclavicular Separation

Acromioclavicular (AC) separation is caused by a downward blow against the outer end of the shoulder that can result from the shoulder being driven forcefully into the boards. Bodychecking another player by accelerating the shoulder into that player or falling on an outstretched arm can also cause the separation.

Immediate Treatment

Using brown tape to tape the AC joint down helps the ligaments and capsule heal in a shortened position. This decreases the chance of a step formation and helps the joint to heal properly. A commercial "Kenny-Howard AC Immobilizer" should be applied as soon as possible (see Chap. 28). On return to the sport, the temporary use of the cantilever shoulder pad helps to decrease the chance of a recurrence.

Medial and Lateral Epicondylitis (Golfer's Elbow and Tennis Elbow)

It occurs because lacrosse requires the ball carrier to cradle the stick. This is a rapid rotation and flexion and extension motion of the wrist in order to maintain control and possession of the ball. This rapid repetitive flexion and extension motion can lead to tendinitis (Fig. 21-1).

Prevention

Stretching programs for golfer's elbow (medial) and tennis elbow (lateral) have proven to be effective, and forearm braces should be used.

Olecranon Bursitis

This commonly occurs from falls on the hard floor. The player can wear lightweight shoulder and elbow pads, but they do not offer much protection and players have an option not to wear them. Figure 21-2 illustrates a large chronic olecranon bursitis in the operating room, just prior to surgery.

Fractures of the Forearm

These often occur from direct stick contact, a cross-check, or slash. These are legal checks. The offensive player will hold the stick and ball in one hand and place the opposite arm in a protective fashion to ward off the opponent's blows. Arm pads are not always used. Thus an isolated ulnar shaft fracture or less commonly a fracture of both bones occurs.

Wrist Injuries

Hand and wrist injuries in the contact sports player are often neglected, and we must emphasize how stoical some of these players are. They may often have a fractured scaphoid that goes unrecognized if they do not complain. If you suspect a fractured scaphoid, put the wrist and thumb in a full scaphoid cast. Dislocated metacarpal, phalangeal, and interphalangeal joints are common, and these are best handled at the time of the accident by traction (pulling the finger into the normal anatomical position) and reduction. This is often difficult in the case of a dislocated thumb at the

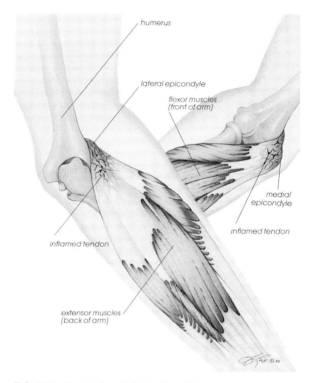

FIG. 21-1 Tennis elbow/golfer's elbow. This condition plagues many a racquet player and golfer, both amateur and professional. Although most common in these sports, the problem can occur when anyone uses the arm excessively. It is basically an inflammation of the tissues in the elbow area.

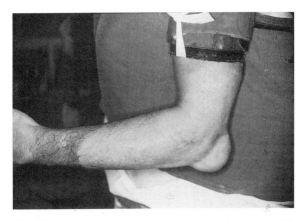

FIG. 21-2   Olecranon bursitis should be prevented by more satisfactory elbow pads. Once it reaches this stage surgery is mandatory. The players say they have "bone chips" in their elbow. The particles in the bursa are fibrous and unrelated to the elbow joint.

metacarpophalangeal (MP) joint because the tendons from adductor pollicis often catch around the neck of the metacarpal in a way similar to the reins of a horse. This prevents the reduction and often makes it difficult, even under general anesthesia (Fig. 21-3).

Fracture of the Hook of Hamate

This is often missed. It is caused by repeated impact from the handle of the lacrosse stick onto the heel of the hand. Protective padding over the heel of the hand in the glove can be an effective preventative but it may limit the technique. Encourage the player to carry the stick up closer to the metacarpophalangeal joints. In some cases this may require surgery (see Chap. 7).

Hands and Fingers

Hands are injured by a slash, contact with an opponent's equipment, and being stepped on. Lacrosse gloves are quite satisfactory, but players often cut out the palms to feel the stick better. This leaves the hands partially unprotected, and contusions, cuts, and fractures occur when they slip out of the gloves.

Gamekeeper's thumb or skier's thumb occurs when a player falls and the thumb is trapped by the stick and forced into hyperexten-

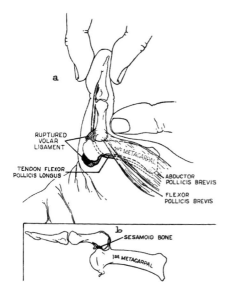

FIG. 21-3 A dislocated thumb may be impossible to reduce due to the adductor tendons catching around the neck of the metacarpal.

sion. This tears the ulnar collateral ligament or fractures a small piece of bone from the proximal phalanx (Stener lesion). Defensive specialists are susceptible owing to their technique of cross-checking.

A cross-check is completely legal and can be done forcefully and repetitively. These injuries are often treated by open reduction and immediate repair of the ligaments. Bennett's fracture of the first metacarpal is another case where immediate open reduction and K-wire fixation are the best treatment.

Prevention is simple. *Do not* allow players to cut all or some of the palm out of their gloves.

Abrasions or Turf Burns of the Knees

These are common from falls or skids on the floor or artificial turf. Deep abrasions can be full of dirt, particularly on natural turf. Preventative measures, such as basketball-type knee pads, are optional but rarely used. Vaseline on bony prominences decreases the friction.

Proper cleansing and antiseptic, antibiotic dressings should be used. Removal of dirt particles using local anesthesia helps reduce "tattooing." Traumatic prepatellar bursitis is very common.

Patellofemoral Syndrome (PFS)

This presents on a regular basis as a result of rapid acceleration, rapid deceleration, repeated pounding, and rotational forces caused by the running nature of lacrosse. PFS is seen particularly in female players between the ages of 12 and 15. This can be aggravated by a multitude of anatomical conditions, including an increased Q-angle, pronated feet, a toed-out knock-kneed gait, and a rotated or tilted patella (see Chap. 34).

Prevention Tips

Correct the anatomical condition through exercises and support techniques. Use brown tape to place the patella in an anatomically correct tracking position ("McConnell taping").

Knee

Knee injuries are one of the key problems in sports. Far more occur than one could ever imagine. One-third of the injuries we have seen at the York University Sports Clinic involve the knee and this is in more than 38,000 patients seen. One has to be aware that there is always more behind a knee injury than is initially suspected. The initial examination in a player with large muscles in spasm is often unsatisfactory.

The player is most apt to sustain a valgus and internally rotated strain, but he or she is less apt to sustain a major knee injury than the football player whose feet are fixed more.

However, anterior cruciate injuries are common in all the contact sports. In most medial collateral ligament injury situations, a cruciate tear has to be suspected. The majority of cases in which there is a hemarthrosis in the knee are also associated with an anterior cruciate tear. We attach a great deal of significance to a pop, crack, or noise at the time of injury and also to immediate swelling, which suggests blood in the joint (Figs. 21-4 and 21-5).

Anterior Tibial Shin Splints

These are caused when the tibialis anterior muscle fatigues and spasms from eccentrically decelerating the forefoot and repeated landings. This causes an irritation to the fascia or the anterior border of the tibia.

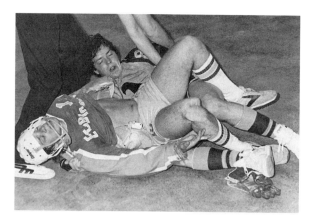

FIG. 21-4   Complete dislocation of the knee results in major damage to the anterior and posterior cruciates, the peroneal nerve, and the popliteal vessels. It is an orthopedic emergency. It should be referred to a very experienced knee surgeon.

Proper prevention involves stretching. Although the players often stretch prior to activity, they often fail to stretch the tibialis anterior. A good stretch is to kneel on the floor with a towel rolled up under the forefoot and to lean back so he or she is sitting on the heels or as far back as possible without pain.

Immediate treatment with a wrap using an anterior shin splint support technique with a pressure pad over the lesion site is beneficial. (Ensure that the wrap pulls the muscle belly into its origin.)

Posterior Tibial Shin Splints

These are caused by the following:

- Weak medial arch supports
- Pounding repeatedly on the hard playing surface, especially in box lacrosse, is a particular problem for people with lax medial arch architecture
- The uneven terrain of field lacrosse also causes problems

FIG. 21-5   *A* and *B* show the major extent of a complete dislocation. Gentle relocation can be attempted at the arena by a skilled practitioner, but otherwise reduce it at the hospital under anesthesia.

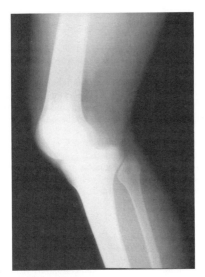

A

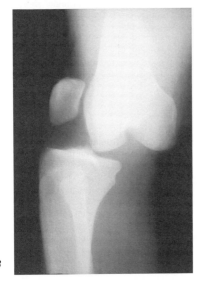

B

- Running on their toes, which typically occurs in preseason when distance is increased for endurance conditioning

Prevention

Prevention includes the following:

- Exercises to strengthen tibialis anterior, tibialis posterior, peroneus longus, and the foot intrinsics that support the medial arch
- Proper shoes that absorb shock, have a strong medial arch support, snug heel counter, and flexibility at the MP joints are important.
- A slow gradual increase in the amount of time spent on hard surfaces at the beginning of training is advised.
- Increase flexibility of the Achilles tendon and deep posterior compartment. Stretching is emphasized. This is helped by running in the reverse direction (backward) during daily training sessions.

Leg, Knee, and Shin Bruises

These are a problem because players do not have any protective equipment on the lower limb.

A direct blow to the unprotected shin bone, commonly from the stick or ball, can lead to a chronic inflammatory state of the periosteal tissue, along with a trapped hematoma under the periosteum. If there is repeated injury, protect the area with a custom-made piece of protective equipment.

Owing to the localized nature of this condition, ice massage has proven to be an effective treatment. Place a felt pad over the lesion site and secure it with a pressure wrap to help control the swelling. Aspiration or subperiosteal injection of cortisone can be done rarely.

Ankle Sprains

There is a high incidence of ankle sprains caused by the running nature of the sport. This is particularly true at the lower levels with poor quality fields, and stepping into divots on the uneven terrain, particularly in field lacrosse, is common. Landing on someone's foot, similar to basketball, is a frequent problem. Twisting when the foot has been fixed into place and decelerating and rolling the foot into inversion is the most common mechanism.

Prevention training includes 2 min of proprioception drills in the player's daily exercise routine. In order to increase the strength of the peroneals and foot intrinsics, towel crunches with the toes, picking up marbles with the toes, and surgical tubing exercises are done. Shoes with upper ankle support and a snug heel counter that does not allow for extraneous movement (three-quarter-cut) are recommended. Several of the new ankle braces offer functional lateral and medial stability and a subtalar stabilizer or orthotic anchor.

One of the most neglected injuries is the sprained ankle. These injuries are usually treated very poorly. A third-degree ankle sprain can occur even when a player is "locked in a boot or skate" and is a common injury in football, basketball, and lacrosse.

If necessary, stress films can be taken at the time of injury under local anesthesia. Most sprained ankles do not need to be put in a plaster cast and even those that are badly swollen can often be treated with AP splints initially and an air cast or brace soon after.

If there is a third-degree tear, most of these injured players can have the splints removed in 3 weeks, and if the ankle is stable no further splinting is necessary, but ankle braces can be used for months if necessary.

When we used to place players in a cast after 8 weeks of inactivity, there was a 40 percent loss of strength in the ankle ligament. This means that it would take up to 12 months before the ligament regains 90 percent of its normal strength, and it never regains 100 percent.

There is enormous force of up to 600 lb transmitted into the knee and ankle of a skater or runner by this type of injury. Thus immediate physiotherapy from day one for ankle sprains and ligament tears is mandatory. Eventually players with such injuries have to do highly specialized physiotherapy using a rebounder, wobble board, springs, weights, pulleys, jumping and agility exercises, and hard running on the equivalent of a golf course fairway. The ankle should be braced and taped up until it regains full strength.

Midfoot sprains and dislocations of the metatarsals and tarsals often require open reduction and are often associated with permanent pain afterward.

A toe fracture can usually be treated by simply strapping the one toe to another. Some football players get a synovitis of the great toe called "turf toe," and this injury responds to rest, ice, physiotherapy, and anti-inflammatory medication.

Turf Toe

The turf shoe sticking to the artificial turf and stopping abruptly while the player's momentum continues forward results in turf toe. This causes the first metatarsal joint to be driven into hyperextension and an inflammatory condition commonly results.

This problem can be prevented by proper shoe size fit with a little space left in the front of the shoe for toe and forefoot movement. A larger toe box is also suggested.

A wrap using a turf toe support technique that limits hyperextension of the first metatarsal phalangeal joint helps reduce excessive motion and usually provides enough splinting to allow comfortable return to play.

Management of Acute Serious Injuries

"Doc, Eddy is bleeding to death!" What do you do? Well, the best motto is "Be Prepared." It is too late to start worrying about what to do when you are on the bench and the injury occurs. For the throat injury you should already have practiced using a large-bore needle in the cricothyroid membrane or have a pocket tracheotomy kit in your emergency bag that is right beside you.

For the "totaled" knee you should have been watching the game closely to see the mechanism of injury. Zimmer or Dupuis splints (Velcro and fabric) should be put in the dressing room or first aid room before the game. A referral system should be set up in advance. First aid for the neck or back injury requires a back board and knowledgeable assistants. All this support has to be available at the side of the field or in the arena's first aid room. Do not take someone's word for its availability. See to it yourself!

Heavy-duty bolt cutters are on the bench to remove the face mask. (Some of the newer masks slip off without cutting, and others have to be cut with a knife.) Do not remove the helmet. Do not move the injured player until your back board and prearranged four-person team is ready. Do not worry about holding up the game. If necessary, take the ambulance (arranged pregame) onto the field. Remember that you are the "boss." Get rid of onlookers and unnecessary helpers.

How do you deal with the "heavy bleeder?" Has the jugular vein or carotid artery been cut? Is he or she unconscious? Have an oral screw and airway in your pocket and know how to use it. Have an ambu bag on the bench with you and oxygen readily available. Apply pressure on the bleeding spot (in this case, the neck) and do not take it off until you are in the operating room.

The mnemonic I use for the shocked patient is A B C D E F:

A. Airway
B. Bleeding
C. Circulation
D. Doctor (notify ambulance, hospital, etc.)
E. Examine
F. Fractures

Airway

If an injured player is not breathing, remove the mouthguard and chewing gum and, if necessary, the face mask. Open clenched jaws with your oral screw. Insert the airway and start mouth-to-mouth resuscitation or use your ambu bag. Use oxygen as soon as possible.

If the player is breathing, simply remove the mouthguard and, leaving the helmet and chin strap in place, slide the airway in under the mask.

Bleeding

Direct pressure with a clean towel is the best means of controlling bleeding. Pressure points are worth a try. A tourniquet can be used if pressure does not work.

I set up my suture tray in the first aid room before the game, and I make sure that the local anesthetic and prep are ready. Various sutures are available. It is important to have proper lighting and assistance arranged beforehand and to make sure that your assistant has had practice in cutting the sutures and is familiar with sterile techniques and other processes.

Take the time to examine the wound and to remove any dirt and debris. Feel for any deep fractures and look for lacerated nerves and tendons and other injuries. Send players with any complicated lacerations to the hospital (see Fig. 21-2).

Circulation

I have IV tubing, needles, and bags of Ringer's lactate available, although I have never had to use this equipment. Nevertheless, it should be kept sterile, and sutures and IV material will evidently stay sterile for years.

Doctor

I have a pickup truck or van on the apron of the field, and I have a car phone handy to the field. At lacrosse games, know where the phone is located and make sure that it is not locked up during the game. Designate someone beforehand to call in case of emergency if you cannot call. Find out before the game how long it takes to get an ambulance and how far the nearest hospital and nearest neurosurgical unit are. "Be Prepared!"

Make sure both teams know that you are "the doctor" and where you are sitting. Obviously you should be within the first two or three rows of the action or on the bench. When I am on the bench I wear coaching shoes, which are waterproof shoes with a good gripping sole for walking on the slippery floor.

Have a back-up arranged in case you have to go to the hospital or to the dressing room. The back-up person should be knowledgeable in first aid or an athletic trainer or physician, and he or she should be prepared to go on the bench automatically when you leave. Tell the coach or trainer roughly what is wrong with an injured player and whether the player will return.

Examine

Keep cool. You have more knowledge about the problem than anyone else present. Carefully console the athlete, but push him or her to be exact about the location of the pain. Examine the area carefully and check the total body carefully and quickly.

I have on hand a good flashlight, laryngoscope, tongue depressors, gauze, scissors, alcohol, stethoscope, and BP cuff. I keep them all in one part of my field bag. This bag is light, has Velcro fasteners, and opens relatively quickly. I also have a back-up bag with ephedrine 1 in 1000, ammonia sniffers, 50% glucose, diphenhydramine (Benadryl), and many other medications. I keep these supplies either on the bench (preferably) or in the adjacent team or first aid room. Someone is responsible for knowing exactly where they are and bringing them to me in case of an emergency.

Fractures

A cervical fracture is the worst type. I try to immobilize the player with such a fracture and, if possible, transport him or her in the position found (Table 21-1). Remember that immediate immobilization of the head and neck unit with two hands is mandatory for any unconscious player. In this circumstance manage the athlete as

TABLE 21-1 Proper Positioning and Removal from Playing Surface or Field

Do not remove helmet.
Do not move head or neck.
Apply cervical collar or immobilize with rolled up towels.
Cut away face mask with sized bolt cutter.
Apply mild traction when lifting onto back board and stretcher in same position as found (on front or back).
Immobilize head and neck with sand bags, rolled towels, or blankets.
Restrain the player if necessary.
If player is face down, immobilize head in position found.
Do not attempt to straighten head.
Apply mild traction when placing face down on back board; do not turn player over.
Use straps or tape to secure player to back board.
Note time of onset.

if a significant neck injury were present. A four-person log-rolling maneuver can be done, followed by a five-person transport procedure. Choose the team leader in advance; either a doctor or an athletic trainer can be designated. From that point, the leader is the boss.

Other limb fractures or dislocations can be straightened on the field or reduced on the sidelines, gently if possible, depending on the physician's expertise. A recurrent shoulder dislocation often goes in easily if it is reduced immediately but is very difficult to reduce later on, once significant muscle spasm has set in.

SPECIFIC ACUTE INJURIES

Head Injuries

Try to be alert to which side of the head the player was hit on, and how the player hit the ice. Be aware of the six grades of concussion (Fig. 21-6). If you are in doubt, have the player sit out. Do not rely on the player for an assessment of his or her own condition.

Again, do not allow your judgment of a player's condition to be overridden by a too-enthusiastic coach. I once had a physical pulling match with a soccer coach who wanted to put a player back in the game even though the player had cerebrospinal fluid (CSF) leaking out of his ear and a basal skull fracture.

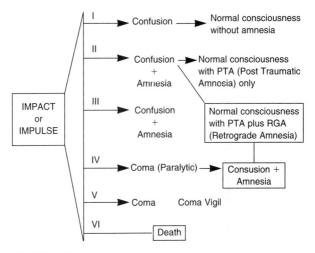

FIG. 21-6   The six grades of concussion.

If the athlete is completely lucid 5 to 10 min after experiencing a brief grade 1 concussion, he or she can probably go back into the play. Do a good neurological exam and check the helmet. The crown cord should be tightened or an old helmet discarded. If there is any indication of a grade 2 concussion, keep the player out, and get him or her to the hospital.

Shoulder Burners

A player with a nerve root contusion or plexus stretch can usually go back into the game if symptoms completely subside in 10 to 15 min. Make sure, however, that all neurological symptoms have subsided (Table 21-2).

Eye Injuries

A consultation with an ophthalmologist is often indicated, since the floor of the orbit of a player's eye may also be damaged. The incidence of eye injuries has been reduced because of the use of the proper face mask. Nevertheless, it is still common for women players to fail to wear facial protection, and regulations to require such protection should be legislated into the league.

Any player with double vision must be referred to a specialist's care. An eye that is sunken is often associated with a fracture of the orbital floor. Do not force the eyelids open if the patient resists strongly. These patients should be referred for ophthalmological care.

All hyphemas demand a consultation, as secondary glaucoma is a possible complication. Even a moderate eye injury can be associated with retinal detachment, and thus an early consultation is important. In some serious soft tissue injuries about the eye with periorbital hemorrhage, the blood supply to the optic nerve can be shut off, and visual loss can occur (see Chap. 2).

TABLE 21-2 Neuropraxia of Upper Trunk or Brachial Plexus ("Shoulder Burner")

Mechanism	
Downward, forward depression of the shoulder.	
Symptoms	
Sensory	Severe, shocklike burning pain and numbness or deadness of the shoulder and arm.
Motor	Inability to lift arm, forearm, and hand. Usually disappears rapidly. Is a concussion.
Treatment	
Return to full activity when all neurologic signs subside.	

Fractures

Mandibular fractures are common. The players have such a high pain threshold that they can actually sustain a mandibular fracture and complain only of altered dental occlusion. In such an injury, x-rays are indicated, and appropriate consultation should be obtained. It is particularly important that x-rays of the condylar process be taken, and intermaxillary fixation is required in most cases.

Laryngeal fractures can present a life threatening situation (see Fig. 15-3). Symptoms are loss of airway, hemoptysis, crepitus, and loss of the Adam's apple prominence. The necessity of a "cricothyrotomy" (tracheotomy) has to be considered. Treatment consists of rest, humidification, and no contact for 6 to 12 weeks. It is basically impossible to protect against this injury. Incidence of cross-checking over the neck or garroting from behind should be decreased by proper applications of the rules.

Mouthguards are mandatory in most leagues, and the intrinsic oral mouthguard made by the player's dentist is the only one that is truly satisfactory. If a player's tooth is broken, take the player and the broken tooth or its pieces to the dentist immediately. Do not clean or wash the tooth.

A fractured nose can be set at the arena with local anesthesia and an internasal pack. A player with a broken nose can play with a face mask in place within 3 to 4 days. It is probably advantageous, however, to wait for a week until the immediate swelling has settled down and then repair the fracture more definitively in the operating room. Again, players can play soon afterward with proper facial protection.

Fractured ribs are common because of cross-checking and little, if any, protective equipment for the rib cage in many players. A quilted kidney protector is allowed. Fractured ribs obviously have to be immobilized initially with a type of Velcro strap that replaces the old type of rib taping. Some players with fractured ribs can play within 10 days of the injury if they wear a flak jacket.

Cardiac Arrest

Cardiac arrest in a young athlete is likely caused by an arrhythmia and may respond to the crisp sternal "thump." CPR principles should be applied. We do not have a defibrillator or cardiac monitor in our first aid rooms, although some advanced support ambulances do have one. Someone trained in basic life support should attend practices and games.

Examining the team at the beginning of the season may make the physician aware of a potential problem. In a loose-leaf book we keep a record of all the players and their initial exam and all treatment given during the season. Thus a new team doctor can become familiar with the patient's history and problems prior to a game.

Pneumothorax

Pneumothorax can occur spontaneously from a rupture of a bleb or from direct trauma. A player in this condition must be taken to the hospital immediately. If cyanosis or hypotension is noted, a large-bore needle can be placed in the second intercostal space 2 inches (5 cm) from the sternal border. The finger of a glove with a hole in the tip can be taped to the needle to act as a one-way valve.

Abdominal Injuries

Blows to the solar (celiac) plexus will "knock the wind out" of a player. This problem is usually transient, and a player can later reenter the game.

Lacerations of the liver, pancreas, and particularly the spleen can occur and be unrecognized. A subscapular hematoma can occur in the spleen, and the patient can be ambulant and seem well until the capsule suddenly ruptures. Then hypotension occurs. Be very careful, therefore, with players who have received abdominal injuries, and transport them to the hospital immediately. This type of abdominal injury has to be thoroughly investigated in a hospital setting. Any player with blood in the urine, even in a microscopic amount, should also be investigated prior to his or her return to contact sports.

RETURN TO PLAY

Before a player can return to play, he or she should have 100 percent strength and 100 percent range of movement in the injured area compared to the healthy extremity or the preseason medical status. If the player has been under a physician's care, the player should only return after consulting with the physician.

Playing hurt is a disservice to the player and the team and could potentially cause further injury and loss of playing time. In many instances the player will know if he or she is able to perform, and as always, common sense rules.

IS THE PLAYER READY TO RETURN?

The team physician will always make the final decision as to whether the player is able to return to play or whether the player sits on the bench. This is a quick checklist to be used when determining whether or not a player is ready to return back into the game. It has been set up in a progression-type manner. If the player encounters pain or is favoring the injured limb, stop. Assess the extent of pain and determine whether or not it is enough for the player to be removed from the game. If the player has successfully completed the step, progress on to the next step.

THE FUNCTIONAL DRILL ASSESSMENT FOR THE LOWER LIMB

1. Jog ahead slowly.
2. Twenty double leg toe raises and single leg toe raises offering support for balance reasons only.
3. Run straight ahead for 10 m half speed.
4. Run straight ahead for 10 m at full speed.
5. Run and shoot at the end of the 10 m at full speed.
6. Run with 45-degree directional changes from the left to the right at full speed.
7. Run a figure eight at half speed over a 10-m course.
8. Run a figure eight at increased speed over a 10-m course.
9. Run a straight line backward at half speed for 10 m.
10. Complete a change of direction drill.

A similar drill can be designed for the upper limb or for any specific joint.

CONCLUSIONS

The lacrosse medical team should be prepared, be on time, be visible, and be alert. Watch the game closely. Be aware of any potential problem. Examine athletes before a game. Be careful not to allow any long-term damage. Be available between periods or quarters. Be thorough. Check the dressing room and opposing team's dressing room after the game. Be cautious. Send any doubtful case to the hospital and follow it up with further investigation when necessary. Be sure that players have reached 100 percent of their capability before they return to their sport after an injury.

ACKNOWLEDGMENT

Illustrations, unless otherwise attributed, are taken from Schneider RC, Kennedy JC, Plant ML (eds): *Sports Injuries: Mechanisms, Prevention and Treatment*. Baltimore, Williams & Wilkins, 1985.

22 | Golf

Peter Welsh   Ben Kern

Gardening was always claimed as "the universal pastime." More recently, however, golf surely must have come to challenge such a claim. The popularity of this avocation has spread from its traditional home in Scotland throughout the entire world. Tiger Woods has become one of the most recognizable figures internationally in nearly every country. At one time the proclivity of the middle-aged middle class in North America, golf's popularity now knows no such bounds, involving both the young and the old and spreading across all segments of society.

The appeal of the game lies in its unique ability to engage all participants in equitable competition regardless of sex, age, physique, and strength capabilities. Golf offers obvious advantages to participants from the health and recreational viewpoints. The exercise of walking in the outdoors in a natural environment offers both physical and mental advantages to participants. Physical demands are not preeminent, for even people with disabilities, including limb loss and sight deficiencies, participate.

Nonetheless, the routine golfer faces injury from time to time that can adversely affect his or her game. In this regard, there are some important fundamentals that can assist the average golfer not only with the game but also in averting such injuries.

Injury to the back can be minimized by attention to general fitness, involving walking rather than riding the course. Lightweight carry bags and stands also help in this regard. Posture and stance are critical to performing well and reducing injury. Grip faults too may predispose to wrist, hand, and elbow problems. Overzealous practice can compound these difficulties if the basic fundamentals of grip, stance, and posture are ignored. Furthermore, as in all sports, failure to warm up adequately can predispose to injury and affect performance.

The opening section of this chapter deals with these important aspects of golf preparation and injury prevention.

THE IMPORTANCE OF THE GOLF SWING

The vast majority of average golfers, in trying to improve their game, set the bar too high for themselves. In attempting to incorporate swing styles and concepts designed for modern tour players who are playing at the highest level, they overtax their capability.

The modern tour player is more of an athlete than those of an earlier era, being more physically fit, stronger, generally leaner, and

453

more healthy. Party boys such as Jimmy Demaret, Bobby Locke, and Walter Hagen have given way to the physical culture exemplified by Greg Norman, Nick Faldo, and Tiger Woods. This is not to say that the "good ol' boys" were not great golfers—they were, but they used radically different swing styles than those used today and relied heavily on finesse, strategy, and gamesmanship to defeat their opponents. Today, tournaments are won with length off the tee, strength out of the rough, and surgical precision with iron shots.

The average golfer is conditioned more like the wiley old-timers than the new crop of tour players and could well learn from their older, classic swing styles as models for their own game.

The modern tournament swing is designed for economy of movement, an absence of moving parts, and a new catch-word, namely, *torque*, that creates the much-sought-after X factor. This is the differential in the amount of rotation between the shoulders and hip turn. The more you can wind up your shoulders without turning your hips, the more torque you can create and still keep your arms connected in the proper position at the same time. Once you have created maximum torque, the idea is to rip your hips around to the target as fast as you can, with your right elbow tucked in front of the right hip bone (for right-handers) without losing any torque. If this happens, the club will not release until the last possible moment, and maximum speed and pressure will be applied to the ball by the club head to compress the ball so much that it travels unheard-of distances.

To the average Sunday golfer, this hurts just to think of it, never mind to do it. However, such golfers want to improve, so try they must. "If it's good enough for Tiger Woods, it's good enough for me. If a 165-pound 20-year-old can hit the ball 350 yards, there's no reason why I can't." Ridiculous!

Why is golf the only sport like this? Can you imagine a person who enjoys ice skating on a pond trying to emulate the technique and style of Elvis Stojko? It would not even be a consideration.

Most average golfers would do better to copy the classic swing style. Rather than trying to restrict the hip turn and leg motion on the backswing by stabilizing the lower body, why not keep the knees and legs relaxed so that the entire pelvic girdle can rotate back, taking the pressure off the spine? Why not soften the right elbow joint on the way back so that the club can swing back more easily rather than create tension in the upper back muscles? On the way down to the ball, let gravity help the club down as you rotate the pelvic girdle through to the target. Relaxing your right knee (right-handers) on the way through will help your legs to react to this rotation without strain. Let your left elbow fold on the way through so that the hands and the club can pass by gracefully without interference. As your pelvic girdle turns through, it will turn your spine as a unit without twisting it. Let your chest and shoulders go with it, and your head too—no need to "keep your head down" long after the ball has been hit. Let it all go—you'll get plenty of club head speed with less chance of injury if you do not twist or stop anything on the way through. If your hips or legs stop and your arms and shoulders keep going, this has a "crack the whip" effect on the body parts that are following it—*ouch!*

In defining the essence of a swing motion that is effective yet attainable by the average person, there are some basic considerations to be adopted.

THE STARTING POSITION

Good posture is the key to the starting position. This position gives you a chance for the body to move gracefully. Note the naturalness: weight evenly distributed, level shoulders and pelvis. The back foot is at right angles to the target, and the front foot is turned out. The left foot must be turned out about a quarter turn to allow the body to finish completely. The ankles are aligned parallel to the flight line.

THE BACKSWING

This part of the swing coils the torso around the spine in preparation for the delivery part of the golf swing. This builds up the potential for creating centrifugal energy. Most of the weight should move to the back foot. The arms, shoulders, pelvis, and spine move back in unison and in balance.

THE SWING THROUGH

Do not call it the downswing because this gives a connotation of hitting down at the ball instead of swinging through it. Maximum power is attained by creating centrifugal force, which means that the power is generated outward from a revolving center. In order to do this, a specific sequence must start from the end of the backswing. The sequence begins with the transfer of weight from the back foot to the front foot. The pelvic girdle (i.e., the pelvis, hip, and lower back muscles acting in unison) turns to face the target. This action turns the chest and shoulders to face the target. The arms, hands, and golf club are moved with this rotation, and the club will follow at a tremendous rate of speed.

THE FINISHING POSITION

This is the culmination of all the movements a golfer makes in the delivery part of the swing. When the force of the golf swing has exhausted itself, one should be completely in balance and relaxed with all the weight on the front foot. The front foot is in its original position as at address. The knees, hips, chest, and shoulders should be facing the target, all level and in good posture, with the spine straight and the head held erect. At all times balance must be maintained.

INJURY PROBLEMS IN THE GOLFER

Golfer's Back

The swing involves a rotation of the spine about a fixed platform with transfer of the weight around a central axis. A smooth swing limits loads on the back; a jerky swing, undue hyperextension, and a reversed-C position all contribute to overload of the low back.

Nonetheless, playing with back pain must to many be a reality of life. Harm will not accrue by continuing to play golf with back pain. Obviously, bending to pick up a club, putting the ball on the tee, or retrieving the ball from the hole may all provoke pain but are not likely to cause harm. Most individuals are afflicted with some component of disk degeneration and mechanical back pain that they must come to live and play with.

Maintaining back fitness with a program of exercises including abdominal-strengthening and pelvic-tilt exercises and protected situps can greatly enhance one's ability to live with a back condition. Flexibility and strengthening of the spine area are aided by McKenzie extension routines with sloppy pushups and back extension drills.

Shoulder Dysfunction

The rotator cuff does not play a significant role in the golf swing, as has been shown on electromyographic (EMG) studies. The larger muscle groups of the trunk and upper body are more important. This is good news for the older athlete, for it is recognized that over the age of 65 years, up to 30 percent of individuals may have rotator cuff tears of greater or lesser degree. This clearly does not preclude playing golf. Individuals, of course, may experience the catching discomfort associated with rotator cuff tendinitis or subacromial bursitis or may be troubled by night pain after activity. Specific treatment may be sought to manage symptoms, or even on occasion surgery may be required, but most shoulder conditions are compatible with being able to maintain golf activity. A somewhat protracted recovery may follow shoulder surgery, but attention to strengthening of the shoulder girdle muscles and restoration of flexibility should ensure a satisfactory outcome.

Golfer's Elbow

The classic description of golfer's elbow is one of pain and point tenderness over the medial epicondyle of the elbow. Pain on impact loading can arise as a result of hitting an obstruction or taking a heavy divot. Overzealous practice, particularly in hitting from an artificial turf mat, also can be a potent contributor to this condition.

The mainstay of management of all elbow conditions has to be in avoiding provocative influences. Local icing, forearm muscle strengthening, and flexibility exercises to stretch the dorsi and palmar flexors can be enhanced by simple drills such as isometric squeezing of a soft rubber ball for the flexors or the spreading of the fingers against the resistance of a rubber band for the extensor group.

Lateral epicondylitis in the golfer is equally problematic. So-called tennis elbow is handled with similar techniques of management, and the use of a tennis elbow splint for the golfer certainly has merit, reducing loads on the tendon origins by shifting the fulcrum of load more distally to the muscle mass.

One form of golfer's elbow that may be more pernicious is the syndrome associated with radial nerve entrapment in the proximal forearm. This will require more careful rehabilitation and does not respond to the use of medication and steroid injection in the same manner as the common bone-tendon junction syndromes.

Other forms of elbow pain include biceps tendinitis and olecranon impaction syndrome, which are also common and should be distinguished from other forms of overuse and overload of the elbow mechanism.

Wrist and Hand

Trauma to the wrist and hand can have a devastating impact on a golfer's performance. The grip and hand function is such an integral part of the smooth execution of the golf swing.

Specific problems can occur from direct trauma, as in striking an obstruction with the club. Fracture of the hook of the hamate can be caused by striking a rock or tree stump with the butt of the club impacting in the hypothenar region. Pain is characteristically incurred locally with every shot and makes play impossible. Diagnosis can be difficult, but a carpal tunnel x-ray can clearly define the fracture, which may require surgical repair. Intercarpal dissociations can arise from a similar mechanism of injury and often will require very specialized review and possible surgical treatment.

Conditions such as de Quervain's tenosynovitis or carpal tunnel syndrome are not specifically golf-related conditions but are injury problems that may certainly have an impact on a golfer's performance. Problems associated with dysfunction of the thumb can be particularly problematic, with partial rupture or strain of the ulnar collateral ligament of the metacarpophalangeal (MCP) joint of the thumb or disease affecting the trapeziometacarpal joint being most debilitating. Simple taping can be very helpful in alleviating symptoms from such sources.

While alterations cannot be made to the shape of the grip of a club because the rules of golf specifically limit such adjustment, accommodation by changing the thickness of the grip can be helpful to those with arthritis of the hand or problems with hand closure.

Disorders of the Hip

Trochanteric bursitis is an irritation of the bursa overlying the outer aspect of the hip where the fasciae latae lay over the underlying bone and can be a source of irritation to the golfer. Fortunately, usually it will respond to local measures, which may include steroid injection and physiotherapy.

Osteoarthritis of the hip is common with advancing age, and golf may be one of the few active recreational outlets that an elderly individual is able to sustain. Arthritis of the hip restricts body turn and weight transfer, markedly limiting the golf swing, quite apart from the obvious restriction in being able to walk the course. For many individuals, the golf cart may become an absolute "game saver." Others may well have to consider total hip replacement surgery. Such intervention may completely rejuvenate the elderly golfer's career, with return to play within 3 to 4 months of surgery. A golf cart may need to be used initially, but ultimately, walking the course again should be anticipated, although carrying a golf bag may not be practical.

Disorders of the Knee

Knee problems can cause major interference with the golf swing, impeding the smooth transfer of weight and restricting body turn. Specific disorders affecting knee function are obviously more completely addressed in other chapters of this book, but for the golfer, minor derangements unresponsive to simple treatment may require consideration of arthroscopic surgery. Following arthroscopy of the knee, a program of simple strengthening exercises with straight leg raise and sideways leg lift and hip flexor strengthening exercises should be encouraged. This generally will allow a return to play within 2 to 4 weeks of intervention depending on the pathology dealt with. Simple flexibility routines for the hamstring, quadriceps, and calf muscle groups also should be maintained.

Many aging athletes injured in the combat sports of youth such as football, soccer, and ice hockey take to golf in their later years only to find their participation hampered by the effects of posttraumatic arthritis. Osteoarthritis of the knee is also common as we age. Fortunately for such individuals, total knee replacement surgery offers an answer that will allow the aging athlete a full return to golf activity. The recovery is necessarily a little longer and the rehabilitation program more protracted than with total hip replacement, but the outcome is no less successful. Early on, walking is to be encouraged, and practice in such skills as chipping, putting, and pitching can be embarked on within a matter of weeks of surgery, even if it takes several months before the full swing is practiced.

Soft Tissue Injuries in the Leg

Soft tissue injuries such as muscle strains of the hamstring and calf can occur when a golfer inadvertently steps in a hole or stumbles and strains himself or herself. Such injuries will respond to physiotherapy with early introduction of a gentle stretching exercise program for the hip adductors as well as the calf and hamstring groups. These exercises should be part of the golfer's warm-up routine in order to prevent injury recurrence.

Achilles tendon rupture is the most serious of the soft tissue injuries, and rehabilitation following surgery and cast protection will take 5 to 6 months before it will be possible to walk the course again. Ankle sprains are not uncommonly incurred on the golf course and will respond to standard treatment measures with the use of an ankle support brace, a useful adjunct to restoring the golfer to active play within a matter of weeks.

Foot Disorders

Just as the feet are the platform on which we stand, so too are they the base for a good golf swing. With walking an integral component of the game, comfortable feet are essential if a golfer is to enjoy his or her round of golf. In this regard, soft spikes are both lighter and much more comfortable to wear. They eliminate the pressure sensation that one experiences with metal spikes when walking on hard surfaces as well as being kinder to the greens.

While appropriately fitting golf shoes are obviously essential, personal accommodation can be further offered by customized foot orthoses. This is especially true for those with persistent foot discomfort from entities such as plantar fasciitis, chronic metatarsalgia from metatarsal prolapse, or chronic arch strain from tibialis posterior tendinitis or midtarsal arthritis.

OTHER HEALTH CONSIDERATIONS IN THE GOLFER

Cardiac Conditions

Following myocardial infarction, walking is an essential component of all rehabilitation programs to improve the overall cardiorespiratory fitness level and circulatory function of the recovering patient. Golf offers an appropriate outlet with a combination of walking and golf cart use.

After Abdominal Surgery

Following abdominal surgery, both general and specific fitness need to be regained. Walking offers such opportunity for general conditioning with specific exercises to strengthen the back, utilizing pelvic tilt and back extension routines to build up the weakened abdominal wall musculature. In the initial recovery phase, an elasticized corset will offer good support until abdominal tone and general fitness are regained. Indeed, this may greatly assist the golfer in his or her return to golf.

Mental and Psychological Health Aspects

The great Scots golf architect Dr. Alistair Mackenzie once said with regard to his practice in his home town in Scotland that patients whom he had seen repeatedly in his surgery with minor ailments were seldom ever seen back in his office again once they had been introduced to golf. Apocryphal perhaps, but nonetheless true. Golf offers an outlet, a recreation that in itself allows for no hypochondriasis or introspection other than with regard to one's own golf game.

CONCLUSION

Golf offers a positive recreational opportunity for individuals of all ages. An absorbing passion for many, a pleasant diversion for others, the combination of outdoor exercise and mental stimulation makes it indeed "the universal pastime."

23 | Track and Field Injuries

Robert Quinn

Track and field, or "athletics," remains immensely popular at all levels in Europe; however, elite level interest has flagged in North America in recent years. Nonetheless, participation in running, particularly distance running and road racing, remains strong with millions of Americans taking to the roads on a daily or weekly basis, participating in road races, triathlons, and other events. The focus of this chapter, therefore, will be on distance running-related injuries; however, it will also address jumping and sprinting injuries. Injuries that arise suddenly, representing acute muscle strains, joint sprains, or fractures, are far more common in sprinting and jumping (frequently involving the large muscle groups of the thighs); conversely, the great majority of distance running injuries reflect overuse and repetitive injuries from training.

As always, assessment of the problem begins with a careful history. This should include constitutional history such as weight loss or gain, fevers, chills or night sweats, and in young women careful attention to history of eating, weight fluctuation, menses, and possible pregnancy.

Past history for indications of inflammatory or joint-related issues should be assessed, including inflammatory bowel disease, psoriasis, and family history of arthritis. Prior sports-related injuries and medical history should be reviewed.

Next, there should be a detailed review of the onset of injury (acute or insidious), the mechanism of injury in detail, and aggravating and alleviating factors. Specific attention should be paid to changes in training: intensity, duration, training surface, shoes, addition or deletion of "cross-training," and use of stretching and weights. Shoes should always be examined with the patient, and if at all possible the patient should be seen performing the activity; I frequently ask the patient to run from my office and return, with the hope of having reproduced the symptoms.

Finally, a number of systemic complications can arise from sports training, and in young or elite athletes the issue of performance-enhancing drugs should be addressed.

MECHANICS OF RUNNING

A brief overview of the biomechanics of running is necessary to understand common injuries. Bipedal ambulation can be analyzed by looking at either leg: the supporting leg on the ground is in "stance" phase; while the other (moving) leg is in "swing" phase.

461

During walking, 40 percent of the gait cycle is in swing, while 60 percent is in stance: therefore, in walking, there is a 20 percent overlap—double stance—when both feet are on the ground. Faster walking decreases double stance and increases swing time, but by definition there must always be a double stance period. Failure to do so results in "lifting"—a penalty in race walking.

Running is defined as ambulation without double stance, that is, both legs are in the air at the same time during part of the gait cycle. (Jogging often represents a running motion but insufficient swing time to eliminate the double stance phase.) Stance phase can be further broken down into stages, starting with heel strike.

Stance Phase

Heel strike is the initial contact of the foot with the ground. The extended leg (hip flexed, knee extended, ankle slightly dorsiflexed) prepares to take the weight of the body. Strike should occur on the outer aspect of the heel (this can be verified by checking sole wear) indicating the foot is slightly dorsiflexed and inverted (the subtalar joint is in slight supination).

Foot flat occurs after heel strike when the foot is plantarflexed by an eccentric contraction of the dorsiflexors (tibialis anterior, toe extensors). The entire foot comes into contact with the ground and the entire weight of the body is transmitted to the foot (while running, forces generated equal two to three times body weight). While plantarflexion is controlled by the eccentric contraction of the anterior compartment calf muscles, the subtalar joint rolls into pronation with increasing weight onto the longitudinal arch. Proximally, the tibia rotates internally with pronation, while the extended knee is controlled into a more flexed position by an eccentric contraction of the quadriceps. Runners will often report maximum soreness with "shin splints" or quads soreness after a long run at this stage. Similarly, iliotibial band pain may initially present with a sharp pain immediately after heel strike.

Mid-stance occurs at the point when the body weight is passing directly over the pronated mid-tarsal area, in front of the neutrally aligned ankle, just behind the slightly flexed knee. Suboptimal arch/pronation support results in excess weight along the medial aspect of the foot, while inadequate heel cup/rear foot pronation support will flatten the arch. This can be seen in the medial arch wear on the sole of the shoe, or a "twisting" of the shoe upper inward over the sole of the shoe.

Heel-off is the stage when the body has passed forward over the foot: weight is shifted forward to the metatarsal heads as the subtalar joint supinates; the ankle is slightly dorsiflexed (and about to powerfully plantarflex); the knee slightly flexed; and the hip extended.

Toe-off initiates the swing phase as the foot plantarflexes and thrusts the body forward; the knee and hip are extended.

Once the foot leaves the ground, the leg is accelerated forward under the moving body by the iliopsoas to be extended in front of the body in preparation for the next heel strike. Injuries also occur in swing phase, particularly in sprinters. Toe-off is also crucial in jumpers, and is modified by the activity; long- and triple-jumpers exaggerate the motions of heel- and toe-off to extend the jump; high jumpers twist during a prolonged heel-off stage to capture centripetal force as part of their acceleration. The "airborne" cycle of the leg can be subdivided.

Swing Phase

In acceleration the toe leaves the ground, the hip flexes the leg forward and upward, the knee flexes, and the foot is behind the body. The powerful iliopsoas flexes the hip; initially the hamstrings help flex the knee, then contract eccentrically as the quadriceps begin to extend the knee.

During "swing through" the hip flexes past neutral, clearing the flexed knee. At this point, the other foot is in mid-stance.

In deceleration, the knee extends and foot dorsiflexes in preparation for the heel strike. Hamstring injuries in sprinters often occur during acceleration or deceleration; the powerful hip concentric actions of the iliopsoas and quadriceps overcome the eccentric contraction of the hamstring, resulting in a "pulled" hamstring.

**SYSTEMIC COMPLICATIONS
OF DISTANCE TRAINING**

In recent years increasing attention has been paid to the total body effect of distance running training. Most frequently, these only occur in elite level athletes running upwards of 100 km per week, with intensity in their training.

Anemia

While anemia is fairly common in distance runners, exact incidence and etiology remain unclear. Suspicion should be aroused when performance begins to tail off, and specific questions such as the presence of hematuria after long runs should be raised. Some "tea colored" urine after a long run is frequently related to muscle breakdown, and 14 percent of runners in the Comrades marathon in

South Africa developed myoglobulinuria.[1] While hematuria is usually not cause for concern, it should invariably clear within 72 h; if not, a work-up is indicated.

Factors contributing to anemia can include microscopic or occult gastrointestinal (GI) loss; some have speculated this can be due to GI trauma on the long run or relative GI vascular insufficiency with shunting away from the splanchnic bed. Mechanical trauma has also been indicated. Use of NSAIDs as a contributing factor should be considered.

Many distance runners are vegetarians or vegans and therefore, appropriate iron, B_{12} and folate supplementation is of concern. Relying on MCV and hemoglobin indices can be misleading as these can change slowly. Any reasonable suspicion should trigger specific iron and iron saturation studies and B_{12} and folate tests. Laboratory B_{12} values may be misleading: Supplemental B_{12} should be given at low normal levels.

Iron supplementation can be given orally: 325 mg PO TID on an empty stomach is ideal but often poorly tolerated, it can be taken with food. IM can be given in those who do not tolerate PO or have malabsorption. Hemoglobin should be rechecked in 3 to 4 weeks, with an appropriate response being a correction halfway to normal; full correction will take 2 months.

Folate can be replaced with 1 mg PO QD. B_{12} 100 mg IM q week $\times$ 4 weeks is usually adequate, but subsequent injections q month may be needed. In both cases reticulocytosis should occur within the week, and hemoglobin should normalize within 2 months.

Menstrual Dysfunction

Altered and absent periods occur frequently in female distance runners, and delayed onset of the menarche and secondary sexual characteristics is common in teenage female athletes engaged in intense training for distance running, ballet dancing and gymnastics. All female athletes should be questioned regarding menstrual status, eating habits, body weight, recent changes in weight, and the use of prescription and over-the-counter medications. One should always be mindful of the "female athlete triad" of disordered eating, menstrual dysfunction, and osteoporosis. The identification of menstrual dysfunction should always trigger a review of thyroid, adrenal, and ovarian function. Pregnancy needs to be rule out. Detailed physical examination including Tanner staging, pelvic exam, and signs of anorexia (lanugo hair, dry skin and nails, hypotension, lower extremity edema) or bulimia (parotid gland hypertrophy, dental caries, conjunctival petechia) should be performed. Relevant labwork includes CBC; electrolytes, BUN and creatinine, Ca^{2+}, Mg^{2+}, cholesterol, protein, albumin, and pregnancy tests.

Although there is no uniform agreement, altered periods during intense training or competition for one or two periods, provided body weight is adequate, is acceptable. Delayed menarche (age > 16 years or 1 year beyond average of mother and sisters); amenorrhea (absence of 3+ periods), any signs of anorexia or bulimia, or a second stress fracture necessitates a thorough review including nutritional status, moderation/cessation of training, body weight goals, and nutritional counseling. Consultation from a counselor with expertise in eating/body image, should be sought early, particularly for teenagers.

In the post-teen athlete suppression of the menstrual cycle can happen with intense training and needs to be monitored; many athletes choose to use the birth control pill in order to maintain "control" over their period, as a menstrual cycle occurring concurrently with a significant athletic event can interfere in some cases with optimal athletic performance.

Osteopenia and Osteoporosis

Weightbearing exercise is paramount during the pre-menopausal years for optimal muscle bulk and bone density, women who have suppressed their menses can have increased risk of osteoporosis, which can be seen in young, fair, amenorrheic distance runners. Amenorrhea as defined above, recurrent stress fracture, stress fracture in an axial bone (stress fractures have been seen in the ribs of a female marathoner), or incidental radiologic findings of osteoporosis are definite indications for metabolic work-up, cessation of training, and calcium supplementation.

Male Fertility

Questions have been raised as to whether or not intensive training suppresses development of secondary male sexual characteristics and negatively impacts on fertility, but recent studies have shown that male distance runners are at no increased risk for sperm count or motility problems.

PERFORMANCE-ENHANCING DRUGS

While these have traditionally been limited to elite and international level athletes, their use continues to grow at national and collegiate levels.

Anabolic Steroids

There is evidence that the use of anabolic steroids continues to grow in high school—both boys and girls. Most commonly, one sees the use of anabolic steroids in sprinters and jumpers to increase muscle mass, decrease recovery time, and enhance performance. These agents carry multiple complications to the user and should be discouraged; the question of whether to medically observe someone using substances illegally remains an ethical "Catch 22." Signs of possible steroid abuse include facial swelling, acne, sudden increase in muscle mass, and irrational temper outbursts.

Side effects are legion, including electrolyte imbalance, liver function test abnormalities, hirsutism, acne, mood disorders, cardiovascular problems including hypertension, altered lipid profile, decreased testicular size and oligospermia.

Recently, other drugs have also begun to appear, including human growth hormone (with the same desired effects as the anabolic steroids), creatinine, and various amphetamine and amphetamine-related substances to increase performance.

Agents to Increase Red Cell Mass

The use of erythrocyte stimulating medications such as erythropoietin (EPO or Procrit) has grown in the distance running and cycling communities. Recombinant hormones can effectively increase red cell mass, thereby increasing oxygen delivery capacity to the tissues. This technology is as effective as "blood boosting" without the risks and difficulty of transfusion. Potential complications include fatal polycythemia due to hyperviscosity, as was suspected in the death of several European international cyclists some years ago.

Autologous transfusion of red cells can increase oxygen-carrying capacity and significantly improve performance. Speculation was widespread several years ago, however, the erythropoeitin has made this obsolete.

Altitude training and "live high-train low" techniques are designed to expose the athlete to lower oxygen concentration; thereby stimulating increased red cell production. Both have been effective.

Clenbuterol

Clenbuterol is a beta-2 agonist used as a bronchodilator. It is used in Europe and Asia, but not approved by the FDA in the United States. Six Olympians were disqualified in 1992 for its use, and Clenbuterol is banned by the IOC and NCAA (and thoroughbred racing). Reputed benefits of Clenbuterol include its anti-catabolic effects which increase muscle mass and reduce fat.

Caffeine

Caffeine is widely used as a CNS stimulant in athletics and elsewhere: many athletes drink coffee before training, and caffeine tablets are widely available. Caffeine is rapidly absorbed and reaches peak activity within 1 h, the half life is 3.5 h. Mechanism of action is by adenosine antagonism and potentiation of Ca^{2+} release in muscle. This results in vasoconstriction, diuresis, CNS stimulation, gastric secretion, and increased lipolysis in adipocytes. Anecdotal evidence is highly suggestive, but published studies conflict.

Caffeine is banned by the IOC at levels above 12 μg/mL; by the NCAA above 15 μg/mL.

Caffeine Equivalency of Common Caffeine Preparations

Substance	Approximate Urinary Equivalency per Dose (μg/mL)
Coffee	1.5–3
Tea	1.5–3
Cola	1–1.5
NoDoz	3–6
Anacin	2–3
Midol	2–3

GENERAL PRINCIPLES OF TREATING THE RUNNER

Specific treatment strategies will be addressed with specific injuries, however, certain overriding principles will allow the sports medicine physician to establish and maintain a therapeutic relationship with the athlete. The desire to stay active or "not lose fitness" is often nonnegotiable. It is imperative that when activities are limited or curtailed, alternate activities be assigned; while this is particularly difficult for sprinters and jumpers, cross-training activities such as weight-lifting, stationary cycling, or water running can be used to maintain muscle strength and fitness (without exacerbating the injury in question). For distance athletes a number of options exist, including swimming, running in the water, stationary cycle, road cycling, and cross-country exercise machines. Most distance runners will have difficulty getting their heart up while swimming due to less-than-ideal swim technique; therefore, some advocate the use of alternate breathing exercises (only breathing every third stroke or twice per lap).

Running in the pool is an extremely attractive alternative or complement to distance running; however, the athlete needs to be familiar with monitoring his or her heart rate as exercising at a subtraining rate threshold is a frequent mistake. A good rule of thumb is to calculate maximum heart rate (220 − age for men; 210 − age for women); then subtract another 10 beats per minute due to increased resistance of water pressure, and calculate target heart rates from there. It requires considerable mental effort to reach training rates running in the water.

When analgesia and inflammation control are needed the use of oral anti-inflammatories is generally safe and effective; their side effects including gastric intolerance should be reviewed in detail. Simple guidelines include the prescription of inexpensive and readily available first line agents: ibuprofen 600 mg TID or QID, naproxen 375 mg BID. If one agent fails, a second agent from another family can be tried. Both efficacy and side effects can vary between agents. Gastric side effects can be reduced by administration with food. Oral sulcrafate 1 gm BID or misoprostyl 200 mg BID are helpful in reducing side effects.

Local steroid injection, usually with a long-acting local anesthetic agent, can be very useful. These injections are best used when an athlete is near peak and cannot afford time off or competition is imminent, earlier in a training program a more methodical approach yields better long-term results. A steroid injection alone (without the identification and correction of aggravating factors, the modification of training and footwear, and the incorporation of appropriate stretching and strengthening) is useless.

The classic paradigm of "RICE" (rest, ice, compression, elevation) should be applied to acutely traumatize all inflamed areas.

Phase 1: Identification of the Problem(s)

Treatment of any injury begins with accurate diagnosis and prognosis. This includes the appropriate lab work and x-rays, identification of contributing factors (physical and mental), and analysis of training and racing schedules. Diagnostic and therapeutic interventions, including injections, should be undertaken. During this time treatment is symptomatic: by avoiding all aggravating activities and by aggressive use of NSAIDs. Arriving at a definitive diagnosis, including necessary investigations, should take no more than a week.

Phase 2: Pain and Inflammation Control

This is usually the period of maximum rest, icing, and physical therapy intervention with ultrasound and assisted exercises. During this phase, correction of training errors and trial of new shoes or orthotics should be learned and done faithfully. Cross-training should be established, with heart-rate training goals established and met.

Phase 3: Resumption of Modified Training

This period consists of return to modified activities as tolerated; that is, up to minor discomfort but NOT reproducing symptoms. The goal of this phase is increasing strength and endurance, testing new training techniques and equipment, and setting boundaries on training. Self-exercise and strengthening, self-icing, and careful monitoring of a gradually escalating program.

Phase 4

This phase consists of reintegration into full activities, monitoring for signs of overtraining or recurrence. Training modifications, stretching, warm-up, and strengthening must be maintained.

Most athletes wish to truncate these stages as much as possible; however, phases 2 and 3 can frequently be done concurrently, provided alternate exercises and activities are prescribed. The transition to stage 4 should not be rushed, as many injuries which become chronic frequently have simply never been allowed to heal. Repetition of the same errors-too much road running, too intense, inappropriate footwear-guarantees another trip to the clinic.

SPECIFIC INJURIES

Low-Back and Buttock Pain

Back pain and *sciatica* are fairly common complaints in both "week-end warriors" and elite athletes, accounting for about 5 percent of complaints. A careful history is needed to determine if, in fact, the pain originates in the lumbar spine or elsewhere; if the pain radiates, and if there is radiation below the knee. The latter, in combination with tingling, numbness, or perceived weakness, strongly suggests a radicular component.

The majority of back pain, however, occurs in the lumbar area and is related to mechanical factors; addressing this issue hinges on careful history and physical. The physical exam should include peripheral joint screen, screen for psoriasis, and special tests, including testing for strength, sensation and reflexes, straight leg raising and femoral stretch, perianal sensation, and palpation of the spinous processes and pelvic brim. Hip and knee range of motion should be assessed and Gaenslen's sign for assessment of the sacroiliac joints and Schoeber's test should be performed.

Finally, the history should focus on whether the pain is inflammatory (worse with rest); or mechanical (worse with activity) in nature.

The majority of low-back pain in athletes, particularly week-end warriors, is related to poor body mechanics and muscle tone. Reminder of body mechanics, appropriate warm-up, and a specific abdominal-strengthening exercise program will often suffice to address most back pain; in athletes with hyperlordotic spines maintenance of excellent abdominal strength is key to preventing low back pain.

While more common in gymnasts and football linemen, spondylolysis with or without spondylolisthesis may represent a stress fracture and cause of back pain. Classically, these injuries are worse with activity and alleviated somewhat with rest; the physical examination may be completely benign or show tight hamstrings; on occasions this injury can lead to nerve root irritation.

Diagnosis hinges on lumbar spine films with lateral looking for the classic "Scotty dog collar". Nuclear bone scan can determine if the bone lesion is "hot" or active, or old.

Treatment, unfortunately, means avoidance of traumatic activities for a period of several months; frequently a bone scan is helpful in determining whether or not the lesion is "hot" or quiescent. In hot lesions a rigid thoracolumbar corset may help provide support.

Sciatica

Athletes will frequently present with symptoms of back or buttock pain with radiation down the leg. A special test as outlined above should be undertaken, as well as palpation in the sciatic notch and tests straining the piriformis muscle as outlined below. Radicular signs can arise from irritation at the nerve root (often due to degenerative changes or disc protrusion); along the course of the sciatic nerve frequently due to the piriformis muscle, or even more distally at the knee. It is always a challenge to separate piriformis muscle strain syndrome from hamstring origin inflammation.

In cases of a radicular component the diagnosis can be confirmed with electrodiagnostic studies or magnetic resonance imaging (MRI). When confirmed treatment should start with a conservative but comprehensive treatment of oral anti-inflammatories, "spinal stabilization" program, and avoidance of running until symptoms are under control; if symptoms do not come under control, then a short first of oral steroids (starting at 50 mg daily and titrating by 5 mg every two to three days) is often very useful (although the literature equivocates on this). Before the use of oral steroids the patient must be informed of all possible side effects including restlessness/agitation. Athletes with radicular signs should be cleared before returning to training. Appropriate alternate training includes swimming and running in the water; stationary cycling in a relatively upright position is appropriate provided symptoms are not reproduced. Weightlifting should be avoided until the etiology is clarified by CT or MRI, or when symptoms resolve. Progressive symptoms, leg weakness, and bowel, bladder, or erectile dysfunction necessitate prompt referral.

The use of epidural steroids has grown in recent years; however, the most recent literature regarding this again equivocates. Epidural steroids can provide effective short-term relief but should be seen as a "bridge" while back strengthening and spinal stabilization are undertaken.

Back pain that seems atypical or does not respond to treatment should always prompt a search for other etiologies, as unfortunately athletes are not "exempt" from other back conditions including Scheuermann's disease, Reiter's syndrome, and ankylosing spondylitis.

Sacroileitis (SI) represents a diagnostic challenge: The history is difficult to tease apart from other types of mechanical back pain. When suspected, SI views should be checked, as well as an ESR, RF, ANA, and possibly HLA-B27. Rheumatologic consultation is needed when an inflammatory etiology is suspected. Nuclear bone scan can detect SI (including from cycling); NSAIDs and the trial of a stabilizing belt, along with intraarticular injections under fluoroscopy, are useful.

Piriformis Syndrome

Buttock pain associated with sciatic symptoms suggests the diagnosis of piriformis syndrome. Usually the pain starts as a dull ache late in the run; with ongoing training the pain comes sooner in the run, becomes sharper, and is associated with a radiating pain or burning down the leg. Pain may be reproduced by prolonged sitting.

The piriformis muscle originates on the ventral side of the sacrum, exits via the sciatic foramen deep to the iliopsoas muscle, and tracks deep to the gluteus medius to insert on the superior aspect of the greater trochanter. The muscle serves as an accessory hip abductor and external rotator. In Grant's series of dissections,[2] the tibial and peroneal divisions passed immediately below the piriformis in 87 percent of dissections; in 12 percent the peroneal division passed through the piriformis; and in 0.5 percent the peroneal division passed above the piriformis.

In addition to the usual physical exam; one needs to measure leg lengths. Palpation in the sciatic notch should reproduce pain, and may cause symptoms down the leg. With the patient lying on the unaffected side, hip flexed to 90 degrees, adducted to allow the knee to rest on the bed, the gluteus muscles must be relaxed. A line drawn from the cephalad edge of the greater sciatic notch (just distal to the PSIS) to the greater trochanter roughly parallels the piriformis, and can be palpated at the one-third and two-third distance for tenderness. Piriformis tenderness can be confirmed by bimanual exam, with the muscle being palpated from within the pelvic floor via rectal or vaginal route. Finally, provocative measures include resisted hip abduction/external rotation from the above position.

Treatment is stepwise. Running should be avoided until symptoms are under control. Stationary cycling often reproduces symptoms by direct mechanical compression; therefore, water exercise during phase 1 is the best. Saddle height and alignment should be checked carefully if the athlete is a cyclist. Correcting half a leg length discrepancy is a good rule of thumb. Return to running must be on LEVEL surfaces.

Topical ice is helpful acutely, as are NSAIDs. A physical therapy program of three to four times daily, prolonged stretching, friction massage, and steroid phoresis is helpful. If these measures fail, direct injection with 1% lidocaine (without epinephrine) and a long-acting steroid can be undertaken. Positioned as above, the tender area is palpated. The "internal" finger localizes the most tender area, and the needle is introduced using the tender area as a target. The needle must be introduced fairly deeply, depending on the amount of soft tissue. Care must be taken not to produce any neurologic symptoms. Surgical release has been described for refractory cases.[3]

Chronic Hamstring Tendinitis

A difficult differential diagnosis is that of sciatica; piriformis syndrome, hamstring injury, and chronic hamstring origin tendinitis, often associated with an ischial bursitis (weavers bottom). The latter is common but often goes unrecognized. Symptoms are insidious in onset but become better defined: a dull pain in the low buttock/proximal hamstring, worse with prolonged activity. Pain may radiate to the knee, not lower. Pain may start to occur with prolonged sitting.

Physical examination reveals tight hamstrings, often reproducing pain. Discrete tenderness can be elicited at the proximal hamstring, often with a palpable band of 'tight muscle." A bursal inflammation is occasionally felt at the ischial tuberosity.

Treatment is rest; cycling with progressive raising of the seat to further extend the hip, or water running; stretching of the hamstring, then strengthening; and local deep heat with ultrasound, and deep friction massage ("crucifixions" per Noakes).

Pelvic Pain

Pelvic pain is a frequent problem in distance runners and sprinters and can arise from a variety of sources including the SI joints, the symphysis pubis, and the origins of the large thigh muscles. Atypical pelvic pain from visceral pathology can occur. When assessing pelvic pain particular attention should be paid to the presence of fevers and chills and changes in bowel and bladder habits, and the possibility of pregnancy or ectopic pregnancy must be addressed.

Causes of refractory pelvic pain in athletes have included subacute appendicitis, fibroids, and even ectopic pregnancy.

Prostatitis

Deep pelvic pain, "fullness," dysuria, and adductor region pain worsened with activity in males is suggestive of prostatitis. The etiology is felt to be "a dirty diaper syndrome": prolonged activity, perspiration and trauma from shorts to the urethral orifice in distance runners and cyclists allows bacteria accumulating in the soiled shorts to ascend the urethra. Typically, onset is associated with rigors, night sweats and chills, then pain.

Diagnosis is based on history, physical examination with a tender prostate, and culture of urethral discharge "milked" from the prostate; and corroborated with an elevated PSA. Treatment is finding a suitable nonstraining activity such as swimming, and 4- to 6-week course of oral ciprofloxacin.

Osteitis Pubis

Irritation and inflammation of the symphysis pubis is seen commonly in distance runners, weightlifters, and football and soccer players. Symptoms include pelvic pain and pain at the base of the penis, or the urethra in females; pain can be reproduced with resisted leg adduction, and with forceful abdominal muscles contractures or endurance activities.

Diagnosis is based on history, physical findings, and investigations. X-rays of the pelvis often show sclerosis and widening at the symphysis pubis, and bone scan may be hot to the area.

Treatment includes avoidance of stressful activities, including weightbearing and running; gradual strengthening of the adductor musculature; and anti-inflammatories. Refractory cases can be injected under fluoroscopy.

Thigh Pain

Quadriceps Rupture

The quadriceps muscle is subject to rupture, particularly with traumatic jumping or landing events. The history is usually straightforward, and usually one finds a palpable "knot" of muscle (most commonly the rectus femoris). Immediate surgical repair is indicated in athletes, however, people can function at a reasonably high level with a chronic rupture, although, this does lead to early fatigability and often muscle pain.

Muscle Soreness

Quadriceps soreness is common after extreme effort, such as a marathon and can be the rate-limiting step in return to fitness. It is felt to arise from damage related to repeated eccentric contractions and damage is to the area near the Z-band of the sarcomere. Cell damage and muscle fiber necrosis may persist for weeks. The following guideline by Martin, apply to muscle soreness.

Grade	Symptoms	Activity
0	No discomfort	Continue training
1	Discomfort with palpation	Reduce train: 1 week; no race: 2 weeks
2	Discomfort with walk, unable to squat	Reduce train: 2 weeks; no race: 1 month
3	Severe pain, walk with difficulty	Reduce train: 1 month; no race: 2 months

Appropriate activities during the "reduce train" period include slow jogging (avoiding hills), stationary bike at low resistance, intermediate speed, and swimming.

Knee Injuries

Approximately one-third to one-half of all running injuries occur around the knee; with the most common being patellofemoral syndrome.

Patellofemoral Syndrome

This describes a condition in which the pain is felt to arise from poor dynamics between the patella and the femur. A variety of terms have been used including "chondromalacia patella," however, pathologic terms should be avoided when the diagnosis remains a syndrome.

Diagnosis: The typical presentation in distance runners is that of a dull aching knee pain; often worse with initiation of the activity, then frequently a period of "letting up" once the person is sufficiently warmed up, but the pain almost invariably recurs if the activity is maintained. Downhill running is particularly problematic. Pain also occurs frequently at rest and the so called "aisle sign" is typical: The patient prefers to sit with the knees in an extended position as flexion reproduces pain and frequently opts for the aisle seat on planes and in movie theaters.

Physical examination includes assessment of the "Q-angle" (the angle between the axis of the tibia and the femur: measured by drawing a line from the ASIS to the midpoint of the patella, and intersecting this line with a line parallel to the patelar tendon to the tibial tubercle. An angle of greater-than-16-degrees is associated with a higher incidence of patellofemoral syndrome.

Standing posture is assessed for "inward looking," high- or low-riding patellae; genu recurvatum; examination of the feet looking for pronation; and inspection of quadriceps muscle bulk, particularly vastus medialis. The patient should squat, watching for pain and patellar tracking; patellar tracking should also be assessed while sitting. A small knee effusion is common, particularly after activity. Pain can be reproduced by pressing the patella into the femoral groove; or by the "apprehension sign": compression of the patella into the femoral groove, then contraction of the quadriceps causing a sharp pain. Imaging is often not needed, but skyline views can be helpful.

Commonly, the pain is due to poor tracking of the patella, with the patella tracking laterally in the groove producing pain. The vastus medialis (VMO) tends to be less developed than other components of the quads, further, the patella is pulled laterally by the vastus lateralis, lateral retinaculum, and the IT tract. McConnell has described measuring distance from the condyles to the mid-patella (should be centered); tilt can be assessed by palpating the relative borders of the patella.

Chronic problems can lead to degenerative changes in the patellofemoral joint.

Often distance runners fail to fully extend the leg during swing phase such that the final muscle contractors for knee extension is underutilized; resulting in deficiency of vastus medialis and asymmetrical tracking.

X-rays are indicated when treatment fails and symptoms persist past 4 to 8 weeks: Standard knee films rule out other causes of knee pain; patella alta or baja can be best seen on lateral view, and axial views with the knee flexed 20 to 45 degrees allow visualization of the patellofemoral joint.

Treatment and rehabilitation start with rest, ice, and anti-inflammatory medications.

Cross training activities include swimming, water-jogging, and cross-country skiing (or a ski machine). Stationary cycling can be done, with care to raise the seat to an appropriate height and with avoidance of pain.

Exercise focused specifically on building the vastus medialis, including extended knee leg raises and resisted individualized hip and knee abduction, adduction, and stretching, are indicated. High repetition, relatively low weight exercises requiring concentric and eccentric quad and hamstring activity are needed, for example, leg presses (controlled rate; flex and extend, avoid flexion past 90 degrees), drop squats, and lunges. Self-mobilization of the patella can be quickly taught by a physiotherapist and done several times daily.

McConnell taping techniques can help with tracking, and hasten return to running. A nonirritating tape is applied to the patella and taped medially, the tape can be moved proximally or distally on the patella based on the riding angle. A strong tape is then applied to hold the patella medially. Some trial and error is needed to find the best taping alignment.

A well-fitted patella stabilization orthosis can hasten return. Surgical options remain for refractory cases.

Bursitis

Many bursae exist around the knee which can become inflamed due to overuse or poor mechanics related to muscle tightness. These are clinical/bedside diagnoses and imaging studies are rarely needed.

Pes Anserinus bursa fills the potential space between the medial hamstrings and their insertion on the medial tibial plateau. History is that of a vague pain becoming sharper with continued activity, usually well localized to the area distal to the medial joint line. Pain can be reproduced by palpation distal to the medial joint line, by following the line of the hamstring tendons to the medial tibial flare. There is often swelling and localized tenderness. Treatment includes local ice, NSAIDs, and aggressive hamstring stretching. Ultrasound and steroid phoresis can be helpful. A local injection of lidocaine and steroid can provide immediate relief, and allow the athlete to train through the rehabilitation stage.

Prepatellar and deep infrapatellar bursae lie in front of, and posterior to, the patellae. Both can present with similar symptoms to patellofemoral syndrome, but usually there is no pain at rest. Prepatellar bursitis can usually be well localized by patient and examiner by a swelling directly in front of the patella; infrapatellar bursitis presents with more distal pain and fewer findings. For both, treatment is local ice, NSAIDs, hamstring stretching. The prepatellar bursae can be easily aspirated and injected if needed. Refractory infrapatellar bursitis may require injection, which needs to be done *behind* the patellar tendon.

Jumper's Knee (Patellar Tendinitis)

This inflammation of the patellar tendon usually occurs at the proximal attachment (inferior pole of the patella). While common in jumpers, it can also be seen in sprinters, but rarely in runners. Often the jumper "comes in having made the diagnosis," the challenge is to identify and correct training errors. Excessive bounding, bounding onto a hard surface, and inappropriate footwear are common triggers. Mechanical knee problems, poor patellar tracking, weak ankle dorsiflexors, tight hamstrings also predispose.

Physical examination revealed tenderness at the inferior patella pole and along the tendon. Assessment of quadriceps and hamstring strength and range of motion, as well as dorsiflexion at the ankle. X-rays may show degenerative changes at the inferior patella pole.

Treatment includes ice acutely, NSAIDs, avoidance of bounding/jumping. Ultrasound with steroid phoresis may be helpful.

Hamstring, quadriceps, Achilles stretching, and flexibility, as well as eccentric strengthening of the quads and ankle dorsiflexors (the major "braking" muscles of heel strike), must be initiated at diagnosis.

Iliotibial Band Syndrome

The iliotibial tract runs from the pelvic brim to the proximal lateral tibia at Gerdy's tubercle, with extension anteriorly to the patella. It is in the tendinous continuation of the gluteus maximus and tensor fascia lata. Lateral knee pain in distance runners often suggests IT band syndrome; with the pain occurring in the last few degrees of extension as the IT band rides over the lateral femoral condyle and the proximal fibular complex. Pain occurs initially as a poorly localized ache, with continued running it becomes sharper and more localized to the lateral aspect of the knee. With more activity, the pain may radiate proximally to the tensor fascia, causing a diagnostic difficulty. Pain is almost always limited to running, with little pain between episodes. Diagnosis is based on the history, and physical exam of the knee which is unremarkable; however, tenderness occurs over the lateral femoral condyle. Pain can be reproduced by pressure over the area while the patient fully extends the knee, a palpable click over the condyle may be felt. Ober's test for IT tightness involves laying the patient on the unaffected side with unaffected limb flexed at hip and knee. The involved side has the hip extended and the knee flexed; failure of the hip to adduct past horizontal indicates IT tightness.

Imaging studies offer little to confirm the diagnosis.

Treatment starts with the usual: rest, ice, and aggressive stretching. Localized ultrasound with phonophoresis, can hasten recovery. Unfortunately, any running must be avoided. Cross training activities to maintain fitness should focus on swimming and stationary bike, with care being taken to have the seat a little lower than normal to avoid the last 15 degrees of knee extension. Localized corticosteroid injection may provide relief and allow the athlete near peak to continue, however, athletes earlier in their training should take the time off, cross-train, and aggressively stretch the area as these injuries can be problematic. Rarely, surgical release is indicated for refractory cases.

Avoidance of running while rehabilitating is key, an aggressive stretching exercise of the IT band should be undertaken.

Plica Syndrome

The plica is an embryologic remnant appearing as a fold of synovium which may impinge on the joint space as a fold near the underside of the quadriceps tendon, or along the free edge of medial patellofemoral joint. The diagnosis is suggested by episodic pain/snapping/instability felt at the anterior edge of the knee. X-rays are of no help. After failing conservative treatment and stretching, consider arthroscopy for definitive diagnosis and treatment.

Posterior Knee Pain

Runners often present with pain localized to the popliteal fossae, poorly localized and occurring initially after the run, and then during the run. History should focus on mechanism of injury and aggravating factors: recalling that both the hamstring (hip and knee) and plantarflexor (knee and ankle) groups span two joints. Pain may be caused by muscle tightness/strain in one of the groups, a posterior strained joint capsule, or Bakers cyst. The latter can usually be easily visualized. This area is difficult to localize and examine. In addition to the usual knee exam, the athlete must be viewed from behind standing, rising on toes, and squatting. Knee extension with flexed hip and dorsiflexed ankle will help determine muscle group tightness.

Bakers cysts are usually self-limited, but can be aspirated and injected with steroids if persistently painful.

Strain of the deep musculature—the popliteus and plantaris—are difficult to tease apart. Treatment is nonspecific: ice and ultrasound to the area, concerted stretching of the gastrocs/hamstrings, and modified training. Sprinting, downhill running, and forceful knee extension are to be avoided.

Shin Pain

Shin pain is common in all track and field athletes; and the differential diagnosis necessitates a thoughtful work-up: "shin splints" can be "trained through"; a stress fracture mandates time off running; and compartment syndrome will prove refractory to conservative measures. "Tibial stress injuries" run the spectrum from periosteal inflammation ("shin splints") to tibial stress reaction or stress fracture. The key determinants of severity of injury are persistence of pain beyond running and imaging patterns on bone scan and MRI (not always needed).

Shin Splints

Beginning runners, and those increasing mileage or intensity are at risk to develop "shin splints" or "tibial stress syndrome." A dull aching pain occurring after running, then at ever-shortening intervals into the exercises, suggests the diagnosis, which if untreated, will lead to a stress fracture. The exact etiology of shin splints is unclear, but is felt to stem from inappropriate loading on the dorsiflexors of the foot (maximally eccentrically strained during the heel strike), inappropriate loading on other calf muscles related to controlling excessive foot pronation, and resultant strain at the origin on the bone. The bone site can arise posteriorly or medially on the tibia, or the lateral aspect of the fibula. Bone scans in asymptomatic high-mileage runners can show increased remodeling in these areas.

Diagnosis is based on the history and physical exam: Unlike stress fractures, there will be bony tenderness and even a rough feel along the medial tibial edge, but no rest pain. Pain may be reproduced by resisting dorsiflexion of the foot. Bone scanning is more sensitive than plain X-ray, although frank stress fracture will show upon plain films. In shin splints, the bone scan may be normal, or show diffuse increased uptake along the tibia, but not the focal hot spot seen in a stress fracture.

Treatment of shin splints hinges on identification and correction of aggravating factors:

- Reduce training, especially downhill running, sprints, and the tendency to overstride.
- Appropriate foot wear with good heel cushioning and pronation control helps minimize eccentric forces needed by the calf muscles. Athletes with chronic/recurrent shin splints should be assessed for orthotics to correct foot strike abnormalities—most often overpronation.
- There is considerable evidence that insuring adequate calcium intake (1000 mg/day) is helpful, particularly in female athletes.
- Adequate stretching of heel cord.

All athletes with shin splints should have calf, anterior compartment and lateral compartment stretching reviewed.

Ice rubs to the affected areas, three to four times daily is indicated.

Shin splints occurring early in a training program or after resumption of intense intervals often require only sorter shoes, "backing off" in training, and time. "Air casts" (pneumatic tibial orthoses) can speed return to running.

Stress Fracture

A dull ache, initially similar to shin splints but occurring with any activity suggests stress fracture. Differentiation from other aches is difficult, and frequent delay to diagnosis (often athletes suspect and fear the diagnosis). Initially described in Army recruits ("march fracture") this type of repetitive, cumulative microtrauma occurs in human athletes, thoroughbreds, and greyhounds. Stress fractures occur in a variety of sports, and the location is dictated by the stress on the bones. In gymnasts, who tend to hyperextend lumbar spine, it can occur in the pars intraarticularis. In runners, it occurs most commonly in the shin (approximately 50 percent in the tibia and

15 percent in the fibula), but also in the tarsal and metatarsal bones (25 percent) , and in the femur, femoral neck, and pubic arch.

Diagnosis is based largely on history: Without trauma, the runner reports a localized ache, initially only after exertion, but quickly with any weight bearing at all. History should focus on recent training with particular attention paid to recent changes in shoes, type of interval, running surface, and the training itself (mileage, intensity, long runs). The final straw can often be identified by the runner.

Physical exam demonstrates point tenderness, warmth, erythema over the area (can be quite normal in deep bone involvement). Tenderness to percussion or vibration is helpful; as is the "standing test" or "hot test" (standing or hopping on the involved leg reproduces pain).

X-rays are helpful to rule out other bony pathology, but are usually normal. A fine periostitis may be seen. Nuclear bone scanning is most helpful in confirming the diagnosis; the scan is hot in all three phases; whereas "shin splints" (periostitis) is hot only in the delayed phase. MRI with fat suppression technique is sensitive and accurate, but costly.

Treatment is frustrating for the athlete, and the most common treatment failure is premature return to the offending activity. Rest is unavoidable.

Phase 1 focuses on establishing the diagnosis and identification of errors to be avoided in the future. Strict rest, ice, NSAIDs, and stretching of the muscles about the affected area. With no stressful activity through the fractured bone, aerobic activity therefore is limited to swimming/water running. For most running injuries, even stationary cycling is initially inappropriate.

Phase 2 often extends out to 2 to 3 months. Running starts with slow-paced, 20-min jogs on a soft surface only after the resolution of bony point tenderness; and ends only when the athlete can resume everyday, near-normal distance/time at a slow pace, pain free. Progressive stretching to initially gentle strengthening, then increasing loads (both concentric and eccentric groups) is guided by pain: and should remain pain free. Alternate activities can be increased, and at two months gentle running on grass 3 days per week can be attempted.

Phase 3 starts 6 to 12 weeks out, when alternate day training on soft surfaces is tolerated, increasing mileage and days per week: Intense interval training is the last activity to be reintroduced for runners, bounding the last for jumpers.

"At-risk or critical" stress fractures have been identified by Baxter, and merit special attention. Navicular, proximal second metatarsal, intraarticular, and medial and lateral great toe sesamoid stress fractures have been identified as fractures requiring a high index of suspicion, aggressive treatment, and close follow up. Navicular fractures are hard to catch early, the nonspecific foot pain can be mistaken for extensor tenosynovitis. Six weeks of nonweight-bearing, with immobilization, is recommended.

Compartment Syndrome

This is a relatively rare condition, and a diagnosis usually reached after a failure of well-designed treatments for other conditions. An inability of the fascia to accommodate the expanding (working) muscle results in abnormally increased intracompartmental pressure, which presumably retards arterial circulation and leads to muscle ischemia; the pain may be due to the pressure phenomena per se, or the accumulation of the metabolic products of muscle activity. This usually occurs in the shin: the anterior, lateral, deep, or superficial posterior compartment may be involved.

History is somewhat similar to shin splints, but more "cramping." The pain is always related to exertion, never before activity, and slowly subsides afterwards. The athlete may report muscle cramping or "spasms," an unusual firmness to the muscle, or foot numbness related to nerve compromise around the affected compartment. Physical exam is normal when the athlete is asymptomatic, with exertion the affected area may be firm and tender.

Intracompartmental pressure monitoring using either a solid state intracompartmental catheter or slit catheter remains the gold standard for diagnosis; but is not widely available. Often the diagnosis is made on clinical grounds and failure of conservative treatment (which will always fail). Treatment is surgical release.

Ankle Pain

The majority of ankle pathology in track and field athletes is due to trauma; most frequently an inversion injury resulting in a first-, second-, or third-degree tear of the collateral ligaments; and in severe cases accompanying injury to the peroneal nerve and/or avulsion fractures of the tibia. Treatment depends on the severity of the injury.

Achilles Tendinitis

This injury dates to the antiquities. Achilles tendon rupture also occurs in sprinters, and treatment (immobilization in a plantar flexed position versus operative repair) depends on the activity level, expected outcomes, and time frame of the individual athlete. Complete rupture can be determined by the immediate onset of pain and swelling, palpable deficit in the heel cord, impaired gait, and failure to move the foot with passive squeezing of the calf. Immediate orthopedic consultation is needed.

Achilles tendinitis can be divided by where the site of inflammation/tenderness is at the location on the os calcis, or more proximal. The Achilles injury is common in runners for a number of reasons: the gastroc and soleus muscle complex is used each step both eccentrically at heel strike and concentrically at toe-off; forces are equal to 10 x body weight. An area of friction can arise at the heel collar (leading to a "pump bump") and in women who wear heels during the day, the calf muscles/tendon are held foreshortened.

Clement described a bowstring effect of the Achilles in runners who pronate with the tendon being further stretched about the os.

Symptoms are usually self-evident to the athlete. The early injury is manifested as pain/tightness in the heel cord first thing in the morning: at this stage NSAIDs, ice for 20 min every 3 to 4 h, stretching, avoidance of intense training and hill running, and new, softer shoes will often suffice. A soft heel insert of less than 10 mm is helpful.

With the pain occurring running, physical therapy for more aggressive stretching, friction massage, ultrasound is added. All intense training is held, and running should be stopped at the point discomfort progresses to pain. At the end of each workout, the athlete should "pinch" the heel cord: decreasing pain reassures, while increasing pain necessitates further reduction in training.

Once pain begins to interfere with running or change gait, running must stoop and cross-training activity begin. Cycling should be done in a high top shoe or ankle immobilizer to minimize movement of the Achilles; even swimming can irritate the ankle with forceful kicking (plantar flexion). Persistence of recurrent problems indicates referral to an orthopedic surgeon.

As soon as the pain is controlled, rehabilitation begins. In addition to calf stretching, eccentric and concentric strengthening is needed. A simple at-home remedy has the athlete stand on the edge of a step with weight on the balls of the feet. Slow toe rises and return to BELOW neutral are done. When this is well tolerated for several sets of 15, three times daily, the same exercise can be done with slowly incremental weight on the leg press: the knees are locked in extension and slow dorsiflexion/plantarflexion is undertaken.

Tenosynovitis

While the Achilles tendon is the most common injury, similar injuries can occur acutely or insidiously at other sites. The patellar tendon has already been addressed. Another frequent site is at the extensor retinaculum across the dorsal aspect of the ankle, laterally where the peroneal tendons track beneath the lateral malleolus, at even proximally at the origin of the large thigh muscles at the ASIS.

The history is usually straightforward: dull proceeding to sharp pain with activity; often well localized. If addressed early, local ice, stretching, and steroid phoresis can prevent time away from training. Gait dynamics and shoe wear should always be checked.

Foot Injuries

Foot injuries are extremely common in all track and field athletes.

Plantar Fasciitis

This typically presents as a well-localized pain at the base of the heel; worst first thing in the morning and then letting up somewhat through the day, presenting again with an exacerbation with any activity. While the history is usually quite diagnostic, physical exam can confirm it with direct local pressure over the heel pad area; and often pain reproduced with forceful dorsiflexion of the toes.

X-ray of the heel is not routinely needed, but in recurrent and refractory cases worthwhile to assess for heel spur; particularly in young men this should trigger a check for other inflammatory symptoms or signs suggestive of more widespread enthesopathy. Excellent results can usually be obtained with supporting the longitudinal arch; exercises of the foot including the "towel roll" and stretching; and anti-inflammatories. Appropriate longitudinal arch support and foot wear cushioning are key to successful management. More refractory cases can be injected locally with lidocaine and steroids.

"Black Toe"

Hematoma beneath the great toe is almost always related to repetitive trauma: Either shoes too small, too loose (with slippage causing the toe to strike against the inside of the shoe) or prolonged downhill running. This seemingly trivial injury can be quite painful and limit therapy; in cases with significant pain drainage by piercing the nail with a sterilized hot lancet (even conceivably a paper clip) allows evacuation of the hematoma and pain-free return to activity.

SUGGESTED READINGS

1. Schiff HB, MacSearraigh ETM, Kallmeyer JC: Myoglobulinuria, rhabdomyolysis and marathon running. *Q J Med* 47:463–472, 1978.
2. Grant JCB: *Grant's Atlas of Anatomy*. Baltimore, MD, Williams & Wilkins Co.

3. Barton TM: Pyriformis syndrome: A rational approach to management. *Pain* 45:347–352, 1991.
4. Martin et al: Muscle Soreness, 1983.
5. Baxter DE (ed): *The Foot and Ankle in Sport*. St. Louis, Mosby-Year Book, 1995:84.
6. McBryde AM. *The Foot and Ankle in Sport*. St. Louis, Mosby-Year Book, 1995:81–93.
7. Clement DB, Taunton JE, Smart GW: Achilles tendonitis and peritendinitis: Etiology and treatment. *Am J Sports Med* 12(3):179–184, 1984.
8. Fredericson M: Common injuries in runners: Diagnosis, rehabilitation and prevention. *Sport Med* 21(1):49–72, 1996.
9. Cumming DC: Exercise and reproduction in women. *J SOGC* Feb/Mar 1991:9–17.
10. Noakes T: *Lore of Running*. Champaign, IL, Leisure Press, 1991.

24 Swimming

Peter J. Fowler   Lorie Forwell

Swimming is enjoyed by an enormous number of participants. While accurate figures are not available, estimates of up to 100 million participants (Americans) at both recreational and competitive levels have been quoted. The current popularity of programs for master swimmers and triathlons contributes to both the continued growth of the sport and to the increasing age range of competitors. Swimming has relatively few inherent risks of injury. However, the intensely repetitive nature of the sport, particularly at the elite level, can result in overuse problems in the shoulder primarily but also in the elbow, knee, foot and ankle, and back.

The fundamental components of an accurate diagnosis and successful management of these problems are a good history, systematic physical examination, knowledge of anatomy and biomechanics, review of the training program, and education of the coach and athlete. The role of an informed coach in treatment and, more important, prevention cannot be overemphasized. Preventative measures are essential to a successful training program and should be incorporated from the outset.

In the majority of athletes with overuse injuries, conservative treatment that includes relative rest, technique modification, and physiotherapy intervention will be sufficient to restore function. Surgical intervention is a consideration when all nonoperative treatments have failed. This chapter reviews the causative factors in swimming injuries, physical examination, treatment options, and a comprehensive discussion of shoulder rehabilitation.

THE SHOULDER

Injury to the shoulder is the most common problem facing the competitive swimmer regardless of age. The term *swimmer's shoulder*, first used in 1974 by Hawkins and Kennedy,[1] describes symptomatology that frequently results from of a combination of anatomic and biomechanical factors rather than from a single causative agent. The contributing factors include overuse, anatomic features, shoulder joint laxity, fatigue, impingement, and stroke mechanics. Recent literature has identified an increase in the incidence of swimmer's shoulder from 3 percent in 1974 and 50 percent in 1981 to between 47 and 73 percent in 1986.[1-3] Rigorous training programs for national-caliber swimmers that typically demand at least nine 4000- to 8000-m sessions per week may be a factor in this increased incidence.

SWIMMING STROKES

In three of the four competitive strokes, the front crawl (freestyle), butterfly, and backstroke, 75 percent of propulsion is provided by the arms. In the breast stroke, the arms and legs contribute equally. With respect to arm action, the biomechanics of all four strokes are deceptively similar. The phases common to each stroke are the reach, the catch, the pull, and the recovery. During the reach or entry, the arm reaches forward to enter the water. In the catch phase, which is alike for all competitive strokes, the swimmer begins to pull or scull the water. Here, the swimmer flexes the elbow to 100 degrees and begins to extend, horizontally abduct, and slightly medially rotate the shoulder. In the pull phase, which is the propulsion or power phase, the glenohumeral joint (GHJ) of the shoulder is in adduction and internal rotation, with the exception of breast stroke. The arm is at maximum elevation at the start of the pull and in full extension at its completion. During the recovery phase, when the arm returns to start another pull, the glenohumeral joint is in abduction and external rotation. Again, excluding the breast stroke, the recovery is performed out of the water.

ANATOMIC AND BIOMECHANICAL FEATURES

The shoulder joint is a highly mobile joint with little bony support. The stability necessary for the arm to function with power and precision through its range of motion is provided by the shoulder capsule, ligaments, rotator cuff muscles (supraspinatus, subscapularis infraspinatus, teres minor), and larger muscles such as the pectoralis major and the serratus anterior.

Dynamic stability for containment of the humeral head in the glenoid fossa is provided by the rotator cuff muscles working in a force couple combination with the deltoid and the long head of the biceps. The supraspinatus helps resist upward displacement of the humeral head; the infraspinatus works in combination with the supraspinatus and subscapularis to depress the humeral head. The subscapularis also resists anterior or inferior displacement of the humeral head in the glenoid fossa. In addition to its role as a humeral head stabilizer, the long head of the biceps is active in forward flexion, a function that should not be overlooked in the shoulder biomechanics of swimming.

FACTORS IN TENDINOPATHY

Overwork

As the most mobile and least stable joint, the shoulder is most vulnerable to injury in the overhead position. To keep up with the continuous, repeated demands of competitive swimming, the muscles of the rotator cuff may be required to work excessively to contain and stabilize the humeral head. Such a workload can lead to fatigue of the muscles and the onset of a chronic condition. Superior migration of the humeral head may occur, and with this, a subsequent increase in subacromial loading is seen that can trigger a tendinopathy. In addition to rotator cuff fatigue, scapular muscle fatigue can alter the mechanics of the entire shoulder complex. The scapular muscles (serrus anterior, rhomboids, and trapezius) work continuously during swimming-arm action. Fatigue and lack of control of the periscapular muscles can alter the glenohumeral joint mechanics and may contribute to the onset of impingement tendinopathy.

Hypovascularity

Rathbun and Macnab[4] demonstrated that the blood supply to the supraspinatus and the biceps tendons is affected by arm position. An area of avascularity occurs close to the musculotendinous junction during adduction and internal rotation. In this position at the end of the pull phase, the tendons are stretched tightly over the head of the humerus. This repeated avascularity, known as the "wringing out" mechanism, occurs in the area of the tendon most vulnerable to loading. Repeated interruption of the vascular supply may contribute to early degenerative changes and increase the potential for rotator cuff damage. Circulation to the area is restored during abduction.

Subacromial Loading

Supraspinatus and biceps tendons insert on or across the humerus directly below the coracoacromial arch, which is formed by the coracoid process, the rigid coracoacromial ligament, and the anterior acromion. The anatomic arrangement of these tendons makes them particularly susceptible to impingement. When the arm is in abduction, forward flexion, and internal rotation, a position assumed in the catch phase of all competitive strokes, the humeral head moves under the arch, where the tendons may be repeatedly impinged. If scapular mechanics have been altered, the tendons may be impinged against the arch, causing a mechanical irritation and inflammatory response that can further compromise the available space beneath the arch. Untreated, this may progress to involve the subacromial bursa and acromioclavicular ligament.

Three acromial shapes have been identified by Bigliani and colleagues[5]: type I, flat; type II, curved; and type III, hooked. A competitive swimmer with a hooked (type III) acromion or a master swimmer with degenerative spurring of the acromion may be predisposed to impingement due to the decreased dimensions of the coracoacromial arch. In these situations, a tendinopathy that is resistant to treatment may develop.

Stroke Mechanics

During the entry phase and the beginning of the pull phase, the shoulder is in forward flexion, abduction, and internal rotation. The head of the humerus is forced under the anterior acromion and the coracoacromial ligament and may impinge the supraspinatus and biceps tendons, particularly if fatigued.

Lateral impingement may be associated with the recovery phase of freestyle and butterfly. To return to the entry position, the arm must abduct. With associated horizontal abduction and internal rotation, the head of the humerus comes up against the lateral border of the acromion. This is particularly true when the shoulder leads the rest of the arm. When the head leads the arm through recovery, there is less potential for lateral impingement. As mentioned previously, during the end of the pull phase, the shoulder is in adduction and internal rotation, a position that leads to the wringing out mechanism.

An analysis of the arm position in the freestyle stroke of swimmers experiencing pain appeared to correlate the occurrence of the pain with the biomechanical factors implicated in rotator cuff tendinopathy. Almost 50 percent of the swimmers experienced shoulder pain during entry or the first half of the pull phase, 14 percent felt pain during the second half of the pull phase, 23 percent during the recovery, and 17.8 percent during the entire pull or recovery. Some swimmers in this last group experienced pain throughout the entire stroke.[6]

Increased Laxity

Increased laxity should not be overlooked as a contributing factor in the athlete with resistant tendinopathy. In the individual with loose or lax shoulders, the rotator cuff muscles are already working excessively hard just to contain the humeral head. The rigor of training makes additional demands on fatigued or fatiguing muscles. In 1982, Fowler and Webster-Bogaert[7] investigated the association between rotator cuff tendinopathy and shoulder laxity. They assessed 188 competitive swimmers between the ages of 13 and 26 years for positive signs of tendinopathy and for posterior, inferior, and anterior instability or increased laxity. Fifty recreational athletes without shoulder pain were used as a control group. A formal history was taken of each subject, and any episodes of shoulder pain were recorded.

The apprehension test was used to assess anterior instability. Any sign of pain or anxiety was recorded as a positive response. Inferior instability was assessed using the sulcus sign. The load and shift test to evaluate posterior laxity was conducted with subjects both sitting and supine. Excursion of the humeral head relative to the posterior glenoid fossa was the index for posterior laxity. In many normal asymptomatic individuals, the proximal humerus can be translated posteriorly 50 percent of the glenoid width; therefore, any movement greater than this was classified as excessive posterior laxity.

Fifty percent of the 188 swimmers had a history of shoulder pain. Some degree of posterior laxity was present in one or both shoulders in 55 percent of the swimmers and in 52 percent of the control group. This suggested that swimming does not predispose an athlete to increased laxity. Twenty-five percent of the swimmers had a history of tendinopathy and increased posterior laxity. The tendinopathy was consistently present in the lax shoulder, indicating that there is a relationship between shoulder pain and increased laxity.

Shoulder Strength Imbalance

Manual testing performed on these same swimmers demonstrated external rotator weakness in one or both shoulders of 40 subjects, with 33 having both weakness and a history of tendinopathy in the same shoulder. Based on these findings, a second study was conducted to measure rotation strength about the shoulder. One-hundred and nineteen swimmers and 51 controls (participants in activities not requiring arm rotation strength primarily) were tested on the Cybex II dynamometer. Internal and external rotation strength was measured in three arm positions: neutral, 90 degrees of abduction, and 90 degrees of flexion. A significant difference was found in the rotation torque ratio between swimmers and controls in neutral and 90 degrees of abduction that was attributed to the greater strength of the internal rotators. External rotation strength between the two groups was not significantly different.

In the pull or power phase of the swimming stroke, the glenohumeral joint is in adduction and internal rotation. Many swimmers selectively train their internal rotators to improve speed and endurance. This may explain the resulting imbalance between the internal and external rotators that may contribute to the onset of shoulder pain.

CLINICAL EVALUATION

An accurate history to define the pain is essential. This should include onset, duration, location, activity causing the pain, and position of maximum pain. A review of the complete training program, including the dry-land and weight-training components, will provide important additional information. A systematic physical examination should include inspection, palpation, and assessment of range of motion, joint laxity, motor strength, and neurologic status. The history and physical examination are augmented by provocative and stability testing as well as appropriate imaging when indicated.

As a tendinopathy progresses, generalized pain about the shoulder is often present at night or at rest. The athlete avoids painful positions and those which aggravate the symptoms. To minimize pain during swimming, subtle changes in stroke mechanics may develop. Over time, a gradual loss of shoulder range of motion along with muscle weakness may occur. Wasting of the supraspinatus and infraspinatus muscles may become apparent. In the mature athlete, this may be an indication of gross degeneration of the rotator cuff tendon or of a partial tear. Such changes are seldom seen in age-group swimmers and, in fact, are rare in athletes younger than 25 years.

Clinical classification of tendinopathy is based on Blazina's categories[8] for jumper's knee that associate pain with level of activity. In grade I, there is pain after the activity; in grade II, there is pain during and after activity, but it is not disabling; in grade III, there is disabling pain during and after the activity; in grade IV, there is pain with activities of daily living.

Physical Examination

Successful treatment of shoulder girdle dysfunction is based on a detailed and thorough assessment. Circumspect observation of the athlete prior to a hands-on assessment will reveal important information. The individual's posture or the resting position of soft tissue structures can affect patient function. The adaptation of muscle and soft tissue to these positions may cause resting and/or functional imbalances in flexibility or strength. In flexibility imbalances, one group of muscles is shortened and the antagonist(s) are lengthened. In strength imbalances, there is a weakness differential between muscle groups. For example, a muscle resting in its lengthened position will be most effective in that position and somewhat weaker in the shortened position. In this situation, because muscles require more energy to function in the lengthened position, they may be prone to fatigue and dysfunction.[9] Similarly, a shortened muscle is weaker in its lengthened position and often will lack the ability to achieve its full length. These imbalances will become more obvious with time and stress. Although we will focus on muscle imbalance, it is important to keep in mind that for every muscle there is surrounding connective tissue that plays an important role.

Posture/Alignment (Table 24-1)

Although the alignment of the entire body should be assessed, the area of primary importance for the function of the shoulder girdle are the cervical spine, the thoracic spine, the scapulae, and the humerus. Following a thorough history, a visual inspection of these areas and a quick screening test will indicate the degree of their involvement in the patient's problem.

The Cervical Spine

In most cases, patients will "correct" their posture if they know that it is being assessed. Therefore, this is best done when the patient is unaware that his or her posture is the focus of the therapist's attention. It is important to keep in mind that the effect of small but habitual deviations such as head tilt or rotation on soft tissue, disks, and vertebrae can become significant.

The cervical spine should be inspected from sagittal, anterior, and posterior views. Sagittally, the presence or absence of a lordosis as well as the location of the curve should be noted. A head-

---

TABLE 24-1 Overview of Shoulder Rehabilitation

• Assess posture (resting position) of soft tissue structures	
• Assess involvment of supporting structures	
• Quality of movement	
Cervical and thoracic spine	Correct alignment
	Instruction
	Stretching, strengthening
	Functional exercises
	Assess joint function
	Quality of movement
	Mobilization
Scapula	Periscapular muscle retaining
	Assess static, dynamic, functional
	Biofeedback
	Control of strength and power
	Training modification
	Involve coach
Glenohumeral joint	Joint function assessment
	Muscle balance NB
	Specific strength training
	Speed
	Type of contraction
	Open versus closed chain
	Joint/muscle position
	Control of movement
	Proprioception

forward position (noted when the ears are in a plane anterior to the shoulders) predisposes to a lengthening of the neck flexors coupled with a shortening of the neck extensors and the posterior cervical-scapular muscles (e.g., levator scapulae and upper trapezius). In this case, since the levator scapulae also elevates and downwardly rotates the scapula, the force may exceed that of its antagonists and influence scapular function. The result may be a weakness and lengthening of the lower trapezius, which depresses and upwardly rotates the scapula. This in turn will exaggerate the imbalance of that force couple.

Anteroposterior (AP) observation may reveal a rotated or side-flexed cervical spine that will result in shortening of the corresponding muscles and lengthening of their antagonists. Unilaterally, the levator scapulae can rotate the cervical spine, and imbalances similar to those cited earlier may be due to an entirely different cause. The assessment of cause and effect is essential. Muscle contour and bulk are assessed anteriorly and posteriorly. Asymmetries can be indicative of problems with the function of the surrounding soft tissue. Comparing paravertebral and periscapular muscle bulk with suprascapular muscle bulk will provide important information. A slight person should be proportionately slight; a muscled person should be proportionately muscled. Asymmetries in this situation may indicate a recruitment preference caused by strength training routines or neurologic deficits.

A cervical spine scan should include quick tests of range of motion, strength, dermatomes, and myotomes, as well as a history of complaints. Any abnormal findings should be followed by further investigation. For instance, if range of motion is limited or excessive, an in-depth assessment of the mobility of the intervertebral joints should be undertaken. Any limitation or pain with mobilization of these joints will affect the function of the cervical spine and those muscles attached to it.

The Thoracic Spine

The thoracic spine should be observed for normal alignment. Lordosis, kyphosis, scoliosis, and rotation can be noted with sagittal and AP observations. As in the cervical spine, any deviation from optimal function of the thoracic spine will affect the surrounding soft tissue. Rhomboids, for example, can be inhibited with pain or dysfunction of the midthoracic spine. As rhomboids downwardly rotate and adduct the scapula, the patient may present with an abducted and/or upwardly rotated scapula. This, in turn, will shorten serratus anterior, pulling the scapula further into the abducted, upwardly rotated position. The thoracic spine is often ignored when treating the shoulder girdle. However, its function and integrity are important to much of the soft tissue that stabilizes the scapula.

Again, a scan similar to that of the cervical spine should be undertaken and followed up as indicated.

The Scapula

The scapula is the base of support for the upper extremity as the pelvis is for the lower extremity. Therefore, its position and stability have a great influence on upper extremity biomechanics. The common scapular movements are elevation, depression, abduction, adduction, upward rotation, and downward rotation. The resting positions of the scapula can be altered in severe cases. However, dysfunction most often is presented with movement. Scapular position will dictate the position of the glenoid fossa and the ability of the periscapular muscles to control its movement.

The position of the glenoid fossa is a critical element to the reloading of the scapulohumeral muscles. If the glenoid fossa is tipped such that it is facing more inferiorly, the humerus will sit in a relatively abducted position, thereby functionally shortening supraspinatus and other abductors. Associated lengthening of teres major and other adductors and rotation of the humerus may then occur. The stronger, shorter muscle will dominate, causing the humerus to rest in a position of most comfort. When movement does occur, the facility of recruitment will favor the shortened muscles and place them at risk for overuse.

Similarly, if the scapula rests in a upwardly rotated position, causing the glenoid to face superiorly, the glenohumeral joint will sit in a relatively adducted position. This, in turn, will shorten the adductors and lengthen the abductors. If at this time the patient abducts the shoulder, there will be recruitment of a muscle that is sitting in its lengthened position. The muscle then goes through a greater range of motion, which increases the eccentric contraction required for the return movement. This creates more work for the muscle, resulting in fatigue and overuse.

It is important to keep in mind that rarely does a joint as mobile as the glenohumeral joint selectively shorten one set of muscles without the added element of rotation. This should be assessed. For example, in many swimmers, in addition to shortened adductors, there is often a shortening of the internal rotators. This imbalance of flexibility and frequently strength between the internal and external rotators of the shoulder has been documented.[10] Once established, such a muscle imbalance can progress due to abnormal stresses on the muscles stabilizing the scapula. This creates a vicious cycle. Patients with an elevated or depressed scapula present a challenge that can to a great extent become an anatomy review for the physician and therapist. If the upper trapezius is tight, the clinician is likely to note an elevated or upwardly rotated scapula or a scapula that elevates and/or upwardly rotates with the initiation of humeral movement. The affect of this on the lower trapezius is one of lengthening and weakening, which again compounds the problem. With this force couple acting on the scapula, its control and stability are compromised. Since the scapula is the insertion for many muscles controlling the glenohumeral joint, these cease to have a stable base, resulting in less than optimal function. The added stress placed on the muscles as they attempt to compensate, especially during sporting activities, can be the source of pathology.

The Glenohumeral Joint

Tenderness elicited by palpation of the supraspinatus tendon medial to its insertion of the greater tuberosity suggests a tendinopathy. If the long head of biceps is involved, there will be tenderness over the bicipital groove. Those with supraspinatus involvement often demonstrate the classic "painful arc syndrome," which causes pain with active abduction between 60 and 100 degrees. Symptoms of a biceps tendinopathy can be reproduced by resisting forward flexion of the straight arm while the forearm is supinated. Biceps tendinopathy can be associated with refractory rotator cuff tendinopathy.

Placing the shoulder in the impingement-aggravated position often will reproduce clinical pain. In the test described by Neer, the examiner resists forward flexion of the raised straight arm while the forearm is supinated. This drives the head of the humerus against the anteroinferior border of the acromion. In a second test, the examiner internally rotates the arm, which is forward flexed to 90 degrees.

It is important to determine if muscle weakness, particularly in the external rotators, is present. With the patient's arm in external rotation and adduction and the elbow flexed to 90 degrees, the examiner applies an internal force, which the patient is instructed to resist. Gross weakness will be conspicuous. Pain may accompany this test.

Increased laxity or frank instability may contribute to the progression of tendinopathy or may be the absolute cause of pain. The relocation test assessing anterior instability has two components. First, the arm is stressed in external rotation and abduction, and the patient is observed for a reaction to pain. Then, the examiner, by applying posteriorly directed pressure on the proximal humerus, either relocates or supports the humeral head, allowing increased external rotation with less pain. The patient with anterior glenohumeral instability will experience apprehension and/or pain when the humeral head is slightly subluxated during external rotation and abduction. When it is reduced or supported, the pain and/or apprehension is lessened.

Anterior and posterior glenohumeral translation is assessed with the patient in both the supine and upright positions. In order to assess the amount of translation, the humeral head must be reduced at the start of the test. In the technique for carrying out the test with the patient sitting, the examiner stabilizes the shoulder girdle with one hand and, grasping the humeral head between the thumb and forefinger, applies anterior and posterior stress, noting the amount of translation. When the test is performed with the patient supine, the arm is positioned in 90 degrees of abduction, and anterior and posterior translation is assessed. With respect to posterior translation, movement of the humeral head to 50 percent of the glenoid width is considered to be within normal limits. Although movement greater than 50 percent is not necessarily abnormal, this would increase the workload of the rotator cuff and influence shoulder mechanics. If the shoulder is unstable, applying an axial load may reproduce the symptoms experienced during swimming. This would be pain caused by instability itself. Inferior instability is indicated by the presence of a sulcus between the acromion and the head of the humerus with inferior traction.

TREATMENT

Treatment is directed at reducing pain and correcting biomechanics. This should incorporate relative rest, which means rest from aggravating factors rather than complete rest. The cornerstone of treatment is to retrain soft tissue and muscle to resume normal function. Patient education, which requires a great deal of time on the part of the clinician, is the key here. In addition, communication with the athlete and the coach will assist in working out a program to minimize the detraining effect of reduced training. If the patient does not understand the importance of correct biomechanics and resting positions, treatment will be only temporarily effective. Much of what the patient is required to do will be in the form of exercise and functional retaining. The function of the spine and scapula is just as critical in activities of daily living as during sport. In most cases, in any given day, individuals spend 1 to 3 h at sport but 12 h or more "at life." This does not take into account positions during sleep! Patient education is the most important aspect of treatment.

Cervical and Thoracic Spine

The first step is to correct the alignment and posture of the cervical and thoracic spine. The use of a mirror and mimicking by the therapist is very effective. In most situations, instruction and demonstration will be sufficient. However, in some cases, muscles are already too tight and/or weak to sustain normal posture. Here, appropriate stretching and strengthening are required before the patient can maintain correct posture successfully for a sustained length of time. Frequency is more important than intensity when performing functional exercises. For example, five times per hour throughout the course of the day is more advantageous than exercising for a 45-min period. The patient should develop a constant awareness of body position, and to this end, work and daily activities must be taken into account when prescribing a rehabilitation program.

If this approach is unsuccessful, a more thorough evaluation of the spine may be indicated. An assessment of joint mechanics may demonstrate a need for mobilization or manipulation of a segment. Not infrequently, a patient presents with all the classic signs of an overuse problem of the shoulder, and the underlying culprit is dysfunction of the cervical or thoracic spine.

Scapula

Scapular function and control directly influence the function of the glenohumeral joint. Retaining the periscapular muscles can be particularly challenging. A muscle such as the lower trapezius, which the patient can neither see nor relate to a specific activity, can be retained using biofeedback. Visual or auditory feedback is provided by means of electrodes when the correct contraction is performed (Fig.24-1). Patients can then repeat the correct contraction until they are able to recruit the muscle with ease. Initial progression will

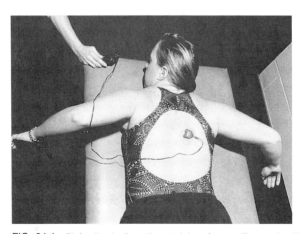

FIG. 24-1 Biofeedback allows the retraining of a specific muscle with visual or auditory input by means of electrodes when the correct contraction is performed.

include exercises to incorporate simple arm movements, such as forward flexion, while receiving feedback. Then a specific point in the range of motion or activities that are more complex or sport-specific can be added. Rehabilitation is completed when exercises for strength, speed, and power can be performed with scapular stability. This final step will ensure that the patient does not return with the same problem in the rear future. Mirrors and videotaping also can be effective teaching tools. Retraining takes time and, more important, repetition. It is essential that the patient understand the process in order to achieve long-term success.

Pathology or habitual improper posture may be due to *or* encouraged by technique that is less than optimal. Coaches and/or parents should be encouraged to observe the patient's swimming stroke for compensation or inefficiencies. Viewing a videotape together with the physiotherapist, coach/parent, and athlete often can shed much light on the problem. This may mean a "back to the drawing board" approach to training in exchange for long-tern gains.

Glenohumeral Joint

As in patellofemoral joint, the glenohumeral joint is largely controlled by soft tissue. Therefore, most pathology is found in these structures, and they should be the focus of treatment. Optimal soft tissue function is paramount if injury during is to be prevented.

Grade I Tendinopathy

A grade I tendinopathy responds well to conservative management. Swimmers are instructed to increase the time spent in both prepractice stretching and in-the-pool warm-up. Stretching to increase blood flow, restore range of motion, and decrease potential for impingement should involve all components of the shoulder, including the anterior structures. In-the-pool warm-up with pain-free strokes should be prolonged and slow-paced. Additional warm-ups should be continued after kicking sets. A swimming warm-down is recommended after the training session. Icing the shoulder with ice cups or bags for a maximum of 15 min after practice often will reduce pain.

Strengthening the external rotators is important to improve control of the glenohumeral joint, which in turn maximizes muscle efficiency and improves performance. The external rotators are initially worked in adduction and then in varying degrees of abduction. If one stroke causes symptoms, it should be discontinued until these subside and then gradually reintroduced with any faulty mechanics corrected. Physiotherapy assessment at this early stage may prevent the inevitable progression of the pathology. If the faulty mechanics are not rectified, pain will likely return. Often treatment will be an independant exercise program for the reeducation of correct mechanics.

Grade II Tendinopathy

In addition to the preceding measures, a grade II tendinopathy requires relative rest, physiotherapy, and medication. Relative rest is not abstinence from the sport. The athlete is encouraged to use strokes that do not cause pain and to emphasize leg work. Kickboards place the shoulder in a pain-provoking position and should not be used. For aerobic training, running and cycling can augment the limited swimming workouts. Anti-inflammatory medication also often will provide symptomatic relief.

At this stage, physiotherapy is indicated. Proper functioning of this joint depends on the optimal soft tissue function. Treatment is based on the therapist's evaluation. All the basic assessments of range of motion, strength, sensation, stability, joint mobility, and neural tension, as well as additional appropriate special tests, must be considered. This will include the cervical and thoracic spines, scapula, and glenohumeral joint mechanics. Any specific findings should be addressed with the specific treatment techniques. For example, if capsular restriction is evident when assessing gleno-humeral joint mobility, it should be treated with mobilization techniques in order for functional activities and muscular exercises to be successful.

Observation is once again an effective assessment tool. Note the resting position of the humerus: abduction, adduction, internal rotation, external rotation, and the position of the head of the humerus in the glenoid. One role of the subscapularis is to stabilize the head of the humerus anteriorly. An anterior position in the glenoid may indicate some subscapularis dysfunction.

At this point, the glenohumeral joint can be addressed in more detail. Full range of motion at the expense of other structures is unacceptable and should be guarded against. When assessing the movement of the glenohumeral joint, it is important to note the presence and degree of any associated movements. For example, normal abduction requires some external rotation of the humerus to allow the head of the humerus to pass under the acromion. No or excessive rotation will necessitate some compensation. Once again, the quality of the movement must be considered.

Accessory movements, i.e., those which cannot be performed voluntarily by a given muscle but must occur for normal joint function, also can be compromised with dysfunction. An example is the inferior glide of the head of the humerus on the glenoid during flexion or abduction of the glenohumeral joint. If this inferior glide does not occur, the subacromial space will be smaller due to the position of the head of the humerus and potentially exacerbate impingement problems.

Muscle Balance

As mentioned earlier, muscle imbalance can be in the form of flexibility or strength. A tight or shortened muscle can greatly influence the integrity of the joint, capsule, and connective tissue as well as its own function and that of its antagonists. Also, in a tight muscle there is a shortened distance between its origin and insertion. The joint will accommodate by rotating the humerus, thereby shortening the functional distance of a given muscle. Eventually, one rotator will be shortened and its antagonist lengthened, thus compounding the problem. The two-joint muscles, such as the biceps, are common culprits. If shortened, the biceps can choose one of many functions (or a combination of all) to alter the position of the scapula, humerus, and forearm. For instance, the biceps is a powerful supinator, elbow flexor, and glenohumeral joint flexor. If tight, especially during forearm pronation, the elbow and perhaps the shoulder will experience less resistance in a slightly flexed position. This, in turn, may elevate the scapula, affecting the function of all scapulohumeral muscles.

With most activities, the prime movers of a given joint can be isolated to allow the task to be performed. However, with every movement an equal and opposite force is required to stabilize the base structure and facilitate optimal movement. In many instances, especially in sport, the movers develop to a greater extent than the stabilizers, creating an imbalance. Swimmers tend to develop the internal rotators of the glenohumeral joint. When this occurs without adequate strengthening of the scapular stabilizers, the internal rotators (many of which have a scapular origin) will pull the scapula into an abducted position. This will disadvantage the scapular adductors that stabilize, and a vicious cycle will be established. Many swimmers augment their training with weights. If poorly designed, these programs can add to the problem and inhibit rather than enhance performance. Programs should be designed with the length and strength balance of the movers and stabilizers in mind.

Strength Testing

Strength testing as part of a complete assessment should address quality and specificity in addition to force. Testing a particular muscle isometrically in neutral may or may not demonstrate normal strength but will not identify deficits through range or at higher speeds. A circumspect history will give the clinician insight as to where attention should be focused. The patient may complain of pain only when force is required in a given position, e.g., in overhead or abduction/external rotation. Eccentric and high-speed testing may be necessary to reveal any biomechanical compromise. Any compromise in scapular action or in the thoracic or cervical spine during testing should be noted. In addition, strength is very specific, and its many aspects need to be considered. These include speed, type of contraction (eccentric versus concentric), type of biomechanical chain (open versus closed), and position of the joint/muscle. For example, a swimmer who rehabilitates the shoulder musculature up to 90 degrees of abduction, at speeds less than 300 degrees per second, and always open-chain concentrically will not have prepared the muscles with adequate specificity to return to the sport. Such a swimmer requires strength and control overhead, at speeds in excess of 1000 degrees per second, both eccentrically and concentrically. This specificity must be addressed in order for the movers and stabilizers to have complete success with no recurrence. Many of these exercises can be incorporated into a home program or training regime using free weights and/or surgical tubing. Pain during strengthening should be avoided at all costs, since the result will be a reflex inhibition of the muscle instead of activation.

Proprioception

The other area of growing importance is the control of movement. In a joint with the mobility of the glenohumeral joint, it is essential to be able to control the joint and its stabilizers through its range of motion and strength/power requirements. This introduces the concept of proprioception of the shoulder girdle. Kinesthesia or proprioception of the glenohumeral joint has recently been given some attention but is difficult to assess objectively. However, providing the patient with controlled tasks may identify specific difficulties. Ease of performance, comparison with the other side, and reproduction of joint position (eyes closed) can be assessed subjectively. Challenging positions, such as overhead or abduction with external rotation, would be a progression. Very little work has been done in this area, but we are becoming aware of its importance. In recurrent dislocators, it has been shown that once visual feedback has been removed, patients perform control tasks much differently from those with a normal capsular structure.[11] This compensation comes at a cost. The measurement of proprioception or kinesthesia is difficult at best, but we must find clinical methods that address these issues. As with the lower extremity, it is important to perturb the stability and force a control reaction of the musculature. This can be done using physiotherapy balls, a Body

Blade, tubing, water exercises, balance boards, and Profitters. Once the concept is defined and understood, the exercises are limited only by the imagination of the therapist. Again, proprioceptive exercises should be progressed through gradations of difficulty of speed, position, and type of contraction required. They also should be progressed to include a functional component that is individualized according to each patient's needs. In swimmers, ball exercises done overhead against a wall are appropriate (Figs. 24-2 and 24-3).

Hydrotherapy

Water as a medium for exercise and retraining is very valuable and underutilized. Buoyancy allows the therapist to devise a variety of exercises and activities to enhance range of motion, strength, and proprioception. In water, resistance is not isolated to one plane, and no muscle can act independently without sufficient trunk stability. The neuromuscular reeducation that occurs when these exercises are performed correctly can effectively accelerate the rehabilitation process. These exercises can be progressed using paddles, water wings, air mattresses, or pool noodles (Fig. 24-4). Unfortunately, the availability of this medium in the clinic setting can be limited. However, with adequate instruction and demonstration on land, compliant patients can benefit from unsupervised pool activities outside the clinic.

Additional Areas

Other important areas are pain, modalities, and neural tension. The topic of pain alone can overtake any discussion of rehabilitation. Pain not only will inhibit activity but also will influence the quality of the movement at any time. Appropriate treatment of pain should be included with the primary purpose of allowing the patient to perform a given task. Once normal function can occur, the pain also will subside. However, it is a vicious cycle that needs to be broken before rehabilitation can be successful.

A number of modalities are available for use by therapists. Ultasound, laser, and electric current are important and effective adjuncts that will help the patient and therapist to successfully perform exercises and activities essential to complete rehabilitation.

Neural tension and connective tissue are other important areas believed to have far-reaching effects on both metabolic and musculoskeletal problems. However, our understanding of these is limited, and while many physiotherapists and massage therapists have treated these areas successfully, more knowledge is needed about their role. It is an ongoing challenge to develop a more complete understanding so that treatment can be more effective. No

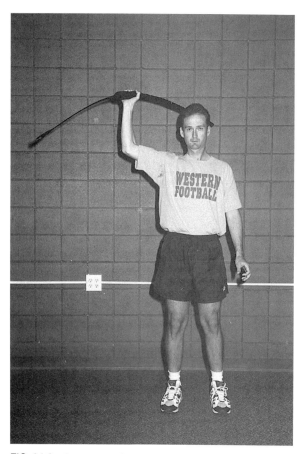

FIG. 24-2 Demonstrates functional proprioceptive training with a Bodyblade.

single structure acts in isolation, and therefore, assessment and treatment of interactive as well as individual function will meet with greater long-term success.

A steroid injection into the subacromial space should be considered only if there is no response to treatment and if impingement-aggravated tests still elicit pain. The swimmer's load should be de-

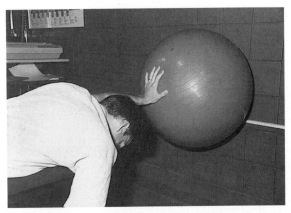

FIG. 24-3 Demonstrates a proprioceptive ball exercise in a functional position for swimmers.

creased after injection, and return to previous levels should take place over a 4- to 6-week period. Steroid injections should not be used routinely.

Grade III Tendinopathy

If tendinopathy progresses to grade III or beyond and becomes refractory despite conservative measures, the swimmer may have to choose between a change of sport and surgical intervention. Most young athletes select the former, a wise decision in most instances. However, if a career at the national or international level is possible, the athlete can be faced with a difficult dilemma. With guidance from both coach and physician, the swimmer can carefully examine the implications of each alternative.

Surgical options may include resection of the diseased segment of tendon along with the involved adjacent subacromial tissue and/or decompression of the same area. Before surgery is planned, the swimmer must understand that the postoperative period demands a commitment to a rehabilitation program and that the success of any procedure is contingent on compliance with this program. Typically, a postoperative regimen is a progressive exercise program geared to restoring range of motion and balanced muscle strength. Return to the pool should begin with slow swimming, which advances to interval training and guided stroke modification. In addition, there should be an overlapping period between formal rehabilitation and return to the sport.

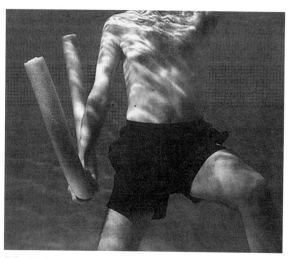

FIG. 24-4   Demonstrates the use of hydrotherapy to train for strength and control of the glenohumeral joint (abduction/adduction) with a pool noodle providing resistance.

This functional rehabilitation stage should include exercises that work the muscles of the shoulder girdle in the position/manner in which they are needed for the performance of the swimming stroke. Overhead exercises with the ball, tubing, pulleys, and wobble boards will incorporate trunk control and specifically retrain the neuromuscular system to accept additional training. Attention to the number of repetitions and sets can mimic the need for anaerobic and aerobic work, which will depend on the events in which the athlete competes.

Grade IV Tendinopathy

A grade IV tendinopathy is seen most often in the mature athlete and may indicate a torn rotator cuff. Imaging techniques such as arthrography, ultrasonography, and magnetic resonance imaging (MRI) will help confirm the clinical diagnosis. Lesions such as partial-thickness tears and a thickened subacromial bursa can be identified by arthroscopy of the shoulder joint and subacromial space. In the younger swimmer, anterior and posterior superior quadrant labral tears can cause pain, although this is not a frequent occurrence. These may be treated successfully with arthroscopic excision. Bursectomy alone followed by appropriate rehabilitation can provide relief in the younger swimmer, but a more radical decompression, which includes resection of the anteroinferior acromion and a portion of the coracoacromial ligament, is generally recommended. Return to preinjury level of participation is unlikely, a fact that should be understood before plans are made for surgery. Postoperatively, range of motion is often low, and muscle strength, endurance, and power, particularly in the abductors and external rotators, deteriorate. Physiotherapy, as described previously, that rehabilitates all the muscle groups and biomechanics of the shoulder girdle plays a significant role in the postoperative period.

PREVENTION

Overuse syndromes of the shoulder in the swimmer are much easier to prevent than to treat. Four components are fundamental to a preventive program: balanced muscle strengthening, flexibility, technique modification, and avoidance of overwork. Again, the importance of an informed coach cannot be overstated. Ongoing stroke analysis, advice concerning stroke errors, careful planning of planning of practice/training sessions, and regular monitoring of performance to prevent rotator cuff fatigue are among the responsibilities of the coaching staff.

Training

Overwork is a primary cause of tendinopathy and is often the result of increased intensity of training sets. Increases in workload should take place gradually. Rigorous training sets before the athlete is ready or "extrahard" practices at the beginning of a training regimen can trigger the onset of shoulder pain. Workouts should be designed so that the difficult portion is completed early in the practice when the swimmer is rested. These should be organized so that there is relative rest for structures at risk. For example, after the difficult work has been completed, the practice can continue with stroke drills, with alternating stroke and leg work or with emphasis on start and turn techniques. With proper instruction, the swimmer will learn to guard against fatigue. Rest days also can be planned to follow a practice with an increase in intensity.

Strengthening

As mentioned previously, in competitive swimming, both pool and dry-land training focuses on strengthening the internal rotators, extensors, and adductors important to propulsion. Little emphasis is placed on strengthening the antagonists that play a significant role in "containment of the shoulder." The imbalance in strength that may result in the two muscle groups can contribute to tendinopathy. Therefore, an awareness and early correction of any imbalance are important in prevention. External rotators are strengthened by performing both isotonic and eccentric exercises to improve power and control primary mover and antagonist muscle action. The training program should not neglect the scapular and triceps muscles. When doing weight training, subacromial loading positions should be avoided. Paddles can produce increased leverage, which may overload the rotator cuff muscles and should be used with caution.

Flexibility

In 1985, a study by Griep determined that regardless of sex or the stroke most frequently used, those swimmers with restricted flexibility were more likely to develop a tendinopathy than those who maintained and improved their flexibility with a stretching program.[12] Stretching should be included in the daily warm-up routine. When teaching and demonstrating stretching techniques, it is important to emphasize that overstretching of the soft tissue can be harmful. For this reason, pairs stretching is not recommended for younger swimmers who may not appreciate the risks of overstretching. Individual stretching is appropriate for this group.

The stretching techniques employed by pairs can be either passive or proprioceptive neuromuscular facilitation (PNF). In the first, the partner very slowly and gently stretches the swimmer to the pain-free limit and then holds this position. In the second, the swimmer stretches to the pain-free limit. This position is maintained by the partner while the swimmer contracts against the resistance provided. These are repeated a variable number of times.

Technique Modification

Poor technique can slow a swimmer down and cause injury. Ongoing stroke analysis and recognition of breakdown in stroke mechanics will help the swimmer adjust technique and limit excessive subacromial loading. It is particularly important to analyze stroke mechanics during fatigue. In freestyle or backstroke, lateral shoulder impingement can be a result of insufficient body roll. A high elbow position during the recovery phase of freestyle must be achieved by body roll. Attempting to force the elbow into a higher position with muscle activity rather than sufficient body roll can induce subacromial impingement.

Overreach with excessive internal rotation during the catch phase of all swimming strokes may result in undue subacromial loading and extra work by the cuff muscles to contain the humeral head. In addition, excessive internal rotation may intensify the wringing out phenomenon. Changes to body roll, reach, and the degree of shoulder rotation will reduce the frequency and length of time that the shoulder is in the precarious position.

Although evidence of the effect of breathing patterns on the incidence of tendinopathy is contradictory, breathing to alternate sides does prevent constant leaning on one shoulder.

SHOULDER INSTABILITY

Anterior Instability: Prevention and Treatment

Anterior instability is not often the cause of pain in competitive swimmers but is usually secondary to a traumatic incident in another sport. Primary conservative treatment of anterior instability is stroke modification and balanced strengthening exercises. If symptoms do not subside, examination under anesthesia and/or arthroscopy will confirm intraarticular lesions such as a Bankart or Hill-Sachs lesion. An anterior stabilizing procedure can provide relief, and the athlete can return to preinjury levels of performance if motion and strength are regained.

Multidirectional Instability: Prevention and Treatment

Swimmers with frank posterior instability may have pain from dislocating their shoulders during the swimming stroke cycle. The at-risk position of forward flexion and internal rotation is a component of all strokes. Pain in swimmers with congenital or acquired multidirectional instability must be differentiated from that experienced by those suffering from tendinopathy who have concomitant increased laxity.

Persistence with a nonoperative program is recommended in swimmers who have experienced instability over a long period. In most cases, stroke modification, correction of biomechanics and strength deficits, as well as adjusting training programs to minimize the magnitude and incidence of abnormal motion can be successful. Surgical intervention such as an inferior capsular shift, "a reefing procedure" to the posterior cuff and capsule, or a glenoid osteotomy should be considered only when all nonoperative treatments have been exhausted. These procedures are intended to provide symptomatic relief for daily activities, perhaps for recreational swimming and other sports, and occasionally for highly competitive swimming.

THE ELBOW

The arm pull in the butterfly stroke and breaststroke and less frequently in the freestyle is the main cause of stress syndromes about the elbow. Most competitive swimmers use a form of "elbow up" pull in which the elbow is bent and held higher than the hand throughout the first part of the pull. This position permits maximal backward thrust of the hand by allowing the swimmer to push the water back at the most efficient angle. The elbow then bends to about 100 degrees as the arm is pulled under the body. The upper arm is rotated medially, and the forearm is pronated. The high-elbow position is likened to reaching over a barrel. Dropping the elbow is a common fault in the swimmer's stroke pattern. This results in less efficient angle to push the water backward, requiring more force in the common extensor muscles.

Lateral epicondylitis, frequently referred to as *tennis elbow* (described in detail by Nirschl) can ensure.[12] There is inflammation of the extensor carpi radialis brevis and extensor communis aponeurosis at the lateral epicondyle of the humerus. The prime etiologic factor in swimming appears to be overwhelming moments of force combined with repetitions. This results in a combination of extrinsic overload in conjunction with excessive muscle contraction.

Treatment

The treatment of this condition includes relief of acute and chronic inflammation; increase in forearm extensor power, flexibility, and endurance; a decrease in the moments of force placed against the elbow by altering stroke; and very infrequently, surgery. The muscles of the forearm are best strengthened by applying eccentric loads to aid in both flexibility and muscular strength and endurance. Relief of acute inflammation is aided by the application of ice and the judicious use of anti-inflammatory medication and physiotherapy modalities such as ultrasound. Stroke alteration is essential in most cases for long-term management.

Physiotherapy intervention will be similar to that for the shoulder. A thorough assessment of the biomechanics of the upper quadrant, muscle imbalances, and local changes to range of motion, strength, and stability will be performed. Not infrequently does the elbow develop an overuse syndrome because of a particular weakness in the shoulder. The elbow therefore will attempt to compensate and become fatigued and overused.

In resistant cases, there is a place for steroid injections. These should be used with caution and infrequently. Kennedy and Willis[13] have verified evidence of collagen disorganization and weakening for up to 6 weeks associated with steroid injections.

In refractory cases, surgical excision of the degenerative lesion most frequently found in the extensor carpi radialis brevis is carried out. Surgery is followed by slow, methodical return to the swimming training program.

THE KNEE

Medial knee pain is not infrequent in breast-stroke swimmers and is related to the whip kick. While this is the superior kick in terms of speed and propulsion, it subjects the knee to abnormal motion. Faulty technique can cause problems; however, because of the nature of the kick, the intensity and number of repetitions performed and even proper execution do not preclude knee injury. Medial synovial plica syndrome, medial collateral ligament stress syndrome, and patellofemoral syndrome are the common diagnoses attributed to the high valgus and outward rotational stresses necessary to achieve the maximum propulsive effect of the whip kick.

In medial synovial plica syndrome, pain is secondary to the inflammation cause by the friction produced as the plica snaps across the medial femoral condyle during repeated knee flexion and extension. The diagnosis is made by eliciting local tenderness and palpating the thickened synovium as it crosses the medial femoral condyle.

During the whip kick there is increased tension in the medial collateral ligament (MCL) as the knee moves from flexion to extension. This is further increased with a valgus stress and dramatically increased when external rotation forces are applied to the knee. Medial collateral stress syndrome is suggested by point tenderness along the course of the ligament. Often this is located at the origin of the MCL at the adductor tubercle of the femur, but just as frequently it occurs where the superficial fibers cross the upper tibial margin. The pain often can be reproduced by applying a valgus external rotation force to the knee flexed to 20 to 30 degrees.

The clinical findings of patellofemoral syndrome do not differ in the swimmer and may include abnormal alignment of the lower extremity as well as hypermobility or frank instability of the patellofemoral joint. This may be associated with patella alta. There will be tenderness when the patellar facets or femoral condyles are palpated. Symptoms may be reproduced by the patellofemoral compression test or by laterally deviating the patella. In our experience, the more serious patellofemoral problems occur in age-group swimmers. This may be due to improper execution of the whip kick. However, an inherently unstable patellofemoral joint, because of the forces generated by the whip kick, often will preclude the achievement of elite levels in the breast stroke.

In the age-group swimmer, other knee pathologies not related to swimming must be ruled out. Chronic ligamentous instability, a torn medial meniscus (uncommon in the stable knee in this age group), and osteochondritis dissecans are among the possibilities. Osteochondritis dissecans should be looked for radiographically, particularly if there is any chronicity to the complaints. It is important to keep in mind that a multifactorial etiology may be present in many knee problems.

Treatment

Identifying the cause is critical to successful long-term treatment. Improper technique should be recognized by the coach and corrected. In many cases this will eliminate the knee pain. However, anatomic problems such as significant patellofemoral or ligamentous instability may be incompatible with the repetitive stress inherent in the whip kick, and a prolonged treatment program in these athletes may be doomed to failure. Physiotherapy assessment of the functional mechanics of the lower quadrant may be necessary. The muscle imbalances around the pelvis, hip, and knee can greatly influence the recruitment pattern of the muscles around the knee. Assessing gait and dry-land function can demonstrate what muscles are short and strong such that the kinetic chain of the lower extremity is altered. Communication among the coach, swimmer, and physician is important to avoid frustration and disappointment and to provide realistic direction. Therapeutic measures depend on the diagnosis and include anti-inflammatory medication and ultrasound to control acute symptoms.

FOOT AND ANKLE

Foot and ankle pain can be a problem in swimmers regardless of the stroke performed. Tendinitis of the extensor tendons of the ankle and foot where they are firmly bound over the ankle dorsum by the extensor retinaculum is the most common cause. In both the flutter and dolphin kicks, the ankle and foot are brought into extreme plantar flexion and then back to neutral. There is little room for inflammation under the tight retinaculum. The diagnosis is obvious in most cases. Crepitation may be palpable and audible as the foot is brought from plantar flexion into dorsiflexion.

Treatment

Local therapeutic modalities such as ultrasound and ice as well as anti-inflammatory medications and wrapping of the foot and ankle are often of benefit. Preventative stretching prior to practices is important. Less vigorous kicking or no kicking will allow swimming to continue. Resumption of normal kicking is achieved gradually. If persistent, physiotherapy intervention may be necessary to assess the biomechanics of the foot. As with the knee, the function of the foot and ankle for the nonswimming hours of the day may predispose the pattern of use of the muscles of the foot and ankle in the water.

THE BACK *(Diagnosis and Treatment)*

During the breast stroke, many swimmers pull with an early elbow flexion and increased arm abduction. This prolongs the elbow-up position and propels the upper torso above the water. In most cases this aggravates the already lordotic attitude of the lower back. This stress can cause a variety of lower back problems, including stress fractures of the pars interarticularis or even frank spondylolisthesis. More often, accentuation of a mildly symptomatic spondylolisthesis or a mechanical low back pain from posterior facet irritation occurs and limits the competitive breaststroker's training. Such back complaints also may occur in butterfly stroke swimmers. Here, inefficient and incorrect mechanics are often the cause.

An accurate and precise diagnosis is important. In most cases the primary complaint is pain with some radiation into the buttocks. Hamstring tightness may lead to a diagnosis of spondylolisthesis. Positive findings that are frequently identified include palpation of a step deformity at the spine of L5 and an abnormal gait with a backward-tilting pelvis. The diagnosis is confirmed radiographically. If x-rays are normal, a bone scan will help in the diagnosis of a pars stress fracture. A recent stress fracture must be treated with a prolonged period of rest.

Spondylolisthesis is treated symptomatically according to the severity of the complaints. Following a temporary rest from training, slow return with a carefully planned program is prescribed. Hamstring stretching and abdominal strengthening are of particular importance in the ongoing treatment and for prevention. The function of the spine is somewhat more complex than that of the peripheral joints. A physiotherapy assessment of the dysfunction should include and in-depth assessment of joint mechanics. The position and function of the pelvis, hip, and lower extremity will complete the story of the kinetic chain. In the water this chain is open. When standing on land, the kinetic chain is closed. The differing mechanics that ensure have to be well understood for full rehabilitation. Once the mechanics are normalized, strengthening and functional retraining to control the pelvis and spine will allow successful return to the pool and prevention of future problems.

Mechanical low back pain often will respond to a similar program. More resistant cases may require prolonged treatment that can incorporate modalities such as transcutaneous nerve stimulation or repeated mobilizations to the affected area. Occasionally, a steroid injection to the inflamed facet is necessary.

The term *adolescent swimmer's back* was coined by Wilson and Linseth. Three adolescent patients with backache aggravated by swimming the butterfly stroke were diagnosed with Scheuermann kyphosis. The authors were not certain whether the forceful contraction of the chest and abdominal musculature during the power phase of the butterfly stroke caused the vertebral abnormalities or merely was an aggravating factor. Two of the three swimmers experienced dramatic relief once they had stopped performing the butterfly stroke, which suggests that these patients should confine their swimming to the backstroke and freestyle.

SUMMARY

Prevention, diagnosis, and treatment of injuries depends on an understanding of the basics of swimming strokes and practice techniques as well as interaction and communication among professionals charged with the care and training of swimmers. With respect to physiotherapy, biomechanics and control of motion are two areas of growth with the potential to enhance and accelerate rehabilitation programs.

REFERENCES

1. Kennedy JC, Hawkins RJ: Swimmer's shoulder. *Phys Sports Med* 2(4):35, 1974.
2. Lo YPC, Hsu YCS, Chan KM: Epidimiology of shoulder impingement in upper arm sports events. *Br J Sports Med* 24(3):173–177, 1990.
3. McMaster WC, Troup J: A survey of interfering shoulder pain in United States competitive swimmers. *Am J Sports Med* 21(1):67, 1993.
4. Rathbun JB, Macnab I: The microvascular pattern of the rotator cuff. *J Bone Joint Surg* 54A:540–553, 1979.
5. Bigliani NU, Morrison DS, April EW: The morphology of the acromion and its relationship to rotator cuff tears. *Orthop Trans* 10(2):216, 1986.
6. Webster-Bogaert SM: Swimmer's shoulder. University of Waterloo, Waterloo, ONT, 1981.
7. Fowler PJ, Webster-Bogaert MS: Swimming, in Reider B (ed): *Sports Medicine: The School-Age Athlete*. Philadelphia, Saunders, 1991, pp. 429–446.
8. Blazina ME: Jumper's knee. *Orthop Clin North Am* 4(3):65, 1980.
9. Astrand P, Radahl K: Neuromuscular Function, in *Anonymous Textbook of Work Physiology: Physiological Bases of Exercise*, 2d ed. New York, McGraw-Hill, 1977, 55–128.
10. Forwell LA: Proprioceptive deficits associated with recurrent shoulder dislocation. Thesis, University of Western Ontario, Department of Physical Therapy, 1994.
11. Griep JF: Swimmers shoulder: The influence of flexibiliy and weight training. *Orthop Trans* 10(2):216, 1986.
12. Nelson M, Leather GP, Nirschl RP, et al: Evaluation of the painful shoulder: A prospective comparison of magnetic resonance imaging, computerized tomagraphic arthrography, ultrasonography, and operative findings. *J Bone Joint Surg* 73(A):707–716, 1991.
13. Kennedy JC, Willis RB: The effects of local steroid injections on tendons: A biomechanical and microscopic correlative study. *Am J Sports Med* 4:11, 1976.

DEFINITION AND IMPORTANCE OF MUSCULAR CONDITIONING

Muscular conditioning implies the growth and development of muscle tissue as well as improvements in the force a muscle is able to exert (strength). The development of muscle tissue and strength is not just important for the elite athlete or for the vain. Clearly, muscle tissue development and its strength are important aspects of physical fitness and wellness.

The main function of muscle is to produce physical movement. However, an often overlooked function of muscle, and one that is very important to the medical professional, is to provide support for our body's posture. Atrophying muscles are unable to support the body's bony structures, and as a result, posture may decline as we age, which may cause injury or pain to occur. Good posture and muscular development have come to represent a fit physique that has become extremely important in today's society. Therefore, more and more people today are beginning to follow an exercise regimen that includes resistance training for muscular development. This chapter will describe the effects and parameters of resistance training as they are currently understood.

PHYSIOLOGIC ADAPTATIONS TO RESISTANCE TRAINING

Muscle Size

The application of overload to a muscle leads to hypertrophic muscular adaptation. The force a muscle is capable of producing is directly related to the cross-sectional area of the given muscle. Therefore, as a muscle is introduced to overload, it will adapt by synthesizing greater and greater numbers of contractile proteins or myofilaments. This leads to a thickening of the myofibrils and thus a cumulative effect of enlarging the diameter of the individual muscle fiber. This phenomenon is known as *muscular hypertrophy*, and it is reversible if the muscle does not continue to deal with overload. There is also a great deal of controversy over the potential for an increase in the number of muscle fibers known as *hyperplasia*. This phenomenon has been exhibited in animal studies; however, there is conflicting literature as to its existence in humans.[1,2]

Neurologic Adaptations

Resistance training affects the neurologic system by improving motor unit recruitment and the firing rate of the motor unit. This improvement in the neurologic capacities of the motor unit is believed to be the reason for the initial increases in strength in a novice weight lifter. In addition, there is improved neuromuscular coordination both within the affected muscle group and in those muscles which may assist in a given movement. Force of contraction will be maximal when all available motor units have been recruited and when they are all firing at their optimal rate.[3] As the weight training experience of an individual increases, there also may be an increase in the synchronization of motor unit recruitment as well as a dampening of the protective mechanisms of a muscle, which will allow for greater strength gains to occur.[4]

Biochemical Changes

With high-intensity training there can be a significant increase in muscle glycogen, creatine phosphate, and adenosine triphosphate substrate stores. There also may be an increase in the quantity and activity of the glycolytic enzyme myokinase and creatine kinase.[5] Participation in low-intensity, high-volume training (endurance training) can improve the oxidative capacity of the muscle. Most of the improvements to the oxidative capacity of the muscle occur only in the type I fibers whose oxidative capacities are already developed; however, there can be some improvement in the type IIa fibers' moderately developed oxidative capacity.[1]

PRINCIPLES OF RESISTANCE TRAINING

Overload

In order to achieve muscle growth and muscle strength increases, the muscle has to receive some sort of overload. This means that a load greater than what the muscle is used to handling must be applied to resist against a muscular contraction. Overload can be achieved in many ways; a weighted implement, manual resistance, resistive machinery, or elastic resistance can represent it. It may even be applied using the weight of the body or its extremities against gravity, and it may be cumulative in its effects.

In order to achieve significant gains in strength and potential muscle growth, there is a level of overload that must be used. In resistance training, overload is achieved by measuring the greatest load an individual can lift through a given movement. For example, how much an individual can bench press for one repetition. This is referred to as the *one-repetition maximum*, and all training overloads are calculated as a percentage of this initial value. Depending on the goal of the training bout, the overload may be applied during one repetition of the movement or over a number of repetitions.

Adaptation

There are specific adaptations to resistance training overloads. These adaptations will be specific to the chosen overload and will not increase or decrease unless the overload changes. Therefore, in order to achieve continued improvement, overloads must be progressive in nature.

Progressive Resistance Training

Continued gains in strength and muscle development will not be observed unless the overload is increased progressively over time. Generally, all loads are lifted an assigned number of times, or repetitions. An individual must perform the desired number of repetitions, with failure occurring on the last repetition. For example, an individual has been asked to lift a weight of 135 lb on the bench press for eight repetitions. When the individual performs the group of repetitions, the eighth repetition must be the last repetition; the person must fail to be able to lift another repetition. If he or she is capable of lifting another repetition, then the load he or she has chosen does not represent sufficient overload to achieve strength or muscular development increases. If this occurs, the person must increase the load the next time he or she performs the lift. This increasing of the load to achieve failure in the prescribed number of repetitions is referred to as *progressive resistance training*.

Individual Differences

Always remember that there are many differences between individuals. What may cause an increase in strength for one person may not for another. What has worked for one group of individuals in a specific situation may not work for another group or individual. When developing resistance training programs, one must be very open to the many methods of achieving a specific goal and apply those which best suit the individual.

Reversibility

All training adaptations are transient and reversible. If one does not continue to do resistance training at the same level of intensity, the improvements made as a result of the training will not last. Resistance training must be a year-round enterprise. Cessation of training will result in loss of strength gains as soon as 2 weeks after cessation.[6]

Variability

Since adaptations occur as a result of training overloads and will not increase without the changing of such overloads, it is important that these overloads be varied. There are both physiologic and psychological factors that contribute to adaptation to training overloads. In order for there to be constant progression, it is best to achieve the most efficient and variable program possible. Without such variability, an individual may drop out of the exercise regime or may observe training plateaus with no improvement.

The Desired Goals of Training

There are essentially four training effects one may be trying to achieve by participating in resistance training. These training effects or adaptations to training stimulus are not isolated, and there may be a great degree of crossover in each of the effects.

The endurance athlete or the athlete who is required to produce strength movements repeatedly during an event may wish to develop the strength endurance capabilities of the muscle. This is to say that this individual wishes to improve the muscle's ability to generate low to moderate forces over and over again. In addition, strength endurance-type training may be the type of training that is attractive to the individual who may wish to lose weight and develop greater muscle tone. Many individuals do not wish to develop great muscle bulk. They just want to feel that the muscle is present and that there is less fat surrounding it. These individuals must combine resistance training with aerobic conditioning to improve muscle tone and increase caloric expenditure so as to decrease body fat percentage.

Other individuals are concerned with the development of muscle tissue. These individuals are often referred to as *bodybuilders*, and ultimately, their goal is to achieve maximum hypertrophy of muscle tissue. Their reasons for doing so may cross from the ability to compete within the sport to achieving the ultimate physique. In addition, there are a number of sports that may require that an individual increase his or her size and strength, such as football or rugby. Increases in hypertrophy result in increases in strength and body weight; this type of strength gain is referred to as an increase in *absolute strength* because there is no concern for the relationship between body weight and muscle strength (this is known as the *strength-to-mass ratio*).

Another group of individuals may be concerned with the strength-to-mass ratio. They wish to increase their strength but wish to limit the potential for the associated mass increases. This type of strength improvement is known as *relative strength development*. It is required most often in sports that demand strength without a great deal of mass development, such as wrestling, boxing, and volleyball, to name a few, and may even be desirable in power lifting.

Power development is the final goal of resistance training that may be achieved. Power is speed strength, or the ability to generate force in the shortest possible period of time. An individual who is powerful is able to generate very large force quantities in extremely short periods of time. An individual who can vertically jump over 30 in. in the air from a standing start is generally considered to have powerful legs. This individual is able to rapidly accelerate his or her body mass into the air to significant heights. Power is desirable for any sport or activity that requires that force be generated rapidly, such as sprinting or jumping, or any sport that contains these.

VARIABLES OF RESISTANCE TRAINING

Intensity: Load

Intensity is the first and most important variable in resistance training. Intensity is represented by the percentage of the individual's one repetition maximum (1RM). The 1RM is representative of the greatest load an individual can lift through a given movement. It is generally agreed on that increases in strength or muscular development require the use of loads or intensities that represent between 60 and 100 percent of the 1RM.[4]

A load that represents 100 percent of the 1RM will require an individual to recruit as many motor units as possible in order to develop the required force. The act of recruiting as many motor units as possible is referred to as a *maximal voluntary contraction* (MVC). As the percentage value of the 1RM decreases, less and less motor units are required in order to handle such a load for one single contraction. However, if done to failure, repeat stimulus using less than 100 percent of the 1RM will require that a number of motor units be activated during each ensuing repetition; thus motor unit recruitment will become maximal at the point of fatigue.[4] In order to develop strength, it is necessary to stimulate maximal motor unit recruitment. This can be done using loads that represent 100 percent or less of the 1RM. It is necessary that all sets of an exercise be performed to failure to ensure that maximal motor unit recruitment has been achieved.

Maximal motor unit recruitment results in physiologic and neurologic adaptations. One of these physiologic adaptations is the development of thicker muscle fibers, or hypertrophy. The force a muscle is able to exert is directly related to its cross-sectional area. Muscular hypertrophy results in increases in body weight. Therefore, an increase in strength as well as an increase in body weight is referred to as an increase in *absolute strength*. Using loads that represent between 60 and 100 percent of the 1RM has been found to cause the greatest gains in strength development.[4] It has been found that bodybuilders who tend to train at an intensity that represents between 60 and 80 percent of the 1RM with a greater volume of training exhibit greater hypertrophy gains, especially of the slow-twitch type I fibers, than power lifters. Power lifters tend to use intensities of 80 percent and greater and lower volumes of training.[1,7] Power lifters have exhibited greater hypertrophy gains in their fast-twitch type IIb muscle fibers.[1,7] These results may be caused by the nature of the recruitment pattern achieved using larger or smaller loads. To achieve increases in strength, endurance intensities of below 60 percent of the 1RM are generally prescribed.

As the percentage value of the 1RM decreases, the number of repetitions an individual may be able to perform will increase. This associated relationship is referred to as the *1RM continuum* (Table 25-1). The 1RM continuum is affected by the level of training experience of the individual, the gender of the individual, the muscle group trained, and individual differences.[4] This means that for any given exercise there is no certain number of repetitions associated with a certain percentage of the 1RM. It is best, then, to assign the intensity of an exercise by the number of repetitions that must be achieved rather than assigning a specific percentage of the 1RM. This method of assigning intensity is also best for the novice because it is not often easy to determine the 1RM with someone who has never lifted a weight before. Since the number of repetitions performed has a general relationship to the percentage intensity of the given load, there will still be a clear indication of the intensity of the workload performed (see Table 25-1).

Volume: Sets and Reps

It is generally agreed that in order for a training stimulus to be effective, it must be applied several times. This concept is of greater importance as the training age (years of resistance training experience) increases. Novices have shown improvements using just a single set of a specific number of repetitions. For the most part, increases in strength require that the stimulus be repeated.[8] The number of repetitions and thus the intensity of the exercise are determined by the goal of the training program. The number of times this training stimulus may be applied or the number of sets of repetitions one should perform is subject to an inverse relationship with the number of repetitions performed.[4] The higher the number of repetitions performed, the fewer the number of sets are required to achieve the required training stimulus. The lower the number of

TABLE 25-1 Relationship between Maximum Number of Repetitions and Training Effect

Maximum Number of Repetitions	Percent of 1 Maximum	Training Effect
1	100.0	Relative strength increases
2	94.3	through enhanced neural
3	90.6	drive.
4	88.1	
5	85.6	
6	83.1	Optimal compromise of
7	80.7	maximal strength and
8	78.6	hypertrophy gains.
9	76.5	Best hypertrophy gains
10	74.4	leading to increased
11	72.3	maximal strength.
12	70.3	
13	68.8	Strength-endurance gains
14	67.5	with less hypertrophy gain.
15	66.2	
16	65.0	
17	63.8	
18	62.7	
19	61.6	
20	60.6	

NOTE: All percentages are only guiding values, since the relationship between the maximum and submaximum loads is influenced by training age/status, gender, muscle group, and the exercise.
SOURCE: Adapted from Poliquin C: *Theory and Methodology of Strength*, NCS Level 4–5, 1990.

repetitions performed, the greater the number of sets that may be performed. The number of sets performed is subject to the law of diminishing returns; at a certain point there will be less benefit from each ensuing set performed so that the energy and time used will not generate any greater return than has already been achieved.[4]

The combination of the number of sets and the number of repetitions performed are referred to as the volume of training. The volume of the training stimulus is similar to the duration of the training stimulus seen in other types of conditioning training and may be manipulated according to the goals of the training program.

Duration of the Workout

The length of the workout is often goal-dependent; however, most agree that the length of the actual resistance training portion of an overall workout should not exceed 1 h. The duration of the program is most often determined by the intensity of the training session. It is difficult to maintain intensity for long periods of time due to energy requirements. The rule of thumb for workout duration would be the higher the intensity, the shorter the workout.

Frequency

How often an individual must train to achieve results depends on his or her training age. The novice can achieve improvements with just two training sessions of a particular muscle group per week. For the more advanced individual, there has been little difference found between the results obtained with three training sessions a week versus five training sessions of the same muscle group.[4] In fact, there is some belief that the increased frequency may lead to tissue breakdown and injury with no greater increases in strength. It is therefore recommended that similar muscle groups be trained two to three times per week. There should be time between training sessions for tissue regeneration and energy repletion; this period is generally agreed on to be 48 h.

Rest

The rest between each training stimulus during a training session depends on the goals of the program. As the goal of training shifts from strength endurance, to muscular hypertrophy, to strength, and to power development, the length of time of rest must increase. In endurance training one wishes to deplete energy stores, fatigue the muscle fibers, and make them work through exhaustion in order to increase the physiologic endurance properties of the muscle. Rest, therefore, is of limited importance and should be short. In hypertrophy training the length of rest increases to some degree so that the larger requisite loads may be used; however, the premise of total muscle fiber fatigue is still the central theme.

In strength and power training one wishes to train the neurologic recruitment patterns of the muscle, attempting to effectively achieve full motor unit recruitment in each repetition. This training of the neurologic system combined with high force output requires that energy stores within the muscle be completely replenished between each set of repetitions. It takes a minimum of 3 min for ATP stores to be replenished within the muscle.[4] Not only is metabolic recovery an issue, but neurologic fatigue requires even longer periods of rest (up to five to seven times as long as ATP regeneration).[6] Therefore, the rest between sets in strength and power training is generally held above 3 min and may extend to even greater periods in some cases.

Rest between exercises is totally dependent on the order of the exercise prescription. If the next exercise to be performed uses a different muscle group, then the length of rest is of little importance. If the same muscle is to be trained, the length of rest between exercises is similar to those times seen between exercise sets.

Tempo

The speed of contraction during an individual repetition is referred to as the *tempo* of the movement. The tempo directly affects the time under tension of the muscle contraction. Tempo is expressed as a three-digit number developed by the Australian strength and conditioning expert Ian King. The first number indicates the length of the eccentric contraction, the second number indicates a pause time between the eccentric and concentric motions, and the third number indicates the length of the concentric contraction. An example would be 413, which indicate 4 s eccentric, 1 s pause, 3 s concentric. If one contraction takes 7 s, as expressed above, a set of 10 of these contractions would take 70 s, which is referred to as the *total time under tension*. Longer time under tension causes greater fatigue of the slow-twitch muscle fibers. Therefore, slower tempos are often used to create greater hypertrophic responses. Higher tempos, especially those which are explosive in nature, are reserved for power development.

TRAINING MODES

Type of Load

All resistance training programs involve the use of loads. The nature of these loads is really determined by their relationship to the natural strength curve of the muscle to be trained and the degree to which they may need to be balanced (stable or unstable loads). There are several types of loads.

Unstable Loads

Free weights Free weights are any load that is free-standing and must be balanced by the body while being manipulated through an exercise pathway. Generally, free weights do not correspond to the natural strength curves seen in the human body. The free weight does not change, so the load lifted must be chosen so that the movement may be accomplished at the weakest point in the range of motion. In most human motions this point is found either at the beginning or at the end of the range of motion. This means that the muscle may not be challenged to its fullest degree through its strongest range. Free weights do, however, mimic the requirements of daily life more realistically, as well as requiring that the load be balanced, which calls on the use of synergistic support.

Elastic resistance Elastic resistance equipment uses the elastic properties of materials such as rubber or other like substances to create a load. The use of elastic resistance is more and more prevalent in fitness programming today because it is an easy and modifiable way of achieving resistance. It is important to note that elastic resistance increases throughout the entire time it is being stretched. This type of resistance does not follow a human strength curve at all, and in fact, elastic resistance is greatest, usually, at the weakest point in range of motion. In addition, one elastic can only achieve a certain level of resistance, so this requires that you have a number of elastics available for different exercises. If the elastic resistance is not located in a fixed equipment package, it does contribute to the development of synergistic support and stabilization.

The body The loading of the body using the body or its limbs can be an effective method of resistance training. The movements are affected similarly as in the use of free weights; however, they are limited by the initial strength of the participant. Some exercises may be modified so that they are easier or harder within certain limitations. For example, an individual may perform a push-up from the knees or with the feet on a chair depending on whether one wishes the exercise to be easier or harder. Some believe that this may be the best way to exercise the body because it develops greater functional strength.

Stable Loads

Fixed resistance A fixed-resistance load is similar to a free weight in that it does not adjust for the changes in force production caused by the strength curve of a human motion. The load is fixed, however, in some form of equipment frame using weight stacks, pulleys, and fixed bearing joints (often referred to as *selectorized equipment* because of the use of weight stacks with pin loading). This fixed or stabilized load eliminates the requirement for the load to be balanced and as such tends to decrease the requirement for synergistic support and stabilization. This type of load tends to be more conducive to beginner programming, where an individual may be intimidated by the loading of a free weight or the requirement to balance the load.

Variable resistance This form of loading is very similar in setup to the fixed-resistance load. It differs from the fixed-resistance equipment in its method of load application. Variable-resistance equipment attempts to adjust the load through a range of motion so that it follows the common strength curve of that motion. The load is adjusted through the range of motion by the use of a cam that has been built to average strength curve specifications. Variable-resistance equipment attempts to resolve the problem of free weights, allowing the muscle to be taxed to its fullest throughout the entire range of motion. A problem with variable-resistance equipment is that it can only be built for the average population. Those with longer or shorter limbs or different tendinous insertion points do not fit into this average category and may not experience a true variable-resistance effect. It also requires that contractions be performed at precise tempos in order to benefit from the full effect of the variable resistance.

Isokinetic resistance True isokinetic resistance requires the use of complex machinery fitted with transmission-like gears that are able to limit the speed of contraction of a muscle through a given range of motion. Limiting the speed of contraction creates a loading situation where the load reacts to the force production of the muscle. It is the only true method of producing resistance that follows the exact strength curve of a given muscular contraction in a given individual. Essentially the resistance will only allow the limb to achieve a specific speed through a specific range of motion, so no matter how hard the individual forces or how the force changes, the limb will only move at the set speed. Isokinetic resistance allows for the full development of muscular strength throughout a range of motion. Isokinetic resistance is fixed in its effects, requiring no synergistic support or stabilization of the load. Some argue that it may achieve true strength curve training; however, the movements performed in everyday human motion are not subject to such resistance, and as such, it does not prepare the body for functional human motion.

Hydrodynamic resistance Hydrodynamic resistance uses liquids or gases housed in cylinder-like chambers to produce resistance similar to that found when moving a limb through water. Hydrodynamic resistance is similar to isokinetics in that the resistance reacts to the initiation of greater forces by producing greater resistance forces. Owing to the nature of the cylinder systems used, this resistance is never perfect and does not achieve the specific effect of isokinetics. In addition, hyrodynamic resistance does not provide eccentric load and requires that in every motion performed there be a push and pull motion. This allows for balanced development of agonist and antagonist; however, the muscles may not benefit from eccentric loading. A lack of eccentric loading may be beneficial for the novice because eccentric loading is believed to cause more damage to the contractile proteins of a muscle, thus contributing to day-after muscle soreness.

Choice of Exercise

There are a diverse number of exercises that may target a similar group of muscles or specific muscle. These exercises may be exchanged throughout the duration of a strength training program in order to achieve variety, as well as full development of a muscle or group of muscles. Exercises should be chosen according to the goal of the program and the experience of the participant and to ensure efficient and effective strength development. Exercise options such as using mode variations, changing the angle of the original exercise, and switching to single-limb movements should all be explored.

PRINCIPLES OF PROGRAM DEVELOPMENT

Strength Endurance Training

Strength endurance development requires that one apply low- to moderate-intensity loads, generally below 60 percent of the 1RM over a high volume of training (usually two to three sets of above 20 repetitions). The desired effect of strength endurance training is to train the muscle's fatigue-resistance capabilities using loads that will stimulate a limited amount of muscle growth. The training stimulus generally affects the muscle's ability to handle lactic acid development as well as improving its oxidative capacities. This type of training may be of significant benefit to the moderate-endurance athlete in whom muscular endurance may be a factor. Increasing the number of sets (two to three), decreasing the length of rest time between sets (45 to 30 s), and using large muscle group exercises (squats, presses), all in combination with aerobic exercise, will achieve improvements in the muscle's oxidative properties, as well as significant caloric expenditure. This type of training may be desirable for the weight-conscious individual.

Absolute Strength

If hypertrophy or absolute strength is the goal of the client, it is best to use loads that represent 60 to 80 percent of the 1RM. Rest periods can vary from as little as 30 s to as much as 3 min but should not be long enough to allow for complete ATP recovery. Generally, the nature of hypertrophic development requires maximal motor unit activation until fatigue with repeated stimuli, requiring that larger volumes of training be used. It is not uncommon to use three to four sets of an exercise of between 6 and 20 repetitions and the use of a large number of exercises (as many as four to six) for one muscle group.

Relative Strength

Relative strength refers to the development of strength with limited increases in body weight. Increasing the strength-to-mass ratio requires that larger intensities of training (80 percent of the 1RM and above) be applied using a lower volume of training (four to five sets of one to six repetitions). The use of extremely heavy loads causes maximal motor unit activation to be achieved very early in the training stimulus. This type of loading has been found to improve the neurologic activation of motor units, leading to significant increases in strength without concomitant increases in muscle mass. It has been observed that athletes who train with very high-intensity loads show a great deal of hypertrophy of the fast-twitch types IIa and IIb fibers, with a limited increase in slow-twitch type I fiber hypertrophy.[8] This finding agrees with the concept that high intensities will increase strength but limit overall muscle fiber hypertrophy, leading to increases in relative and not absolute strength.

Training with high intensities requires that long rest periods be used between each set of an exercise. It is not uncommon to use rest periods of between 3 and 5 min. This long rest period allows for complete regeneration of ATP and neurologic recovery so that the second bout of exercise may be performed at maximal potential, since the goal is to train the neurologic capacity of the muscle. The tempo of the exercise should be slow to moderate so that neural recruitment is complete and synergistic stabilization is encouraged.

Power

Power development requires that the speed of contraction be increased. Power training affects motor unit activation and firing rate in order to produce smooth and explosive force production. In addition, it calls on the training of the neurologic reflex patterns within the body that allow for quicker force production. Because of the nature of the exercises that must be performed such as plyometrics or Olympic-style lifts, there may be potential for injury. Therefore, it is recommended that a significant strength base be achieved prior to attempting the exercises involved in power development.

Generally, the intensity and volume of training may be manipulated within a very broad scope; however, it is important that the speed of contraction or the attempted speed of contraction be explosive in nature. Rest time should be maximized in order to observe complete ATP recovery between sets (Table 25-2).

TABLE 25-2 Loading Parameters in Relation to the Desired
Training Effect

Variables	Strength Endurance	Hypertrophy	Relative Strength	Power
Intensity	Less than 60%	60–80%	80–100%	60–100%
Sets	2–4	2–6	5–12	3–10
Repetitions	20 and above	6–20	1–5	1–12
Rest	10–60 s	10–240 s	180–300 s	120–600 s
Tempo	Moderate	Varied	Slow	Explosive

SOURCE: Adapted from Poliquin C: *Theory and Methodology of Strength*, NCS Level 4–5, 1990.

PERIODIZATION OF TRAINING

Periodization refers to the manipulation of training variables within specific periods and phases for the purpose of achieving specific training goals.[6] Periodization is usually applied over a period of a yearly plan; however, the principles may be extrapolated for application within any specific training period. Periodization can be as simple as changing the exercises of a client's program in order to prevent boredom to as complicated as the diverse manipulation of all training variables that can be seen in the development of sports-specific programming. It is difficult within the context of this book to offer a complete education on the performance of periodization; however, I will attempt to introduce the reader to most of the basic principles.

In order to periodize, one requires that there be an end-range goal that the client wishes to achieve. This goal may have a number of aspects to it, or it may be very specific. The developer of a training program must identify the goal(s), the time frames, the resistance training experience of the individual, and a number of other aspects. This investigation is referred to as a *needs analysis*. The information attained in the needs analysis is extremely important because it will define the type of training program that must be developed, as well as its time frames and complexity.

Cycles

The base element of periodization is the cycle. A cycle may be as short as a week (microcycle) or as long as 1 year (mesocycle). Each cycle has a specific training goal, and the training variables are manipulated in order to achieve that goal. Usually cycles are grouped into periods and phases that have specific training goals according to their timing. There are many ways of periodizing and many ways of organizing a training schedule. All of these depend on the information attained in the needs analysis. The following are some common training phases one may employ.

The General Preparatory Phase

This phase is usually an introductory phase of training; usually it uses parameters of training that are characteristic of the strength endurance format of training, low-intensity/high-volume resistance training. It may be coupled with aerobic training or other forms of cross-training to initiate the individual to the training program. The exercises should be multimuscle oriented and nonspecific. This type of phase may be employed with the novice or may be used as a reintroduction to a long-term training program for a high-performance athlete. It represents a reasonable method of introducing or reintroducing resistance training to an individual that will yield results with limited muscle soreness. This phase usually will last no longer than 8 weeks but may be longer or shorter if necessary.

Specific Preparatory Phase

This phase of training defines the goals of an individual more specifically with respect to the training regime. Usually the intensity of the training increases, with moderate to high volumes of training. Exercises must become more specific to the requirements of the individual's goals or the sport he or she may be preparing for. This phase should last between 6 and 8 weeks but may be longer or shorter if necessary.

Precompetition Phase

When preparing a client to compete in a sport, there are additional phases to consider. The first of these is referred to as the *precompetition phase* and is marked by an increase in intensity and a dropoff of volume. In addition, exercises and training must be very sports specific, with little time wasted on peripheral types of training. This phase usually lasts no longer than 6 weeks but may be longer or shorter if required.

Taper Phase

This phase usually lasts no longer than 1 week and represents a dropoff in intensity and volume of training to base levels in order to achieve full recovery and regeneration for competition.

Competitive Phase

In longer-season sports it may be necessary to address a competitive phase that will maintain strength levels as much as possible throughout the length of the competitive season. The use of moderate intensities and low volumes of training usually occur during this time.

Cyclic Progression

Periods and phases are the base organizational groupings that may be used in long-term periodization. Within these periods and phases are a series of microcycles that are cyclically manipulated to prevent stagnation of the physiologic adaptation process as well as to prevent boredom and provide motivation.

At the center of cyclic progression is the observation that a program that does not change will only yield results during its initial stages. If a program continues with limited variation, strength improvements will plateau, and the individual may become bored of the program. In addition, all tissues that are subjected to a training stress require opportunities for rest and recovery, where significant regeneration may occur. Since intensity is the most important factor in the improvement of strength, a technique of manipulating training intensity has been identified that is known as *staired progression*.

Staired Progression

Staired progression refers to the manipulation of training intensity within the framework of a training phase over a series of microcycles. Staired progression attempts to initiate a physiologic state known as *supercompensation* within the muscle tissue of the body. Generally, if one is introduced to a new training stimulus or load at the beginning of a microcyle that is higher than anything handled previously, this training stimulus will cause fatigue to occur. If the same load is maintained over the period of this same microcycle during ensuing training sessions, the body will begin to adapt to this new training intensity by midcycle and potentially feel capable of handling even heavier loads by the end of the microcycle. This new level is referred to as a new *ceiling of adaptation*.[6]

At the beginning of the following microcycle, the individual may be feeling both physiologically and psychologically capable of handling a greater load. The intensity should then be increased to challenge the body to adapt even further. This progression of intensity may continue through a period of two to four microcycles, at which point an unloading period should be initiated.[6] The unloading period or microcycle represents an opportunity for the body to regenerate after a series of intensive training microcycles. The unloading period should not return to initial levels of intensities; rather, it should be reduced to the level of intensity reached at the midpoint of the staired progression phase[6] (Fig. 25-1). The unloading period allows for tissue regeneration and synthesis as well as

The Concept of Staired Progression of Intensity

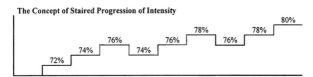

FIG. 25-1   The concept of staired progression of intensity. (Reprinted with permission from Bompa T: *Periodization of Strength.* Don Mills, Ontario, Veritas, 1993.)

the replenishment of energy stores that will have been depleted over the period of staired progression. This replenishment of energy stores during the unloading phase may exceed the previous levels attained before the training stimulus was initiated.[10] This gain in energy replenishment is commonly known as *supercompensation*, and it may leave the individual in a heightened state of preparedness for another successive series of increasing training intensities.[10]

MANIPULATING INTENSITY AND VOLUME

When one describes the number of sets times reps and their intensity, there are a number of ways they may be presented or prescribed. The simplest of ways is a fixed presentation; this indicates that the repetitions are associated with a specific intensity and that they remain constant over the desired number of sets (e.g., six sets of five repetitions at 85 percent intensity). It can be presented in a number of ways also: $6 \times 5 \times 85\%$, $6/5 \times 85\%$. Another way of prescribing the volume and intensity is to describe them as unfixed, e.g., three sets of 10 to 12 reps at 70 to 74 percent intensity, or 3×10 to 12 at 70 to 74 percent. The difference between these two methods is that generally over a period of three to five sets using the same load one should not be able to maintain the same number of repetitions if one is lifting to failure on each set. The unfixed presentation takes into consideration that the first set may be performed to 12 repetitions, and the last set may be performed to 10 repetitions. This type of presentation takes into consideration the variability of the repetition continuum, describing the associated intensity as a range rather than a specific number (Fig. 25-2).

Other methods of prescription may include pyramid presentation or split-set presentation. An example of the pyramid style (which allows one to cover a greater range of intensities in one workout) would be 1×10 at 75 percent, 1×8 at 78 percent, 2×6 at 83 percent. This type of prescription is fairly advanced and should not be directed at the novice. The split style may look as follows: 2×10 at 75 percent, 2×6 at 83 percent, 1×12 at 70 percent.

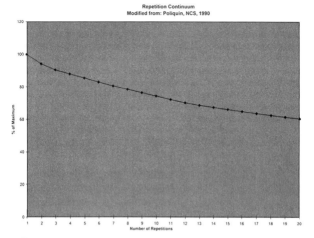

FIG. 25-2   Repetition of continuum. (Modified from Poliquin C: *Loading Parameters of Strength Development*. NCCP National Coaches Seminar, Level 4/5, January 1990.)

There are any number of ways that the pyramid or split style may be applied, and there are very few rules associated with their application.

SPECIAL CONSIDERATIONS IN RESISTANCE TRAINING

Core Development

Always make certain that a program addresses the need for good core strength. The muscles of the low back and abdominals must be well prepared to provide support for the use of the limbs in strength movements. For some individuals, this may mean attending to core strength first before any other training begins or before any significant strength training begins.

Balanced Exercise Prescription

Always design strength training programming so that it prevents strength imbalances from occurring. The "mirror effect" of strength training often causes individuals to concentrate their efforts on the muscles they can see instead of training with a balanced approach. Training imbalances may lead to postural imbalances that may in turn lead to injury. The safest rule of thumb is that for every exercise one assigns for the agonist, there must be an exercise assigned for the antagonist.

Flexibility

Make sure that the exercises that are assigned are demonstrated and performed through a full range of motion through a correct exercise path. Many times individuals will adopt efficent exercise patterns using incorrect musculature to perform a motion, or they may cheat the exercise of its full range of motion. It is of absolute importance that the exercise be performed with correct technique in order to prevent the development of inflexibility that may contribute to joint or muscle/tendon injuries.

Synergistic Support

Always begin strength training programming slowly in order to allow the synergists to be prepared for increased loading. When dealing with a young individual or a novice, pay close attention to exercise technique and prevent individuals from compromising technique in order to lift greater loads. The synergists must be given time in order to be prepared for large degrees of loading; otherwise, joint injury may occur.

TYPES OF RESISTANCE EXERCISES

In conventional resistance training there are really only seven motion patterns that occur. These are the press motion, the pull motion, the squat motion, the lunge motion, flexion/extension motion, adduction/abduction motion, and rotation. These motion patterns may be combined to provide variation. Variation also may be attained by changing the angle of the motion, the start or finish position of the motion, or the position of nonaffected joints above or below the joint of motion or by using dumbbells, barbells, or other modes of training. It is imperative that one clearly understands these motion patterns, the muscles involved, and the effects of the exercise modifications. For too long exercises have been known by a gym name given them by the many bodybuilders and weight lifters who have developed them. The development of exercises requires that one understands the concept of motion patterns and functional anatomy; once this is true, one may be free to create any exercise that may affect any muscle. The following known exercises follow the motion patterns reflected above:

The press motion: Bench press, decline press, incline press, military press, behind the neck press, the dip, the push press, etc.
The pull motion: Upright row, low row, pull-down, the chin-up, the clean, etc.

The squat motion: Leg press, squats, hack squats, dead lifts, power cleans, etc.

The lunge motion: The lunge, the split squat, the step-back lunge, the step-up, etc.

Flexion/extension motion: The bicep curl, the tricep extension, the kick back, the push down, the crunch, the curl up, the cobra, roman chair extensions, hip extension, hip flexion, leg extensions, leg curls, etc.

Abduction/adduction: The fly, the lateral abduction, adductions, lateral leg lifts, etc.

Rotation: Shoulder rotation, hip rotation, rotary crunches, rotary extensions, etc.

When designing resistance training programs it is extremely important to understand the concept of motion patterns so that one's program achieves balance while being as efficient and as effective as possible. For example, if one were to set out to design a program that improves upper body strength, it is important to identify those muscles which need to be trained and the motion patterns that affect those muscles. Once this is known, then exercises should be chosen to develop strength in a balanced fashion, leaving room for variation using various angles and training modes.

TYPES OF DAILY PROGRAM ORGANIZATION

Aside from the overall periodization effect of a training program, there are particular methods of program design specific to the daily workout. The daily program design relies heavily on the training age of the participant, the type of training goals, and the time available for training. Several methods of daily program design are available.

The Full Body Routine

This style of programming is most often used with the novice or those individuals with time constraints, either due to lifestyle or other training requirements, as in the case of an athlete. This type of program is demonstrated by the body being broken down into several regions with each of these regions receiving at least one training stimulus during the program. Commonly these areas are divided into the chest, the upper back, the shoulders, the arms (biceps/triceps), the abs, the low back, the hips and thighs, and the calves.

I would suggest that this method of body division does not adequately reflect the best method of program development because it does not challenge one to define the anatomic considerations of each exercise. Clearly, it is important that one develop a balanced program that remains functional in nature. I would suggest the following method of division: upper body, core, lower body. Within these divisions there would be further division: upper body, press motion, press motion above the head, pull motion, pull motion from above the head; core, flexion motion, extension motion, rotation motion; lower body, squat motion, lunge motion, ankle flexion/extension motion.

The full body program should be repeated no more than four times a week with 1 day's rest between sessions; however, it must be repeated a minimum of three times a week to be effective. Usually it is best to keep exercise prescription from motion to motion to a minimum because the cumulative effect of multiple exercise prescriptions will be a long, low-intensity workout.

The following program is an example of the full body program:

The upper body

The press motion	The pull motion
The press motion above the head	The pull motion above the head
	Bench press
	Dumbbell military press
	Cable row
	Cable pulldown

The core

The flexion motion	The rotation motion
The extension motion	Crunch
	Cobra
	Rotary crunch

The lower body

The squat motion	Leg press
The lunge motion	Smith machine split squats
The ankle flexion/ extension motion	Heel raises/toe lifts

This form of programming rarely should exceed 10 total exercises, so it becomes extremely important that the program be both efficient and effective. As the preceding program demonstrates, each of the major muscle groups and their synergists receive equal stimulus throughout the program, with few single-muscle-specific exercises included. More specific flexion/extension exercises and adduction/abduction exercises cannot be performed in the full body style program or it will become far too long and cumbersome. These muscle groups are effectively trained in the combined press/pull/squat motions.

The Upper/Lower Two On, One Off Split Routine

This type of program setup is best suited to the intermediate- to advanced-level participant or the athlete. It is defined by the separation of the body into two component training days. The first training day involves training of the upper body, and the second training day involves training of the lower body. Core group training may be fractured or grouped into a separate training session or during only one of the training sessions depending on the degree of focus. The upper body and lower body programs should then be broken down as follows: upper body, press motion, overhead press motion, pull motion, overhead pull motion, shoulder abduction/adduction (various planes), elbow flexion/extension core training flexion/extension; lower body, squat motion, hip flexion/extension, hip abduction/adduction, knee flexion/extension, ankle flexion/extension, core rotation. Each upper body/lower body split is to be followed by 1 day off, and then the cycle must begin again. This ensures that adequate rest is observed without the loss of potential training effects. A sample program is as follows:

Upper body day

The press motion	The overhead pull motion
The shoulder adduction/ abduction motion	The elbow flexion/ extension motion
The overhead press motion	The core flexion/extension
The pull motion	Incline dumbbell press
	Flat bench flies
	Bent over laterals
	Military press
	Barbell bent over row
	Close grip front pull-down
	Incline dumbbell curls
	Tricep push downs
	Reverse crunch
	Roman chair extensions

Lower body day

The squat motion	Front squats
The hip flexion/ extension motion	Four-way hip
	Leg extensions
The hip adduction/abduction	Leg curls
Knee flexion/extension motion	Heel raises
The ankle flexion/ extension motion	Toe raises
	Rotary crunches
The core rotation motion	Crossover cable crunch

Once again, each session includes approximately 10 exercises and covers all the required muscular training efficiently and effectively.

Multiple Split Routines

Multiple split routines are designed for the advanced weight lifter and are usually reserved for the bodybuilding participant. The desire to train with higher volumes in order to create greater muscle growth stimulus requires that the body be broken down into even more sections to concentrate on specific muscle group training. Quite often similar movement patterns are combined so that large volumes of training may be effected on one or two muscle groups at a time. Using the old system of training, one might have observed sessions that trained the back and biceps and the chest and triceps. With the newly suggested system, multiple splits might appear as follows:

Three Day On, One Day Off Split

Day 1

Upper body press motion	Shoulder abduction motion
Upper body overhead press motion	Elbow extension motion
Shoulder adduction motion	Core extension
	Bench press
	Incline dumbbell press
	Military press
	Cable crossovers
	Bent over laterals
	French press
	Dumbbell kick backs
	Roman chair extensions

Day 2

Upper body pull motion	Elbow flexion
Upper body overhead pull motion	Core flexion
	Wide grip cable row
	Dumbbell row
	Front pull-down
	Close grip chin-up
	Barbell curls
	Preacher curls
	Crunches

Day 3

Lower body squat motion	Leg press
Lower body lunge motion	Hack squats
Hip adduction/abduction motion	Step-forward lunge
Knee flexion/extension motion	Four-way hip
Ankle flexion/extension	Leg extensions
Core rotation	Leg curls
	Heel raises
	Toe raises
	Rotary crunches

With this style of training, the number of exercises may vary from day to day between as low as 5 exercises and as high as 10 exercises, depending on the desired volume of training. The multiple split may take many shapes and forms. Some individuals advocate the use of agonist/antagonist type training on the same day. They point to the fact that an inhibitory mechanism present during exercise that involves the limitation of force production due to an antagonistic inhibitory mechanism will be limited if the antagonist is fatigued prior to an agonistic exercise. Still others feel that it is most efficient to train all those muscles involved in common motions on the same day, as was done in the preceding example. Modification of this area is certainly not limited to these two methods. Just make sure the program developed is suited to the needs of the participant.

Training for a Weight Lifting Sport or Specific Sport

A differentiation must be made between the daily routine in sports preparation and fitness or aesthetics training. Generally, when one trains for fitness or to improve appearance, one should work within the framework of a balanced training program that affects all the major muscle groups of the body during a training microcycle or week.

When training for sport, the daily routine of the training program is affected by the current goal of the program. For example, if one were training a volleyball athlete for the season, the off-season would be broken down into several periods and phases. During the general preparatory phase, the athlete may work on overall muscular development using a basic style program. However, during the specific preparatory phase, the time available to resistance train may be more limited, and the program must reflect the muscular development goals specific to that sport. A power lifter, for example, should not spend more than 45 min to 1 h on any one specific preparation session. The exercises he or she performs must be specific to the goals of power lifting and must leave room for high-intensity training. A power lifter may only be assigned three exercises to perform during the course of 45 min. This is necessary so that rest time between sets and intensity level remain where they must be to achieve maximal strength gains.

CONCLUSION

It is most important to realize after having read this chapter that there are many ways to construct a successful resistance training program; however, there are many key ingredients that must be included so that the program remains efficient and effective. The most important of these ingredients are intensity and variety. As long as the program one develops has these two ingredients, one will observe some degree of success. Always remember that there is no perfect program, so stop looking!

REFERENCES

1. Gollnick P, Armstrong R, Saltin B, et al: Effects of training on the enzyme activity and fiber composition of human skeletal muscle. *J Appl Physiol* 34(1):107–111, 1973.
2. Gonyea WJ: The role of exercise in inducing skeletal muscle fiber number. *J Appl Physiol* 48(3):421–426, 1980.
3. MacDougall D: *Principles of Strength and Power Training.* NCCP National Coaches Seminar, Level 4/5, January 1990.
4. Poliquin C: *Loading Parameters of Strength Development.* NCCP National Coaches Seminar, Level 4/5, January 1990.
5. MacDougall D, Ward GR, Sale DG, Sutton JR: Biochemical adaptation of human skeletal muscle to heavy resistance exercise and immobilization. *J Appl Physiol* 43:700–703, 1977.
6. Bompa T: *Periodization of Strength.* Don Mills, Ontario, Canada, Veritas Publishing, 1993.
7. Schmidtbleicher D, Haralanbie G: Changes in contractile proteins of muscle after strength training in man. *Eur J Appl Physiol* 46:221–228, 1991.
8. McDonach MJN, Davies CTM: Adaptive response of mammalian skelatal muscle to exercise with high loads. *Eur J Appl Physiol* 52:139–155, 1984.
9. Harris RC, Edwards RHT, Haltman E, et al: The time course of phosphocreatine resynthesis during recovery of the quadriceps muscle in man. *Pfluegers Arch* 907:392–397, 1976.
10. Zatsiorsky V: *Science and Practice of Strength Training.* Champaign, IL, Human Kinetics Publishers, 1995.
11. Poliquin C: Variety in strength training. *Sports* 8:8, 1988.

26 | **Figure Skating**

Sandra Fielding   Robert Lee

Figure skating is a popular sport with participants ranging in age from 3 to 90 years. It is an activity that can be pursued both recreationally and competitively. Traditionally, the sport consists of the disciplines of free skating, pairs skating, and ice dancing. Because the routines are performed to music, the skaters must demonstrate creativity and musicality. Recently, precision skating, which involves groups of 16 or more skaters performing complex routines on the ice, has become more popular in many countries around the world. Like many sports, figure skating has evolved over the years and continually offers the skater new creative and technical challenges.

COMMON FIGURE SKATING TERMINOLOGY

Edges.   There are two edges of the skate blade. The inside edge is medial; the outside edge is lateral. A figure skating blade has a curve called the *rocker*. In forward skating, the balance point moves towards the back of the blade within balance range. In backwards skating, the balance point moves towards the front of the blade within balance range.

Stroking.   Forward and backward skating involving straight-ahead strokes or crossover stokes.

Connecting Steps/Footwork.   A series of edges of varying depth, changes of edge, turns, dance steps, and small jumps used to link free-skating skills together.

Spins.   Different spins on either foot with different body positions at the knee or back. Four basic spinning positions: upright position, layback position, sit position, and camel position.

Lifts.   In pair skating and ice dancing (with limitations), male partner lifts up female partner.

Figures.   Footwork skill tracing patterns on the ice with the blades (no longer judged or tested).

Jumps.   Different jumps named by the takeoff position of the feet and the number of revolutions. These are commonly called flip, lutz, axel, salchow, loop, and toe loop.

Neutral Position.   A position where the shoulders are square to the hips.

Field Movements.   Skills connecting jumps, spins, and footwork, e.g., spirals, arabesques, spread eagles, pivots, and Ina Baurer.

CATEGORIES IN COMPETITIVE FIGURE SKATING

The U.S. and the Canadian Figure Skating Associations have established four distinct disciplines in competitive skating, and they supervise the structure and skill testing levels.

Singles Free Skating: Women and Men

Competitive free skaters perform a short and a long free-skating program to music. The long program varies from 2 min for prenovice skaters to 4-1/2 min for senior men. The specific skills involve footwork, spins, jumps, and connecting moves. Skaters require a high level of aerobic fitness. Their maximum oxygen uptake ($\dot{V}_{O_2}$max) in one study ranged from 54.7 to 68.8 mL/kg per minute, and work intensity during simulated competitive figure skating corresponded to 89 percent of the $\dot{V}_{O_2}$max.[1] This study indicated that figure skaters had quite high associated aerobic power. It also studied the incidence of injuries among the elite Danish figure skaters over a 1-year period. The skaters trained from 15 to 41 h per week, 60 to 95 min of this time being spent on warm-up activities. The injury incidence rate during competitive skating was recorded as 1.4 injuries per 1000 h of training, which is low compared with other sports.

Pair Skating

Male and female partners perform a short and a long program to music. Not only are the same technical skills as in free skating required, the partners coordinate every move together in extreme precision and unison. There is a higher risk of injury than in other skating disciplines. Athletic and aerobic lifts and throws require a strong male partner and often a small, light female partner. The females hit the ice with an impact up to eight times their body weight. They do extensive off-ice training together in a gym setting.

   In one variation of the pair camel spin, the women spins more slowly than the man so that her head actually passes under his extended leg while they are both spinning. If either slips, or if the man holds his leg too low, the woman may suffer a laceration from his blade. The lifts are most dangerous in pairs skating, and in the one-handed triple overhead axle lift, the man lifts the woman well over his head for three and one-half rotations, supported only by one hand. When the pair falls out of this lift, the women falls at least 6 feet.[2]

Ice Dancing

Male and female partners perform a series of different routines to different types of music. The moves are limited to footwork, small lifts, and short spins. The emphasis is on intricate, close footwork, and often the partners become entangled due to the rapid velocity and high sequence of the steps, and falls occur at all levels of performance. No lifts, jumps, or spins of the kind used in free and pair skating are allowed. Aesthetic, creative aspects and interpretation of music are emphasized, and there is a recent trend toward more athletic and technically difficult skating. The constant complex footwork puts more pressure on the knees and back and demands endurance, strength, and flexibility. There are often lacerations from skate blades, and the use of protective gloves can prevent potentially serious lacerations. On-site first aid facilities at the arena help reduce the demand for local accident services.

Precision Team Skating

This unique form of synchronized team skating is evolving rapidly at the recreational and international competitive level. Around 20 skaters are on the ice at the same time and perform choreography that involves footwork, speed, and close complex connecting moves. There are no jumps or spins, but the risk of collision with a teammate is the highest of the four forms of skating. Upper body and arm strength are required in addition to endurance.

DEMOGRAPHICS AND UNIQUE SITUATIONS FOR THE COMPETITIVE SKATER

Predominantly Preadolescent/Adolescent Females

Competitive skaters often train at a high level before the age of 10 and often compete at the national or international level by age 13 or 14 years. In managing the injured figure skater, the sports medicine practitioner must be familiar with a variety of sports medicine issues unique to this population. These include growth and development, nutrition, pediatric and adolescent medicine concerns, and sports psychology.

The female athlete triad of disordered eating, amenorrhea, and osteoporosis is usually not a problem in figure skaters. A study by Slemenda and Johnston[3] noted that although skaters were thinner and significantly more likely to have oligo- or amenorrhea, and had similar skeletal densities in upper body sites to nonathletic control subjects, they had significantly greater density in the pelvis and legs. These differences were not evident until the midteens. Also, another study by Sovak and Hawes[4] regarding the anthropologic status of international-caliber speed skaters noted an additional muscle mass located in the entire lower extremity in speed skaters as well as in male and female figure skaters.

Winter sports athletes also had diminished iron status. Hemoglobin and serum ferritin levels were studied in the competitors at the

1992 Winter Olympics by Clement and associates,[5] and they concluded that Nordic skiing participants had the highest incidence of suboptimal iron status. A total of 50 percent of the Nordic women skiers had prelatent iron deficiency, and 7 percent were anemic. This should be checked in the women speed skaters, who were low in serum ferritin, as well as the ice skaters.

Ice Rink Conditions

The environment of an ice rink or arena provides many challenges for the competitive skater. Rinks are poorly heated, resulting in very cold training conditions. There is usually a lack of space to stretch and warm up, and the floor is wet and dirty. A lot of a skater's stretching has to be done on the wooden bench in the dressing room. Since ice time is limited and expensive, on-ice warm-up is often rushed.

The ice surface itself is often not ideal for figure skating, either being "hockey ice" (too cold, hard, and brittle) or ice that is too warm, soft, and slow. Sometimes the thickness of the ice varies at different parts of the arena, and this can affect all the skaters. Singles skaters performing "pick" jumps (driving the toe pick of the skate blade into the ice to elevate the skater into the jump) can pick right through the ice onto the hard concrete surface, causing injury. In fact, skaters frequently have relatively long picks for maximum jump perfection.

Competitive figure skaters are at risk of carbon monoxide and nitrogen dioxide exposure in ice arenas as a result of the internal combustion engines of Zambonis and the poor ventilation systems in most indoor arenas. Vigorous exercise, increased length of exposure, and underlying pulmonary or cardiovascular disease increase the risk toxicity.

Symptoms of high CO and NO_2 exposure may include the following. For CO, headache, dizziness, weakness, tachypnea, nausea, vomiting, and incoordination are common. For NO_2 cough, hemoptysis, chest pain, dyspnea, profuse sweating, dehydration, weakness, anxiety, and nausea are common. Recognition and treatment of the cause of exposure symptoms are imperative.

INJURIES TO FIGURE SKATERS

Like many sports and activities, the frequency and severity of injuries rise with higher levels of competition. This is due to the greater difficulty of the moves, the higher speed at which they are performed, and the greater number of hours spent daily on the ice by the competitors. Injuries in skating at all levels have a lower frequency than in ballet and gymnastics. Roughly 50 percent of injuries that do occur are repetitive and overuse injuries in nature; the other 50 percent are traumatic, suffered from falls from landing or spills from collisions with other skaters or the arena boards.[6]

Traumatic Injuries

Falls

An important skill a skater learns early in training is how to fall on the ice. As soon as a fall is developing, the skater should bend the knees and sit down. Most skaters fall frequently without causing any injury, but sometimes an awkward fall, landing on the outstretched hand, for instance, can cause significant injuries. These include the following:

Hand and upper extremity injuries such as scaphoid and wrist fractures are common.

Despite the strong support from the boot, ankle and foot injuries occur, such as severe sprains or fractures.

Knee ligament injuries are common, and overuse conditions such as jumper's knee and Osgood-Schlatter's apophysitis are also common.

Patellar subluxation and dislocation occur due to the large axial and rotational forces on the knee during a jump. These high-impact jumps also damage the growth plates (epiphyses).

Although falls are frequent, trochanteric hip bursitis can occur but is not common.

Traumatic back injuries including spondylolisthesis due to the hyperlordotic postures and tight lumbosacral fascia and muscles occur, but associated sciatica is almost nonexistent.

The sports medicine practitioner approaches the treatment of trauma to the skater in a similar fashion to any other sports injury with this important additional concept: One should allow skaters to go back on skates for stroking and other low-stress skills (if the injury permits) while undergoing rehabilitation and recovery from the injury. This allows the skaters to preserve their balance and form on the ice, as well as work on their choreography and maintain mental focus.

This is extremely important when a serious figure skater has to stay off the ice. Competitive skaters, like long-distance runners, develop significant withdrawal symptoms. This is important because most of their close friends are in the skating or running world, and they lose that peer support. This also keeps the skater from seeking medical care early on. They are sure that the doctor will tell them to "stop skating." Thus the injury can become more advanced after delaying initial treatment and demand rest.

The approach should be judicious or "relative rest"; the skater should swim, cycle, and do upper body cardiorespiratory work, and usually he or she can be allowed on the ice for simple, nonharmful skating skills. As soon as the skater is allowed to improve physically and be with his or her peers, the psychological stress diminishes.

Overuse Injuries

Single skaters will suffer predominantly lower extremity overuse injuries. Pairs, dance, and precision skaters also have upper extremity overuse injuries that occur from lifting, holding, throwing, or catching partners.

Common overuse injuries to skaters include shin splints, patellofemoral syndrome, patellar tendinitis, Osgood-Schlatter's apophysitis, and jumper's knee. Rehabilitation must be tailored individually, based on the athlete's growth and development, muscle strength, and flexibility. Closed kinetic chain eccentric loading exercises are important. Pool therapy using a body harness for pool exercises, if necessary, is also a good approach.

Groin and Abdominal Strains

Similar to the hockey players, figure skaters place high rotational and eccentric stresses about the groin that can lead to chronic groin and abdominal strains and osteitis pubis. Abdominal and trunk stabilization exercises help alleviate these injuries.

Back Injuries

Stiff boots limiting ankle and knee motion can result in hypermobility of the lumbar spine and instability. Also, similar to gymnasts, figure skaters often incorporate extreme lumbar hyperextension positions into their routines (Fig. 26-1). This can predispose the skater to facet-type injuries that may progress to spondylolysis or spondylolisthesis injuries. It is important to be suspicious of any skater who presents with low back pain.

The skater should refrain from practicing jumps, layback spins, lifts, or any other element that causes pain until a definitive diagnosis is made and a treatment plan is implemented. The most common cause of low back pain is muscular strain associated with microscopic tears. This is due to tight lumbodorsal fascia and muscles. Daily stretching and spinal stabilization exercises should be instituted and continued throughout the year. Flexibility work such as aerobics and ballet stretching with a bar in the basement at home should be encouraged.

"Landing Leg" Injuries

Figure skaters "take off" a jump on either leg, depending on the jump. However, figure skaters always land jumps (if done prop-

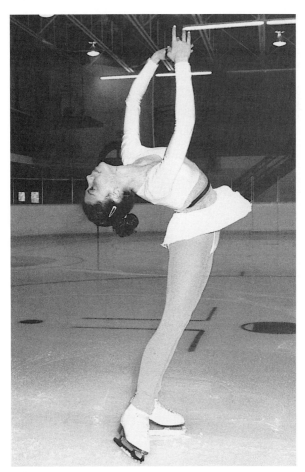

FIG. 26-1 A skater doing "a layback spin," demonstrating excessive hyperextension forces, which can lead to instability of the lumbar spine.

erly) on the same side. Most skaters are right-side dominant and learn to land jumps on the right leg. For the typical single skater learning to master jumps, there is increased stress on the right lower extremity, up to three to five times the skater's weight (Fig. 26-2). The load is particularly on the knee extensor mechanism with in-

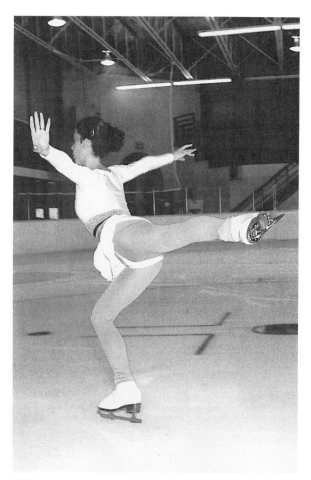

FIG. 26-2   A skater landing jumps demonstrating stresses through the patellofemoral and ankle joints, which can be up to five times the skater's weight.

creased torque on the ankle. This leads to overuse injuries. However, an exception to this occurs with stress fractures in figure skaters. A paper by Pecina and colleagues[7] studied 42 skaters, and

9 had stress fractures. In all instances the fractures occurred in the takeoff leg. The skaters were training 3 to 8 h daily six times a week. All the skaters were able to resume a preinjury level of activity 3 to 7 months after treatment began.

Landing skating jumps places eccentric forces on the lower extremity, and the amount of force of this stress can be magnified by several *extrinsic factors* (hard ice landing surface, steel skate blade, and rigid boot). Some *intrinsic factors* include rapid long bone growth, tight extensor muscles, joint inflexibility, and lower leg malalignment. The more difficult double, triple, and quadruple jumps require very rapid revolutions in the air. This adds additional torsional stress to the takeoff and landing legs. Compounding this issue is the tendency in recent years for skaters to continuously practice more difficult jumps more often and at a younger age. This is due to the trend in judging the sport that rewards attempts and completions of the difficult elements. Careful assessment of lower leg alignment is important. A visit to the rink and discussion with the coach using slow motion videotaping are very helpful.

Ballet dancers are not allowed en pointe until both age and experience permit. Young figure skaters should have a similar time and complexity concern with regard to jumps. If sufficient height is achieved to complete the revolutions with ease, then continued practice is allowed.

A study by Podolsky and associates examined 18 junior figure skaters with Cybex-2 strength testing and concluded that the heights of the jumps were significantly correlated with strength data. Knee extension at 240 degrees per second and shoulder abduction at 300 degrees per second were shown to be the most important strength parameters in determining the height of a jump. Therefore, off-ice strength training is an important part of successful progress.

Boot-Related Injuries

The competitive leather skating boot traditionally has been heavy, stiff, and always requires a break-in period. It is often fitted one full size smaller than the skater's street shoe. The best boots are custom made from either computerized measurements or a mold of the skater's foot, and these can be extremely expensive because of the thicker leather involved and the need for replacement every 9 to 12 months.

These boots also require a break-in period, and this can be hastened by the skater wetting his or her feet when he or she puts on the new skates. Skaters also can get the boots without the blades on and wear them at home to allow the boot to conform to the shape of the foot. When the leather dries, it tends to shrink slightly. Even in handmade boots, skaters complain of painful pressure points, calluses, numbness, and large bursae on both the medial and lateral malleoli, and these swell up quite prominently after each skating session. These problems should be drawn to the attention of the bootmaker, and he or she often will modify the boots by punching out the leather with a stretching device that reduces the pressure points. Skaters often supply their own foam pads, but the padding often can be done more satisfactorily by the bootmaker or a qualified brace maker or skate fitter with more resilient low-density foam or sorbothane-like materials.

Thus skaters often present to the sports medicine clinic complaining of foot pain. It is important to determine if the skating boot is contributing to the cause of the foot pain. Important questions to ask include

Does the pain occur *only* while skating? Does it occur with walking or playing other sports?
Was the onset of the pain related to wearing new or different boots?
If the boot has been the same for some time, have the skater's feet been growing? If so, are both feet the same size?
If the boots have been the same for some time, are the boots wearing down and losing ankle support?
Are the boots custom made or second hand?

The blades are also important, and they differ according to the discipline. Figure blades have greater rocker (curve) and lack the toe picks closest to the ice. Dance blades are shorter posteriorly to permit closer footwork. Free-skating blades vary more, and some skaters have less rocker but larger toe picks. The design of toe picks varies in contour and length.

Also, in less expensive boots the blades are riveted to the boot, and in more expensive boots the blades are screwed to the sole of the boot to permit adjustments for balance. A very small error in blade mounting can affect the skater's performance and potentially perpetuate an overuse injury.

Forefoot pronation can be modified by moving the blade medially, similar to canting a ski boot on the ski. Sharpening is also important. Free-skating and dance blades are ground with a deeper hollow and sharper edges.

The skates should always accompany the injured athlete to the sports clinic. For sports medicine practitioners who see figure skaters frequently, consultation with the skater's coach and with a boot fitter from the skate store will help with a diagnosis and treatment plan for the injured skater. Boot-related injuries of note are discussed below.

Posterior Ankle Pain

Pump Bumps   This is a common complaint among figure skaters. Superficial bumps on the back of the heel overlying the attachment of the Achilles tendon to the calcaneus are often called *pump bumps* because women who wear a style of shoes called *pumps* also get this injury. Note that in most cases there is no bony or Achilles tendon involvement. It is caused by a combination of friction and pressure on the back of the heel because the boot is either too big, causing friction, or too small, causing pressure, or the contour of the heel cup of the boot does not match the shape of the heel. Local therapeutic modalities such as ice, ultrasound, and medication often provide only temporary relief.

Treatment involves removing the source of pressure, and this is important even for small bumps, since these tend to grow larger over time. Unfortunately, in a figure skating boot, this is easier said than done. Placing cushioned foam donuts or gel pads in the skate boot is the first intervention a skater will do, but this does not work for larger bumps because the pressure point may be very slightly reduced but not eliminated. Because of the seam on the back of the skate boot, it is difficult to "punch out" that part of the boot. The way to eliminate pressure is either to construct an orthotic that pushes the whole foot forward slightly or to get new boots. Pump bumps almost never need to be operated on. They will settle down once the pressure is reduced.

Achilles Tendinitis   To get as much height into a jump, the skater must plantarflex the takeoff foot. Unlike other jumping sports, such as basketball, the rigid skate boot will restrict and limit the degree of plantar flexion. This restriction, combined with the rigidity of the back of the ankle boot, can cause an overuse Achilles tendinitis.

Treatment is to restrict the frequency of jumps in practice. Also a heel lift placed in the boot (1/4 in sorbothane) and in all the skater's shoes as well. In many cases the boot maker has to refit or repad the skate boot.

Note that skaters can develop an Achilles tendinitis from the off-ice training activities of running, jumping, aerobics, and other sports. It is important to ask the skater what he or she does in addition to skating and modify those activities appropriately.

Medial Ankle Pain

When a skater complains of pain, tenderness, swelling, or redness on the medial side of the foot and ankle, it is important to locate specifically the source of the symptoms. The differential diagnosis includes tibialis posterior tendinitis, medial malleolar bursitis, tarsal tunnel syndrome, symptomatic bipartite navicular bone, and stress or avulsion fractures.

Again, as with pump bumps, relieving pressure in the boot may be just as important as treatment and rehabilitation in the sports medicine clinic. If the skater's foot is pronated in the skate boot, orthotics designed to wedge the medial aspect of the foot or a blade adjustment, can help.

Anterior Ankle Pain

Constant or repetitive dorsiflexion of the foot in the skate boot while stroking or landing jumps can cause an anterior tenosynovitis. Unfortunately, the injury often occurs at the location where the skate boot must be laced very tightly to provide support, and the laces cannot be loosened significantly without affecting the boot function. The skater usually laces the boots loosely over the toe box, firmly over the instep, and loosely again over the upper hooks to allow ankle dorsiflexion while maintaining circulation in the foot. Adjusting or modifying padding on the tongue of the skate may help, and if the skate boot is too stiff or does not flex much, getting new boots may be the only option.

Orthotic Use in Figure Skating Boots

Biomechanical correction of lower extremity malalignment with orthotics is an accepted treatment option, although physiotherapy to correct muscle imbalances and boot modifications should always be done first. The orthotist or podiatrist must be quite skilled in fabricating a smaller orthotic with the appropriate heel lift.

PREVENTION OF INJURIES TO FIGURE SKATERS

Education

Early detection of and intervention for aches and pains are imperative in preventing chronic overuse injuries. The sports medicine practitioner has an important role in preventative issues. This is especially so in figure skating, which is a predominantly individual sport. The athlete has less frequent exposure to the team trainer, physiotherapist, or team doctor. However, almost all competitive skaters and coaches are involved with each other at a local club level or at the regional or sectional level. Thus educational workshops; preventative counseling on nutrition, stretching, warm-ups, etc.; and preparticipation screening can be done with support from the club or groups of clubs in specific geographic regions.

Cross-Training

Figure skating is an art as well as a sport; therefore, structured off-ice training must incorporate visualization skills, strength, flexibility, balance, and coordination training as well as rest time. Figure skaters have a tendency to spend far more time training on ice than off. For the competitive skater *daily* cross-training is necessary, alternating more physically challenging days (i.e., running, weights) with more "mind focusing" days (i.e., meditation, relaxation, artistic components).

Strength training should incorporate the principle of progressive resistance; the stress placed on a muscle must be continually increased as it becomes capable of producing greater force. Key areas are ankle peroneal muscle strengthening, abdominal stabilization, and shoulder girdle strengthening (especially for pairs and precision skaters). Flexibility of the quadriceps and hamstrings is important to alleviate and/or prevent anterior knee pain. Running (provided education is given to avoid stress fractures) and in-line skating are excellent forms of cardiovascular cross-training. Likewise, ballet is often encouraged because it perfects form, tone, and flexibility.

It is important that every skater's program is tailored individually to suit his or her body structure and composition, psychological well-being, and growth and development. Thus a skater, like other athletes, may be dealing with many health care professionals to simultaneously give him or her the best program possible.

Rest Period

Many sports are evolving into a 12-month-a-year commitment for the athletes. Figure skating is no different, and many skaters—unless they're injured—skate year round, placing their bodies at risk for "burnout." With skating clubs offering summer school skating, it is possible to skate almost every week of the year. Young skaters should rest from training on the ice for a period of time in the summer off-season or take 2-week break periods once or twice during the winter season. Two weeks is sufficient, since muscle strength will not diminish. However, dizziness may occur with the first few spins on return, until the vestibular apparatus readjusts.

THE RULES

The International Skaters Union (ISU) has outlined specific elements to help rule out dangerous activities that may be rewarded by higher marks from the judges. The ISU disallows the horizontal jump or back somersault from competition and limits the number of jumps and triple overhead lifts.

It is also important to have more honest and consistent, reliable judging. Judging figure skating is difficult because of the artistic considerations. This also leads to frustration and lack of the appropriate safety measures.

THE FUTURE

The trend in competitive figure skating is to perform more difficult technical elements and to master them at a younger age. In singles and pairs skating, younger athletes are encouraged to learn, practice, and attempt more difficult jumps more frequently. In dance and precision skating this means more complicated footwork and elements with an emphasis on speed and athleticism. In the sports medicine setting, will this parallel the experience of competitive gymnastics? If so, then the trend will be toward even more overuse injuries seen in even younger athletes. To stem this theoretical increase in injuries, the recreational and competitive figure skating community should involve sports medicine physicians, physiotherapists, and trainers to provide advice on stretching, strengthening, conditioning, and nutrition counseling. On-site medical coverage at skating competitions is important for both injury diagnosis and management.

Although the figure skating boot has lagged far behind the new technologies incorporated into hockey skates and speed skates that help improve performance and reduce injuries, there has been research and development into new figure skating boots and blade designs. Some of these designs have already been made into prototypes and are undergoing on-ice testing by figure skaters. New skates called *articulated skating boots* are synthetic molded boots incorporating a hinge that allows flexibility at the ankle while maintaining structure and rigidity. They are also 25 percent lighter than the current leather boot. Researchers suggest that an articulation skate could reduce impact loads by 30 percent.

REFERENCES

1. Kjar M, Larsson B: Physiological profile and incidence of injuries among elite figure skaters. *J Sports Sci* 10(1): 29–36, 1992.
2. Smith A: Figure skating, in Schneider RC (ed): *Sports Injuries*. Baltimore, Williams & Williams, 1985, p. 518.
3. Slemenda W, Johnston CC: High-intensity activities in young women: site specific bone mass effects among female figure skaters. *Bone Miner* 20(2):125–132, 1993.
4. Sovak D, Hawes: Anthropological status of international caliber speed skaters. *J Sports Sci* 5(3):287–304, 1987.
5. Clement DB, et al: Iron status in winter olympic sports. *J Sports Sci* 5(3):261–271, 1987.
6. Smith A: Skating injuries: A guide to prevention and management. *J Musculoskel Med* 14(12):10–29, 1997.
7. Pecina M, Bojanic I, Dubravic S: Stress fractures in figure skaters. *Am J Sports Med* 18(3):277–279, 1990.
8. Podolsky A, Kaufmann KR, et al: The relationship of strength and jump height in figure skaters. *Am J Sports Med* 18(4):400–405, 1990.

27	**Cycling**
	Gloria C. Cohen

Cycling is a relationship between the cyclist and the bicycle, both of which can undergo various modifications to enhance this union. It is important to understand this relationship in order to prevent and treat bicycle injuries effectively.

As bicycling becomes increasingly popular among various age groups so, unfortunately, does the incidence of injury. Many recreational riders, from children to adults, are experiencing overuse injuries resulting from improper bike fit, poor riding technique, or doing too much too soon. Elite cyclists or racers often sustain injuries from crashes and collisions from cycling under conditions of high velocity and force. They too succumb to overuse injuries and muscle strains and sprains.

THE BICYCLE

The bicycle is composed of a frame with various components—handlebars, brakes, wheels, pedals, gears, and saddle (Fig. 27-1). Although each bike comes with a set of components, many of the more experienced or elite cyclists tend to use components from various manufacturers on their bikes, thereby individualizing the bike. A bicycle will vary in geometry, stiffness, and weight, depending on its primary function, such as road or track racing, touring, or downhill or cross country mountain biking.

The proper bicycle fit for the cyclist is essential for injury prevention as well as enjoyment. Modifications to this fit are often part of the treatment regime. The frame may be the correct height, but the distance between the seat post and handlebars, that is the length of the top tube, may need adjustment (Fig. 27-2). There should not be more than a 45-degree forward lean. Often riders lean too far forward because of poor sizing and can suffer from neck, back, or hand symptoms from this posturing. Correction may require modifying the handlebar stem or moving the saddle forward. The fore and aft position of the saddle is determined with the rider on the bike with the pedals at the 3 and 9 o'clock positions with the ball of the foot on the pedal.[1,2] A plumb line dropped from the mid-anterior forward patella should fall on the axle of the pedal (Fig. 27-3). For some individuals, a different frame may be the only solution.

The key to a proper bike fit is that different bikes are for different people. The older rider might prefer a beach cruiser or "comfort

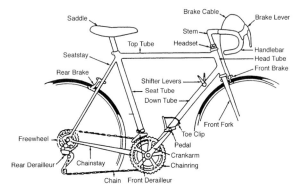

FIG. 27-1 Anatomy and terminology of a "generic" bicycle.

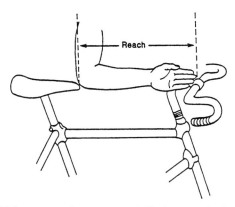

FIG. 27-2 Diagram of handlebar reach. The frame may be the correct height, but the distance between the seat post and handlebars may need adjustment.

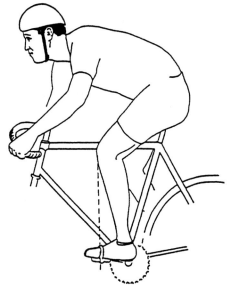

FIG. 27-3 The fore and aft position of the saddle is determined with the rider on the bike with the pedals at the 3 and 9 o'clock positions with the ball of the foot on the pedal.

bike" with a bigger, more comfortable saddle and wider handlebars. The competitive mountain bike racer would be more efficient on a "downhill bike" with more suspension that takes up the bumps for downhill mountain biking.

MUSCULOSKELETAL INJURIES

Musculoskeletal injuries can be divided into two categories: overuse and traumatic.

Overuse Injuries

Overuse or repetitive stress injuries are the more common type and can be further subdivided into particular ailments according to the area of contact the cyclist has with the bicycle—pedal, seat, and handlebar.

The Pedal

Pedal contact describes the relationship of the pedal to the cyclist's lower extremity. There are several types of pedals to choose from, ranging from a platform pedal for recreational riders, to the use of the clipless variety used by competitive and avid cyclists. Toe clips and straps are also used as a way of securing the foot to the pedal.

The forces under the foot during cycling vary with the type of shoe. A stiffer cycling shoe allows for a more even distribution of the pressure than the flexible running or aerobic shoe, as well as a significantly increased index of effectiveness.[3] The first metatarsal head and the hallux tend to contribute the most force in the foot. As the cyclist increases the power output, there are higher peak pressures imparted to the medial forefoot. This may be symptomatic if pronation is present.

The most common problem area in this category of pedal contact is the knee joint, followed next in frequency by ankle and foot injuries. There is considerable compressive force imparted to the patellofemoral joint in cycling. Patellofemoral contact is maximum at 90 degrees of flexion, and then decreases as the knee enters extension.[4]

Patellofemoral pain syndrome (PFPS), referred to as "biker's knee" in cycling, can result from the range of motion of the knee involved in cycling and the pressures exerted across the knee while riding. The rule of the road for many cyclists is "if the knees hurt, gear down." A high gear means a slower spin, and thus a longer period of increased compressive forces across the patellofemoral articulation. Biomechanical malalignment, such as patellar tracking problems and pronating feet with subtalar or rearfoot valgus can contribute to the etiology of this ailment. Improper foot position and incorrect seat height can also play a role.

Management of this problem involves adjusting the pedal system, and correcting for pronation. This may involve either special pedals, or the use of custom-made lightweight orthotics which fit into the cycling shoe. Some cyclists use a Velcro system to secure the device in the shoe. Others might use a fixed cleat system with the alignment assessed using a Fit Kit, which is offered by many cycling stores. It is a system that measures the best position of the various bike parts in relation to the rider's anatomy. A trained individual determines the correct position for the cycling cleats with the rider on the bike using mobile templates in place of the pedals. If this adjustment does not remedy the situation, then the rider may need to switch to a rotating pedal system.

There are several different systems with a good amount of float 5 to 10 degrees of rear heel movement. The foot will move a significant distance without pulling out of the pedal. It will accommodate body abnormalities better than a fixed pedal system. A fixed pedal system demands a perfectly smooth pedaling style. In addition, it may be necessary to adjust the seat height if the seat is too low or too far forward.

Treatment involves use of ice, nonsteroidal anti-inflammatory medication (oral or topical), and physiotherapy (local modalities such as ultrasound, laser, and muscle stimulation, as well as a strengthening and stretching program for the quadriceps and hamstrings), and modification of riding—avoiding hills, long rides, and high gears—until the symptoms have subsided.

Other anterior knee problems are patellar tendinitis, and lateral retinaculuum tightness or plica syndrome. Treatment is as for PFPS, with emphasis on eccentric quadriceps exercises in the case of patellar tendinitis. Although most injuries will respond to the conservative approach to treatment, in some cases of plica syndrome surgery may be required for release of the lateral retinaculum.

Iliotibial band friction syndrome (ITBFS) presents as lateral knee pain, caused by friction of the band over the femoral condyle with each pedal stroke. This is frequently seen with inadequate conditioning and increased hill riding. Biomechanics of the lower extremity and bike fit can also play a role and should be addressed in the management of this problem. The medical protocol previously described applies for this injury.

Hamstring tendinitis presents as pain at the biceps femoris insertion at the posterolateral aspect of the knee. This is increased with hill climbing and with resisted hamstring flexion. Hamstring strain or "pull" tends to be of gradual-onset in cycling, although acute injuries can occur with a sudden hard effort in a deconditioned muscle. In the slow-onset type the rider complains of tightness and discomfort in the upper third of the posterior thigh, especially with climbing. Treatment consists of progressive stretching and strengthening of the hamstring and physiotherapy modalities. Lower back flexibility exercises should be included in the treatment regime. Some find the use of compression shorts beneficial.

Achilles tendinitis can result from improper technique (such as excessive ankling involving exaggerated plantarflexion; or exerting too much force on the pedal in hill climbing), biomechanical malalignment, or inadequate warmup. There is localized tenderness of the tendon, and swelling or crepitus may be present. Along with correction of the preceding factors, medical treatment consists of local physiotherapy, Achilles, gastrocnemius and soleus stretches, ice massage, and nonsteroidal anti-inflammatory medication (NSAIDs). A heel pad placed in both shoes for all activities may be helpful to relieve some of the stretch on the tendon, and to provide some shock absorption. If there is a nodule and swelling present within the tendon, then the cyclist should be referred for an orthopedic consultation for assessment for tenolysis.

Foot problems often present with paraesthesia, commonly in the forefoot, as well as metatarsalgia. The foot numbness usually occurs after a long ride, and will be transient, resolving within 1 h off the bike. It is caused by tight shoes, be it from inside the shoe or outside pressure from shoe straps or clips. This can be aggravated by riding with high pedal resistance. Adjustments to the shoe fit, toe clip size, and cleat position are important to remedy the situation. In some cases placement of an oval metatarsal pad in the pressure area is required. Once again the rider should be advised to ride in a lower gear to decrease the pedal resistance.

The Saddle

The seat or saddle can have an effect on the areas discussed above, but it is the direct contact the cyclist has with this component of the bike that presents its own set of problems. Ischial bursitis may result from constant friction on the ischial bursa. Using a saddle with a proper fit and allowing for an initial "breaking in" period for a new saddle can prevent this condition from occurring.

The "Gel Saddle" made by "Spenco" has a shock-absorbing gel fluid that acts like human tissue. It adds more natural padding. It keeps its shape and this allows extended riding time and comfort. There is also a saddle to lessen problems for patients with prostate trouble. It has no nose and two pads that work independently to remove pressure from the prostate area.

If despite these precautions the saddle soreness does progress to ischial bursitis, then treat with ice massage; physiotherapy with modalities such as ultrasound and laser, as well as stretches, nonsteroidal anti-inflammatory medication; and in persistent cases a cortisone injection into the bursa, preferably under fluoroscopy if available. If the symptoms persist despite the preceding treatment protocol and rest time off the bike, then refer to an orthopedic surgeon for assessment regarding excision of the bursa. Other saddle-related ailments are discussed in the sections on gender-specific conditions and on dermatologic problems.

The Handlebar

The third area of contact to consider between the cyclist and the bicycle is the handlebar. Ulnar neuropathy, or "cyclist's palsy," presents with symptoms of numbness, tingling, and sometimes motor limitation along the course of the ulnar nerve in the ring and little finger. It is usually the superficial sensory branch of the nerve rather than the deep motor branch that is affected. The pressure transmitted by the hands on the handlebars, particularly when riding for long hours or on rough terrain, can irritate or compress the nerve as it passes from the wrist to the hand in the canal of Guyon. Riding with the hands in a hyperextended position on the handlebars can also contribute to the etiology of this neuropathy. The symptoms are usually transient, and can take weeks or months to disappear. The median nerve is not commonly affected in cycling and so carpal tunnel syndrome does not usually occur.

The best initial treatment for these neuropathies is prevention, but implementation of the following steps even after symptoms are present, is beneficial. Use of padded handlebars and padded cycling gloves is effective in cushioning the pressure points and providing shock absorption.

There are also "gel gloves" made with a similar material to the "gel saddle." This material is similar to the normal padding on the hand. It doubles the normal padding and the material is more dense than the usual foam padding.

The cyclist should be encouraged to frequently change hand position on the handlebars to avoid applying constant pressure on the hands. It is important to check the frame fit to ensure that the rider is not leaning too far forward with added weight on the hands. In some cases a switch from drop handlebars to upright ones may remedy the situation.

In downhill mountain biking, the cyclist has a firm grip on the handlebars while descending the variable terrain. This often produces forearm extensor muscle strain from the vibrations incurred while riding. It is helpful to ice the area after the ride. In some instances a supportive band of flexible tape or wrap of a couple of inches in width around the proximal forearm musculature may limit these vibrations during a ride. Regular stretching and strengthening of the extensor muscles, including eccentric contractions, help decrease the severity of these symptoms.

Neck and low back strain can result from incorrect positioning of the handlebars, in addition to improper frame fit. The rider may overreach to the handlebars, thereby forcing the neck into hyperextension and the low back into hyperflexion. Often a cyclist will extend the neck to prevent an improperly fitted helmet from slipping forward. This combined with increased weight onto the upper extremities can cause muscle spasm in the trapezius and levator scapula muscles producing persistent neck and back symptoms.

Proper bike fit and positioning for the individual must be assessed. Changes may include adjusting the handlebar height for an easier reach or moving the seat forward. The elbows should be slightly flexed when the hands are on the handlebars, and the rider should be encouraged to change hand position often. Maintenance of strength and flexibility for the spinal musculature with specific exercises is important. Ice massage, nonsteroidal anti-inflammatory medication, and physiotherapy treatment may also be indicated. A preexisting leg length discrepancy can contribute to low back pain, particularly to symptoms related to the sacroiliac joints. True leg lengths are measured from the anterior superior iliac spines to the medial malleoli, although some measure to the lateral malleoli.[5] Correcting for this leg length difference by addition of a lift inside or outside the shoe, or modification of the pedal/cleat system can alleviate this problem.

The presence of pelvic asymmetry on the bike without a true leg length difference may cause one side of the pelvis to be rotated anteriorly in relationship to the opposite side. This gives the impression that the anteriorly rotated side is longer. The resulting apparent leg length discrepancy is visualized with the cyclist lying supine and observing the uneven levels of the medial malleoli. Manual therapy is usually an effective treatment for the pelvic malalignment along with appropriate spinal stabilization exercises.

If the neck or back symptoms persist, then radiographs should be taken to rule out any underlying bone or joint abnormality. If radicular signs are present initially, this would not be included in this overuse category and should be assessed and managed accordingly.

Traumatic/Impact Injuries

Traumatic and impact injuries range from minor abrasions to fractures to fatal head injuries. The high risk of injury among children emphasizes the need for improved safety measures.

It is well recognized that the use of an approved helmet (one that complies with accepted safety standards) reduces the incidence of head injuries and the number of fatalities occurring from a blow to the head. The two accepted standards for bicycle helmets are the American National Standards Institute (ANSI) one and that of the Snell Memorial Foundation, the latter being the stricter of the two. There is an ANSI or Snell sticker attached to the inside of a helmet that meets these standards. A helmet without a sticker provides a false sense of security to the rider. In order for a helmet to be effective, it must be worn at all times for recreation, training, and competition, regardless of the distance to be traveled. It is estimated that 75 percent of cycling related deaths are a result of head injury.[6]

An approved helmet consists of:

1. A stiff smooth outer shell that distributes the effect of a blow to the head, and protects against penetration from sharp objects.

2. A nonspringy foam liner made of expanded polystyrene that absorbs shock by crushing. It should be at least 1/2 inch thick. Size-adjustment pads can be attached by velcro for a secure fit for proper head protection.

3. A strong retention system that ensures that the helmet is properly and comfortably positioned on the head. One should not be able to displace or remove the helmet without unfastening the buckle. Only about half the forehead should be visible.

Once there has been an impact to a helmet, with or without any visible damage to the inner or outer shell, it is recommended that the helmet be replaced with a new one, as it may not perform its function a second time.

The guidelines regarding return to activity depend on the severity of the injury and the presence of any subsequent symptoms. "Second impact syndrome" can occur if the rider suffers a second blow when there has not been complete recovery from a previous concussion.

Traumatic injuries to the musculoskeletal system are contusions, sprains, and fractures. These injuries tend to occur on the left side of the body.[7] This may reflect the fact that most cyclists find right-hand turns easier than left-hand ones, and tend to slow or hesitate when making fast left turns. With the derailleur and "drive train" or working parts of the bike on the right, cyclists prefer to fall to their left to protect these components. In competitive cycling, track races are counterclockwise, whereas road races are in both directions.

The most common fractures sustained in cycling are those involving the upper extremity. Clavicular fractures usually occur from a fall on the point of the shoulder or on the outstretched arm. Most fractures occur in the middle third of the clavicle. The diagnosis is usually obvious with a visible deformity, pain, crepitus, or fracture motion. The proximal portion is displaced superiorly to the distal fragment. X-rays confirm the diagnosis. Clavicular fractures are described by the location of the fracture (middle, distal, or proximal third), amount of angulation, and displacement.

Treatment for the nondisplaced or minimally displaced fracture consists of symptomatic treatment with a sling or a figure 8 strap/harness for 4 to 8 weeks (until the fracture is healed), analgesics as needed, and early rehabilitation with gentle range of motion exercises of the shoulder to maintain mobility. The athlete should not ride or train for at least 1 week postinjury. Once the pain has subsided, he or she may train on a turbotrainer or stationary bicycle while continuing to wear the figure 8 bandage. Road riding can be resumed about 3 weeks postinjury, providing it is on level terrain. Use of a mountain bike on the road may allow more shock absorption at this stage. A follow-up x-ray should be taken at

6 weeks postinjury to confirm fraction union. The cyclist may return to competition at that time.

Prevention is important. The cyclist should learn to fall with the arms tucked into the body and a tuck and roll motion. Beginners can practice this on soft grass with their coach. If there is significant displacement or severe skin tenting resulting from the angulation of the fracture, then open reduction is recommended.

Acromioclavicular joint (AC) separations usually result from a direct blow to the point of the shoulder from a fall from the bike. The impact usually causes the acromion to be forced downward. Occasionally this injury can occur from a fall onto an outstretched arm, transmitting the forces up to the AC joint. The cyclist presents with pain, tenderness, swelling, possible deformity, and drooping of the arm and shoulder on the affected side.

The AC joint injuries are graded in three stages according to the extent of ligament injury. Radiographs are required for accurate diagnosis. Fracture of the distal end of the clavicle or avulsion of the tip of the coracoid process must be ruled out. An anterior view of both AC joints may show a mild joint separation. An additional stress or weighted x-ray determines the measurable separation of the joint and compares the coracoclavicular space to that of the unaffected side.

Grade 1

A grade 1 sprain is a mild sprain of the acromioclavicular (AC) and coracoclavicular (CC) ligaments with no separation of the joint. There is tenderness and swelling over only the AC joint with minimal decrease in shoulder movement. The clavicle is stable.

Treatment is conservative with ice, analgesics, and anti-inflammatory medication, a sling for support and physiotherapy (local modalities as well as range of motion and strengthening exercises). Road riding can resume as tolerated, preferably on smooth level terrain initially. The cyclist can return to racing when the AC joint is nontender and shoulder range of motion is full, usually 2 to 3 weeks postinjury. As a safety precaution when returning to cycling, the athlete should tape a rubber doughnut pad about 1 inch thick over the AC joint to protect the area.

Grade 2

A grade 2 sprain is a severe sprain of the AC ligament, with little or no injury to the CC ligament. Injury to the CC ligament may present as a partial tear or stretching of the ligament. There is considerable tenderness and swelling over the AC joint and some tenderness over the CC ligament. Shoulder range of motion is significantly limited secondary to pain and slight elevation of the distal clavicle. Reinjury at this stage could aggravate the injury to a grade 3 injury.

Treatment is as above, but immobilization is for a longer period, usually 3 to 4 weeks, with a modified Kenny-Howard sling (Fig. 27-4). Cycling on the road is not recommended until about 3 to 4 weeks postinjury, but the athlete can use a stationary bike or wind trainer until then. Then he or she can train on level road, avoiding climbing. Normal upper body weight training can resume at 7 weeks, and racing by 7 to 8 weeks, according to the preceding guidelines.

Grade 3

A grade 3 sprain is a complete tearing of the AC and CC ligaments, often with damage to the deltoid and trapezius muscles. There is marked swelling, tenderness, and obvious deformity of the AC

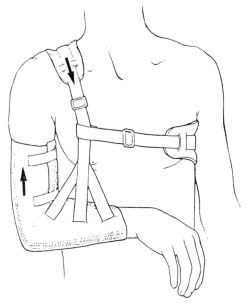

FIG. 27-4 Diagram of modified Kenny-Howard sling consisting of a strap across the chest and elbows sling to support and maintain the AC joint.

joint with upward displacement of the distal clavicle. This category can be expanded to include further compound injuries.

There is some treatment controversy depending on the extent of the injury and the situation. Usual treatment is the conservative approach with a progression of that described for grade 2 in the preceding. Return to riding may take as long as 10 to 12 weeks. The operative approach has often been supported for manual workers and elite athletes. These injuries should be referred to an orthopedic surgeon for assessment and management. Possible prevention is a tuck and roll when you fall.

Possible complications from this injury include degenerative changes of the acromion with osteophyte formation, soft tissue calcification, and osteolysis of the distal clavicle.

Wrist injuries occur from a fall on an outstretched hand. Fracture of a carpal bone, particularly of the scaphoid (navicular), must be ruled out in the initial assessment of a possible acute wrist ligament sprain.

Tenderness on palpation over the scaphoid in the "anatomical snuffbox" is highly suggestive of a fractured scaphoid. Radiographs of the wrist must include scaphoid views. Oftentimes the initial x-rays are negative despite clinical findings suggesting a fracture.

Treatment is immobilization is a scaphoid plaster or fiberglass (lighter) cast. This extends from the interphalangeal joint of the thumb to just below the elbow with the wrist in slight radial deviation and dorsiflexion. Healing time depends on the fracture site, commonly at least 8 to 12 weeks, but can be 12 to 20 weeks. Repeat radiographs to be taken at 2 and 4 weeks postinjury. A bone scan is helpful in confirming the diagnosis and may be positive within 48 to 72 h of injury. It is certainly positive by 2 weeks postinjury. There is a high risk of complications from this injury such as delayed union, nonunion, and avascular necrosis. The athlete should be referred to an orthopedic surgeon for all displaced fractures, fractures of the proximal third, persistent clinical findings despite negative investigations, and any complications.

Acute wrist ligament sprains are treated with initial ice, nonsteroidal anti-inflammatory medication, wrist support, gradual range of motion and strengthening exercises, and physiotherapy if indicated.

Spoke injuries occur when a body part is trapped between the frame and the spokes of a bicycle. This can result in laceration, crushing, and shearing injuries. Sometimes the true severity of the injury is not apparent for several days, so monitor closely. The bicycle should be equipped with a spoke guard if there is a child carrier attached to the bicycle. "Doubling," or giving another person a ride on a bicycle, should be prohibited.

ABDOMINAL INJURIES

Injuries to the abdomen can occur from bicycle accidents. It is important to be cognizant that handlebar trauma has been responsible for various abdominal injuries, sometimes involving the viscera. Insidious symptoms may delay the diagnosis. A traumatic "handlebar hernia," although rare, can occur from the impact of a bicycle handlebar on the abdominal wall.[8] A CT scan of the abdomen is important in confirming diagnosis along with physical examination.

Intimal tearing of the external iliac artery can occur after blunt trauma to the groin or abdomen.[9] The cyclist may present with subsequent symptoms of claudication in the ipsilateral thigh. This requires cardiovascular referral for assessment and management. If Doppler examination and angiography demonstrate arterial occlusion the cyclist requires surgery for external iliac artery resection and placement of a Dacron graft.

There have also been nontrauma cases of intimal thickening of the external iliac artery where the lesions were unilateral and the cyclist experienced symptoms of claudication only during very intense efforts.[10] It is postulated that repetitive kinking of the artery with the rider in a tucked position might contribute to the arterial wall damage.

DERMATOLOGICAL INJURIES

Skin problems can be of acute or chronic origin. "Road rash," the term used for abrasions sustained while cycling, is the most common cycling injury. The severity of the wound is graded similar to that for burns: first degree, superficial; second degree, partial thickness; third degree, full thickness.

It is imperative that the wound be thoroughly cleansed and embedded dirt particles removed soon after the injury has occurred to prevent infection and tattooing. Sterile water and antibacterial solutions or water-diluted hydrogen peroxide can be used. If the preceding are unavailable, then use tap water and simple soap. If the cleansing is done within the first few minutes after the injury, there is often decreased pain possibly owing to numbness in the area from the trauma. As time from the injury elapses, there is increased pain and edema that develops. Topical analgesic such as lidocaine gel (Xylocaine 2%, 4%) or local injectable lidocaine are then used to enable proper cleaning of the wound with the spongy side of a prepackaged surgical sponge brush. Many cyclists keep a sponge brush in their kit bag for cleaning themselves when immediate medical attention is unavailable. When the sponge is not sufficient to remove the embedded dirt, then a sterile nailbrush or toothbrush may be needed.

After the wound is cleaned, a topical antibiotic ointment and a nonadherent dressing, such as a Telfa pad, are applied. Antibiotic gauze mesh tends to stick to the abrasion and should be avoided. The wound should be kept moist to promote healing and a hydroactive dressing, such as DuoDerm, Tegaderm, Op-Site, or Second Skin, applied. Neosporin or Polysporin is readily available. An elastic tubular netting (such as Surginet) holds the dressing in place while still allowing the rider movement of the extremities. Tetanus prophylaxis status should be determined and updated if required.

For follow-up care the dressing should be changed once to twice daily for wound inspection for any signs of infection, and further cleansing and application of antibiotic. The wound may be left open to air after about 5 to 6 days when healing is apparent. Complete healing takes place by 10 to 12 days. To prevent further scarring and blistering, sunscreen should be applied over the healed area.

Abrasions are usually associated with contusions so the area should be treated with ice. Be aware of the possibility of an underlying muscle contusion with a large or third-degree abrasion, and monitor for signs of compartment syndrome or myositis ossificans. Wearing a thin layer of clothing underneath the usual cycling attire can reduce the risk of road rash as the two layers of fabric slide over each other.

Chafing and other dermatologic problems can arise from improper saddle fit and long hours of cycling. This can lead to saddle sores (folliculitis, furuncles) from direct friction and irritation of the skin and hair follicles in the perineal and inner thigh regions and the buttocks. These lesions can range from trivial to severe.

Treatment is symptomatic involving warm soaks and topical antibiotics with or without nonfluorinated corticosteroid cream if indicated. Preventive as well as therapeutic measures include good personal hygiene; padded cycling shorts that are washed frequently (to avoid chafing they should be worn without underwear and there should be no seam in the chamois); padded saddle of appropriate shape; and lubricating cream (zinc-based; Cramer's Skin Lube) applied to the skin as well as the chamois. In some cases it may be necessary to shave the perineum to prevent traction on the perineal hair and subsequent folliculitis.

If deep boils, furuncles, or folliculitis with abscesses develop, incision and drainage, oral antibiotics, and time off the bike to allow healing may be required. If the sores tend to be unilateral, or continually recur on the same side, examine for leg length discrepancy and pelvic malalignment. Deep painful fibrous nodules may develop which warrant surgical excision.

FEMALE CONCERNS

Yeast vulvitis and vaginitis may be a recurring problem for women riders. The importance of good personal hygiene, including early change of clothing after riding and washing of cycling shorts after each use are advised. Appropriate antimycotic creams and tablets, and thorough drying of the perineum after cleaning the area often achieve satisfactory results.

Vulvar hematoma may result from blunt or sharp trauma to the vulva. This must be closely monitored as the bleeding can extend along tissue planes to involve the broad ligament. Ice is applied frequently for the first 48 h, then heat. If the hematoma is expanding, or if it is large initially, arrange for a gynecologic referral for assessment and possible surgical exploration. There is a concern that a vessel may need to be ligated. If there is a stable, large, anterior hematoma, hospitalization may be required for the first 24 to 48 h for catheterization.

Most moderate size hematomas can be managed on an outpatient basis, but observe for any signs of infection. In some cases a short course of prophylactic antibiotics may be indicated. The rider should remain off the bike until the swelling, tenderness, and erythema have resolved. When she returns to riding, it is suggested that she wear padded cycling shorts or add saddle padding to cushion the area. Some women apply a zinc-based cream to the area before riding to decrease friction and irritation.

There is a special saddle with a nose area with an oval shape, which can be hollow or very soft. That area bends down to alleviate pressure. A company named "Terry" specializes in women's products.

MALE CONCERNS

Anterior saddle cant in men can cause pudendal neuropathy with symptoms of transient numbness and tingling in the penile shaft and scrotum. This is caused by compression of the dorsal branch of the pudendal nerve between the symphysis pubis and the saddle. To alleviate the problem check the saddle position. The saddle should be level or minimally slanted upward, and of the correct height. The rider should be encouraged to change his position on the bike and stand at times. If the symptoms persist despite adjustment to the cant, increasing the padding in the cycling shorts or on the saddle may be helpful. Sometimes the solution is a wider saddle, or one with a longitudinal furrow to decrease the pressure concentrated on any one area of the anatomy. If symptoms persist despite these modifications, then refer for urologic consultation (Fig. 27-5).

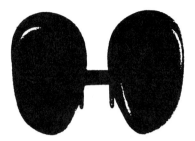

FIG. 27-5   Easy saddle relieves prostatic pressure.

Although not commonly seen, male impotence can result from continued pudendal nerve compression after repeated or multiday rides. The cyclist complains of inability to attain an erection. The rider is advised to stop riding until the symptoms resolve, then to reevaluate the bike fit and make the necessary adjustments as discussed for pudendal neuropathy. As in the preceding, urologic referral is indicated for persistent symptoms.

Traumatic urethritis and prostatitis can present with symptoms ranging from asymptomatic microscopic hematuria to gross hematuria and dysuria. The chronic pressure in this region with cycling may aggravate chronic prostatitis in older males. Benign prostatic hypertrophy must be ruled out. Management is mechanical as discussed in pudendal neuropathy, as well as medical. The indication for nonsteroidal anti-inflammatory medication and antibiotics needs to be assessed on an individual basis.

ALTERNATE FORMS OF CYCLING

The use of a stationary bicycle or a recumbent bicycle, are alternatives to cardiovascular conditioning when the athlete is recovering from an injury, provided the use of these bikes does not aggravate the symptoms. The seat should be adjusted in both types of cycles so that there is no stress on the knees, avoiding full extension and hyperextension. Improper positioning on the recumbent bike, and increased resistance on the stationary bicycle can lead to patellofemoral pain syndrome.

TRIATHLONS

This endurance competition involves swimming, cycling, and running in succession. Thermoregulation is important to avoid hyperthermia and hypothermia. Appropriate hydration and nutrition intake before, during, and after the race must be followed to prevent dehydration and nutritional and electrolyte imbalance. Triathletes are not permitted to follow another cyclist too closely, that is the "no drafting" rule, which decreases the risk of multiple cyclists crashes (Fig. 27-6).

SAFETY AND PREVENTION

Safety plays a significant role in injury prevention and has been discussed under several sections in this chapter. Cyclists of all ages must be aware that the bicycle is a vehicle that commands proper cycling skills and careful behavior. Safety promotion programs starting as early as kindergarten, are now being offered through several schools and community centers. Other preventive measures being developed are motorist education and increased availability of bicycle paths.

It is imperative that the bike be kept in proper mechanical order, with particular attention to brake wear and adjustment, tires, derailleurs, and spokes. A helmet should always be worn when cycling, and reflectors (bike reflectors and reflective tape) and lights used when riding at night or in the city. As previously discussed, various types of protective clothing and equipment are beneficial. Protective eyewear should be of an unbreakable material such as polycarbonate.

Various environment conditions can present problems for the ill-prepared cyclist. Cycling on a warm or hot day can lead to dehydration if appropriate efforts are not made to maintain adequate

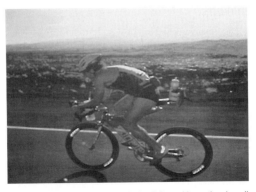

FIG. 27-6   An ideal, durable, triathalon bike, with resting handle bars and water bottle holder.

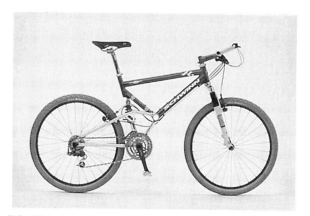

FIG. 27-7 This is a competition racing mountain bike with shock absorbing frame.

hydration. A standard bicycle water bottle holds 20 ounces (600 mL) of fluid and that quantity would not be sufficient fluid replacement for a long ride. The cyclist should be able to pass clear urine every 1 to 2 h.

Sunscreen should be applied to prevent sunburn and development of skin cancers, including melanomas. This includes application to the often forgotten, but very much exposed, external ear.

CONCLUSION

In summary, many cycling injuries result from overuse. This can be partially remedied by assuring proper frame fit and correct cycling technique and equipment for the individual. Accidents, however, will still occur, so it is important to be prepared for assessment and management of these injuries (Fig. 27-7).

REFERENCES

1. Mellion MB: Common cycling injuries: Management and prevention. *Sports Med* 11(1):52–70, 1991.
2. Mellion MB, Hill JW: Bicycling, in Mellion MB, Walsh WM, Shelton GL (eds): *The Team Physician's Handbook*, 2d ed. Philadelphia, Hanley & Belfus, 1997, pp. 785–789.
3. Henning EM, Sanderson DJ: In-shoe pressure distributions for cycling with two types of footwear at different mechanical loads. *J Appl Biomech* 11:68–80, 1995.

4. Leadbetter WB, Schneider MJ: Cycling injury, in Kraus J (ed): *The Bicycle Book*. New York, Dial, 1982, pp. 195–214.

5. Reid DC: *Sports Injury: Assessment and Rehabilitation*. New York, Churchill Livingstone, 1992.

6. Burke ER: Safety standards for bicycle helmets. *Phys Sports Med* 16(1):148–153, 1988.

7. Bohlmann JT: Injuries in competitive cycling. *Phys Sports Med* 9(5):117–124, 1981.

8. Mitchiner JC: Handlebar hernia: Diagnosis by abdominal computed tomography. *Ann Emerg Med* 19:812–813, 1990.

9. Scheerlinck TAM, Van den Brande P: Posttraumatic intima dissection and thrombosis of the external iliac artery in a sportsman. *Eur J Vasc Surg* 8:645–647, 1994.

10. Rousselet MC, Saint-Andre JP, L'Hoste P, et al: Stenotic intimal thickening of the external iliac artery in competition cyclists. *Hum Pathol* 21(5):524–529, 1990.

11. Cohen GC: Cycling injuries. *Can Fam Phys* 39:628–632, 1993.

12. Hopkins SR: Bicycling, in Agostini R (ed): *Medical and Orthopedic Issues of Active and Athletic Women*. Philadelphia, Hanley & Belfus, 1994, pp. 419–429.

13. Burke ER: *Science of Cycling*. Illinois, Human Kinetics Publishers, 1986.

14. Garrick JG, Webb DR: *Sports Injuries: Diagnosis and Management*. Philadelphia, Saunders, 1990.

28 | Racquet Sports, Tennis, and Squash

Marlene Nobrega   *R. Charles Bull*

Tennis originated in the 1100s or 1200s in France; it was called "jeu de paume," meaning the game of the palm. The players batted the ball back and forth over the net with the palm of the hand, similar to handball.

The modern version was developed in England in 1873 when Major Wingfield patented the tennis racquet, and it became known as "lawn tennis," since it was played outdoors on grass. This spread quite quickly to the United States; the U.S. National Lawn and Tennis Association was established in 1881. International tennis became a professional sport in 1968.

Squash originated at Harrow in England in 1850 and became popular in the United States in 1880. There are two forms, American and English. The English court is slightly wider at 21 ft (6.4 m), whereas the American court is $18\frac{1}{2}$ ft (5.6 m).

In the American game, a 15-point score wins, whereas in the English rules, the server must score 9 points to win. The first player to win three games wins the match. The American ball is more solid and bouncy, and the English ball makes a "squash" sound when it hits. The player has more time to retrieve the ball in the English game.

Squash is a faster game than tennis and more taxing on the joints. Sudden deaths occur in squash, rarely, owing to the intensity of the cardiovascular workout. More recently the number of elite junior tennis programs worldwide has grown. Germany, Czechoslovakia, Canada, and Sweden have produced stars and overtaken the United Kingdom and the United States.

Also, the equipment has changed dramatically. Initially, the surface was closely trimmed grass, and small wooden racquets were used. This progressed to steel and now graphite and titanium racquets are available.

Tennis is a very versatile game that allows people of all ages to play satisfactorily against their peers, and players of different ability can rally well, although minor skill differences can result in large score differences in a game. Conditioning is vital for singles play, whereas doubles is more forgiving. To play well in singles, one usually needs additional cardiovascular training, that is, interval running, whereas doubles play does not need that additional work. It can usually give senior players a satisfactory workout over the course of 1 h.

INJURIES

Most injuries in tennis are classified as overuse. Some series report injuries as high as 74 percent in men and 60 percent in women in world-class players. The most common injuries are to the rotator cuff (impingement syndrome), in biceps tendon in the shoulder, lateral and medial epicondylitis in the elbow, tendinitis in the wrist, low back and abdominal muscle strains, leg muscle cramps, and plantar fasciitis.

Rupture of the medial head of gastrocnemius (tennis leg) often occurs, as does Achilles tendon rupture. Ankle sprains are common, especially on the hard court.

The mechanics of the racquet stroke, and body movements in serving (overhead) are different in the club players and elite level players. Elite players use their legs and trunks as much as their arms to generate power and speed. The recreational player tends to overuse the shoulder and arm.

The serve is broken down into four stages.

1. *Windup* from the serving stance to the toss of the ball, and this showed very low EMG activity.
2. The serving, or *cocking phase*, which begins after the ball toss and terminates at the maximum external rotation of the glenohumeral joint. This also requires rotation and hyperextension of the back. Muscular activity is moderately high in supraspinatus, infraspinatus, subscapularis, biceps, and serratus anterior. The stabilizing effect of the rotator cuff is clearly shown in this cocking phase.
3. The third phase of the tennis serve is *acceleration*, and it begins at maximal external rotation and hyperextension and terminates at ball impact. This is similar to the acceleration phase in throwing and has the highest muscular activity (see Chap. 4). The muscles involved in the shoulder are pectoralis major, subscapularis, latissimus dorsi, serratus anterior, as well as deltoid, trapezius, and triceps.
4. The fourth and final phase occurs after impact. This is *followthrough* and derotation to return facing the net. This is characterized by moderate activity of the posterior rotator cuff, serratus anterior, biceps, deltoid and latissimus dorsi, and there is flexion of the spine. In unskilled players, the contribution of the lower extremity and trunk muscles is less, and they are apt to have more stress on their shoulder girdle muscles. The degree of abduction and extension in the second or cocking phase often leads to impingement.

Many club players roll over the ball to achieve topspin, and this increases the shoulder impingement. The other strokes include volley and forehand and backhand ground strokes—each causes mechanical problems in the shoulder, elbow, wrist, and back, and certainly hyperextension and rotation of the back creates problems.

STROKE MECHANICS

In the authors' opinion, poor stroke technique is the most important predisposing factor of upper extremity injury in the recreational player. This is not true in the elite or professional player.

The following are important principles in understanding tennis biomechanics.

1. To be successful at tennis, a player must develop control, consistency, depth, and power. The successful player must not sacrifice control, consistency, or depth for increased power.

   This is a common error in all players. The professional game has certainly become a slugfest both on the men's and women's tour. Professional players spend as much time in the gym as they do on the court. Pros are bigger, stronger, and more powerful than ever. The advances in technology provide players with powerful racquets. The difference is that professional players can control the power and do not produce as many abnormal forces for the body to absorb. Recreational players want to hit like their favorite pro, so they often purchase a much too powerful weapon for their ability and then try to hit the life out of the ball.

   More Control, Less Power = Fewer Injuries

2. Any golfer will tell you "it's all in the grip!" and faulty grip biomechanics in the amateur golfer (females in particular) are the leading cause of upper extremity injury.

   The grip on the racquet is just as important. It becomes confusing, as there are three variations of tennis grip. The Western, Eastern, and Continental (Fig. 28-1). In the past, most players used one grip (Continental) for all strokes. At present most tennis coaches teach different grip styles. The grip type depends on the player's ability, style of play, and shot selection.

   In patients complaining of any upper extremity injury, in particular wrist and elbow pain, the grip should be evaluated by their teaching professional. A common error seen in the amateur player is the attempt to place a lot of topspin on the ball in the forehand and to slice the backhand. These shots can produce tremendous forces on the elbow and wrist at the best of times, let alone when the grip mechanics are faulty. Wrist pain in the professional players is a common complaint and is the result of the heavy topspin being placed on their shots.

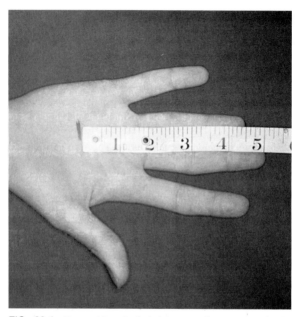

FIG. 28-1 Racquet handle "grip." Larger grips are more forgiving when elbow and wrist problems are present. A comfortable size can be selected by measuring the distance from the middle of the palm to the tip of the middle finger (shown here as 5 inches or 12.7 cm).

In those players wishing to continue to play or train while injured, recommend that they return to hitting the ball flat while recovering.

3. "Tennis is a lower body sport." What happens to the ball when it leaves the racquet starts at the ground. The forces begin at the ground, to lower limb, to hips, to trunk, to upper limb, to racquet. This is the kinetic link principle. When you leave one part out of the "linked" system or the links occur in the wrong order, the athlete will place forces on other links, and the result is *injury*.

The most common example of this error in the recreational player occurs in the one-handed backhand stroke. The player contacts the ball late and leads with the elbow and then "flicks" the wrist in an effort to move the ball off the racquet.

Biomechanically, a one-handed backhand requires more links working in sequence. The two-handed backhand requires fewer links as the trunk and upper extremities all move together as one segment. It is simple—the fewer parts to worry about, the lower the percentage of error and abnormal force production.

In reality, the two-handed backhand is a forehand with the arm at the back of the racquet acting as the dominant force. The player must use body rotation to hit the ball, thereby reducing the chances of leading with the arms before the trunk. The essential body rotation also generates the much wanted power of the stroke.

ANATOMY

For our purposes, the shoulder girdle is made up of four separate articulations. These are the glenohumeral joint, which is by far the most important; the scapulothoracic articulation; the sternoclavicular joint; and the acromioclavicular joint.

The shoulder is a very mobile joint, because the glenoid itself is only approximately 50 percent of the size of the humeral head, but the bony contact is augmented by the glenoid labrum, which is a fibrocartilaginous rim or collar that attaches around the labrum. The ball is held in the socket by a capsule of tough tissue that is attached close to the humeral head, except at its most inferior margin, where it is 3 cm below the edge of the articulation.

There are thickened areas in the capsule that form the glenohumeral ligaments—superior, middle, and inferior. There are four muscles in the anterior and posterior shoulder girdle. There are two muscles anteriorly, subscapularis, which inserts into the lesser tuberosity, and supraspinatus, which comprises the most important superior aspect of the rotator cuff. This muscle initiates abduction or the ability to pull the arm away from the side of the body, and if this motion is weak or supraspinatus does not contract properly, it is pathognomonic of a ruptured or torn rotator cuff. Supraspinatus attaches the upper part of the greater tuberosity and is often torn at the part or in the body of the tendon.

The posterior shoulder girdle muscles are infraspinatus and teres minor, which play a lesser role in the subacromial pathology.

The acromioclavicular, or AC, joint at the latter end of the clavicle has a wedge-shaped meniscus, and this is often torn. The coracoacromial ligament forms the subacromial or coracoacromial arch; the subacromial bursa lies between this arch and the humeral head, and it is often compromised. The amount of clearance can be altered by degeneration, spurring, muscular hypertrophy, inflammation, and so on.

Impingement of the bursa most commonly occurs between 60 and 120 degrees in the painful arc, and pain in that area is pathognomonic of a shoulder bursitis syndrome.

The most important factor in the diagnosis is the patient's history. The athlete should be able to point directly to the area of maximum tenderness, that is, the biceps tendon, coracoacromial ligament, posterior biceps tendon area, and so on. Other factors, such as dead arm symptoms or complete numbness and inability to use the arm, often suggest nerve root irritation or brachial plexus impingement. The thoracic outlet syndrome is often suggested when the pulse disappears when you raise the arm in abduction past 90 degrees or have a positive Wright's or Adson's test (see Chap. 6).

A thorough examination is important, and you have to check the athlete muscle by muscle and work your way down from the neck, throughout the shoulder, into the wrist, and down throughout the back, and so on. Squash players often have a hypertrophied dominant shoulder and forearm musculature, and hypertrophy is commonly seen in the forearm of the dominant racquet arm (Fig. 28-2).

Also, glenohumeral instability is very important. It is assessed by grasping the humeral head and moving it in the glenoid. Obviously you should test the opposite shoulder. Some athletes become so lax they can freely sublux their shoulders.

Once the rotator cuff is inflamed or torn or the patient has tendinitis in the biceps or bursa, quality players will exhibit muscle activity patterns similar to amateurs.

Common findings on examination of the shoulder include the following:

1. Excess external rotation of the glenohumeral joint (dominant arm) tested in 90-degree abduction. This extra rotation is required in the service motion.
2. Reduced internal rotation
3. Weakness of the external rotators or decelerators, especially eccentrically
4. Tightness of the internal rotators (rounded shoulders)
5. Weakness of the scapular stabilizers
6. Tight posterior capsule glenohumeral joint

Another injury that is created in the deceleration phase is the "snapping scapula." This is a painful discomfort owing to an inflamed bursa beneath the medial border of the scapula where it moves on the thorax. This can give a grinding and crunching, and it gradually subsides with rest, physiotherapy, and good follow-through and an altered serving and stroking pattern.

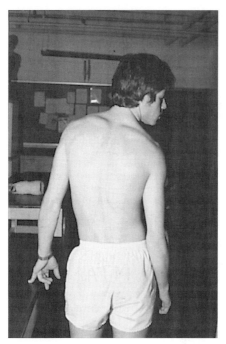

FIG. 28-2 Tennis shoulder. Early one-sided training and excessive loading lead to "tennis shoulder." The racquet arm has an increased size of bones, muscles, and increased laxity of the joint capsule occurs. The shoulder is lowered and the arm is relatively lengthened. Also note an "S" shape scoliosis off the thoracic spine.

To prevent and rehabilitate the tennis player's shoulder syndromes:

1. Improve glenohumeral internal rotation;
2. Stretch the posterior capsule; and
3. Strengthen the decelerators and scapular stabilizers.

If progress is not made by 6 weeks in a player with a shoulder injury, one has to assume that there is a significant rotator cuff or labral tear, and an MRI should be ordered. In most cases, arthroscopic repair can be done, and in some cases of severe impingement syndrome, an anterior acromioplasty or partial resection of the acromion is indicated.

Common Elbow Injuries in Tennis

Tennis elbow is the most common affliction occurring in recreational tennis players. It is much less common in professional players. The pathology involves the elbow, wrist, and finger extensors. The pain is at the external epicondyle and the origin of extensor carpi radialis brevis and is caused by improper backhand strokes. The wrist should be firm during the backhand stroke, and a two-handed backhand should be emphasized.

The player complains of pain and weakness, and in extreme cases there is atrophy of the extensor muscles of the forearm. When the pain is quite acute, physiotherapy is usually beneficial. Three steroid injections right into the periosteum over the lateral epicondyle and adjacent to the extensor tendon can be done, each 1 month apart. There are a number of braces available that vary from the clasp to the full elbow, forearm (Lastrap), and upper arm type.

This lateral compartment type of tendinitis often involves the wrist and finger extensors, which are particularly vulnerable during the deceleration or follow-through phase.

Flexor tendinitis of the wrist and finger flexor tendons is often referred to as "golfer's elbow." This is more apt to occur in professional players from hitting too hard. Again, stretching of the flexors and pronator teres is recommended, bracing and steroid injections are also effective. Surgery is almost never effective in the medial aspect, whereas a lateral tennis elbow release is usually a satisfactory procedure in the 10 percent of cases that are resistant to conservative therapy.

Wrist and Hand Injuries

Wrist and hand injuries are multiple and differ in tennis from squash injuries. In tennis, the ball is hit with a stiff wrist, whereas squash requires a snapping of the wrist.

Wrist injuries can occur from direct, blunt trauma such as a fall or sudden uncontrolled force with a serve and most often from repetitive, controlled, persistent play. Wrist tendinitis is commonly caused by hitting topspin strokes. The racquet should be altered, and a consultation with the pro is often beneficial.

De Quervain's tenosynovitis occurs at the level of the radial styloid where abductor pollicis longus and extensor pollicis brevis pass through the fibro-osseous canal. This can be treated by cortisone injection but often needs surgical release.

"Squeaker's" wrist, or tennis wrist, often occurs just proximal to that in the bursa, involving those two tendons as they pass over the radius. This swelling is quite dramatic and often improves with splinting, anti-inflammatory medications, and cortisone injection.

Tennis players also get a swelling and thickening at the base of the second and third metacarpals, called a "carpometacarpal boss." This can be mistaken for a ganglion, but usually it is just inflamed tissue at the insertion of the wrist extensors and responds to rest and physiotherapy.

Fractures of the hook of the hamate can occur in tennis players when the handle of the racquet is jammed against the hamate, and this is diagnosed by local tenderness over the hook of the hamate and tendinitis of the fifth finger flexors. It is important to order special hamate x-ray views (see Chap. 7).

Scapholunate dislocations can occur in tennis from a fall on the courts or in squash from a trauma against the wall. It is important to order special carpal x-ray views. In this case, arthroscopy of the wrist can often be helpful (see Chap. 7).

Tears of the triangular fibrocartilaginous complex (TFC) of the wrist also often occur in racquet sports. This can also be diagnosed and treated arthroscopically. We do a debridement of the triangular flap tear and a synovectomy, which usually returns the tennis player to the sport within 4 to 6 weeks.

There is also a rare condition in racquet sports called chondromalacia of the pisiform, or "racquet player's pisiform." This can respond to simple excision of the pisiform.

Carpal tunnel syndrome and ulnar nerve compression both occur frequently in tennis and squash, and these can be surgically decompressed.

Back Strain

Back strain is quite common in tennis players, both acute and chronic. During the service, motion hyperextension and extreme torque of the lumbar spine occur. Abdominal muscle strengthening is the key to avoiding and rehabilitating this.

Abdominal Injury

Abdominal rectus muscle tearing results when the player tries to hit the ball when it is behind him or her, and the player reaches back and snaps his or her body forward. This can be quite severe, and the diagnosis of acute abdomen is sometimes made. Basically, this is difficult to treat, but rest, swimming, and gradual resumption of abdominal exercises, such as crunches and so on, are beneficial. Strengthening the upper and lower abdominal muscles concentrically and eccentrically is important (see Chap. 33).

Tennis Leg

Rupture of the medial head of gastroc, called "tennis leg," frequently occurs in tennis and squash. The player plants the foot and extends the knee and feels very severe pain at the medial head of gastroc and a tearing sensation. There is early swelling, usually the next day, and marked immobility. This can often take 4 to 6 weeks to settle, but the player usually returns to full competition without the need for surgical intervention.

Achilles Tendon Injury

Achilles tendon rupture also occurs in tennis and squash, and the player thinks that his or her opponent has hit him or her with the racquet. Manually squeezing the calf should cause the foot to dorsiflex, and the player should be able to do a one-legged toe stand. Often you can feel the gap in the Achilles tendon. If in doubt, this type of injury should be referred, as this is one of the most commonly missed injuries in sports.

Ankle Injury

Ankle sprains are also very common in tennis, and these are very difficult for the elite player to overcome as he or she loses proprioceptive and stereotactic reflexes (see Chap. 16). The elite player must be rehabilitated aggressively, with closed kinetic strengthening and proprioceptive drills. Many players wear ankle supports and braces postinjury.

Plantar fasciitis and calcaneal fasciitis are major problems in tennis; these are dealt with well in Chaps. 10 and 16.

EQUIPMENT

There are two factors that contribute to injury: an increased shock load owing to "off-center" hits, that is, not hitting in the sweet spot, and frame vibration.

Racquets

The size and the composition of the racquet are crucial.

Size

Oversized racquets are best. Oversized racquet heads have larger sweet spots and therefore reduce the number of off-center hits, thereby reducing the vibration and shock load. Wide body racquets generate more power. They allow players with slower swing mechanics to enjoy playing a more powerful game. With a thin body racquet, the player must generate his or her own power from the swing mechanics. As the average recreational player has several swing mechanic faults, the more help he or she can get from the racquet the less strain there will be on the body.

Composition

Frames are made of graphite, fiberglass, kevlar, ceramic, and now titanium. Graphite frames are more forgiving; they are lighter and produce less frame vibration than aluminum frames.

Tennis equipment manufacturers are now introducing new lines of racquets that are titanium and graphite weaves. Titanium is a strong, durable material that weighs more than graphite but less than aluminum. The combination has produced some of the lightest and most powerful racquets on the market. The technology is new, and the manufacturers feel that its appeal with the senior, female, and injured player should be great because of its "weightlessness," power, durability, and superior antishock properties.

Grip

Cushioned grips counterbalance shock load with "off-center" hits. Larger grips are more forgiving when elbow and wrist problems are present. Handles are being designed to reduce the shock load of off-center hits. (NOTE: When purchasing a racquet, buy within your playing ability and try the demo first.) (See Fig. 28-1.)

Stringing

Tennis guidelines The low range of the manufacturer's recommended tension range increases the "sweet spot," decreases the shock load, increases the power, and decreases control of the ball.

Type of string Natural gut is very resilient and forgiving in injuries. It is, however, more expensive, fragile, and affected adversely by moisture. Multifilament, thinner-gauge strings are most forgiving on the arm. Manufacturers are researching and introducing "arm-friendly strings" to the market, that is, GAMMA TNT Rx. String vibration dampeners have been found to have little value.

Frequency of stringing It is most important to have your racquet restrung at the beginning of each season and again midway through your season by a certified racquet technician. The stringer can help you select the appropriate string type, tension, and racquet type for your game style.

Balls

Pressureless balls, old balls, and wet balls are heavy and increase the shock load on the upper extremity.

GENERAL FITNESS

Tennis is a sport that combines several fitness parameters.

1. Aerobic endurance

2. Anaerobic capacity
3. Balance
4. Coordination
5. Agility
6. Flexibility
7. Strength, power, and endurance

Deficits in any of these areas, especially over several categories, will certainly predispose the tennis athlete to injury. When attempting to return the injured player to sport, the practitioner must identify which of the preceding parameters require more rehabilitation in order to lessen the chance of recurrence, that is, the unfit player with generally poor flexibility will be slower getting to the ball and will tend to reach and lunge and hit the ball late. This in turn will result in poor swing mechanics and potential injury. Remember, the majority of patients play tennis to get fit, and we must promote good fitness in order to play tennis.

ENVIRONMENT

Playing Surface

Hard courts are the most common playing surface in North America. The Australian Open and U.S. Open Grand Slam Championships are played on hard courts. Hard courts are cement and are generally fast-playing courts. They favor the serve and volley player as well as the power hitters.

From an injury perspective, these courts are extremely hard on any lower extremity problems, as they provide no shock absorbency and limited ability to slide to the ball. The faster pace of the ball requires better foot work, earlier preparation, and better timing by the athlete to produce quality shots. Upper extremity problems such as rotator cuff tendinitis and tennis elbow may be aggravated in the athlete who consistently hits the ball late. The faster pace of the ball also increases impact forces on the arm.

Clay courts are the most common surface in South America and Europe. The French Open Grand Slam is played on red clay. Clay courts can be red or green clay. Green clay, or "Har Tru," is most common in North America. Clay courts play slowly and are soft and slippery. With the pace of the ball being considerably slower, the athlete has increased reaction time getting to the ball and in preparing the racquet to hit the ball. The athlete's stroke mechanics are generally better when playing on clay.

Lower extremity injuries, such as plantar fasciitis, shin splints, and knee problems, are less common and less aggravated when playing on clay. Muscle strains, especially of the groin, and ankle sprains are common because of the slippery texture of the clay.

Other court surfaces, such as Omni carpet and artificial grass, are cushioned and also play slowly. Few average recreational players have a choice of court surface, but we as practitioners should be aware of the significant differences between surfaces and how they may help or hinder the tennis athlete.

HEAT AND HUMIDITY

Heat disorders are a common problem in both the recreational and professional tennis athlete. Of the four categories, heat cramps, heat syncope, heat exhaustion, and heat stroke, heat cramps are the most common heat injury sustained by the tennis athlete. The calf and quadriceps are the most frequently affected muscle groups. Heat cramps are painful muscle spasms that occur because of excessive dehydration and electrolyte loss during sweating.

PREVENTION OF HEAT DISORDERS

1. Identify susceptible individuals.
2. Gradually increase the practice time in the heat (conditioning).
3. Hydration is the most important preventative measure. You cannot overhydrate an athlete, so drink cool fluids such as water, electrolyte drinks, and diluted fruit juice before, during, and after a practice or match. In match situations, the athlete should drink approximately 1 cup of fluid at each changeover. Do not use thirst as a guideline for hydration, as it will be too late. Avoid or limit caffeine and alcohol intake, as they act as diuretics. Athletes should monitor their body weight and urine (which should be as clear as possible) when training and competing for several days or weeks in the heat. Dehydration most definitely leads to decreased physical performance.
4. Remember that cooling occurs by evaporation; therefore, expose skin to air and avoid restrictive clothing, dark colors, nylon, spandex, and poly blends.
5. Evaluate weather conditions in advance. The greater the humidity, the harder it is for the body to cool itself.
6. Towel off sweat. In match play, a player should towel off all exposed skin every changeover. The player must regularly change shirts and wear a hat. Fanning the athlete or using ice towels or packs on the neck, armpits, and abdomen will quickly cool the player's core temperature.
7. The loss of emotional control in a match or during practice expends needed energy. Hyperventilation prevents the lungs from efficiently exchanging oxygen into the blood. An increase in sweating dehydrates the body, and anxiety causes muscle contractions that may lead to cramping.

8. Educate athletes, coaches, and professionals. Certain issues are sensitive, and they should certainly be treated with respect and confidentiality.

TREATMENT OF MUSCLE CRAMPS

This is one of the most devastating problems in tennis. This is owing to a buildup of metabolites in the muscle, associated with losses of salt and potassium, and dehydration. Poor conditioning also plays a major role in cramping. Emphasis must be on prevention through adequate hydration, nutrition, and conditioning.

Cramping of the calf muscle can often be lessened by altering footwear and using heel lifts. If cramping occurs, the player should drink plenty of fluids, gently stretch the muscle, and apply ice to the muscle to help reduce the pain and spasm. Often gentle massage helps. The recreational player should stop playing until the cramp stops completely. The competitive player, particularly the elite player, may continue to play but must understand the following:

- Their performance will decrease as the cramping progresses.
- They risk injury to the cramping muscle or to another muscle or joint owing to the compensation, that is, the player will not want to explode with the legs in the service action and will therefore begin to serve more from the arm.
- Their performance will be reduced the next day.
- The more severe the dehydration and cramping, the greater the requirement for medical intervention such as intravenous treatment.
- The player must be educated as to why cramping occurs and make changes to his or her hydration and nutrition routine in order to prevent this most disabling tennis injury. Conditioning also plays an important role in prevention. On the professional tennis tour, a trainer may assist a cramping player only once during a match.

CONDITIONING

The key to avoidance of injuries in tennis and squash is the proper off-court conditioning. The player should have a full facility with Cybex, Kincom, and so on, machinery and access to a trainer, a coach, or physiotherapist who can watch him or her hit into a net and hit on the court. The therapist and coach can then recommend proper rehabilitation and cross-training in times of stress and injury.

Exercises

Posterior Capsule Stretch

The back of the shoulder is stretched by gently pulling your shoulder across your body and under your chin. Hold 30 to 60 s and repeat several times.

Band Exercises

One of the best ways to exercise is with a rehabilitation band or surgical tubing. Ideally exercises should be done with a 2-2-4 count (2 s forward, 2 s hold, and a slow 4-s return to the starting point). You should do three sets of 10 to 15 repetitions with a 30-s rest in between. These should be done three to five times a week (Fig. 28-3).

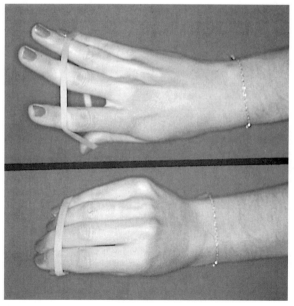

FIG. 28-3 Dynamic finger and hand exercise. Put an elastic band over the ends of the fingers and spread the fingers as widely as possible. Do this to the 2-4 count: 2 s spread and 4 s slow return. Do three sets of 15 repetitions.

Abduction

Stand straight and step on tubing end. Start with your arm at your side. Work against tension by raising your arm. Initially raise your arm no higher than halfway (45 degrees) (stage 1). As your pain diminishes, progress to shoulder level (stage 2). The exercise should be varied by using various hand grips on the tubing to use different muscles. The three grips are: palm forward, palm backward, and thumb down (Fig. 28-4).

External Rotation

Attach tubing to a doorknob. Stand sideways to the point where the tubing is attached. Start with forearm across the body, elbow at a right angle. Rotate the arm out against resistance, keeping your

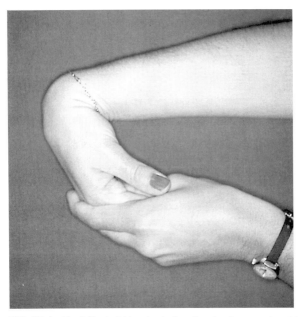

FIG. 28-4 Flexibility stretching. Lock elbow in extension; pronate wrist, palm down; and flex wrist joint with opposite hand past 90 degrees until you feel the stretch in the extensors in the upper forearm. Hold for 10 s; repeat 15 times; and do this three times every day and before you play.

elbow tucked against the body. If helpful, hold your elbow with your other hand.

Internal Rotation

From the preceding position, turn around 180 degrees. Start with your arm bent at a right angle and pointing away from your body. Rotate your arm in across your body while keeping your elbow tucked in.

Wall Push-Out

Stand several feet from the wall. With your hands approximately shoulder width apart, do a push-out against the wall. Keep your back straight. Go as close to the wall as possible, and do the push-out slowly and controlled, both toward and away from the wall. Do three sets of 10 to 15 repetitions.

The best preventative for injuries is overall fitness, and most competitive tennis players should have a fitness test evaluation and an on-season and off-season program written out. The program has to emphasize power and endurance, anaerobic and aerobic conditioning, balance, agility, and flexibility.

Stationary bicycles are good because they train the same leg muscle groups that are employed in tennis. Varied muscle strengthening programs, both for overall conditioning and endurance, should be employed (see Chap. 16).

A psychological profile of the competitive tennis player is also important, and the sports psychologist is often very important in the development of a tennis player.

Flexibility

Flexibility is an important part of injury treatment and prevention. For stretching to be effective, it must be done on a regular basis. Always stretch when you are warmed up. It is important to stretch before and after activity. Stretching should not be painful. All stretches should be done in a slow static manner, with *no bouncing*. Hold stretches for at least 30 to 60 s and repeat several times. For difficult problems, a therapist may have to assist you to improve your flexibility.

Weak or inflexible muscles of the arm are a major contributor to the problem of golfer's and tennis elbow. The exercises shown here will not only strengthen the damaged muscle tendon unit to prevent injury but will also help improve your game.

Some of the exercises will be too painful to do in the early painful stage. Your physician will advise you when to initiate the exercises.

Elbow Stretch

Lock the elbow and bend the wrist, using the other hand until you feel the muscles in your forearm stretch. Hold for 10 s and relax. Repeat fifteen times. Do this three times a day and always before you play your sport.

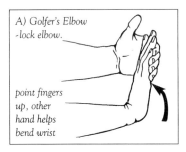

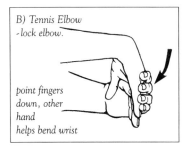

Band Exercises

Obtain a rehabilitation band or surgical tubing (approx. 2 ft) at a medical supply store or use a bike tire innertube. Ideally, exercises should be done with a 2-2-4 count (2 s forward, 2 s hold, and a slow 4-s return to the starting point). You should do three sets of 10 to 15 repetitions with a 30-s rest in between. These should be done three to five times a week.

Wrist Curls

Sit at a table with forearm supported and wrist over the edge. Loop the tube under the knee and tie tight enough to provide enough tension against movement.

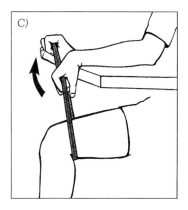

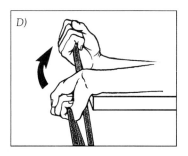

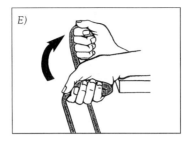

Extension

Hold the loop with the palm down and extend the wrist.

Flexion

Hold the loop with the palm up and flex the wrist.

Radial Deviation

Hold the loop with the thumb up and curl the wrist upward.

Squeezing a rubber ball will also strengthen the injured area. Carry one with you and squeeze it as often as you can.

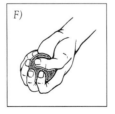

RECOMMENDED READINGS

1. Chandler TJ, Kibler WB, et al: Shoulder strength and endurance in college tennis players. *Am J Sports Med* 29(4):455–458, 1992.
2. Cohen D, Mont M, et al: Upper extremity physical factors affecting tennis serve velocity. *Am J Sports Med* 22(6):746–750, 1994.
3. Easterbrook M, Cameron C: Injuries in racquet sports, in Schneider RC (ed): *Sports Injuries.* Baltimore, Williams & Wilkins, 1985, pp. 553–571.
4. Ellenbecker T: Shoulder injuries in tennis, in *The Athlete's Shoulder.* New York, Churchill Livingstone, 1994, pp. 399–407.
5. Gray B: Racquets. *Tennis* 58–60, 1998.
6. Groppel J: The biomechanics of tennis strokes, United States Tennis Association Sports Science Conference, Saddlebrock Florida, Conference Notes, April/May 1993.
7. Leach R, Lewis T: Tennis injuries, in Schneider RC (ed): *Sports Injuries.* Baltimore, Williams & Wilkins, 1985, pp. 450–461.
8. Leach R, Miller JK: Lateral and medial epicondylitis of elbow. *Clin Sports Med* 6(2):1987.
9. Leach R: *Sports Med Sci Tennis* 1:4–6, 1996.
10. Lehman R: Racquet sports, injury treatment and prevention. *Clin Sports Med* 7(2), 1988.
11. Nicola T: Tennis, in Mellion (ed): *Team Physician's Handbook,* 2d ed. St. Louis, Mosby, 1997, pp. 816–827.
12. Tennis Canada Coaching Certification System, Course Conductor Manuals Coach 2, Coaches Guide, 1994. Coach 4–5, Influence of the Environment on Training and Performance, 1993.
13. Conversation with Dan Kerr, Certified Racquet Technician, Stringer, Canadian Davis Cup Team

| **Strength Training
and Weight Lifting**

R. Charles Bull

Body building, weight lifting (Olympic type), and strength training
are three different disciplines.

Most men and women in the gym today do strength training for
overall physical fitness and conditioning. *Strength training* is often
a means to enhance performance in a specific sport. It is versatile
and can provide the athlete with an optimal resistance program that
addresses any form of strengthening. The Said Principle, "Specific
Adaptation to Imposed Demand" allows the golfer to do wrist curls
with a 4-lb or 2-kg dumbbell, and the discus thrower to do the same
exercise with a 50-lb or 20-kg dumbbell (Table 29-1). *Body
builders* are also building strength and conditioning to tone their
muscles and shape their muscles more for appearance's sake and
compete for titles such as "Mr. or Ms. USA" or "Mr. or Ms. Universe."

True power lifters and Olympic weight lifters are in one of the
most popular sports internationally. They are trained and need extensive coaching in order to compete.

Power lifting events consist of three maximal lifts: the hack
squat, the bench press, and the dead lift.

Olympic lifting is performed with two lifts: the snatch, in which
the barbell is lifted from the floor to an overhead position in one
movement; and the clean and jerk, in which the barbell is first lifted
from the floor to the shoulder level and then jerked overhead in the
second movement (Fig. 29-1). Modification for Olympic use is the
power clean, in which the bar is moved to midthighs, then the shoulders, and then overhead. These Olympic weight lifters and the big
shotput athletes and discus throwers develop their muscles differently. They tend to peak every 7 to 10 days and go to maximum
lifts. When they do this maximum lift, they tear tissue microscopi-
cally and then they start over again and gradually build up to a
greater peak. They usually do fewer reps, for example, seven or
even three when the weights get very heavy, and fewer sets, for example, five.

The advanced body builders training for physique contests usually require eight to 10 reps for five or more sets.

Both the body builders and power lifters train five to six times
per week, using a split training program, that is, abs, neck, pecs and

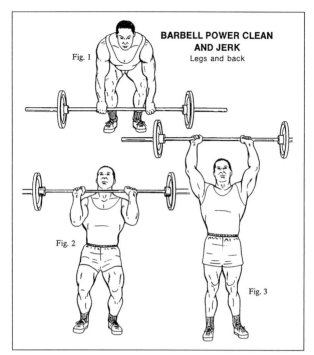

FIG. 29-1 Barbell power clean and jerk. Place a barbell in front of you. With your feet about 16 in. apart, step up to the bar until your shins are nearly touching the bar. Bend down and get a palms down grip on the barbell with your hands placed about 26 in. apart. Bend your legs until your upper thighs are nearly parallel with the floor. Keep your arms straight and your head up. Your back will be at about a 45-degree angle. Inhale and pull the bar straight up as you stand erect until the bar is nearly as high as your shoulders. Then flip the bar over and back until it is resting on your upper chest and exhale. Inhale again and squat down about 12 in., keeping your back straight and your elbows forward. With the power from your legs and back, thrust the barbell overhead to arm's length, locking out the weight and holding it there and exhaling again. From this position lower the weight back to your upper chest and then to the floor to complete the repetition.

shoulders, and arms on Monday, Wednesday, and Friday. Then back, hips, legs, and calves on Tuesday, Thursday, and Saturday.

They vary the intensity also, for example, Monday heavy, Wednesday moderate, and Friday light. One reason they take the anabolics is to train more intensely, heavy, heavy, light.

There is no exact formula in weight training and each person has to discover what works best for him or her. Basically, you have to *listen to your body*. The regime can vary, and there should be a built-in rest day. However, this does not necessarily have to be every Sunday. If there is a day when training seems to be at an incredibly low or inefficient level, it is best to have a light aerobic workout—cycle, skip, or swim, and then shower and go home. Then you will be twice as good the next day.

The average strength training athlete does not have to abide by the arms and upper body one day, legs and lower body the next day principle religiously. Alternating an arm machine and then a leg machine is probably sufficient, once the athlete is in good shape.

For the average person, the tendency to overdo things and just fatigue the muscle is a big problem. Once the muscle is fatigued, it is more likely to be injured. Thus, the motto, "Train, don't strain" is of maximum importance.[1] The average person should do the following:

1. Try to exercise all of his or her muscle groups.
2. Change sets and repetitions for variety.
3. Use different exercises for the same muscle.
4. Train for pleasure. Your workout should be exhilarating.
5. Work around an injury (avoid exercises that irritate the injury).
6. Set realistic goals and work hard to achieve them. Don't quit!

(Modified from Bill Pearl *Keys to the Inner Universe*. Typecraft, Pasadena, CA 1982.[2])

All three disciplines usually have training cycles for 6 to 8 weeks and then either increase the weights or add different machines to their regimen. The main indication of progress is the way you feel. Your workout should be exhilarating, and you should leave with a muscle burn and the typical feeling that you have done something worthwhile but not significant postworkout pain.

If an injury occurs, such as a strain, you usually do not have to stop. You should just avoid the exercises that irritate that injury, for example, divorce the left leg, use the right leg, and continue on.

Also, the average athlete should set realistic goals and work hard to achieve these goals. It is surprising how little setbacks can make the athlete quit training. Consistency is the rule. Remember, "slow and steady wins the race."

GETTING STARTED

The warm-up can be active: 10 to 15 min on the exercise bike and the Schwinn-type bike with a combination leg and arm component is the best for overall warm-ups. Stretching can start when you are on the bike, with your shoulders and neck. Then you can work down from your neck through to the calf muscles. Running stretches are satisfactory (see Chap. 34). You should be in a light sweat when you start your weight workout. Begin with the abdomen and chest and work to the lower abdomen. Then triceps, biceps, and finish with the legs.

The leg exercises require more weights, and you are less apt to strain the low back if you warm up more prior to the heavier exercises. The low back is the weakest link in the human body, according to Bill Pearl.[2]

When the body builder is quite facile and adept with the leverage and proper weight lifting methods, the last two repetitions of each exercise should be done at about 80 to 90 percent of maximum effort and strength. Once this becomes relatively easy, the poundage can be increased. Be careful to increase the weights very gradually; 5 lb is sensible.

Assessing the amount of weight lifted depends on maximum strength (1 RM = the maximum amount of weight lifted for one repetition). When an athlete can complete two or more repetitions above the usual number in the last two workout sessions, it is time to increase the load.

PROPER BREATHING

Bill Pearl emphasizes, "Never hold your breath while lifting."[2] Power lifters and Olympic lifters always exhale while the exertion is greatest. For example, in the bench press, inhale deeply as you lower the weight and exhale as you push the weight back to the starting position above the chest.

The accompanying diagrams of the proper way to use free weights are from a book by the lifting guru, Bill Pearl.[2] His work has stood the test of time, and the principles are used now in much of the weight lifting equipment—Cybex, Paramount, David. However, the free weights allow you more versatility, as you can see in the following figures.

There are approximately four exercises for each section and each affects the muscles slightly differently. Obviously, the exercises do not have to be done in this order or with the three sets of 10 principles. However, they do have to be done progressively, and the heavier exercises should not be done until you are fully warmed up. The following exercises are adapted from Bill Pearl.[2]

Abdominals

1. The conventional classic sit-up is fine for the well-conditioned athlete. Make sure your knees are bent.
2. For the more mature athlete or anyone with back trouble, "crunches" are better (Fig. 29-2).
3. "Jackknife sit-up" (Fig. 29-3). This is a moderately difficult abdominal exercise that gets the fast-twitch muscles.
4. "Dip stand leg pull-in" (Fig. 29-4). This is an excellent abdominal exercise. It can also be done with left or right rotation. A full leg raise, with hips flexed to 90 degrees and legs straight and parallel to the floor, is more difficult.

Chest, Pectorals

1. "Barbell bench press" (Fig. 29-5). This is the classic bench press exercise. It is often used as a guide for the athlete's overall strength. It can also be done on an incline bench for upper pecs and a decline bench for lower pecs.
2. The bench press is easier, safer, and more controlled on a "universal" but somewhat less effective. This can be done sitting or lying down.
3. The pec deck (Fig. 29-6) is a great machine for confidence building. The leverage is quite satisfactory, and athletes usually make good progress.
4. Dumbbell flys are a classic chest and lung exercise. Expand your chest with maximum inhalation and then forced expiration at the top. Lower the dumbbells out to each side of the chest until the weights are even with your chest.

Shoulders, Deltoids, and Trapezii

1. "Standing dumbbell press" (Fig. 29-7). This type of military press is well-controlled with dumbbells, and this alternate left-right sequence needs to be done with perfect concentration.

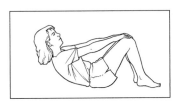

FIG. 29-2 Knee reach. Lie flat on your back, legs bent. Stretch arms out toward knees. Lift shoulders off floor using stomach muscles. Hold for 5 s and then relax. Repeat 10 times.

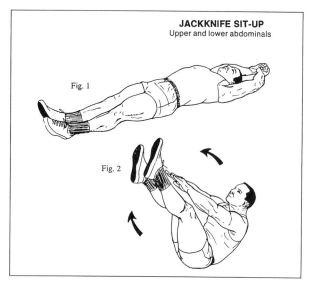

JACKKNIFE SIT-UP
Upper and lower abdominals

Fig. 1

Fig. 2

FIG. 29-3 Jackknife sit-up. Lie on the floor in a supine position. Place your arms behind your head at arm's length. You then bend at the waist while raising your legs and arms up at the same time, coming together vertically above your waist. Lower your arms and legs back to the floor to complete the repetition. Inhale as you commence the exercise and exhale as you finish. Keep your elbows and knees locked out during the exercise.

2. The upright rowing exercise affects the whole chest, shoulders, and upper body. It can also be done with a bar, either free or on the rack. Keep the weights in close to the body.
3. The military press (Fig. 29-8) shows the traditional military press with free weights. A modification on the Universal can be done frontward and backward. This suggests front and back use of other machines, such as the pec deck, stair stepper, and treadmill.
4. The classic military press with bar (Fig. 29-8) is also used as a guide to upper body strength. It can be modified to behind the neck for posterior, deltoid, and traps.
5. Upright rowing with pulleys is safe and affects front deltoids and chest. Pull the weight straight up until it is almost under your chin.

Legs and Back

1. The split clean (Fig. 29-9) requires instruction as timing and breathing is very important. It is very important for quick IIa and quick IIb fibers.
2. The clean and jerk (see Fig. 29-1) gets more quads muscle power into the action.
3. Front and rear pull-downs (Fig. 29-10) can usually be done with good progression of weights and builds enthusiasm by tangible results. Be careful with the rear pull-down as it can lead to shoulder impingement problems if overused.
4. The lat pull in "rowing" can be done with or without the assistance of your legs, but do not arch your back. Pull the cables to the sides of your chest just below the pecs.
5. Dumbbell pull-up is also a good eccentric exercise. Let the weights down slowly and have a partner help you lift them up.

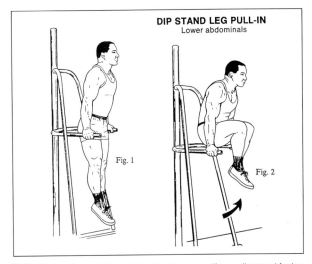

DIP STAND LEG PULL-IN
Lower abdominals

Fig. 1

Fig. 2

FIG. 29-4 Dip stand leg pull-in. Position yourself on a dip stand facing away from the machine with your body being supported by your arms, having your elbows locked out. Hanging in a vertical position, inhale and bend your knees while pulling your upper thighs into your midsection. Return to starting position and exhale. Concentrate on your lower abdominals during the exercise. Note that your lower legs are vertical to the floor at the halfway point of the exercise.

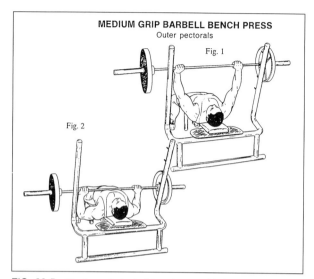

FIG. 29-5　Medium grip barbell bench press. Lie in a supine position on a flat bench with your legs positioned at the sides of the bench and your feet flat on the floor. Using a hand grip that is about 6 in. wider than your shoulder width, bring the barbell to arm's length above the chest but in line with the shoulders. Lower the barbell to a position on the chest that is about an inch below the nipples of the pectorals. Note from the illustration that the elbows are back and the chest is held high. Inhale as the barbell is lowered to the chest and exhale as you push the barbell back to arm's length. Do not relax and drop the weight on the chest but lower it with complete control, making a definite pause at the chest before pressing it back to starting position. Keep the head on the bench and do not arch the back too sharply as to raise your hips off the bench.

Lie face down on a bench and pull the weights straight up until they are at your sides, even with your chest.

Triceps

1. Triceps curl (Fig. 29-11). It is very important to have the elbows point to the ceiling to isolate triceps. This can also be done with your back supported against a chair.
2. Dumbbell triceps. This is easier to control than the bar. Elbows to the ceiling and alternate right hand on top, then left hand on top.

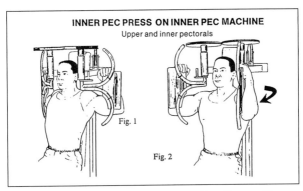

INNER PEC PRESS ON INNER PEC MACHINE
Upper and inner pectorals

Fig. 1

Fig. 2

FIG. 29-6 Inner pec press on inner pec machine. The way this exercise is performed will depend a great deal on how the inner pec machine you use is constructed. Some are more elaborate than others and have adjustable seats and arms. The main thing to remember while performing this exercise is to keep the upper arms fairly high and about in line with your shoulders. You should keep the forearms in a vertical position so as not to bring any more of the triceps and deltoids into play than necessary. Concentrate on squeezing your forearms together by concentrating on the pectorals doing the work. Inhale as you are squeezing and exhale as you return your arms back to starting position.

3. Seated assisted triceps (Fig. 29-12). Note how the left arm supports and holds the right arm in against the head. This is the best triceps exercise.
4. Press downs on lat machine is another good eccentric exercise. Go back up slowly.
5. Reverse grip dips with palms out are very difficult and require practice. Start with a conventional palm in dip and alternate for biceps in and triceps out.

Biceps

1. The biceps curl is another mainstay of weight training. Start out against a wall so you do not arch your back. As you progress, move out and cheat slightly, but *do not* arch the back. Just rock back gently.
2. Pulley curls can be done with palm up for biceps medialis and palms down for biceps lateralis. Use a Scott bench.
3. Preacher curl is the *best* way to completely isolate the biceps and do your maximum. Use a low preacher bench.
4. The easy bar also isolates biceps very well (Fig. 29-13).

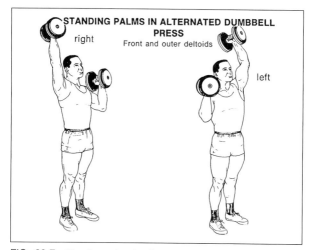

FIG. 29-7 Standing palms in alternated dumbbell press. Clean two dumbbells to shoulder height. Lock the legs and hips solidly. Keep the elbows in slightly and have the palms of your hands facing each other. Take a deep breath and press the right arm straight up over your right shoulder. As you commence to lower the right arm, begin to press the left arm to arm's length above your left shoulder, letting the air out as the left arm is raised. Be sure to keep the palms of the hands facing each other during the entire exercise.

5. The seated dumbbell curl gets the biceps medial fibers and deltoid (Fig. 29-14).

Thigh

1. The half-squat on a 2 × 4 is a safe exercise if you get proper instruction. The athlete needs spotters and a power belt to handle heavier weights. This can also be done on the rack.
2. The leg press machine is a good "closed chain" exercise (Fig. 29-15). Lock the machine at 90 degrees knee flexion if possible. Make sure your back is well supported.
3. Thigh extension or the quads machine is another benchmark machine (Fig. 29-16). Be careful of the midrange if you have preexisting knee problems.
4. Hamstring or biceps curl is very important, because most people develop the quads and neglect the hams. There should be a

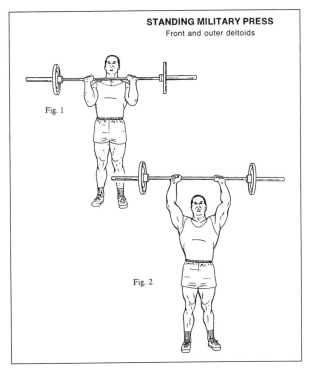

STANDING MILITARY PRESS
Front and outer deltoids

Fig. 1

Fig. 2

FIG. 29-8 Standing military press. This is the standard military press. Clean the weight to the chest. Lock the legs and hips solidly. This will give you a solid platform from which to push. Keep the elbows in slightly and under the bar, press the weight overhead, lock the arms out. When lowering the barbell to the upper chest, be sure it rests on the chest and is not held with the arms. If the chest is held high, it will give you a nice shelf on which to place the barbell and to push from. Inhale before the press and exhale when lowering the barbell.

60/40 ratio, that is, 60#s quads and 40#s both hams. The exercise can be done with both legs, but it is important to do one-leg quads and hams too, particularly after an injury. Lie face down on a leg extension machine. Place your heels under the top foot pads. Curl your leg or legs up to 90 degrees.

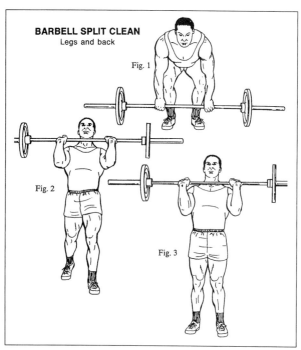

BARBELL SPLIT CLEAN
Legs and back

Fig. 1

Fig. 2

Fig. 3

FIG. 29-9 Barbell split clean. Place a barbell in front of you. With your feet about 16 in. apart, step up to the bar until your shins are nearly touching the bar. Bend down and get a palms down grip on the bar with your hands placed about 26 in. apart. Bend your legs until your upper thighs are nearly parallel with the floor. Keep your arms straight and your head up. Your back will be at about a 45-degree angle. Inhale and pull the bar straight up as you commence to stand erect. Continue the pull by raising up on your toes after you have come erect and have pulled the barbell about as high as your lower pectorals. Then throw your right leg straight back about 32 in., trying not to bend your knee. Your left leg should travel straight to the front about 8 in., enabling you to lunge under the bar, catching it on the top of your upper chest by flipping the bar over and back with your wrists. From this position bring both feet in line with each other to complete the movement. Exhale as the bar reaches your upper chest. Return the bar to the floor, and one repetition of the exercise is completed.

Calf

1. Toe raises can be done on the leg press machine. It is the classic eccentric exercise when you go to the position with your ankle flexed and toes are up on the power rack using a dumbbell at shoulder height.

Neck

1. Do isometrics North, South, East, and West. Using both hands, push your head and hold forward, back, and sideways. Also push the chin against the palm for left and right rotations. Hold on each for 10 s and repeat three sets of 10. Resist your neck muscles with your hand and arms.
2. Bridging is still done as part of training in football and wrestling. It has a lot of criticism and must be done with careful supervision. It should not be done before maturity or after age

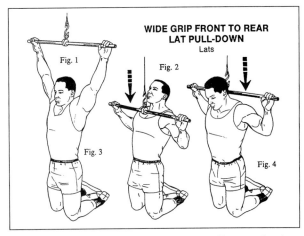

FIG. 29-10 Wide grip front to rear lat pull-down. Place your hands on a lat machine bar about 36 in. apart. Kneel down on your knees until you are supporting the weight stack with your arms while they are extended overhead. Inhale and pull the bar straight down until it is even with your upper chest. Return to starting position and exhale. Now inhale and pull the bar straight down until it touches the back of your neck just above your shoulders. Return to starting position and exhale. Continue going from front to rear until the prescribed number of repetitions are completed.

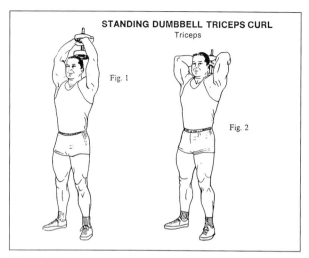

FIG. 29-11 Standing dumbbell triceps curl. Grasp one dumbbell with both hands and raise it overhead to arm's length, vertical with the floor. As you are raising the dumbbell rotate your hands up and over until the top plates are resting in the palms of your hands while your thumbs remain around the handle. Stand erect with your back straight, head up, and feet about 16 in. apart. Keep your upper arms in close to the sides of your head during the exercise. Inhale and lower the dumbbell behind your head in a semicircular motion until your forearms and biceps touch. Return the weight to starting position using a similar path and exhale.

40. Your head should be on a mat and your body raised upward to a pyramid position with your legs.

Wrist

1. Wrist curls are very important for golfers, hockey players, and baseball players with light weights (2 to 4 kg) maximum (5 to 10 lbs) (Fig. 29-17). The heavier interior football lineman and discus throwers can do them with much heavier weights.

FREE WEIGHTS

According to Falkel and Cipriani, free weights allow sports-specific movements and pattern as well as speed of movement.[3] They can provide the athlete with an optimal resistance from any

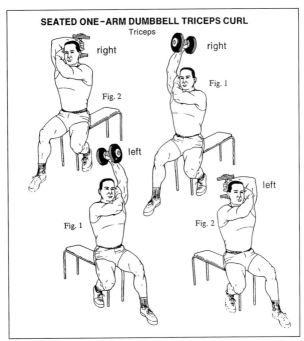

FIG. 29-12 Seated one-arm dumbbell triceps curl. Grasp a dumbbell in your right hand and press it overhead to arm's length as you sit at the end of a bench with your feet about 16 in. apart and planted firmly on the floor. Keep your head up, back straight, and right upper arm in close to the right side of your face. Inhale and lower the dumbbell straight down in a semicircular motion by bending your arm at the elbow but keeping your upper arm vertical throughout the exercise. The dumbbell should be lowered until your forearm and biceps touch. Press the dumbbell back to starting position using the same path and exhale. Do the prescribed number of repetitions with your right arm and then change positions repeating the same number with your left arm.

program to address any form of strengthening that is required for a specific sport or activity.

SYSTEMS OF RESISTANCE TRAINING[3]

The initial system for resistance training was developed by De-Lorme and Watkins in 1948 based on a 10-repetition maximum.[4]

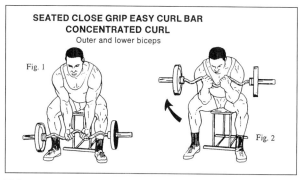

FIG. 29-13   Seated close grip easy curl bar concentrated curl. Grasp an easy curl bar with both hands using a palms up grip and the closest hand spacing curves possible. Sit at the end of a flat bench. Bend forward at the waist keeping your back straight, head up, and feet planted firmly on the floor about 16 in. apart. Place your upper arms against the sides of your upper thighs while holding the easy curl back straight down at arm's length. Keeping your upper arms against your inner thighs, inhale and curl the easy bar straight up in a semicircular motion until your biceps and forearms touch and your hands are directly under your chin. Return the easy bar to starting position using a similar path and exhale.

DeLorme suggested the first 10 reps would be at 50 percent of the 10 RM resistance, the second at 75 percent, and the third at 100 percent.

First 10 reps, 50 percent
Second 10 reps, 75 percent
Third 10 reps, 100 percent

These three sets of 10 principles have stood the test of time, both in strength training and remedial physiotherapy rehab.

In papers published in 1979 and 1985, Knight and Merrick detailed the Daily Adjustable Progressive Resistance Exercise (DAPRE) system that consisted of four sets.[5]

The first set was 10 reps of a "working weight," which was handled safely by an athlete reconditioning from an injury. The second set was six repetitions at approximately 75 percent of the working resistance. The third and fourth sets were against the full working resistance.

In the third set, the maximum number of repetitions are attempted, and based on this, the fourth set would be done at an adjusted level. This system is changed daily depending on the athlete's response.

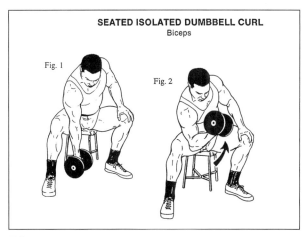

SEATED ISOLATED DUMBBELL CURL
Biceps

Fig. 1

Fig. 2

FIG. 29-14 Seated isolated dumbbell curl. Grasp a dumbbell in your right hand and sit on a stool or a flat bench. Put your left lower leg to the rear slightly to get it out of the way and place your left hand on your left lower thigh to help support your upper body. Position the dumbbell in front of you hanging at arm's length between your legs with a palms up grip. Your arm should not be resting against any part of your leg. Inhale and curl the dumbbell upward in a semicircular motion by bending your arm at the elbow and keeping your upper arm vertical with the floor. Continue the curl until your biceps and forearm are touching. At the top position the dumbbell should be shoulder height. Return to starting position using a similar motion and exhale. Do the prescribed number of repetitions with your right arm and then change positions doing the same number of repetitions with your left arm.

First set, 10 reps "working weight"
Second set, six reps at 75 percent
Third set, maximum number of reps at full working resistance
Fourth set, adjusted weight for five to six reps depending on third set

There are many other systems of weight training, particularly among the body builders. This is well-documented by Falkel and Cipriani.[3]

The most popular systems of resistance training are as follows:

1. *Single-Set Systems.* One set per exercise session performed with 8 to 10 repetitions maximum.

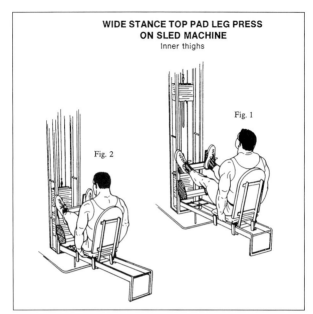

**WIDE STANCE TOP PAD LEG PRESS
ON SLED MACHINE**
Inner thighs

Fig. 1

Fig. 2

FIG. 29-15 Wide stance top pad leg press on sled machine. Sit on the back-supported chair and hold on to the sides of the seat under your buttocks. Place your feet on the two top pads provided and press the weight stack out as the seat moves backward until your legs are straight and knees lock. Inhale and bend your legs toward your upper body until the weight stack nearly touches the remaining plates and your upper thighs are to the sides of your torso. Keep your knees pointing outward. Press the stack out again until your legs are straight and exhale.

2. *Multiple-Set Systems.* Two to three warm-up sets with increasing resistance, followed by two to five sets at 5 to 6 RM. This is the body builder's usual routine.
3. *Light-to-Heavy-Systems.* This is the DeLorme system.
4. *Heavy-to-Light Systems.* Sets of three to six repetitions performed with heavy weights, followed by sets with lighter weights, keeping reps the same.
5. *Temple or Pyramid Program.* Successive sets in which the resistance is increased and the number of reps decreased, to a maximum of 1 RM, which is then reversed, and the weight is decreased, and reps increased (5, 4, 3, 2, 1 then 2, 3, 4, 5).

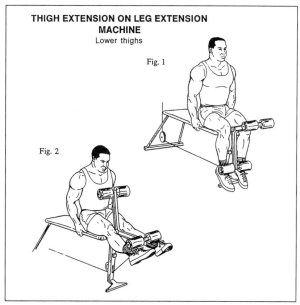

THIGH EXTENSION ON LEG EXTENSION MACHINE
Lower thighs

Fig. 1

Fig. 2

FIG. 29-16 Thigh extension on leg extension machine. Sit at the end of a leg extension machine placing the top part of your ankles and feet under the lower foot pads. Back up far enough on the seat to keep the end of the seat against the rear of your knees. Hold on to the seat with both hands just behind your buttocks. Point your toes slightly downward. Inhale and raise the weight stack until your legs are parallel with the floor. Return to starting position and exhale. Keep your upper body in a fixed position during the exercise.

6. *Super Sets*. Two distinct exercises performed with the same body part, one right after the other, with no rest between the two exercises.
7. *Circuit Program*. This series of resistance training exercises is performed with minimal rest and 10 to 15 reps are performed, in order to establish 1 RM. The circuit on different machines is repeated two to four times. This can also be done in an aerobic cardiovascular fashion.
8. *Multipoundage System*. This requires one or two assistants to remove a set amount from the bar or dumbbell after each set of repetitions. This is good for eccentric negative exercises where

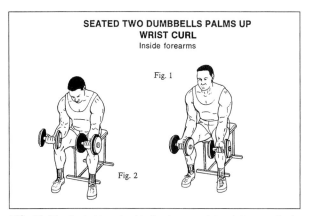

FIG. 29-17   Seated two dumbbell palms up wrist curl. Grasp a dumbbell in each hand. Sit at the end of a flat bench and plant your feet on the floor about 12 in. apart. Lean forward and place your forearms on your upper thighs keeping your palms facing up. Have your hands over your knees just at your wrists. Lower the dumbbells to the lowest possible comfortable position by bending your wrists downward but keep a tight grip on the dumbbells throughout the exercise. Inhale and curl your hands upward as high as you possibly can. Do not let your forearms raise up from your upper thighs. Lower the weights to starting position and exhale.

the dumbbell is lifted by the two assistants and the athlete lets it down.

9. *Forced Repetition System (Stripping)*. After completion of a set to exhaustion, a coach assists the lifter with just enough help to allow for several more repetitions. This is often done about 2 weeks prior to a body building competition, similar to an exhaustive run prior to carbohydrate loading for a marathon race (see Chap. 33).

Probably the most beneficial of these systems are the Multiple-Set System,[4] the Light-to-Heavy (DeLorme) System,[5] and the Pyramid Program.[6]

Overtraining is often manifest by increased muscle soreness and stiffness (more than normal postworkout stiffness, lasting into the next day). An inability to complete the usual program, at the same intensity, and lack of a normal high or exhilaration from the workout is noted. These are progressive signs. If this happens, cross-train more, swim, cycle, and decrease the poundage. Reassess your diet: Alcohol decreases serum testosterone and growth hormone. Lack of sleep, stress, increased anxiety, and nicotine are all detrimental to maximum "peak" training.

At this point a gym instructor or personal trainer can help. The instructor can modify your workout. You can do more eccentric type of training, which works on types IIa and IIb white fibers that contract the quick muscle fibers. It can produce higher force outputs at lower metabolic cost. Compared with concentric or conventional exercises, it is 25 percent less taxing. Isokinetic machines with optimal rest periods, alteration of intensity exercise sets, and fewer repetitions can directly affect your results (see Tables 26-2 and 26-3; see Chap. 26).

Resistant exercises and progression in children is documented in Table 29-1. A child can do basic exercises when he or she has the proper instruction, encouragement, and desire. Significant increases in strength will occur, but no hypertrophy. Increased

TABLE 29-1 Basic Guidelines for Resistance Exercise Progression in Children

Age (years)	Considerations
≤7	Introduce child to basic exercises with little or no weight; develop the concept of a training session; teach exercise techniques; progress from body weight calisthenics, partner exercises, and lightly resisted exercises; keep volume low.
8 to 10	Gradually increase the number of exercises; practice exercise technique in all lifts; start gradual progressive loading of exercises; keep exercises simple; gradually increase training volume; carefully monitor toleration to the exercise stress.
11 to 13	Teach all basic exercise techniques; continue progressive loading of each exercise; emphasize exercise techniques; introduce more advanced exercises with little or no resistance.
14 to 15	Progress to more advanced youth programs in resistance exercise; add sport-specific components; emphasize exercise techniques; increase volume.
≥16	Move child to entry-level adult programs after all background knowledge has been mastered and a basic level of training experience has been gained.

Note: If a child of any age begins a program with no previous experience, start the child at beginning levels and move him or her to more advanced levels as exercise toleration, skill, amount of training time, and understanding permit.

From Kraemer WJ, Fleck SJ: *Strength Training for Young Athletes*. Champaign, IL, Human Kinetics, 1993, p. 5. Copyright 1993 by William J. Kraemer and Steven J. Fleck. Reprinted by permission.

strength is owing to improved coordination of the muscles and more efficient use of the varied muscle groups.

Female athletes have improved their performance in all sports, particularly in weight training. They also do body building and power lifting. Generally, muscle strength in women is two-thirds that of men, and women are definitely weaker in the chest and arms in pretty well all sports, even gymnastics. They can be equally as strong in the lower extremities, however. Women definitely achieve increased strength following resistance training, but only minimal muscle hypertrophy in the majority of studies. This is owing to the hormonal levels, men have 20 to 30 times higher levels of androgen testosterone, which has the strong anabolic function of tissue building of muscles.

The aging athlete and weight training in the elderly are also much more popular now. In 1990, there were 31 million people over the age of 65 in the United States. This is 12 to 13 percent of the population. It is predicted that by the year 2020, there will be 52 million Americans over the age of 65 years. Octogenarians are the largest growing segment of the entire population.

Canadian statistics document 3.2 million, or 11.7 percent of Canada's total 27 million population, were over the age of 65 in 1991. It is predicted that this number will be 5 million out of 35 million in the year 2011, and 9 million out of 41 million in 2031, accounting for 22 percent of the total population.

Athletes reach their maximum strength between the ages of 20 and 30 years, and this in essence peaks at the age of 25.[7] The athletes tend to plateau through to the age of 50 years, with a small, yearly, progressive decline of approximately 4 percent per decade. After the age of 50, the loss is 10 percent per decade. At around the age of 65, the progress is even more rapid owing to a change in fiber type brought about by aging itself and also a lower level of physical activity.

There is more loss of muscle mass and reduced size in the fast-twitch type II fibers particularly. The neural function and ability to coordinate motion also deteriorate. There is an increased connective tissue in the muscle, and this causes increased stiffness in the aging process. Thus, warm-ups and stretching have to be modified proportionally.

Also, in the United States, between 400,000 to 500,000 hip and knee replacements are performed yearly. These patients usually have marked relief of pain and increased mobility, and they want to exercise and train. (See Chap. 9 for suggested training after a prosthetic joint.)

Professor James Zachazewski has proposed the use of a *Progressive Velocity Flexibility Program (PVFP)* whenever ballistic stretching is considered.[3] This is for the elite athlete who is already superbly conditioned (Table 29-2).

The athlete progresses from slow controlled stretching with close monitoring, to fast full-range stretching over days or weeks. The stretching program must be performed three to five times a week to maintain the stretching and flexibility gains, and it can be done even at home prior to going to the gym. With some body parts, tight calves, for instance, gentle stretching can be done five or six times a day.

The end-stage ballistic stretching is a dynamic, rapid action, bobbing motion imposed on the muscle to be stretched. James Zachazewski states that these actions have fallen out of favor because of possible injury; however, it can be effective for increasing flexibility in athletes.[3] It is particularly important in weight training where quick fibers can be stimulated by 20 repetitions in 20 s on a Hydragym machine, for instance, but again, this must be carefully monitored.

Note to the weight lifter on muscle strain: It is not unusual to strain a muscle at times. The cause is usually an inadequate warm-up and improper lifting or trying to lift too much weight.

In most cases you *do not* have to stop your workouts, just avoid using that part, for example, back or shoulder. The key to treatment is gentle stretching five or six times a day.

The difference between exercise-induced muscle change and trauma resides in the absence of bleeding following exercise-induced muscle change, according to Dr. William T. Stauber.[6] Fibers are torn at a microscopic level. The delayed onset muscle soreness (DOMS), according to Professor George Davies from the University of Wisconsin, occurs in all patients when they begin eccentric isokinetic rehabilitation programs, and this stiffness following a muscle program may have an adverse effect on the

TABLE 29-2 Progressive Velocity Flexibility Program

STATIC STRETCHING
↓
SSER—SLOW, SHORT, END-RANGE STRETCHING
↓
SFR—SLOW, FULL-RANGE STRETCHING
↓
FSER—FAST, SHORT, END-RANGE STRETCHING
↓
FFR—FAST, FULL-RANGE STRETCHING

From Zachazewski JE: Flexibility for sports, in Sanders B (ed): *Sports Physical Therapy.* Norwalk, CT, Appleton and Lange, 1990, pp. 201–238.

muscle.[6] Dr. Stauber also suggests nonsteroidal anti-inflammatory drugs (NSAIDs) for delayed-onset muscle stiffness and soreness following a vigorous workout or minor muscle strain; however, this may have an adverse effect on the muscle.[6] NSAIDs are antiprostaglandins, and prostaglandin does play a role in muscle remodeling and repair. Thus, the best method of decreasing pain from muscle strain is more stretching and regular exercise [transcutaneous electrical nerve stimulation (TENS)], as well as hot showers, whirlpool, swimming, and massage. If the stiffness persists for more than 5 days, a doctor should be consulted to decide if formal physiotherapy or rehabilitation treatment will help. Modalities (TENS) can reduce muscle swelling at that stage, and NSAIDs may be necessary. The greater the strength and fatigue resistance capacity of a muscle, the less likely it is to be injured.

Muscle strength does not limit muscle flexibility, provided the athlete pursues an active flexibility program. Thus, weight lifting does not make the athlete "muscle bound." The key is to stretch before and after.

WARM-UPS

The critical temperature is 39°C (103°F), and this is best reached through therapeutic exercise that takes 10 to 15 min in a normal warm-up, but it can vary on any given day.

A warm-down when the muscles are at their highest temperature is also the best way to avoid postexercise soreness.

The best prevention for "DOMS" is sensible, regular exercise. They are much more apt to occur after a layoff, owing to the "too much, too soon" principle and the "no pain, no gain" philosophy.

ECCENTRIC EXERCISES (NEGATIVES)

These produce higher force outputs at lower metabolic costs. Eccentric to concentric percentages of quadriceps range from 146 percent to 300 percent, the elbow flexors 112 percent to 200 percent, and ankle plantar flexors about 178 percent. Optimal repetition for concentric isokinetics is 10, based on Davies' research, and because eccentrics can generate 1.2 to 1.8 times more torque, six to seven reps would perform the same total work.[6] This can be accomplished with free weights or on the Cybex, Kincom, and other machines.

A good example is with the leg extension machine (see Fig. 29-16), the athlete should lift whatever he or she can handle easily with both legs and then gradually adjust his or her one-leg maximum (1 RM). When this is established, the athlete can lift 10 lb more with both legs and then bring it back down slowly with one leg. The athlete should be careful to protect it with the opposite leg, particularly through the dangerous arc.

This can be done with different muscle groups and usually needs an instructor or a partner. When it is done with the Cybex or Kincom machine it is computer-driven. The dynamometer can control the speed, and it is a combination of concentric and eccentric isokinetic exercise.

DROP SETS (NEGATIVES)

This is a combination of eccentric (negative) 3-s drops and explosive 1-s concentric exercises with a diminishing load.[6]

Most body builders are familiar with the concept of drop sets, in which the athlete performs several sets of the same exercise but with little or no rest between sets and with each subsequent set using lighter weights than the previous one. However, for best results, one needs to take into account how efficiently one's nervous system recruits fast-twitch fibers.

Two of the primary factors that determine neurologic efficiency are training experience and an individual's ratio of fast- to slow-twitch fibers. Beginner trainees, particularly women, tend to be less neurologically efficient than advanced body builders, which means they are able to perform more repetitions with weights closer to their 1 RM. For example, at 80 percent of his or her 1 RM, the average body builder will be able to perform about 10 repetitions, whereas an advanced body builder will probably be able to perform only three to five repetitions. As you can see, just because a person's nervous system is not efficient does not necessarily mean he or she is not strong.

DROP SETS FOR THE NEUROLOGICALLY INEFFICIENT BODY BUILDER

Here is an example of how a body builder who is neurologically inefficient (i.e., a beginner) should perform drop sets. The exercise is the bench press, and this body builder's 1 RM is 200 lb.

1. Warm up
2. 140 lb × 12 to 15 repetitions
3. No rest; drop the weight 40 lb
4. 100 × 12 to 15 repetitions
5. No rest; drop the weight 40 lb
6. 60 lb × 12 to 15 repetitions
7. Rest 2 min, repeat steps 2 to 6 two times

All repetitions are performed with a 2-0-2 tempo (lower the weight for two, no pause, raise the weight for two). Aim at constant tension in these repetitions to recruit primarily the type IIa fibers. You'll also notice there is no pause between drops in weight, because this type of body builder is more suited for muscular endurance.

DROP SETS FOR THE NEUROLOGICALLY EFFICIENT BODY BUILDER

Here is an example of how a body builder who is neurologically efficient (i.e., an advanced body builder) should perform drop sets. Again, the exercise is the bench press but the body builder's 1 RM is 350 lb.

1. Warm up
2. 265 lb × 5 repetitions
3. Rest 4 min
4. 300 × 3 repetitions
5. Rest 10 s while your partner removes 10 lb from each side of the barbell
6. 280 lb × max repetitions (normally one or two)
7. Rest 10 s while your partner removes 10 lb from each side of the barbell
8. 260 lb × max repetitions (normally one or two)
9. Rest 4 min
10. Repeat steps 4 to 9 three times

Notice that there is a 10-s pause between drops in weight; this will allow the advanced body builder enough time to be able to activate the higher threshold fibers.

All repetitions are performed on a 3-1-X tempo; that is, a smooth descent of 3 s for the eccentric contraction, a pause of 1 s, and an explosive contraction to tap into the high-threshold fast-twitch fibers. Even though the desired speed of the bar displacement is explosive, because of the amount of weight, the bar may not actually move that fast. However, one must concentrate on accelerating the bar through the concentric range. Of course, near the end of the movement, you will decelerate to prevent injuries. For long-range movements such as squats and deadlifts, you may want to use 4 to 5 s for the eccentric lowering.

The pause should be taken where leverage is favorable (i.e., the lockout position in the bench press), so the muscles can relax and the blood supply can be replenished. According to Australian strength and biomechanics expert Dr. Greg Wilson, this will permit one to access more of the high-threshold fast-twitch fibers.

PERFORMANCE-ENHANCING DRUGS

The muscle magazines usually have two or three interesting articles wedged between pages and pages of ads for all sorts of natural and hormonal products. These are accompanied by truly unbelievable "Before" and "After" photos of people who took ABC pills and lost pounds and gained superb muscles. Most of them are a waste of money. However, one natural product really does work. It is creatine monohydrate. Make sure the market preparations are quite pure. A reputable company is Optimum Nutrition (Coral Springs, FL 33065 [954-755-9822] US $25 for 2 lb [908 g]). You must load for 5 days to get performance improvement. This requires one scoop, 43 g, four times daily. Then maintenance is one or two 43-g servings daily, depending on your size and the intensity of training. Obviously, you have to be training near your "peak" for maximum benefit.

Studies suggest increased muscle volume and strength. It also enhances aerobic and anaerobic running training. It has been used by the Canadian Army with good results (Ira Jacobs, personal communication).

However, cases of hypertension after 8 weeks of steady use have been reported. Thus, do not take this steadily for more than 8 weeks. Stop taking it for 4 weeks and then reload and start another 8-week cycle. There is a letdown when one stops. The weights get heavier and the aerobic machines are harder, but this disappears quickly. Muscle gain and fat loss are permanent, provided one continues to train effectively.

This has no relationship whatsoever to anabolic steroids ("the roids"). Creatine is a natural substance and a source of carbohydrate energy enhancement.

PROPER NUTRITION

Body builders and marathon runners often have bizarre dietary habits known as "reverse anorexia." They do not eat conventional meals or eat at mealtimes. They take large amounts of protein and health foods and eat and drink a lot of fruit concoctions from a blender.

A typical diet might be pineapple, egg whites, protein supplements, and rice. Their goal is to reduce body fat to about 4 percent so they can be "ripped" for a competition.

Home Exercise Equipment

There are more exercise bikes, walkers, rowing machines, Nordic Tracks, power gliders, and weight sets used as coat racks than are actually used for exercise.

The Saturday and Sunday morning TV channels that feature superbly conditioned men and women on a power walker or rider, for instance, are impossible. Those models cannot get into that kind of shape on that type of equipment. The cheaper equipment breaks easily, and once the athlete gets into moderate shape, that equipment is not satisfactory. The cheaper treadmills, for instance, break down when you try to jog on them.

The best home exercise machine is the one you will use. It is very important to try out the treadmill, rowing machine, Nordic Track, cross-country ski machine on your own, in your gym clothing. See if you like it, and make sure it satisfies your goals and needs.

The old adage, "You get what you pay for" is very true in this type of purchase. Home gyms are fine, but you do need a set of weights, and of course you do need to use them in order to gain muscle and get in shape. The addition of an elliptical exerciser for instance (Precor), is worthwhile, but it is much more expensive than the Health Rider or Nordic Track, which both broke down when *Consumer Reports* tested them.

Thus, at least a trial membership at the local gym, or attendance as a guest with one of your friends, is the best way to start strength and weight training. Once you are in shape, augmentation of the exercises at home is quite satisfactory, and a large number of machines, walkers, or riders is unnecessary.

RECOMMENDED READINGS

1. Brewer B: Marco Island Fitness Club. Personal Communication.
2. Pearl W: *Keys to the Inner Universe*. Phoenix, OR.
3. Zachazewski JE, Magee DJ, Quillen WS: Physiological principles of resistance training and rehabilitation, in Falkel J, Cipriani D (eds): *Athletic Injuries and Rehabilitation*. Philadelphia, Saunders, 1996, pp. 206–226.
4. Knight KL: Techniques of progressive resistance exercise. *Arch Phys Med* 29:263–273, 1948.
5. Knight KL: Quadriceps strengthening with DAPRE technique. *Med Sci Sports* 17:646–650, 1985.
6. Davies J, Ellenbecker T: Eccentric isokinetics. *Orthop Phys Ther Clin North Am* 1:2, 1992.
7. Hopkinson WJ: *The Aging Athlete*. Loyola University Medical Centre, 23rd Annual Meeting, AOSSM, 1997.
6. Garhammer J: *Strength Training: Sports Illustrated*. Lanham, MD, Madison Books, 1994.
8. Baechle T, Conroy B: Pre-season strength training in Mellion, Walsh, Shelton (eds): *The Team Physician's Handbook*, 2d ed. St. Louis, Mosby, 1997.
9. U.S. Weightlifting Federation: *Coaching Manual*, Vol 1, 2, and 3. Colorado Springs, COUSWF, 1986 to 1991.

30 | **Dance Injuries**

D.J. Ogilvie-Harris   Penny Fleming

There are many types of dance, such as modern, jazz, character, ethnic, tap, and aerobic. In addition, there is classical ballet, which is a major art form. Dance requires not only great athletic prowess and flexibility but also the ability to interpret music rhythmically, an aesthetic presence, and the appropriate body frame (Fig. 30-1).

Dancers are noted to sustain substantial injuries to the musculoskeletal system. An epidemiological study of ballet injuries in one large professional ballet company covering 3 years showed that the insurance payouts for medical costs were close to US $400,000.[1] It was noted that roughly 25 percent of the dancers had five or more injuries and accounted for over 50 percent of the costs. The foot was most frequently injured (over 25 percent of cases), in

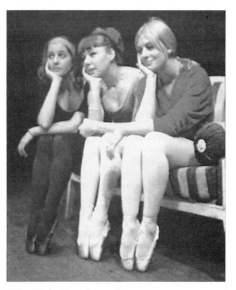

FIG. 30-1 The dancers become accustomed to keeping their "on pointe" even at rest.

about 25 percent of cases the lumbar spine was injured, and other common injuries were to the ankle and knee. In addition to biomechanical abnormalities in the dancers, environmental factors, such as the dance surface itself, affect injury rates.[2]

Dancers themselves indicate that most, at some time or other, have had significant injuries and problems from those injuries.[3] The dancers were asked if they have had musculoskeletal problems in the past 12 months. Seventy percent complained of back pain, 65 percent with problems of the ankles or feet, and 54 percent neck problems. Interestingly enough, there were no differences between sexes. Ankle and foot problems had kept dancers from their daily work in over 50 percent of the cases, and low back problems had prevented them from working to a lesser extent. Although a lot of them had neck pain, only one in five reported that the neck trouble interfered with their activities. Most of the problems related to poor training. Ways of decreasing trouble were mostly related to therapeutic treatments.

CAUSES OF DANCE INJURIES

Anthropometric Variables

Both male and female dancers are required to have a specific physique. Most notably in classical ballet, aesthetics have demanded a thin body type.

This can lead to significant problems with eating disorders in ballerinas. Much has been written about professional dancing and dietary insufficiency. Studies across the world have shown that female dancers in general have inadequate nutritional intake. People training rigorously for ballet have delayed puberty compared to controls. There is significant decrease in bone density in professionally trained women dancers and a high incidence of amenorrhea. Differences across countries may reflect the eating habits of the various dance companies. For example, in the Netherlands, there is a lower prevalence of amenorrhea compared to U.S. dancers.[4] This may directly reflect the different aesthetic values placed by different dance companies.

This area requires constant monitoring. In the prepubertal stages of development, decreased bone density owing to inadequate calorie intake will lead to problems in later life. Intensive dance practice, which is a prerequisite for professional dancing, can in itself lead to eating disorders and weight control in early childhood.[5] The weight and height statistics of children who practice individual sports must be monitored. Early abnormalities can then be detected and treated. This minimizes the chance for the development of osteoporosis, associated menstrual disturbances, and long-term complications. Eating disorders have not been a significant problem among male dancers. They need to be light and muscular. Their build is similar to that of a gymnast.

Flexibility has been assessed specifically in dancers to determine if it plays a role in injuries. Although dancers who have had injuries to the ankle have decreased dorsiflexion, no definite correlation has been found between decreased flexibility and recurrent injuries. However, dancers who have had previous injuries are significantly at risk of sustaining further injuries. This would suggest therefore that intensive rehabilitation efforts should be made following the first injury to prevent reinjury.[6]

Proprioception has been studied extensively in dancers. It is better than in the normal population. Dancers perform superiorly under sensory challenged conditions, such as on foam and dome tests.[7] In one study of classical ballet dancers, using a computer-assisted force plate, male and female dancers had a better perception than active control groups. Following ankle injury, the postural stability was decreased. Even after the dancers returned to their professional activities, they still had abnormalities in perception.[8]

Muscle strength in dancers is similar to that for gymnasts but significantly different to other active athletes. On average, eccentric endurance in professional dancers was 30 percent greater than active control groups. Concentric endurance was only 7 percent greater. A significantly greater eccentric to concentric total work ratio was observed in ballet dancers and greater eccentric and concentric peaks.[9] Repetitive loading of the lower extremities in dance leads to higher eccentric knee extensor stresses and subsequently endurance. Interestingly, no differences were noted between males and females.

Many high-performance athletes tolerate pain well, including professional ballet dancers. Dancers have higher pain and pain tolerance thresholds than age-matched controls. Despite the increased thresholds they have a more acute experience of the sensory aspects of pain. This may be owing to the greater experience of pain by the dancers and also perhaps because they are more in tune with their body image.[10] This is important in treating dancers because, although these patients are "tough," they are also very sensitive to their pain and to their body function. The psychological and emotional as well as the physical aspects need to be addressed.

Technique

As in all sports and athletic activities, correct technique is of paramount importance. Among dance injuries, ballet carries the highest risk of injury to the foot and ankle. In one study, two out of three of all foot and ankle injuries in dancers were in the group doing ballet.[6] Classical dancing "on pointe" puts the foot at risk. In this position, the talus is almost vertical within the ankle mortise.[11] Significant force is placed on the plantarflexed toes. The toes are placed in special pointe shoes, and ballerinas pad these shoes so as to evenly distribute the force across their toes. In the long term there is a significant increase in arthritis of the ankle, subtalar joint, and first metatarsophalangeal joint in ballet dancers. However, there is little change in the incidence of arthritis of the hip.[12] A lot of the degenerative changes were explained by repetitive microtrauma; repetitive injury is also a factor.

The positions during standing and demi-plié are different in ballet dancers and other modern professional dancers. In ballet dancers, there is genu recurvatum at the beginning and end of a demi-plié that is not seen in modern dancers. Associated with this are significant differences in the use of lower extremity muscles. Techniques vary depending on the type of dance but are critical in minimizing the chance of injury.

Dancers are required to perform extensive and repetitive jumps. These jumps lead to repetitive loading of the ankle and knee joint. The jumping distance compared to the maximum jump distance for each individual is critical in determining the amount of joint forces. As the jump distance increases from 30 percent to 60 percent to 90 percent, so does the ground reaction force. This corresponds with increased quadriceps peak magnitudes. In addition, this increases the reaction force at the knee joint and ankle. High-impact situations with jumps of 90 percent of the maximum jump distance create significant magnitudes across joints. This can exceed 14 times the body weight. It is vitally important that the takeoff and landing are precisely controlled. Jumping techniques should be practiced at less than maximum jump distance until technical perfection is achieved.[13]

Overuse and Repetitive Stress

Dancers in general work long hours. In addition to their performances, they also have to be active in rehearsal and class. The vast majority of the time is spent in dance-related activities. They have little time or energy to spend on basic body maintenance activities, such as weight training and concentric or eccentric muscle strengthening. As a result of this they are at risk of repetitive stress injuries. Female dancers in addition often suffer from osteoporosis or decreased bone density and maintain stress fractures. These are commonest in the second metatarsal of the foot. They are also recognized in the tibia, causing shin splints, and may also occur in the spine as spondylolysis.

Overuse injuries to the soft tissues are extremely common with tendinitis of the patella tendon, the Achilles tendon, and flexor hallucis longus. The hip and low back soft tissues are subject frequently to pain and discomfort from overuse. Some of these factors are exacerbated by poor nutritional status and cigarette smoking. Both of these factors lead to decreased bone density.

Trauma

Dancing is an athletic pursuit. The body is subjected to tremendous forces, with choreography often demanding unusual and extreme ranges of motion at very high speeds. Thus, the risk of injury from incorrect landings or takeoffs, misplaced steps, or subsequent falls is extremely high. The commonest of all injuries is a twisted ankle.

TYPES OF DANCE INJURIES

The Lumbar Spine

Dancers have great flexibility compared to many other athletes. Their flexibility is similar to those of gymnasts. Choreography often involves many movements of the spine to extremes of physiologic range of motion. Thus, there is a high incidence of both acute and chronic lumbar problems. Specific strategies should be included in their regular routine to minimize the risk of lumbar trauma; for example, strengthening of the abdominal and small rotating muscles of the back, pelvic stabilization, and Pilates training. Pelvic stabilization, in particular, is often poor and accompanied by imbalances of muscle groups in the area. This needs to be assessed and addressed in the dancer.

Specific strategies should be followed to try and minimize the risk of lumbar trauma. These include specific strengthening of the abdominal muscles, the lumbar muscles, and pelvic stabilization. Pelvic stabilization in particular is often poor and there may be an imbalance of muscle groups. This needs to be assessed in dancers and especially those who have lumbar symptoms or injuries.

Disk herniations are well recognized, more so in males than females. This is related to pas de deux, or the lifting of the female, and the large jumps they must perform. In the overhead position there is excess lumbar lordosis, and this may lead to premature disk herniation.

The management is fairly standard. Initially following a disk herniation there should be a suitable period of rest. Neurologic symptoms need to be thoroughly investigated. Rarely is surgical intervention necessary. Management of disk injury is fairly standard. Rest with proper positioning instruction and a suitable exercise regime are essential initially. Often physiotherapy includes manual mobilization, myofascial release techniques, traction, and muscle balancing instruction.

With the decrease in symptoms, a graduated physiotherapy program will continue to restore movement and strength to the lumbar spine. Pelvic stabilization is critical in these patients. It may take many months until there is sufficient spinal control to return to rehearsals and then performance. Specific use of isokinetic training is probably of great value in restoring power throughout range of movement.

Alternative medicine, although frequently used for spinal injuries, has little scientific proof. Nonetheless, considerable emphasis is given to treatments such as acupuncture, homeopathy, reflexology, shiatsu, and similar modalities. These may have merit, but individual response can be quite varied.

Of particular importance is the development of spondylolysis. A young dancer presenting with acute back pain should always be thoroughly investigated for this condition. There may be a traumatic break in the pars intraarticularis. In the early stages this is best recognized on a bone scan that will be positive in this area. A CT or magnetic resonance scan may later show the lesion.

In some cases, the use of a spinal orthosis allows such lesions to heal. Many now prefer simply to treat them symptomatically and to take them away from the stressful routines for a relatively prolonged period of time, such as 6 months to a year. Then with careful muscle rehabilitation and restoration of flexibility, the individual can return to dancing. However, ongoing care must be taken not to put the spine in a hyperextended position.

In very rare circumstances, the dancer may have ongoing excruciating pain and may even develop spondylolisthesis. This then would lead into the realm of surgical treatment. There is considerable variation in this surgical procedure depending on the extent of the lesion and surgical preference. This may vary from local bone grafting of the pars intraarticularis to decompression of the nerve roots to a fusion of the involved segments, either from anterior or posterior or both. In such an event it is unlikely that the dancer will resume his or her career.

The Pelvis and Hip

In ballet technique, a turned out position is achieved by turning the hip into maximum external rotation such that the feet point outward. Dancers often force this position. This may be a problem because the range of external rotation and abduction is limited at the point where the greater trochanter contacts the outer wall of the pelvis.

It was thought that ballerinas had increased femoral anteversion. However, recent studies have shown that this is not true. This means therefore that the position of turn out is determined mainly by the soft tissue constraints and by the actual contact of the greater trochanter on the pelvis. Once a dancer has achieved maximal soft tissue stretch in training, the turn out therefore cannot be significantly increased.[14] Attempting to force this position leads to a rotation strain on the feet. This tends to make the feet move forward into eversion and predisposes to tendinitis and other similar problems.

Dancers may present with a clicking hip. It is important to determine whether this is the psoas tendon that snaps across the front of the hip joint or a torn acetabular labrum with intraarticular pathology in the hip itself.

A test specifically for the psoas tendon with the hip flexed will reveal weakness but will not be affected by acetabular labrum or articular cartilage problems. In glenoid labrum tears, the clicking can characteristically be reproduced by internal and external rotation of the hip when it is flexed to 90 degrees. Sometimes the clicking may be caused by the fascia lata snapping over the greater trochanter, and this can be palpated clinically. The key to proper diagnosis is to be able to reproduce the click and to try to determine the biomechanics of what produces the click. Magnetic resonance scanning is the best investigation, as it can reveal the precise pathology, which is usually in the soft tissues.

If it is determined that the problem is a tendinitis or a mild effusion in the hip joint from overuse, then a structured program of avoiding stress to the injured area, anti-inflammatory medication, and appropriate stretching and strengthening will usually allow the condition to resolve. Many soft tissue techniques, such as myofascial, trigger point, strain-counterstrain, massage, and muscle energy, to name a few, are essential to any physiotherapy program for these individuals.

If it is determined that it is a torn glenoid labrum or chondral loose body in the acetabulum, then arthroscopy and arthroscopic removal of the damaged area can successfully relieve the symptoms. When fascia lata produces "snapping hip," this can be released surgically through a small incision. On some occasions the fascia lata split longitudinally, but I prefer a cruciate incision in the fascia lata. This relieves the symptoms in the vast majority of cases without significantly weakening the ileotibial band.

Knee Problems

Chondromalacia of the patella with the patellofemoral syndrome is extremely common in dancers. This is owing to: (1) subjecting the knees to high eccentric loads; (2) turnout or extreme external rotation of the hip; and (3) often performing dance movements on their knees. Most professional dancers do have patellofemoral crepitus on examination, but this does not necessarily signify major pathology.

It is uncertain as to why some dancers with chondromalacia have symptoms and others do not. It may be that overuse of the joint produces secondary changes in the subchondral bone or the small fragments of the articular cartilage excite an inflammatory response in the joint. Certainly in those knees that have a small effusion as well as a patellofemoral syndrome, inflammation is a definite cause for the ongoing pain. Those patients where there are signs of inflammation will respond well to anti-inflammatories but, in the majority of cases anti-inflammatories play little role in the management of this condition. Our experience has found that a graduated concentric and eccentric program significantly helps these patients. Isokinetics also play a primary role in rehabilitation.

The knee joint needs to be carefully assessed when presenting with patellofemoral symptoms. Recent studies indicate that ileotibial band tightness was definitely related to patellofemoral pain. The degree of tibial external rotation used in the dance demi-plié was significantly increased in dancers who had ileotibial band tightness.[15]

One of the commoner causes of patellofemoral pain is excess lateral pressure syndrome. The patella may be very tight on the lateral side with decreased patella tilt to manual testing. This would be contributed to by a tight ileotibial band. In this situation, treatment is directed toward mobilizing the patella on the lateral side and specific stretching of the ileotibial band. Self-mobilization by the patient is key.

If the condition is refractory to treatment and the symptoms are limiting, then an arthroscopic lateral retinacular release may significantly improve the situation. I have had good success in both male and female dancers in performing the arthroscopic lateral release specifically for the excess lateral pressure syndrome. Careful rehabilitation is necessary afterward because there is an initial loss of quadriceps strength. Initially, concentric training and subsequently eccentric training of the quadriceps is necessary. It is essential to regain a high level of strength before resuming impact activities such as jumps.

Patella instability with lateral subluxation or dislocation is commonly found. It is more common in females than in males. In most cases, this may be controlled by exercises specifically focused on strengthening the vastus medialis obliquus (VMO). Biofeedback with surface EMGs can be used to specifically trigger the VMO during dance activities. Many dancers with episodes of subluxation or dislocation have significant weakness of the quadriceps muscle in eccentric loading and this can be specifically improved. In rare circumstances, surgical reconstruction is necessary, but the loss of flexibility and power following the surgical intervention may preclude the dancer from returning to a professional career.

Patella tendinitis is particularly common in dancers. The pain is at the origin of the patella tendon at the inferior pole of the patella. Recent studies have suggested that this may be an impingement lesion and that the inferior pole of the patella may in fact impinge on the patella tendon as it courses distally.

Initial treatment for patella tendinitis consists of rest, stretches, and the use of ice and anti-inflammatories. Although anti-inflammatories have not conclusively been shown to be of benefit, a short-term course of 7 to 10 days probably does have some value. Prolonged use of anti-inflammatories is not to be condoned.

One of the most important features of tendinitis is the associated muscle weakness. This is particularly so in eccentric activities. Concentric activity probably does not develop sufficient force to cause tendon ruptures. However, eccentric activity may generate forces many times the body weight and beyond the tensile strength of the tendon. This may cause microruptures at the tendon–bone interface in the area of Sharpey's fibers.

Tendinopathies of this nature have been shown to be histologically characterized by reabsorption of bone around Sharpey's fibers. This is often associated with new bone formation and inflammatory tissue.

In order to restore the tendon to full function, eccentric muscle training is needed. The eccentric load is progressively applied to the tendon in order to rebuild strength of the muscle and of the bone–tendon interface. This must be done in a carefully controlled fashion avoiding the limits of movement so as to allow the tendon and bone to react positively to the stress with increased strength. If the extreme limits of movement, such as full flexion or full extension of the joint are reached and stressed, this may cause further damage to the tendon. Midrange eccentric activities are the essential component for therapy following tendinitis.

A patella tendon strap around the inferior pole of the patella may help to relieve symptoms. Many dancers find this awkward, and find it either falls off their knee during dance activities or gets in the way, particularly when they are doing knee flexion routines.

In refractory cases, judicious use of an injection of cortisone into the area of maximum pain can be considered. The injection is put into the painful area down to the bone. There is a small theoretical risk of tendon rupture, and therefore it is recommended that dancers do not return to high-impact activities for 6 weeks or so following the injection. Scientific evidence is lacking to support the use of cortisone for such tendinopathies but nonetheless there is a large anecdotal body of evidence to suggest it works.

The ultimate solution in resistant cases is surgical decompression. A small incision is made over the distal pole of the patella and the patella tendon itself is split in length with its fibers. At surgery it is often possible to see tears of the tendon where it attaches to the bone and often there is granulation tissue in the area of the tendinitis. More recently, it has been suggested that a small piece of bone is removed from the inferior pole of the patella. At the inferior pole of the patella there is not actual tendon attachment. This bone can therefore be removed. This inferior pole has been suggested as being the cause of the impingement of the tendon rather than damage to the tendon–bone interface itself.

Dancers are also subjected to major traumatic injuries of the knee, such as a torn anterior cruciate ligament or torn menisci. These require standard orthopaedic investigation and management. In the rehabilitation of patients following such injuries, it is essential to stress the role of eccentric activity and flexibility in dance.

In modern dance and ballet, a lot of the movements may take place with the dancer on his or her knees. This may lead to prepatellar bursitis. The initial management of this is to try and unload the knee. Practices may be carried out with the use of knee pads. If the bursa is persistent, an injection of cortisone into the bursa may help to eliminate it. In a few cases, the bursitis may be resistant to treatment and may persist. Surgical excision of the bursa can then be carried out. This is best done arthroscopically, which leaves minimal scar formation and is quite effective. The arthroscope is inserted into the bursa itself and then the bursa is removed from within until no bursal sac remains.

The Foot and Ankle

Achilles Tendinitis

Achilles tendinitis is extremely common in dancers. It is seen clinically as thickening of the tendon. There is often crepitus around the tendinous insertion into the bone. Careful examination is necessary to determine what is the actual anatomic structure causing pain in Achilles tendinitis. The problem may be at the muscle-tendinous junction, within the tendon itself with a partial tear, or a chronic tendinitis. Sometimes it may be at the insertion of the tendon into bone, which is an enthesopathy. It may lie deep to the tendon in the retrocalcaneal bursa. Careful clinical examination with localization of the site of tenderness is probably the best method to determine the source of pain. Magnetic resonance scanning is the ideal way to determine the precise pathologic diagnosis.

When there is persistent pain in the myotendinous junction or the tendinous portion of the Achilles tendon, surgical decompression and repair of the partial tear will often benefit the dancer. An incision is made over the tendon, and the tendon sheath is completely excised. This is done meticulously to minimize the formation of any further scar tissue. The tear in the tendon can often be localized, and painful nodules can be removed. If the tendon is split lengthwise, to remove a tear or a nodule, then it should be repaired with sutures.

Following this operative procedure, the rehabilitation consists of gentle stretching and mobilization. The tendon is not to be subjected to significant concentric or eccentric loads for 6 weeks after the surgery. Then a graduated progressive resistance exercise program is carried out focusing on strength and flexibility. Ultimately, return to dance activities will depend on redeveloping concentric and eccentric muscle strength.

The pain at the distal end of the Achilles tendon may be caused by impingement of the posterior aspect of the os calcis, best known as pump bumps or Hagalung's deformity. This is a bony impingement of the tendon. The posterior portion of the os calcis can be excised to decompress this area.

If the source of the pain is actually at the enthesis where the Achilles tendon joins the bone, there is no surgical treatment. Treatment must consist of trying to minimize the ongoing inflammation. This involves the use of ice, stretching, and strengthening activities in the midrange, focusing particularly on eccentric strength. Pilates exercises which can strengthen the muscles in a nonstressful situation are particularly useful.

In Europe, electromagnetic shock treatment has been used for such tendinopathies. This technology is similar to the lithotripter that uses soundwaves to break kidney stones. The machinery consists of a plastic dome filled with water through which thousands of small shock waves are passed. The dome focuses the shock waves in a very small area of 1 to 2 mm. This is applied to the tendon–bone interface. Over a period of 20 minutes, several thousand shock waves are applied to this area. This results in microstress fractures of the bone. This stimulates new bone formation or callus. This in turn will strengthen the tendon–bone interface or enthesis. Initial clinical results, especially in Germany, have been quite encouraging with 75 to 80 percent positive results. However, the technology has not been subjected to rigorous scientific investigation up to this point in time.

Flexor Hallucis Tendinitis

This is a specific injury in dancers (also in gymnasts). The flexor hallucis longus travels behind the ankle joint and deep to the sustentaculum tali. It travels in a fibrous sheath at the posterior aspect of the joint. In the "en pointe" position, or with the ankle fully plantarflexed, the tendon is impinged. The tendon may well go on to develop chronic tendinitis or a partial tear. The dancers will then find that on plantarflexing the foot, they will have pain in the posterior aspect of the ankle and often a click.

The key point to diagnosis is to place the examiner's fingers directly over the flexor hallucis longus tendon. This can be felt behind the medial malleolus at the midpoint between the medial malleolus and the Achilles tendon. By keeping the foot in neutral and just flexing and extending the great toe, the tendon can be felt coursing in the sheath. If there is significant tendinitis or a nodule, crepitus or clicking can be felt.

A magnetic resonance scan will show the pathology clearly. There will often be fluid within the sheath of the flexor hallucis longus. Splits in the tendon or signs of chronic tendinitis may often be seen.

Conservative treatment is usually not successful for this condition. Once there is actual entrapment within the sheath, then nonoperative treatment usually cannot relieve it. The surgical approach is to make a medial incision and dissect down behind the medial malleolus to the flexor hallucis longus tendon. The sheath may then be opened and the tendon decompressed. The pathology, with a split or nodule, can be seen. The split or tear in the tendon does not have to be removed. However, the tendon must be thoroughly decompressed.

Results of the surgery are generally very successful. Initially, the dancers may have some posterior stiffness from scar tissue formation. However, with the appropriately directed therapy working on flexibility, proprioception, and muscle strength, they should be able to return to professional activities. Following surgery, it will be at least 6 weeks before they can resume any impact activities. They do need a progressive resistive program including elastic tubing and plyometrics before returning to full performance.

Posterior Impingement

Posterior impingement of the ankle is usually owing to either an elongated posterior tubercle or an "os trigonum." The "os trigonum" is an unfused portion of the posterior tubercle of the talus. It arises from a separate ossific center. However, there is a view that this may be fractured in childhood from the repetitive posterior impingement caused by plantarflexion of the foot. This is what produces the loose piece in the posterior aspect of the ankle.

The "os trigonum" is found in the general population. In most athletes, it does not cause problems because they are not required to assume the full plantarflexed position of the foot. In dancers required to go on pointe or demi-pointe, this causes particular problems with impingement. It causes similar problems in gymnasts.

Clinical examination demonstrates pain at the posterior aspect of the ankle on full plantarflexion. X-rays show the "os trigonum." In the presence of persisting symptoms, the "os trigonum" may be removed. If it is still attached by fibrous tissue or if it is a large bony prominence, this can be removed. It is excised through either a medial or a lateral incision deep to the Achilles tendon. At the time of surgery, it is important to make sure that there are no residual bony prominences at the posterior aspect of the talus, which will continue to impinge.

Postoperatively, the major problem is the posterior scar formation from the surgery. It takes a long time for the dancers to restore their full plantarflexion. It is essential that most of the flexibility and all of the strength is restored before going back to full performance. Physiotherapy always includes scar tissue and ankle joint mobilizations, soft tissue massage, modalities to reduce inflammation, and a progressive resistive program.

The Sprained Ankle

The sprained ankle is the commonest injury in dance. In most cases simple conservative treatment with rest, ice, compression, and elevation will result in significant decrease in the pain and swelling. A Jobst pump is highly successful in the first 24- to 72-h management of this injury. Functional restoration programs are essential if the dancer is not gong to be reinjured.

The key areas to rehabilitation following an ankle sprain are the restoration of strength and proprioception. Studies have shown that after an ankle strain, the reflexes in the peroneal muscles are significantly longer in duration than in an uninjured limb. That means that when the ankle suddenly goes into inversion, the peroneal muscles cannot correct the abnormal position and the patient has recurrent ankle sprains. In addition, the peroneal muscles themselves are essential as a proprioceptive device in stabilizing the ankle. Studies have shown that the mechanoreceptors in the lateral ligaments of the ankle are not of great importance. Putting local anesthetic into the lateral ligaments of the ankle did not in any way increase instability or cause problems.

The key areas for restoration of ankle function are to restore the flexibility of the joint and specifically strengthen the peroneal muscles. They should be trained both concentrically and eccentrically. Specific plyometric training of the muscles should be carried out. This could be as simple as a skipping program with the use of a tilt board for proprioception. It could also be much more involved with dance-specific activities on balance boards, trampolines, or in water or the use of elasticized bands, weights, or pulleys. The Kincom or Cybex is another helpful tool when retraining the dancer.

Prospective studies on dancers have shown that after an ankle sprain their proprioception is significantly diminished. It often remains diminished for a considerable period of time after they resume their performances. This will therefore tend to put dancers at risk of reinjury. It has also been noted in dance companies that one of the most significant risk factors for injury is previous injury of the same limb. This suggests that inadequate rehabilitation may lead to return to performance in less than optimal condition.

A certain percentage of ankle sprains will go on to develop chronic problems. When the pain persists for more than 6 months, it may be owing to specific pathologic conditions that lead to chronic ankle pain. These have been divided into three groups of conditions. There are two instabilities, two impingements, and two sets of chondral pathology.[16]

Chronic lateral ligamentous laxity is owing to repetitive inversion injuries (Fig. 30-2). Clinically the patients will have a very lax lateral side of the ankle with an anterior draw. X-rays are not par-

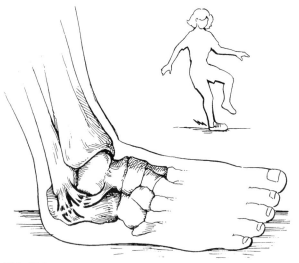

FIG. 30-2   Lateral instability of the ankle caused by an inversion and supination injury.

ticularly helpful because all dancers have increased flexibility and have increased talar tilt. I feel that clinical examination is the most effective. If, in producing lateral instability, the patient's symptoms are reproduced, this is good evidence that the lateral instability is the cause of the problem.

Surgical repair of lateral instability consists of a primary repair of the ligaments. I favor dissecting out the anterior talofibula ligament with the extensor retinaculum and the fibulocalcaneal ligaments and reattaching these directly back to the fibula with suture anchors. Alternately a cruciate incision may be made over the lateral structures, and these can be repaired primarily (known as the Brostrom repair).

Following this type of repair, the patient is in a cast for 6 weeks. They require extensive rehabilitation to regain the flexibility, strength, and proprioception. This type of repair is favored over the more traditional Evans repair that sacrifices the peroneus brevis tendon. In addition, the Evans repair extends across both the subtalar joint and the ankle joint and leads to limited subtalar movement.

Syndesmotic instability is caused by an external rotation injury of the ankle (Fig. 30-3). The patients present typically with pain at the syndesmosis rather than over the tip of the fibula. The external rotation test in which the foot is externally rotated on the calf pro-

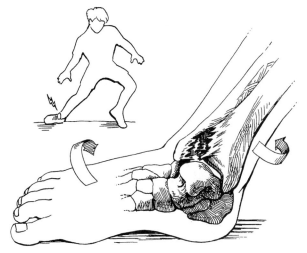

FIG. 30-3 Syndesmotic instability is caused by an external rotation injury.

duces pain at the syndesmosis. A squeeze test to compress the syndesmosis is usually positive. Taking the medial and lateral malleolus and translating them anteriorly and posteriorly produces the pain and instability. A bone scan is the best test and often shows localized increased activity at the syndesmosis. Magnetic resonance imaging may show disruption of the syndesmotic ligaments.

Initially this injury takes twice as long to heal as the lateral ligamentous injury of the ankle. There is no known way of effectively bracing the syndesmosis. If the symptoms persist then arthroscopic treatment can be effective.

At arthroscopy, there is commonly found associated intraarticular pathology. The interosseous ligament is usually ruptured and dangling down within the joint. In addition there is a characteristic chondral fracture of the posterolateral tibial plafond. Removing these areas of pathology seems to relieve the patient's pain in upward of 85 percent of cases. It is therefore the associated intraarticular pathology that seems to cause the pain in chronic syndesmotic strains rather than any residual instability in the syndesmosis itself.

The two impingement syndromes are anterolateral and anterior impingement. The two instabilities are chronic lateral ligamentous instability and syndesmotic instability. The two chondral injuries are osteochondral and chondral fractures of the dome of the talus, and loose bodies.

The anterior impingement syndrome is characterized by painful, limited dorsiflexion of the ankle (Fig. 30-4). It is often associated with bone spurs on the anterior tibia and on the anterior talus. It comes about from repetitive forced dorsiflexion of the foot. It was originally described in soccer players.

The bone spur and anterior scar tissue can be removed arthroscopically. The bone spur is removed with a high-speed burr. Adhesions and anterior scar tissue are removed with a soft tissue resector. Excellent clinical results have been achieved with increased range of dorsiflexion and minimal pain. The condition, however, must be distinguished from osteoarthritis of the ankle, which is also common in dancers. If there is significant narrowing of the joint space, especially anteriorly, then the results are not good.

The anterolateral impingement syndrome is characterized by pain on the anterolateral aspect of the joint (Fig. 30-5). It is owing to chronic inflammation of the anterior-inferior tibiofibula ligament and the anterior talofibula ligament. These are often compressed over the lateral dome of the talus and there may be associated chondral damage in this area. The pain is in the anterolateral aspect of the ankle characteristically on plantarflexion.

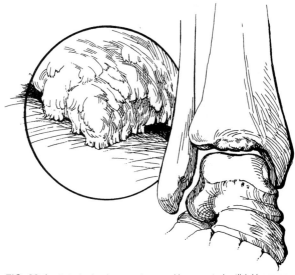

FIG. 30-4   Anterior impingement caused by an anterior tibial bone spur that can be removed arthroscopically.

Arthroscopic removal of the scar tissue at the anterolateral corner of the ankle and resection of the scar tissue back to the underlying ligamentous structures will relieve the pain in about 75 to 80 percent of cases. If there is associated damage to the articular cartilage of the dome of the talus the results are not as good.

Chondral and osteochondral lesions of the talus are commonly found when there is persistent pain after ankle sprains (Fig. 30-6). The key to distinguishing chondral injury and osteochondral injury from simple lateral instability is the fact that, in the former, the pain persists between episodes of instability. Clinical examination is not usually helpful. The magnetic resonance scan is particularly useful for identifying osteochondral lesions and for determining the stage of the lesion.

These conditions can be treated arthroscopically. Chondral lesions are treated by removing the damaged area of articular cartilage. Loose bodies can be extracted from the joint successfully (Fig. 30-7).

Osteochondritis dissecans is generally considered to be a traumatic injury. It probably represents an osteochondral fracture.

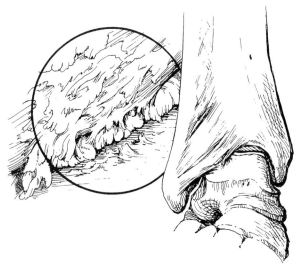

FIG. 30-5 Anterolateral impingement is caused by scar tissue formation after ankle sprains. The pathologic tissue can be successfully debrided arthroscopically.

When the lesion is relatively small, it can be excised arthroscopically with excellent long-term results. Sometimes a defect in the articular cartilage with a crack in the subchondral bone will lead to a posttraumatic cyst of the talus. This appears some weeks or months after the original injury. X-rays show a cystic lesion. The bone scan will usually be positive. A CT scan or magnetic resonance scan can clearly define the cyst, which is usually in the lateral portion of the talus. The treatment for this is to remove the roof of the cyst arthroscopically and debride the cystic material. In most cases the cyst will go on to heal without long-term problems.

Stress Fractures

Stress fractures of the metatarsals are particularly common in dancers. In addition, many other bones in the foot may be subject to stress fractures. The key to the diagnosis is the history of sudden onset of pain with or without swelling. Clinical examination should be able to pinpoint the area of pain. Plain x-rays often are not helpful, but the bone scan is extremely useful in precisely delineating which bone is involved. MRI will show the fracture at the earliest date.

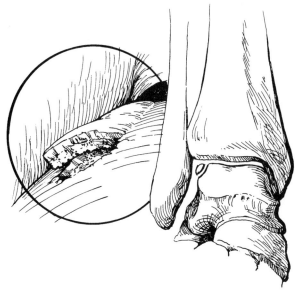

FIG. 30-6 Chondral and osteochondral fractures can be excised arthroscopically.

Stress fractures of the metatarsals require judicious rest with appropriate muscle strengthening and rehabilitation subsequently. Stress fractures of the midfoot, such as of the cuboid or navicular, probably require a period of immobilization and protection of the foot. I favor using a walking cast boot. We have had particularly good results and patient acceptance from using one with air bladders for support. This means the boot can be removed to retain flexibility of the foot and also to work on muscle strength in the midrange. The foot should be protected until the pain and tenderness go away. A graduated return to activities is then necessary. Exercises, including towel scrunches, foot rollers, and therabands are essential in the non-weight-bearing phase of rehabilitation. Often dancers can be returned to pool barre prior to class and rehearsals. Replacement of one cardiovascular activity with another is also critical to any program.

Any dancer with a stress fracture should have bone mineral density checked. This may be a warning sign of inappropriate nutrition. Careful dietary advice may then be necessary.

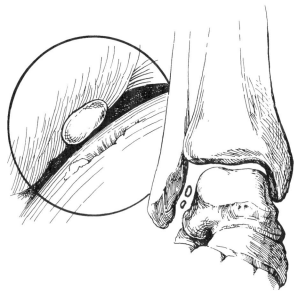

FIG. 30-7 Loose bodies cause locking and should be extracted.

Sesamoiditis

Under the great toe there are two sesamoid bones, a medial and a lateral. The medial bone usually gives dancers difficulties.

Sesamoiditis often develops after a poorly executed jump and landing. The dancer may land on the ball of the foot instead of using muscles in the eccentric mode to absorb the impact. There is often significant force placed on to the sesamoid causing inflammation or fracture.

The sesamoid may fracture. This can be difficult to distinguish from a bipartite sesamoid. A bone scan is most useful in detecting acute injury to the sesamoid.

If it is an acute injury, then the appropriate treatment is rest and relieving pressure from the sesamoid. This can be done with a felt doughnut underneath the sesamoid. Impact loading activities should be avoided until the pain ceases, but the dancer can continue with flexibility exercises and midrange strengthening exercises. Given the fact that many dance movements will not be possible, the dancer should be actively involved in the gym to maintain the rest of the lower extremity strength. Cross-training, swimming, and Pilates are extremely useful at this stage.

In extreme circumstances the sesamoid may need to be removed. This may be due to a painful nonunion of the sesamoid following a fracture. There can be damage to the articular cartilage of the sesamoid (chondromalacia). In rare circumstances there may be osteochondritis dissecans with a small osteocartilaginous loose body coming from the sesamoid.

The sesamoid is removed through a medial incision. Removing the sesamoid, however, does lead to laxity of the attached ligaments, and these need to be tightened. Although the pain may be relieved in classical ballet, it may result in weakness of the foot and great toe that limits the dancer's performance. This, therefore, is only to be undertaken as a last resort.

The Big Toe

Investigations of dancers' feet have shown that they do have significant pain in the big toe. In my own paper on the subject, we found signs of inflammation in the first metatarsophalangeal joint in all 59 dancers in the National Ballet of Canada. Male dancers in particular had hallux rigidus with loss of dorsiflexion of the great toe. It had been shown that in barefoot male dancers, there is five times more pressure on the great toe than on the second toe. This can be related to the fact that the majority of their movements are performed on demi-pointe, taking stress primarily through the metatarsophalangeal joint and then the first ray, whereas ballerinas dance on pointe, padding and taping their toes and distributing forces throughout the midfoot, first ray, and first metatarsophalangeal joints.

It was felt that dancers had a higher incidence of hallux valgus. However, recent studies have shown that it is not in fact correct. There was no increase in the valgus angulation of a hallux in dancers versus nondancers.[17] However, there is no doubt that dancers have a significant increase in the incidence of osteoarthritis of their great toes. They also have significantly decreased movement of the first metatarsophalangeal joint.[12]

Significant hallux rigidus may be a career-ending condition in dancers. Under these circumstances, surgery may be attempted. The favorite procedure would be a cheiliotomy. In this operation, the dorsal bone spur is removed along with approximately half of the metatarsal head. This allows the proximal phalanx to resume its dorsiflexion.

The problem with the operative procedure is that it is hard to control subsequent scar tissue formation. The range of movement may not return to the toe. The additional surgical trauma may increase the stiffness and the posttraumatic arthritis. If the surgery is carried out, aggressive physiotherapy with mobilization is necessary following the operation. In this way an attempt may be made to regain motion and to maintain it.

Plantar Fasciitis

The plantar fascia acts as a major support for the arch of the foot. The origin of the plantar fascia at the medial tubercle of the calcaneus is subject to a lot of stress. If this area becomes painful, then plantar fasciitis with its associated symptoms of pain, morning stiffness, and inability for the foot to absorb impact load becomes a major clinical problem.

The initial treatment is ice, anti-inflammatories, and local modalities of treatment to try and decrease inflammation and improve the blood flow to the area. In walking shoes, orthotics may be of help in relieving the stress on the plantar fascia. However, it is not possible to fit suitable orthotics to dancing shoes or to bare feet.

Stretching is an essential component of the treatment. This involves stretching the Achilles tendon, the plantar fascia, and the toes. Specific exercises to strengthen the intrinsic muscles of the foot are needed. A carefully constructed rehabilitation program is required with specific strengthening of the muscles of the calf (both eccentric and concentric) and of the foot. An isokinetic course, plyometrics, and Pilates are all of value.

Judicious use of cortisone injections into the area of inflammation at the medial tubercle can be quite helpful. If the plantar fasciitis is intractable, then electroshock treatment has been shown to be effective in 50 to 60 percent of cases. As a last resort, endoscopic plantar fascia release can be carried out. Although this does relieve the pain in the majority of patients, it results in a slight decrease in the arch and also hypermobility of the midfoot.

Dancers may suffer from a plantar fascia rupture. This characteristically occurs as they are landing. They experience a sharp pain in the sole of the foot and often an audible snap.

The treatment for this is conservative. Initially, it requires ice, elevation, and gentle stretching. Over a period of 6 to 12 weeks, the injury will go on to heal, although care must be taken that the arch does not drop. They should wear orthotics in their usual shoes and should not be involved heavily in impact activities during this period of time. As the dancers often have had episodes of plantar fasciitis prior to the rupture, an accessory benefit is that their plantar fascial symptoms disappear, following healing of the rupture.

REFERENCES

1. Garrick JG, Requa RK: Ballet injuries. *Am J Sports Med* 21(4):586–590, 1993.

2. Milan KR: Injury in ballet. *J Orthop Sports Phy Ther* 19(2):121–129, 1994.

3. Ramel E, Moritz U: Self-reported musculoskeletal pain. *Scand J Rehab Med* 26(1):11–16, 1994.

4. Fogelholm M, Van Marken Lichtenbelt W, Ottenheijm R, et al: Amenorrhea in ballet dancers in the Netherlands. *Med Sci Sports Exerc* 28(5):545–550, 1996.

5. Keay N, Fogelman I, Blake G: Mineral bone density in professional female dancers. *Br J Sports Med* 31(2):143–147, 1997.

6. Wieslar ER, Hunter DM, Martin DF, et al: Ankle flexibility and injury patterns in dancers. *Am J Sports Med* 24(6):754–775, 1996.

7. Crotts D, Thompson B, Nahom M, et al: Balance abilities of professional dancers on select balance tests. *J Orthop Sports Phys Ther* 23(1):12–17, 1996.

8. Leanderson J, Eriksson E, Nilsson C, et al: Proprioception in classical ballet dancers. *Am J Sports Med* 24(3):370–374, 1996.

9. Westblad P, Tsai-Fellander L, Johansson C: Eccentric and concentric knee extensor performance. *Clin J Sports Med* 5(1):48–52, 1995.

10. Tajet-Foxell B, Rose FD: Pain and pain tolerance professional ballet dancers. *Br J Sports Med* 29(1):31–34, 1995.

11. Hamilton WG, Geppert MJ, Thompson FM: Pain in the posterior aspect of the ankle joint in dancers. *JBJS* 78A(10):1491–1500, 1996.

12. Van Dijk CN, Lim LS, Poortman A, et al: Degenerative joint disease in female ballet dancers. *Am J Sports Med* 23(4):295–300, 1995.

13. Simpson KJ: Jump distance of dance landings. *Med Sci Sports Exerc* 29(7):916–927, 928–936, 1997.

14. Bauman PA, Singson R, Hamilton WG: Femoral neck anteversion in ballerinas. *Clin Orthop Rel Res* 302:57–63, 1994.

15. Winslow J, Yoder E: Patello-femoral pain in female ballet dancers. *J Orthop Sports Phys Ther* 22(1):18–21, 1995.

16. Ogilvie-Harris DJ, Gilbart MK, Chorney K: Chronic pain following ankle sprains in athletes: The role of arthroscopic surgery. *Arthroscopy* 13(5):564–574, 1997.

17. Einarsdottir H, Troell S, Wykman A: Hallux valgus in ballet dancers, a myth. *Foot Ankle Int* 16(2):92–94, 1995.

31 | Gymnastic Injuries and Prevention

Craig McQueen

Gymnastics has grown dramatically in popularity and in numbers of participants over the past several years. The competition has changed the sport so that more difficult maneuvers have led to an increase in acute injuries, and longer training hours have led to an increase in chronic or overuse injuries. Although most experts who have studied gymnastic injuries have noted increases in the injury rate of gymnasts at any level who train more than 15 hours per week, almost all gymnasts train from $4\frac{1}{2}$ to 5 hours per day, 5 to 6 days per week. This is necessary to develop the skills required at higher levels.

Prevention of injury should be paramount in the minds of coaches, parents, and physicians. Although it may be impossible to prevent accidental injury, proper equipment, padding, and spotting during difficult techniques should minimize accidental injuries. Chronic or overuse injuries, on the other hand, may be lessened by the following:

- Flexibility of both upper and lower extremities, as well as the lumbar spine, is essential. Strength of the preceding has been shown to be important in prevention of overuse injuries.
- Periodization of training and modifying training schedules to accommodate symptoms of pain may be necessary.
- Taping and splinting of wrists and ankles may be helpful in alleviating and preventing injuries.
- Flexibility of the upper and lower extremities in gymnasts is essential to prevent overload syndromes. Gymnasts in general do most of their training while still growing. Bone grows at a more rapid rate than muscle and tendon, and therefore during a rapid growth spurt a gymnast may become relatively tight in areas that were previously flexible. Attention must be paid to gymnasts during this time of rapid growth, to ensure that flexibility and strength are maintained. It may be necessary to spend more time on flexibility during a growth spurt.

Strength training is also an essential part of a gymnast's daily program. Therapy and exercises can be very helpful in strengthening both the upper and lower extremities. Strengthening of the peroneals on the lateral aspect of the ankle is helpful in preventing ankle sprains, especially if there is some instability present. Strengthening of the posterior tibial muscle on the medial side of the ankle is helpful in preventing shin splints. Strengthening of the extensors and flexors of the wrist is also important in prevention of wrist injuries, which is also true for the shoulder musculature. Strengthening of the abdominals and the extensors of the spine is also important in prevention of injuries to the lower back. Tightness of the lumbodorsal fascia has been associated with back pain and can be helped by stretching the fascia. Hamstring flexibility is also essential in the prevention of back pain. Classic slow gradual stretching is preferred, and although most stretches are familiar, we will illustrate those for the shoulder and the lumbodorsal fascia.

MEN'S GYMNASTICS

Men's gymnastics is essentially the same in floor exercise and vaulting as is women's; however, it differs significantly in rings, parallel bars, high bar, and pommel horse. With six events in men's gymnastics in contrast to four in women's gymnastics, there are differences in injury patterns with more lower extremities in women, and more upper extremity injuries in men. Wrist problems occur with the pommel horse, rings, and high bar. Elbow problems occur with triceps, especially with the parallel bars and high bar. Misses from releases on the high bar can lead to significant injury. The same forces exist in men's and women's vaulting and floor exercise, with similar injury risks.

Pommel Horse

This consists of continuous motion of trunk and legs while maintaining support on hands and arms. It requires good balance and upper body strength. This event has the lowest risk of injury of all the men's apparatus. Overuse of wrists is the primary risk, occasionally traumatic injury to wrists occurs. Also common is bruising of lower extremities from contact with the pommels.

Rings

This event combines swing and strength elements with strength becoming increasingly more prominent. There is a great deal of stress on the shoulders with this event. Gymnasts are required to have enough strength to lift and hold their body weight through various positions while still maintaining the flexibility to perform "inlocates" and "dislocates" for the swing elements. Shoulder tendinitis and back problems are common in both the elite and lower level athletes. There is also some risk of injury to the lower extremities from dismounts on this apparatus, which is already 255 cm from the top of the mats.

High Bar

This apparatus consists of a single metal bar placed 255 cm from the top of the mat. Elements consist of continuous motion around the bar with various directions of swing. It also incorporates release elements that require the gymnast to release the bar and recatch after performing a somersault, twist, or both. These are the elements that make high bar the riskiest of all events. The most traumatic and serious injuries occur on this event. This is owing to the height of the bar as well as the fact that the gymnasts are often still rotating or twisting on contact with the ground if the bar is not recaught. There is also some risk of injuries to the lower extremities associated with dismounts from this height. It is also common for skin to be torn from the hands. However, these "rips" are considered of minor importance to the gymnasts.

Parallel Bars

The parallel bars are two fiberglass rails located parallel to the ground at a height of 175 cm from the top of the mat. This event consists of swing, balance, and strength elements. The greatest risk of injury seems to be contact with the bar. Bruising is common around the upper arm from landing somersaulting elements in an underarm position. Injuries are not common, but can occur to lower extremities from incorrect landing or dismounts.

Floor

This exercise is 50 to 70 s long, performed on a 12 × 12 m carpeted wooden floor with springs, or more commonly foam cubes underneath. This event combines tumbling with at least one balance and strength element. Tumbling sequences should consist of both forward and backward tumbling. Overuse and traumatic injuries to the lower extremities are common in this event, owing to the force of the landings and some improper landings.

Vault

The sheer velocity in this event makes injuries common, especially for the lower level athletes who do not have the experience to control falls. Lower extremities are once again the most affected because of the speed and height. The horse is set at 135 cm from the floor but most vaults are performed 2 to 4 feet above the horse.

WOMEN'S GYMNASTICS

Female gymnastics involves activities of high velocity, impact, and torsion. Scoring is based on a system of 10 and involves the following:

1. Expression
2. Extension
3. Difficulty
4. Dance
5. Deductions

Four basic activities constitute women's gymnastics, floor exercise, uneven parallel bars, vault, and balance beam.

BALANCE BEAM

The balance beam routines, performed on a 4-inch wide, 4-foot high apparatus, require intense precision and balance. There is a time limit for each routine of 1 min 30 s. Skills performed on the beam are similar to floor exercise. The difference is in the exact placement of the foot on the beam. The skills are also performed at a lower speed than the floor exercise. This event has the *highest frequency* of injuries, most of which are from falls or dismounts. These injuries, for the most part, are less severe because of the lower velocity in which they occur.

FLOOR EXERCISE

Floor exercise combines tumbling skills with dance skills. Each routine has a time limit of 1 min 50 s. The routines are done to music and need to have varying tempos within.

The gymnast has to have three passes (one mount, one dismount, and one middle pass). In between these passes, there have to be different speeds, heights, directions, and difficulties of skills. Most injuries in this event are owing to miscalculations of landings. Lower extremities are those most affected. This event has the highest rate of injuries. McNitt-Gray did a study on peak vertical reaction forces. A vertical jump landing exerts two to four times body weight. Double backs (two backward somersaults in the air) exert on the gymnast a force of 18 times body weight and here they have to stop at 0 velocity.

UNEVEN PARALLEL BARS

This event requires a continuous fluid motion from one bar to the other while the gymnast executes various twists, releases, and hip rotations. It requires extreme upper torso strength, more so than any other event, but the momentum within the routine usually masks this. Injuries occur from falls or faulty dismounts. Other factors that the gymnast has to overcome are rips of the protective callus on the palms and bruises of the pelvis and thighs from contact with the bars. Injuries owing to apparatus failure are also seen in this event.

VAULT

Vaulting is very high velocity. The potential for injury is extremely high and combines the speed of the vault with the difficulty of the skill. This event is less demanding on the gymnast in terms of duration, fewer moves, and so on. However, the injuries tend to be more serious because of the speed with which it is exhibited. The lower extremity is the most affected because of the landings and the speed at which the gymnast hits the springboard. The spotter is always available in any event, but in this one they are not in a good position to do anything if something goes wrong.

GYMNASTIC INJURIES

According to Pettrone, gymnastic injuries rank behind football, wrestling, and softball; however, this varies with the nature of the competition. Injury rates increase as a gymnast goes from club to high school, to collegiate, to elite competition. Many high schools are dropping gymnastics because of the high injury rates.

Some of the causes of high injury rates are as follows. There are only six to ten gymnasts per team, so the relative rate is higher. Studies of injuries per participant hour are also high. Equipment failure, such as forgetting to tighten the beam, vault, or bar hinges, leads to injury. Mat thickness is a problem. It is thin during competition for easier landing techniques, but this leads to higher impact on the lower extremities. It is thick during practice for softer landings, but the foot may become caught during twisting skills with resultant injury.

In today's times, one must not evade the nutritional and psychological issues related to gymnastics. Striving for thinness may lead to nutritional deficiencies, decreased metabolic rate, and disordered eating. Low iron stores, electrolyte disturbances, and in extreme cases, multiorgan pathology may occur from anorexia and bulimia. There is a need to make gymnasts, coaches, and parents aware of unhealthy methods of weight loss and their prevention. Striving for the perfect "10" may be difficult psychologically.

Gymnastics shares many common injuries with other sports. These include ankle sprains, knee injuries, strains, overuse injuries, fractures, and so on. However, there are injuries more or less unique to gymnastics, and it is this group that we will examine.

The uniqueness stems from two factors.

1. Gymnasts, primarily female, start training at a very early age, usually 5 or 6 years.
2. Larger stresses are placed on the upper extremities and lumbar spine that other sports, and both upper and lower extremities are weightbearing.

These factors lead to abnormal stresses on an immature, growing skeleton. Gymnastics involve activities of high velocity, high impact, and high torsion. Combine these three with the immature growing skeleton and you have the high risk of chronic as well as acute injuries. Female gymnasts begin training at age 5 or 6 and train up to 5 to 6 h daily, 5 days per week, reaching peak performance at age 15 or 16 years. This amount of training places unusual stresses on the growth plates of the wrist and on the pars interarticularis of the lumbar spine. Eating disorders, amenorrhea, and subsequent osteoporosis may aggravate this. The emphasis on smallness in gymnastics tends to promote this triad. There is evidence to show that such a training schedule may affect skeletal growth. Intensive gymnastics over 18 h per week beginning before, and continuing throughout puberty, has been shown to reduce adult height.

Stresses to an immature skeleton may lead to several orthopedic problems. Repeated hyperextension of the lumbar spine in floor exercise and on the dismount lead to stress on the pars interarticularis of L5–S1. Stress fractures can occur in this area, either unilateral or bilateral. Repeated stress on the distal radial epiphysis leads to changes in the growth of the distal radius with retardation and positive ulnar variance. This is related to the pronation and extreme dorsiflexion of the wrist, common to gymnastic activities and has several different but related entities. Positive ulnar variance refers to a disorder of the wrist in which the radial growth has been affected, leading to shortening of the radius. This makes the ulna either equal to or longer than the radius. This contrasts with the normal situation in which the radius is longer at the wrist than is the ulna.

Compression forces to the wrist that occur in vaulting, beam, and floor exercise can lead to damage to the distal radial physis (growth plate). There is disagreement as to whether or not distraction forces lead to stress injury, and although this may occur the injuries owing to distraction seem to be less common and less serious than those owing to compression.

We will first consider the progression of overuse or stress injuries of the wrist. With increased training of growing gymnasts, increased stresses have occurred in the wrist. Symptoms of wrist pain occur in specific areas of the wrist according to weightbearing and torsional activities such as pronation and ulnar deviation. With torsional stresses, symptoms of ulnar impaction syndrome predominate on the dorsal ulnar side of the wrist. Repetitive loading of the distal radius, which occurs with vaulting and floor exercise, can lead to a stress injury of the distal radial physis. Subsequent growth of the distal radius may be affected, leading to a series of wrist problems.

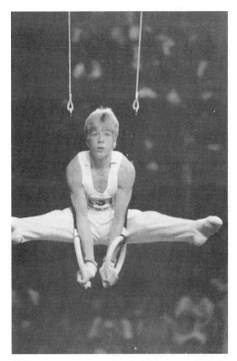

FIG. 31-1 Repetitive stress injuries of the wrist. Repetitive loading of the distal radius may alter subsequent growth or damage the triangular fibrocartilage.

When a young gymnast presents at the office with wrist symptoms, a careful history and physical examination are essential. Age of onset of training, present age, duration and intensity of training, type of training, recent changes in training schedule, site and duration of symptoms, as well as when symptoms occur, are all important in determining the diagnosis and treatment. Careful examination of the injured extremity is necessary. Palpation of the distal radial physis, radial-ulnar joint, distal ulna, and collateral ligaments should be done carefully to localize the area of maximal tenderness. With a stress injury of the physis, there is usually limitation of dorsiflexion, mild swelling, and tenderness of the physis to palpation. X-rays may or may not be helpful in the diagnosis since the injury may be to soft tissue only. The main reason for x-ray is to rule out changes in the distal radial physis. These changes include irregular widening of the distal radial physis. This may be difficult to assess in a gymnast because the changes may be bilateral, and there is no normal wrist with which to compare.

However, widening should be readily appreciated if present and is evidence of a longstanding stress injury. If signs and symptoms of a stress injury of the epiphysis are present but x-rays are normal, the injury is of shorter duration and the prognosis is generally better. Treatment consists of relative rest with restriction of vaulting and floor exercise until the patient is pain free and nontender to palpation. This may be as long as 3 months with the more severe injuries.

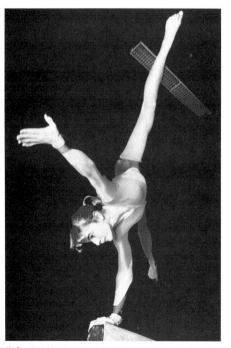

FIG. 31-2   The Rankin. Puts considerable load on the entire upper extremity. *(Courtesy of Janine Rankin, Canadian National Gymnast)*

In many cases of stress injury to the physis, distal radial growth is impaired, resulting in a positive ulnar variance. This may lead to other wrist problems if the athlete continues in gymnastics.

Positive ulnar variance and a subsequent malalignment of the distal radiocarpal joint may lead to an overload of the triangular fibrocartilage complex, or TFCC. The TFCC fills the space between the radius, ulna, and carpus. Chronic overload leads to degeneration and tearing of this complex. Diagnosis is made by a history of ulnar-sided wrist pain, with tenderness and clicking with motion over the TFCC. Weak grip strength is often present and should be measured. Wrist arthrography and MRI can confirm diagnosis. Initial treatment consists of rest, NSAIDs, forearm strengthening, and splinting to eliminate maximal dorsiflexion on return to sports. Surgical intervention may be necessary in light of failed conservative management. There are many surgeons experienced in wrist arthroscopy and diagnosis and treatment can be done arthroscopically, thereby shortening rehabilitation considerably.

Another rather unique injury to gymnasts is triceps tendonitis. This is characterized by elbow pain localized to the olecranon tip. Tenderness is present over the distal triceps insertion, and is an injury analogous to jumper's knee. Treatment consists of relative rest, triceps flexibility and strengthening with oral antiinflammatories as needed. Injections of steroids should be avoided. Dorsal wrist ganglia are more common in gymnasts than in other athletes. Diagnosis is made by palpation of a tender mass of the dorsal wrist. Aspiration and steroid injection may give temporary relief, but ultimately surgical excision may be necessary.

LUMBAR SPINE

Lumbar spine problems are common in gymnasts, figure skaters, and ballerinas because of the hyperextension activities common to these sports. However, it is most common in gymnastics, especially in floor exercise, balance beam, vaulting with associated hyperextension during dismount, which loads the posterior elements of the spine, especially the pars interarticularis of L5–S1. Initial treatment consists of avoiding hyperextension dismounts, back walkovers, and back handsprings for 4 to 6 weeks.

Spondylolysis is now considered to be the result of a stress fracture of the pars interarticularis. This is owing to the repetitive microtrauma seen in gymnastics. Spondylolysis can be differentiated from a stress fracture of the pars, not visible on x-ray, with the use of a bone scan. A single photon emission computerized tomography (SPECT) bone scan is most effective in diagnosing a stress fracture of the pars.

The young gymnast who presents with low back pain will usually have a normal range of motion with no pain on straight leg raising to 90 degrees. Neurologic examination will be normal. There may be lower lumbar tenderness, but the most reliable test is the one-legged lay back test.

This is done with the athlete standing on one leg, opposite knee flexed. Then, while supported, the patient is asked to do a lay back, or hyperextend the lumbar spine. If this reproduces low back pain it is considered positive. If this is positive, or if low back pain has been present for longer than 3 weeks, then x-rays, including AP, and lateral and obliques of the lumbar spine are indicated. If plain films are normal, then a SPECT bone scan may be indicated. If spondylolysis is present, this is the end result of a stress fracture. Treatment of a symptomatic spondylolysis or scan positive stress fracture is the same.

Treatment consists of hamstring flexibility exercises and lumbar bracing. Bracing is done with a molded polypropylene brace with 0 degrees lordosis. Initial rest is necessary until the athlete is asymptomatic in the brace. Then gradual return to practice and competition is allowed. It may take 6 to 9 months for complete healing to occur. X-rays often show healing of the pars defect. If a grade 1

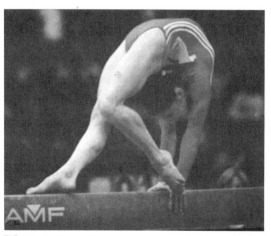

FIG. 31-3 Hyperextension injuries. Repetitive hyperextension injuries of the lumbar spine may cause a stress fracture of the pars, or "spondylolosis."

spondylolisthesis is present, treatment is the same. However, at times the patient will not become symptomatic and a lumbar fusion may be necessary.

Recent studies have shown a high incidence of degenerative disk disease in young male and female gymnasts, so in the event that sciatic symptoms are present or studies for pars interarticularis defects are negative, then MRI studies may be necessary to evaluate disk degeneration or herniation.

Prevention of lumbar injuries is important in gymnasts, and there seems to be a direct correlation between the number of training hours per week and lumbar problems. Those athletes training more than 15 h per week are at risk for developing spine problems. Also, at times of rapid growth, attention must be paid to hamstring tightness and tight lumbodorsal fascia.

It should be noted that, in female gymnasts, a 1991 study showed MRI abnormalities of the lumbar spine in the following categories: pre-elite (9 percent), elite (43 percent), and olympic (63 percent). The most common change was that of disk degeneration, owing to the continued stresses on the lumbar spine; hence, more common in the more advanced gymnast.

Another injury that should be mentioned because of its frequency in gymnastics is that of elbow dislocation. This is common because of the use of the upper extremities in many of the gymnastic maneuvers, and in a fall or miss, the elbow is at risk. Treatment consists of reduction as soon as possible, careful x-ray exam to rule out associated fractures, careful checking for instability of the joint following reduction, and early mobilization. Splinting is usually necessary for 7 to 10 days, but then gentle range of motion should be started. Once full painless range of motion with good strength has been achieved, then return to gymnastics may be allowed. This may take 6 to 12 weeks. If a suspected fracture is present, then comparison films with the opposite elbow may be helpful. Anatomic reduction is necessary to ensure the peak performance of gymnasts. This generally requires an open reduction with internal fixation, followed by early mobilization and rehabilitation. In the growing child an MRI may be indicated to identify a medial epicondylar fracture that is mainly cartilaginous.

There are other injuries to the lower extremities that deserve mention. Shin splints are a common problem in gymnastics, and deserve careful differentiation. The classic shin splint syndrome is caused by inflammation of the origin of the posterior tibial muscle on the medial edge of the tibia, and is referred to as a posterior tibial periostitis. This can be confused with a stress fracture of the tibia or with an anterior compartment syndrome. A careful history and physical examination should give the examiner clues as to the correct diagnosis. A history of increasing pain with swelling of the anterior compartment, and tenderness with relative tightness of the anterior compartment after activity point to a diagnosis of intermittent anterior compartment syndrome. Definitive diagnosis can be made with greater than 30 mmHg pressure in the anterior compartment after exercise. If conservative measures such as ice, rest, and flexibility are not helpful, then a formal compartment release may be necessary.

A tibial stress fracture gradually worsens with time. Pain is progressive, constant, and may make walking difficult. Tenderness is present over the front of the tibia very often at the junction of the middle and distal 1/3 of the tibia. X-rays are often negative, but a bone scan will localize and define the stress fracture. Absolute rest of the extremity is necessary to heal the fracture and the athlete should not be allowed back to practice until the bone is symptom-free and the tibia is nontender. Strength and flexibility should be continued during the rehabilitation phase.

Shin splints or posterior tibial periostitis is characterized by medial tibial aching pain that gets progressively worse as the season progresses. There is significant tenderness over the medial tibia at the origin of the posterior tibialis. X-rays are negative and a bone scan may show some uptake along the medial tibia, but this is markedly different from a stress fracture. Treatment consists of ice, interferential and Theraband strengthening of the posterior tibialis, and if possible, orthotics for the pronated foot. Vaulting shoes with orthotics may be used to continue training.

In backward tumbling, springboard vaulting, and dismounts, if a gymnast underrotates, the landing occurs with the ankle hyperdorsiflexed or at times with the great toe hyperdorsiflexed. This can lead to an anterior impingement syndrome of the ankle or to a turf toe.

The anterior impingement syndrome of the ankle is owing to chronic irritation of the anterior capsule and other soft tissues. Rest, ice, and oral anti-inflammatories are helpful. Turf toe can be more difficult to treat and is often disabling. It is owing to a capsular strain, which may also involve the flexor tendon of the great toe. Rest, ice, taping, and oral anti-inflammatories are again helpful. Immobilization of the toe may be necessary until pain is relieved.

In the treatment of shin splints and turf toe, consideration should be given to the use of a vaulting shoe in practice, with the addition of an orthotic. The orthotic can be designed to support the foot in a neutral position for those gymnasts with a pronated foot and posterior tibial periostitis, and with a more rigid forefoot support for those with a first metatarsal phalangeal joint synovitis or sprain. This would be worn during practice, but not during competition.

ANKLE SPRAINS

Ankle sprains, as in many other sports, constitute the most common injury in gymnastics. Because of time demands and the need for more or less constant training to achieve success in gymnastics, the injury is often treated too lightly or not treated at all. Since various degrees of injury occur to the lateral ligaments of the ankle, a sports medicine specialist should evaluate all ankle sprains. Sprains are graded as 1, 2, or 3. A grade 1 sprain is an injury to either the anterior talofibular or calcaneofibular ligament, which is incomplete, and the ankle is stable to inversion stress with a negative drawer test. Grade 2 is a complete injury to either the anterior talofibular or calcaneofibular ligament, with subsequent instability to either inversion stress, or a positive anterior drawer test. A grade 3 injury occurs with complete disruption of both ligaments. Therefore, there is instability to inversion stress and a positive drawer test.

Too commonly, athletes are seen at emergency rooms or emergent care facilities where proper evaluation of an ankle sprain is unavailable. Also, the coach or athlete may elect to treat a sprain without evaluation. A proper evaluation should consist of a visit to an experienced sports medicine physician.

Proper evaluation by a physician consists of a careful history of injury, hands-on testing, and evaluation of the anterior talofibular ligament, calcaneofibular ligament, and the deep portion of the medial deltoid ligament. Also, attention should be paid to the base of the fifth metatarsal to rule out an avulsion fracture. If instability is suspected after hands-on testing, then stress x-rays should be done, including inversion and possibly an anterior drawer. It may be necessary to compare clinical testing x-rays with the opposite side in order to ensure proper diagnosis.

Proper treatment of an ankle sprain in a gymnast may be difficult, and should be discussed with the athlete, coach, and at times the parents, especially if the gymnast is a minor. With a grade 1 injury, rest, ice, interferential, taping, and gradual use is appropriate. With a grade 2 injury, the same treatment applies with the addition of a double upright rigid splint such as an air cast. This is to be worn 24 h a day for 3 weeks. Activity can usually be resumed at 2 to 3 weeks. With a grade 3 injury, a comparison of the opposite side is important to determine if this is a new injury or if a natural ligamentous laxity exists. If laxity is present bilaterally, then minimal treatment may be necessary, but if unilateral, then the same treatment as that for a grade 2 injury is necessary. Protection, such as taping, bracing, or a combination, may be necessary over several months or on a permanent basis if instability is present.

A rather common but somewhat unknown syndrome may develop after an ankle sprain. The gymnast will complain of continued discomfort in the injured ankle, at times severe enough to interfere with training. The pain is aching in nature and aggravated by activity. It generally gets worse with time in contrast to a sprain, which generally improves with time. On examination, the key finding is tenderness over the sinus tarsi of the foot. This is in the soft spot just anterior to the lateral malleolus. This does not usually respond to PT or oral antiinflammatories. This is a syndrome that responds to a steroid injection deep into the sinus tarsi. This is done with a mixture of 4 cc of Bipuvicaine and 1 cc of Methylprednisolone with a 22-gauge 1.25 in. needle. The gymnast can usually return to practice within 1 week.

Type I and Type II Fractures

These are safe fractures, which usually reduce readily and heal without incident. They are usually stuck by 3 weeks and can take full stress by 6 to 8 weeks, depending on the site and clinical and x-ray union.

Type III Fractures

These involve the epiphyseal plate and are serious. Type III injuries damage the growing cells and can cause a growth arrest. They also often lead to incongruity of the articular surface. They are usually treated with an open reduction and pin fixation.

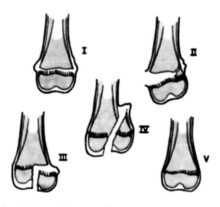

FIG. 31-4   Epiphyseal fractures with growth plate damage. Salter-Harris Classification. Reprinted with permission from Salter RB, Harris WR: Injuries involving the epiphyseal plate. *J Bone Joint Surg* 34:711, 1952.

Type IV Fracture

These are even more serious because they cross the epiphyseal plate, with even greater damage to the growing cells. It is important to reduce these accurately, most frequently with open reduction.

Type V Fracture

These are crushing of the epiphyseal plate, which may cause permanent damage, requiring late correction.

THE FEMALE ATHLETE TRIAD

The term "Female Athlete Triad" was introduced at the American College of Sports Medicine Conference in Washington, D.C. in 1992. The problem has been studied since the 1970s and involves excessive training regimes, and increased thinness, which has led to amenorrhea and subsequent osteoporosis secondary to eating disorders.

Eating Disorders

Eating disorders in gymnasts can take the form of 800-calorie diets, bingeing and purging by vomiting, overuse of laxatives and diuretics, and anorexia nervosa and bulimia nervosa. Diet pills, stimulants, and obsessive exercise also contribute to the problem.

Amenorrhea

The average age of menarche in nonathletes is 12.8 years $+/-$ 1 to 2 years. The average age in athletes can be delayed 0 to 4 years for each year of premenstrual training.

Diagnosis of Primary Amenorrhea

The diagnosis of primary amenorrhea at age 14 consists of: secondary sex characteristics *absent*, no menses, and at age 16, secondary sex characteristics *present*, no menses.

Many female gymnasts have a prepubertal physique until ages 16, 17, or even 18 years.

Secondary Amenorrhea

Absence of menstrual periods for 3 to 6 consecutive months, in a woman who had previous established cycles.

Prevention involves a team approach—athlete, parents, coach, and team psychologist, family doctor, specialist referral, and investigation are advised if decreased training and increased calories and weight do not solve the problem.

Behavioral clues   Behavioral clues include intense fear of becoming fat, self-criticism, anxiety, hyperactivity, and inability to relax.

Physical clues   Physical clues include variable athletic performance, fat and muscle loss, dry thin hair and dry skin, cold hands and feet, enlarged parotid glands, swelling of ankles, knuckle scars, and bloodshot eyes from repeated self-induced vomiting.

Osteoporosis

Osteoporosis is a decrease in bone mass and strength, which leads to bone pain and an increased risk of fractures. Women reach peak bone strength at age 25 to 30 years and then decrease gradually until menopause, and then decrease more rapidly.

Treatment consists of oral calcium; avoidance of nicotine, caffeine, alcohol, and steroids; and after age 16, low-dose contraception.

PYSCHOLOGICAL MAKEUP OF GYMNASTS

One of our best Canadian gymnasts, Elfi Schlagel, dislocated her big toe at a meet at Maple Leaf Gardens in Toronto in front of 18,000 people. This was reduced under local anesthesia and she was told that she was through for 3 or 4 weeks. However, she wanted to continue and went back on for the beam. She was awful, because she could not feel the beam properly with her toe and she fell off several times. Then she said, "Watch me do the vault, it is my best event." And she went out and won the vault.

Gymnasts as a group have astounding maturation, dedication, and confidence. They are capable of phenomenal zeal in their training. Because of their skeletal immaturity, their growing bones are subjected to stresses beyond normal tolerance. This can lead to irreversible complications. Thus, prevention of serious injuries is the key factor in dealing with gymnasts.

SUGGESTED READINGS

1. United States Gymnastics Safety Association: *Certification Course Instructor's Guide*. Reston, VA, United States Gymnastics Safety Association, 1997.
2. Weiker G, Ganim R: *Cleveland Clinic Gymnastics Injury Survey, 1982*. Cleveland, OH, Cleveland Clinic, 1982.
3. Wettstone G (ed): *Gymnastics Safety Manual*, 2d ed. University Park, PA, Pennsylvania State University Press, 1979.
4. Wettstone G: What is gymnastics safety? *Int Gymnast* 36, 1982.
5. Nutzenberger F, Nutzenberger K: Men's gymnastics. Personal communication.

III | OTHER

Athletic Therapy
In Sports Medicine

Ann Hartley   Joe Rotella

Sports injuries fall into two categories, injuries that are caused by a direct mechanism (e.g., trauma, overstretch) and injuries without a direct mechanism that have an insidious onset. This chapter offers advice on injury care for both categories.

INJURIES WITH A DIRECT MECHANISM

These injuries have specific tissue damage that goes through several phases of healing. These phases are inflammation, demolition, healing, and long-term goals (Table 32-1). The therapist must recognize the phase of the injury so that appropriate modalities, exercises, and manual skills can be used to enhance the healing process.

Inflammatory Phase

The inflammatory phase is recognized by the injured structure being warm to the touch and painful, even at rest. Often swelling and redness are present at the injury site.

Inflammation generally occurs from the time of injury to the first 24 h after the injury, but this is not always the case. Even a chronic injury of long duration can suddenly become inflamed just through overuse and be found in the inflammatory phase. So anytime a structure displays heat, redness, sharp pain, and sometimes swelling, we term it *inflamed*.

In this phase of healing, the therapist must try to decrease the inflammation through the use of pressure, ice, elevation, and rest (PIER). Depending on the type of structure damaged and the degree of injury, there is different emphasis on each element of the PIER principle.

Injuries to all the blood-carrying structures, such as muscle strains or contusions, require pressure as soon as possible with a pressure pad and tensor. Elevation, ice, and rest are also indicated. The application of ice is most significant for structures with a poorer blood supply in this phase of healing. Tendons that suffer from overuse paramountly need rest and ice and elevation to a lesser degree. Severe ligament sprains and tears most importantly require rest through the use of immobilization and elevation, especially if the injury is to the lower extremity. For best results, immobilization should be removable so that icing and motion can

665

TABLE 32-1 Aims and Objectives of Rehabilitation Program

	Inflammatory Phase (acute) (days 1–5)		
Aim	When	Why	How
1. Decrease inflammation	Whenever the tissue is inflamed Direct trauma: hematoma Overstretch: strain, sprain, subluxation Overuse: tendinitis, tenosynovitis, synovitis Joint dysfunction Arthritis Infection Any histamine reaction During treatment at home	Prevent further cell damage Decrease secondary complication Increase speed of recovery Decrease hemorrhaging Decrease metabolism Decrease circulation	PIER: Pressure-tensor, pad Ice pack, crushed, hydropack, Jobst Elevate injured tissue higher than heart Increase lymphatic drainage and venous return Decrease bleeding into area Rest collar, brace, air cast: immobilize, splint, tape, crutches, sling, bed rest, proper posture to rest injured tissue Anti-inflammatories (oral)
2. Decrease activity level	Immediately if acute From aggravating movement if overuse At home	To allow for tissue repair To prevent secondary complications	Rest, bed rest Decrease mechanism of injury if overuse Change mechanics Decrease training

3. Decrease the swelling (intermuscular, intramuscular, extracapsular, intracapsular)	Immediately During treatment and at home	Prevent further secondary joint or muscle problems Decrease articular cartilage degeneration	PIER Anti-inflammatory If joint intracapsular: put joint in resting position Direct current (HVGs) IEC (80–150 pps) US pulsed or low-intensity nonthermal
4. Relieve the pain	During treatment and at home	To decrease muscle spasm around site that limits range and strength Allow for athlete to sleep Comfort of athlete	Ice (PIER) Bed rest, immobilize TENS (80–100 pps) IFC (80–200 pps) Painkillers
5. Protect the injured site	Throughout treatment and throughout the day and night	Prevent reinjury Promote a speedy recovery Time for new fiber formation	Tape, brace, pad Alteration of activity NWB, crutches
6. Educate athlete	During treatment daily	To make athlete understand condition To make athlete responsible for recovery also	Home advice Demonstrate PIER and give home program

(continued)

TABLE 32-1 Aims and Objectives of Rehabilitation Program (*Continued*)

	Demolition phase (subacute) (days 3–15)		
Aim	When	Why	How
1. Decrease residual inflammation	Early in rehabilitation program	Prevent secondary complications Ensure not reinflame	PIER before and after treatment or rehabilitation Interferential (80–150 pps) US pulsed or low-intensity nonthermal, 20% duty cycle
2. Prevent secondary complications (adhesions, scar tissue, exudate)	During healing	Prevent loss of range of motion Prevent muscle atrophy Speed recovery process Promote laying down of new collagen synthesis	Active pain-free exercise Ultrasound pulsed or low-intensity nonthermal NMES: muscle pump or joint pump IFC: 80–150 pps Cold WP with gentle range work Cryotemp Massage
3. Relieve pain	When pain limits range or strength	Prevents secondary complications	Joint (traction and distraction) Exercise, joint traction TENS (~100 pps) Ice pack Massage, ice massage Ultrasound Interferential Painkillers (oral)

4. Maintain ROM in joints around the lesion site Increase ROM in restricted ranges (pain-free)	When range is limited Home program and clinic To maintain ranges and assist in movements in surrounding joints	Prevent capsular adhesions Nutrient to hyaline cartilage Prevent scar tissue Promote laying down of collagen in correct lines of stress	Active gentle range of motion pain-free exercises stretch NOT stress joint (4 × 30 s) (6 × daily) Contract/relax Joint traction Gentle oscillations
5. Gentle contraction if muscle injured Maintain other muscles around area	When muscle contraction is affected, i.e., reflex inhibition	Get laying down of collagen in lines of force Prevent adhesions in joint or muscle Muscle pump Relieves muscle spasm	Isometric pain-free (muscle pump) (1–3 ranges) NMES (muscle pump), 10 on, 10 off Isotonic if possible
6. Maintain or increase CV fitness, be sport-specific if is possible	Whenever CV fitness may be lost	To allow early return to sport To motivate athlete	Bike/run/walk/ swim, etc., as sport-specific as possible
7. Educate athlete about home advice and prevention, posture, etc.	Throughout treatment and rehabilitation	The athlete can exercise several times daily	How to do program and why they need it Posture Alleviating activities No aggravating activities

(continued)

TABLE 32-1 Aims and Objectives of Rehabilitation Program (*Continued*)

Healing phase (day 10–8 weeks)

Aim	When	Why	How
1. Increase circulation	When no inflammation present During healing phase As often as possible in both clinic and home	Increase nutrients to lesion site Increase lymphatic and venous drainage Increase tissue extensibility Decrease secondary complications Promote reabsorption of exudate Increase cell metabolism Increase blood flow	Exercises: whole body and local injury site Ultrasound continuous Transverse friction Interferential Massage IFC Warm WP with exercise
2. Increase range of motion (in joints or muscles with limited range) Maintain existing range in joint above and below Stretches for lesion site minimum, then other muscles or joints (surrounding)	Whenever joint range is limited, i.e., joint hypermobility, loss of joint play, muscle injury, bone chips, meniscal tear, joint dysfunction after capsule or ligament injury	To keep hyaline cartilage healthy Lubricate the joint Prevent osteoarthritis changes Prevent capsular adhesions Prevent muscle contractions Laying down of collagen in line of stress	Exercise active ROM Active stretch (4 × 30 s × 6) Muscle and joint stretch Traction, mobilization Hold/relax PNFs Spray and stretch, myofascial TPs

670

3. Increase strength (in muscles that are weak) Maintain existing strength in muscles around area Strengthening exercises minimum specifically for the lesion site	Throughout the treatment and daily clinic and home When muscle strength is down Following periods of immobilization After strain, tendinitis, tenosynovitis, muscle transfers To reeducate the muscles	To prevent joint instability To strengthen injured muscle fibers To correct muscle imbalances To correct posture To prevent recurrence	Sometimes 1–3 ranges isometric Isotonics Isokinetics: slow speed, fast speed, small arc PNFs Eccentrics: late healing Increase muscle strength and power and endurance Bilaterally Pliometrics: late healing Open chain progression to closed chain activities
4. To relieve pain or muscle spasm	Whenever present	To allow better rehabilitation Gentle stretch To relieve muscle ischemia	Active exercise Massage: vigorous Transverse frictions/TENS or ultrasound on a trigger or acupuncture point Interferential (80–150 pps early, 0–10 pps middle, and late healing phase)
5. Maintain or increase CV fitness, must be sport-specific here	See midterm		

(continued)

671

TABLE 32-1 Aims and Objectives of Rehabilitation Program (Continued)

Aim	When	Long-term goals — Why	How
1. Maintain or restore skin and connective tissue	Whenever skin surface is cut or torn	Prevent scar tissue adhering to connective tissue	Transverse friction Massage Ultrasound (3 MHz) Vitamin E cream Myofascial release techniques
2. Ensure that full range and strength of the lesion site are achieved Maintain or increase overall flexibility	If time allows	Helps prevent further injury Reduces pressure on joint and tissues Increases freedom of movement	Stretching routine Specific for sport and individual needs
3. Correct mechanical cause of injury whole quadrant kinetic chain	When overuse condition When posture adding to condition	Prevents recurrence	Coach or professional analysis mechanics Arch support pad Posture Work place posture Daily correct (ADL) Balance pelvic or pectoral girdle
4. Correction of training habits or equipment	When training habits or equipment add to injury	To prevent recurrence	Therapist advise coach, etc. Drills, skating, throwing Progression for sport return
5. Maintain or increase proprioception	In all muscle ligament, capsule, and joint injuries	Prevent recurrence	Proprioception activities and sport-specific exercises Wobble board

6. Protect injury site	For return to play Whenever chance of injury	Injured site can take 6 months to 2 years for full 100% recovery Prevents reinjury If does reinjure, knows what to do	Balance beam Drills Pliometrics Slow to high speed Closed kinetic chain work concentric and eccentric Modification of equipment, taping, strapping, braces, padding
7. Educate athlete	Throughout treatment and with articles		Talk, demonstrate, illustrate, explain condition, treatment, and rehab fully What to do if recurrence

Prioritized order: Lesion site, joint above and below, surrounding muscle group(s), balance pelvic or pectoral girdle, whole quadrant, whole body, whole athlete.

Contraindications to ice: Cold allergy, cold hypersensitivity, Raynaud's disease, impaired sensation, impaired circulation.

Contraindications to heat: Decreased or impaired sensation, decreased or impaired circulation, inflammation, active tumor.

be initiated at the earliest date. Immobilization may be in the form of a splint, tape, brace, crutches, cervical collar, or sling. Generally, in this phase the use of a crushed ice pack, pressure with a tensor and/or pressure pad, elevation so the limb is higher than the heart, and rest, whether it be immobilization or just resting the injured structure from stress, are all important. The emphasis changes according to the severity of the injury and the structure injured. Home advice includes *icing every waking hour for 15 to 20 min and then letting the structure rewarm for 40 min*. A frozen bag of peas or crushed ice is the best, with a damp cloth underneath to prevent frostbite.

Demolition Phase

We teach the analogy of the demolition phase as the phase when the injured tissue is no longer inflamed. The injured structure can be stressed to the end of its range before pain is elicited. The goal in this phase is to move the waste materials caused by the injury so that new tissue can be laid down to heal. The best way to move the waste materials from the lesion site is with interferential current, gentle effleurage massage to the injured site (elevated) or around it if it is too painful, pulsed ultrasound on the 20 percent duty cycle, cold compression units that pump the area, and movement of the joint above and below the injury. It is very important that a home program stresses self-massage, movements of the surrounding joints, icing if still painful, and appropriate posture in standing, sitting, lying, and the activities of daily living.

Continuous Passive Motion

Continuous passive motion (CPM) may be successful here if available, especially when the articular cartilage is involved or the injury is serious and recovery is expected to be lengthy. The CPM machine cycles a joint through a preset range to restore mobility or prevent postoperative immobility. This is best with knee and shoulder injuries and possibly in elbow, wrist, hip, and ankle injuries. These machines are available in hospitals and physiotherapy clinics and may be rented for home use.

Healing Phase

This is the phase where we try to assist nature itself in laying down more new collagen and augmenting the circulation to bring in the raw material oxygen and increase metabolism to allow more regeneration. This phase can be subdivided into early, middle, and late healing.

Early Healing Phase

In early healing, the goal is to gently warm the area to about 40 to 41°C (100°F) with low-intensity, continuous ultrasound (0.1 to 0.4 W/cm^2), gentle exercise on a treadmill or stationary bike, or active range work in a warm whirlpool.

When the target temperature is reached, there is a general body vasodilation that can be seen as the patient begins to sweat and the skin begins to redden. At this temperature, the collagen will have increased metabolism, nutrition, and oxygenation. The collagen will stretch, since it has increased viscoelastic properties. At this temperature, the pain level also decreases. In this early phase, the motions should be pain-free, and the healing structure can be moved but not stressed, especially if it is a healing ligament or capsule. The key is to *keep the motion pain-free.*

Interferential and TENS can be used for swelling and pain on a high rate setting: IFC at 80 to 150 Hz for 20 to 30 min; TENS at 80 pps, less than 250 μs, and a pulse duration of 20 to 30 min.

Neuromuscular stimulation can be used to muscle pump the swelling out (50 pps, 330-μs pulse width, 8 to 10 s on, and 8 to 10 s off for 20 min). Infrared laser can be used on a direct application at 2 J/cm^2 on healing ligaments, tendons, and superficial capsules. The HeNe laser can be used on the local acupuncture points to help decrease pain.

Biofeedback Electromyography and skin temperature thermometers measure responses of nerves, muscles, etc. The patient learns to control these by way of an auditory or visual signal, and then the stimulus is removed.

George Sheehan again said it best. "Everyone," he said, "should run 30 minutes each day and this will alter your body. After that you must proceed with great caution because the next 30 minutes will alter your life."

Biofeedback can be used to retrain joint or muscle function, if necessary, at this point in the athlete's rehabilitation. A good diet meeting all nutritional requirements is paramount at this time, and oral *Arnica montana* also can be used to decrease inflammation. Vitamin E cream and laser can be used to decrease scar formation if the dermis or epidermis is involved. A few exercises can be done often at home and can enhance the area's healing potential. Gentle cardiovascular work, especially pool therapy, is beneficial here.

If the spine is involved, Tai Chi, yoga, or Pilates exercises can augment the athlete's home program. Tai Chi is a 500-year-old martial art that uses a system of body positions to increase health and overall flexibility. The athlete must be responsible for his or her own welfare and must feel committed to working at home, not just in the clinic.

The Pilates technique, invented by Joseph Pilates in the 1920s, consists of repetitive, rhythmic exercises that use the whole body and work on strength and flexibility from the central muscles outward.

The helium-neon laser is light energy created by combining two gases in a vacuum chamber. These gases are excited with a special light called a *flash gun* that excites the helium and neon atoms. When the atoms return to their ground state, they emit light energy. This energy is of wavelength 632.8 nm (within the red band of visible light), and when applied to the skin, it penetrates 0.8 mm directly or 10 to 15 mm indirectly. The physiologic effect of the light energy allows tissue healing and decreased pain.

The infrared laser is light energy produced using gallium-arsenide (GaAs) in a diode. The infrared laser has a wavelength of 905 nm. This wavelength penetrates 5 cm into the tissue. Its physiologic effects can be used for deeper tissue injuries.

Middle Healing Phase

In the middle healing phase, the tissue can be warmed to 43 to 44°C (112°F). During this phase, the secret is to start to stress the healing tissue in the functional role that it is to perform. Therefore, if muscle is injured, you want to encourage the healing area to contract and stretch in both length and width. The strengthening component must be gentle isometrics or short-arc isotonics or isokinetics without pain. These exercises must be executed with careful supervision so that they are done successfully in the clinic and at home.

Isokinetic machines are successful at this stage, especially if the athlete has a sufficient isotonic base or is only partially weight bearing. For the stretch component, you want to take the muscle to the end of range and hold a gentle stretch for 30 s for four repetitions. The origin should be stretched from the insertion and vice versa for the best results. To regain the width of the muscle belly, gentle transverse friction and massage can be used to break up the cross-links in the muscle fibers. The tendon at this stage of healing needs body warming to the same temperature of 43 to 44°C, but the tendon also should be warmed locally with ultrasound on a continuous setting (approximately 0.2 to 0.5 W/cm^2). A ligament or capsule injury should be stressed gently pain-free, with emphasis on regaining normal range of motion but not stressing to produce hypermobility of the joint. A healing ligament after a tear is weakest 5 to 11 days after injury. The ligament and especially the capsule are enriched with mechanoreceptors, so early proprioception exercise is also important. If the injury allows, cardiovascular fitness that replicates the athlete's sport can be pursued. The joints above and below the lesion site should be worked, and overall flexibility work that is needed for the athlete's sporting event should be carried out. Modalities such as muscle stimulation for retraining and interferential and transcutaneous electrical stimulation for pain and swelling can be used.

Late Healing Phase

In the later healing phase, the tissue should be heated vigorously to 44 to 45°C (115°F). This is best achieved with a vigorous sport-specific exercise such as the treadmill, skating, stationary bike, stairclimber, or swimming. The key at this phase is not only to stress the injured tissue along the lines of stress but also to return it to its full potential. The muscle injury should be advanced to *eccentric work* once there is full range and a good isometric base.

The injured muscle must be able to function in synergy with the other muscles of that limb, so proprioceptive neuromuscular facilitation and the Feldenkrais techniques can be started.

Proprioceptive neuromuscular facilitation (PNF) (*A*) Proprioception. Proprioception is the interaction between the nervous system, muscles, tendons, ligaments, and joints. It orients the body part to space and objects. Proprioceptive exercises are balance, "wobble" board, minitramp, etc. (*B*) Neuromuscular: pertaining to the muscles and the nerves that serve these muscles. Facilitation: the promotion or hastening of any natural process, specifically the effect produced in nerve tissue by the passage of an impulse that lowers the resistance to transmission so that a second stimulus may evoke an easier response. (*C*) PNF stretching. Proprioceptive neuromuscular facilitation is a contract-relax sequence, that is, hold, relax or contract against resistance (by the therapist), and then a stretch and further stretch with therapist's assistance.

Feldenkrais method The Feldenkrais method utilizes manual and verbal directed movement patterns that retain the inherent motor patterns lost through injury or dysfunction. These programmed movements expand the neuromuscular capabilities and motor control of the whole body. They increase functional abilities, balance, and body awareness.

The strengthening exercises must be progressed to weight-bearing positions using rebounders, fitter, shuttles, etc. For tendons, eccentric and pliometric work is imperative because this stresses the ligament the most. Any adhesions in the tendons must be broken down with vigorous transverse friction or thermal ultrasound. Biofeedback for muscles that have difficulty firing synchronously or as a stabilizer can be useful here. The athlete should be starting some activities related to his or her sport. For example, the hockey player may start to skate, the runner start to jog, and so on.

In the remodeling stage, the goal is to stress the structure to the demands of the sport to which the athlete is returning. The muscles must have full range and strength, and the joints must have full range of motion and stability. The key in this phase is to have explosive strength, and the joints must be able to withstand abnormal joint forces. The exercises for the athlete should include cutting

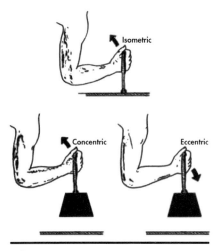

FIG. 32-1   *A.* Isometric (static) exercise: muscle contracts, weight does not move. *B.* Concentric exercise: muscle contracts and weight travels upwards. *C.* Eccentric exercise: muscle contracts and weight travels downward slowly. Not pictured are isotonic exercise, where muscle contracts through range with the weight, and isokinetic exercise, where muscle contracts against a device or machine and weight varies with the effort.

drills, jumping, figure eights, *explosive pliometrics* (Fig. 32-2), and vigorous sports drills.

If a ligament or capsule was torn, then the athlete must brace the joint for 2 years after injury. If there was a muscle injury, then the muscle must be warmed and stretched before challenging it.

Appropriate sport mechanics must be addressed at this time with a qualified coach or trainer for the sport involved. Shoe wear, training schedule, and proper protective equipment also may need to be reviewed. The athlete must be emotionally and psychologically ready for a return to sport. Professional help may need to be pursued in this area. Before a full return to sport, the therapist must

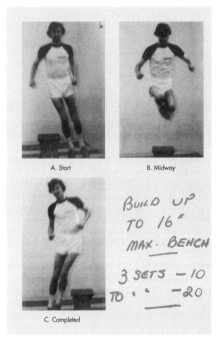

A. Start   B. Midway

C. Completed

BUILD UP TO 16" MAX. BENCH

3 SETS — 10 TO " — 20

FIG. 32-2 Pliometric exercises. "Jump training." Movements of an explosive and reactive nature. Rapid eccentric stretching followed by shortening and concentric contraction. Maximum of one to three sessions per week. Recovery between sets is critical (i.e., 10 s to 2 to 4 min), e.g., box jumping, medicine ball throwing. Enables muscle to reach maximum strength in as short a time as possible.

fully test the joint ranges and strength bilaterally not only statically but also with sport-specific challenges (Fig. 32-3). The athlete's posture and pelvic alignment must be symmetrical. The athlete must be educated to recognize the first signs of a recurrence so that preventative measures may be taken. Pre- and postseason exercises may be necessary.

INJURIES WITHOUT A DIRECT MECHANISM

As indicated earlier, sports injuries can fall into two categories. The first category can be identified as injuries sustained by an obvious episodic trauma, such as a soft tissue contusion. The other category involves a much more complicated mechanism, and these injuries are often insidious in onset. This category involves many factors, all of which contribute to the injury. These injuries also can be

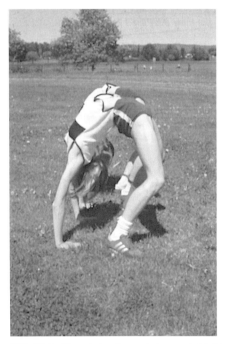

FIG. 32-3 These twins demonstrate remarkable joint range like a lot of good gymnasts and dancers. (Courtesy of Dr. John Porter, Thunder Bay.)

identified as injuries that are chronic in nature and seem to involve recurring episodes of pain and dysfunction.

These injuries without a direct mechanism represent a challenge for the therapist. The therapist's goal will be to determine the cause of the problem so that an appropriate rehabilitation program can be designed. Aches and pains that develop with an insidious onset can come from many sources: a biomechanical alignment, overuse or training error, a visceral or organ dysfunction, an underlying systemic disorder, a kinetic chain problem manifested at a different site, a facilitated segment, or a spinal problem. If the dysfunction persists or recurs, it can be identified as chronic in nature.

Indirect Factors that Can Lead to Chronicity and Their Treatment (Table 32-2)

1. Joint Type and Biomechancial Alignment Problems

A biomechanic problem is the result of a type of trauma. Trauma implies that an injury has occurred due to a mechanical force that has been applied externally to the involved tissue causing structural stress or strain and resulting in cellular or tissue response. These mechanical forces have two components: *stress*, which involves the internal load of tissue resistance and leads to deformation of that tissue, and *strain*, which represents a tissue deformation from an external load. Both these forces are involved in chronic, insidious onset of soft tissue injuries. There is another critical component that must be included in this category of injury, which is the *time factor or use*. Use implies the accumulation of load over time. In many chronic injuries, this component is a critical factor. For example, an athlete who begins to train harder and/or longer can predispose body tissues to become fatigued due to cyclic loading. Therefore, the effects of load on tissue are described by strain and stress. Strain is the deformation of a structure in response to external load, whereas stress is the internal resistance to such deformation.

Structural vulnerability can arise from many different situations. If a joint is *malaligned* (i.e., subtalar valgus, femoral anteversion), the structures that cross the joint (ligament) or support the joint (muscles) may be subject to unusual stress or strain. Day-to-day

TABLE 32-2 Factors for Chronicity

1. Joint type, biomechanical malalignment, hypermobile, hypomobile
2. Kinetic chain, cyclic repetitive
3. Visceral and organ dysfunction
4. Systemic pathology, autonomic
5. Overgrowth syndrome, growing pains
6. Overuse, training error
7. Spinal mechanism

function may not create tissue inflammation in the malaligned joint, but overuse or overtraining may result in microtearing or microtrauma, which may lead to an inflammatory response. The concept of structural vulnerability is one that can be complicated and at the same time lead a practitioner to possible solutions when it comes to chronic injuries. There are two groups that we have chosen to identify. The first is a group of connective tissues (e.g., joints, muscle, fascia, nerves, fibrocartilage, etc.) that move excessively in relation to normal functioning. This group is identified as a *hypermobile group* of tissues. The structural vulnerability of this group is that it may lack the ability to control itself dynamically, and it has the ability to move in varying degrees and with greater amplitude than it normally would. Such tissues require a treatment plan to help (1) strengthen the tissues, which for whatever reason have lost the ability to control themselves dynamically, and (2) limit excessive movements, perhaps by using braces and/or surgical intervention to minimize excessive motion. Strengthening this group of tissues should be done using neuromuscular facilitation, stabilization exercises, and/or strength training exercises that identify the activity and train the athlete in terms of his or her sport and potential deficiencies with which he or she may be confronted.

A joint has excessive laxity, or *hypermobility*, such as foot hyperpronation. In this situation, the tissue that helps to control the joint must work excessively to maintain the structural integrity of that joint. This places a lot of stress and strain on these tissues, which may again lead to tissue vulnerability and tissue failure, whether it is due to focal overload or chronic overuse.

The next factor, as it relates to structural overload, is at the opposite end of the spectrum. In this case, the joint and/or tissue is characterized as *hypomobile*. The second group of connective tissues that relate to structural vulnerability is the group of tissues that do not move well. This group obviously can be identified as the hypomobile group. This group is much more difficult to identify and can become quite complicated. This area seems to be one of the poorest areas of rehabilitation in terms of results. Identifying potential areas of hypomobility is very important. If tissues are limited from moving within a full range of motion, the mechanics of the joint/tissue that are associated with that movement are altered. With the altered movement comes altered function, and slowly, stress and strain are placed on that tissue, which is not able to absorb forces properly, and tissue dysfunction and failure may be the result. In the case of altered function, a single tendon, muscle, or joint that loses the ability to move through a full range of motion affects not only the tissue directly, relating to its movements, but also the mechanics of the joints above and below and eventually of the whole limb. For example, a tibiofemoral joint that lacks full extension in a dynamic gait pattern obviously will place a lot of strain on the knee as well as the structures that cross the knee. It also has the ability to affect the talocrural joint, subtalar joint, tibiofibular joint, and patellofemoral joint below by changing the mechanics of the lower kinetic chain. The sacroiliac and hip joints must adapt due to altered mechanics of the tibiofemoral joint, which does not allow full extension at the tibiofemoral. This concept is an integral part of orthopedic assessment. Orthopaedic assessment involves assessment of the joint involved, plus addressing the joints above and below. In addressing the joints above and below, it should be noted that we are looking at a full range of motion without pain or discomfort. In many instances, assessing the joints above and below may not elicit any pain, and for this reason, it is assumed that the joints have been cleared orthopedically. It must be stressed that a full range of motion is also required for a joint to pass an orthopedic assessment.

Joint inflexibility may lead to muscular imbalances and therefore places an incredible amount of stress and strain on the tissue that crosses the hypomobile joint. In the case of an inflexible group of tissues, such as a group of muscles and their associated fasciae, the joint that they cross is also limited in terms of arthrokinematics and osteokinematics. A joint that loses its ability to move in a full, unrestricted range of motion does not have the ability to ensure proper nutrition to the joint surfaces and help to maintain healthy articular cartilage. Inflexibility can be looked at more globally in terms of its effects. For example, an inflexible hip joint and/or inflexibility of the muscles that cross the hip joint obviously affects the hip and potentially may cause tissue vulnerability, which can lead to tissue failure. To rehabilitate these malaligned, hypermobile, or hypomobile joints involves functional testing of the joints involved and their accessory movements. Joints that are malaligned may require orthotics or proprioceptive retraining to help strengthen the structures involved. For example, a poorly aligned patella may require retraining of the vastus medialis obliquus, the adductor muscles, and the gluteus medius on the opposite side to prevent hip dropping. It may involve retraining the quadriceps muscles to achieve correct muscle timing. A joint that is hypermobile requires excessive retraining with concentric, eccentric, and pliometric work that is sport-specific to reinforce the instability. If the joint is extremely lax, then bracing may be required. To treat the hypomobile joint, the therapist must regain the joint's accessory or joint play movements with joint tractions and mobilizations. Home mobilization exercises should be given, and return to sport should be limited until full joint range is regained.

2. Kinetic Chain Mechanism

Dysfunction in a joint or structure can lead to pathology anywhere along the kinetic chain. The kinetic chain of the upper extremity can include the temporomandibular joint, cervical spine, shoulder joint (acromioclavicular, sternoclavicular, first rib, clavicle, glenohumeral joint, scapulothoracic joint), elbow (humeroulnar, humeroradial, proximal radioulnar joint, distal radioulnar joint), wrist (radiocarpal, ulnar carpal, midcarpal, carpal joints), and hand (metacarpal, metaphalangeal, phalangeal joints). Any pathology of a structure (muscle, ligament, bone, fascia) or joint along the chain can affect one or more of the other joints distally or proximally. The lower extremity kinetic chain includes the lumbar spine, sacrum, sacroiliac joint, ilium, hip, knee, superior tibiofibular joint, inferior tibiofibular joint, talocrural joint, subtalar joint, and foot (metatarsal, tarsal, and phalanges). The hip and pelvis, for example, are not single entities in themselves, especially as they relate to dynamic activities such as occur in sports. The hip is part of the lower extremity and part of a chain of connective tissue that affects the kinetics of the entire lower extremity. Therefore, it can be easily understood that problems that occur in any one area of the body can affect other parts of the body, especially when cyclic repetitive activities occur. These repetitive activities place a strain and stress on the tissue of the whole extremity. When a tissue, group of tissues, or even a joint becomes less mobile, the effects can be seen in tissue a distance away. In the case of altered function, a single tendon, muscle, or joint that loses the ability to move through a full range of motion affects not only the tissue directly relating to its movements but also the mechanics of the joints above and below and eventually of the whole limb. For example, a tibiofemoral joint that lacks full extension in a dynamic gait pattern obviously will place a lot of strain on the knee as well as the structures that cross the knee. It also has the ability to affect the talocrural joint, subtalar joint, tibiofibular joint, and patellofemoral joint below by changing the mechanics of the lower kinetic chain. This situation also may affect the structures above. The sacroiliac and hip joints must adapt, due to altered mechanics of the tibiofemoral joint, which does not allow full extension at the tibiofemoral joint. To effectively treat injuries that are related to dysfunctions of the kinetic chain, arthrologic testing of the whole chain must be carried out to determine which joint or joints along the chain are the cause of or are contributing to the problem. In some cases, if there is muscle weakness, paresthesia, or signs of a neurologic component, a neurologic scan may be called for as well. Treat the whole kinetic chain or quadrant. Start with exercises to regain the necessary motion at the restricted or problem joint or the function of the involved dysfunctional structure. Once full function of this segment is restored, then start retraining work that includes the whole kinetic chain. For example, proprioceptive neuromuscular retraining exercises, Feldenkrais techniques, proprioceptive work, and pliometrics for the whole kinetic chain are appropriate. The progression should be gradual, beginning with open chain work and moving to closed chain work, i.e., quarter squats, with the emphasis becoming more and more sport-specific (Fig. 32-4).

The kinetic chain is a series of links in a mechanical system. An open kinetic chain consists of end segments moving freely in space and not necessarily producing predictable movements from one segment to the other. A closed kinetic chain consists of a pattern of motion in other segments of the mechanical system.

3. Visceral and Organ Dysfunction

Often as therapists our attention is focused on the musculoskeletal system when an athlete arrives at the clinic. We should always be sensitive to the anatomy and physiology of the autonomic nervous system and its segmental innervations to organs. For example, chronic left shoulder pain that does not respond to normal therapy practices and seems to be at its worst with exertion should trigger a query regarding the athlete's heart, diaphragm, or left lung function. The differential diagnosis of shoulder pain is very difficult

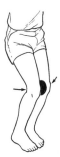

FIG. 32-4   Quarter squat (closed kinetic chain). Squeeze a towel roll or pillow between your knees. Slowly lower down into a quarter squat. Keep your knees pointing straight with your knees directly over your second toe. Do three sets of 15 repetitions. This can progress to a single-leg quarter squat with your injured knee. Remember to keep your knee pointing straight ahead.

because visceral pain may be directed right to the shoulder joint itself. Myocardial ischemia and pancreas pathology both can cause left shoulder pain. Right shoulder pain can come from a peptic ulcer, myocardial infarction, liver disease, or gall bladder pathology. With the aging population, which is becoming more health conscious and more aware of nutrition and exercise, we must be aware of the differential diagnosis for a visceral or organ cause, especially with insidious onset. Treatment involves a general practitioner referral or consultation to rule out underlying organic pathology.

4. Systemic Pathology

The therapist also must be concerned when pain begins in or around a joint without a mechanism yet will not abate. Hip pain, for example, can be caused by bone tumors, appendicitis, pelvic inflammatory disease, femoral hernia, and ankylosing spondylitis, to name a few. We must take a very complete history and conduct a thorough orthopaedic assessment with every athlete to avoid missing underlying pathology. The red flags in the history are that the pain may be present even while resting or sleeping, more than one joint has pain, the pain is not exacerbated by a certain movement, the pain is vague in nature or very acute without cause, or the patient does not feel well in general (e.g., fatigue, malaise, fever) when the pain is present. A good differential diagnosis text is imperative to identify specific systemic pathology. If the therapist suspects an underlying problem, then referral to a general practitioner for the necessary laboratory testing is indicated.

5. Overgrowth Syndrome

Overgrowth syndrome and *growing pains* are terms emphasizing potential muscular imbalances and inflexibility associated with or coincidentally occurring during skeletal changes during maturation. These changes in skeletal proportions can create potential dynamic overloads of soft tissue and again lead to stress and strain placed on a tissue that may lead to tissue vulnerability and perhaps tissue failure. Treatment involves testing muscle groups and connective tissue for tightness, especially in the two joint muscles, and preparing a stretching program and implementing myofascial release techniques. The stretching program must be done after a warm-up, and sport-specific exercises should be given so that the stretching can be done at home and at practice. The muscles also should be tested for resisted strength to correct the imbalances between the muscle groups. A strengthening program that addresses the weaknesses should be given for the clinic and for a home program.

6. Overuse or Training Error

Many chronic injuries are attributed to improper training methods. If an athlete trains too intensely and does not allow tissue to regenerate properly, which is accomplished by an appropriate rest period between training sessions and competition, the tissue vulnerability may contribute to fatigue and eventual tissue breakdown or tissue failure. Prolonged motion and insufficient rest may create a situation where collagen is unable to repair the resulting microtrauma and inflammation. If this situation continues, obviously the potential result could be tissue failure. Chronic injury typically most often affects tendons and is distinguished primarily by degenerative changes. The degenerative changes are thought to be the result of a hypoxic degenerative process involving the cell matrix of the tendons. Many studies have investigated degenerative tendinopathy. In many of the tendon ruptures, previous pathogenic conditions existed. In fact, this number is as high as 97 percent of the tendon ruptures having had previous existing conditions. The degenerative changes that occur from a histologic perspective in chronic injuries are important to note. The changes include alterations in size and shape of the mitochondria, which are essential for energy and oxygen serving the cells. They include alterations in the nuclei of the internal fibroblasts or tenocytes. Alterations also include mitochondrial calcification and tissue hypoxia as well as longitudinal splitting, disintegration, angulation, and changes in the fiber diameter of the collagen.

It is interesting to identify a classification of chronic injuries, to be able to identify this situation when it occurs, and to be able to recognize the potential dangers that could arise from chronic injuries. The classification is as shown in Table 32-3. Classification of chronic injuries helps the practitioner decide what is best at that time to help eliminate the problem and, perhaps just as important, to decrease the potential for the injury to progress. Grades 1 to 3 injuries usually require some modification of activity to allow the tissue rest time to facilitate proper healing. Grades 4 and 5 injuries usually require discontinuation of specific aggravating activities. Grade 5 injuries may require surgical intervention. Indications for surgery are listed in Table 32-4.

While surgery may be a viable option at some point, it is important to determine that the so-called cause of the problem may not have been identified. This may cause mixed results from surgical intervention.

TABLE 32-3 Chronic Injury Classification

Symptoms	Possible Treatment
Grade 1	
Pain after activity	Modification of activity
Does not interfere with performance	NSAIDs
Pain disappears prior to next event	Assess training
	Treat structural vulnerability
Grade 2	
Minimal pain with activity	Modify activity
Pain does not interefere with activity	Assess training schedule
Localized tenderness	NSAIDs off and on Pennsaid (Dimethaid-D)
Grade 3	
Pain interferes with activity	Modify activity
Pain decreases between activity sessions	NSAIDs
	Assess training schedule
Grade 4	
Pain does not disappear between activity sessions	Decrease aggravating activities
Seriously interferes with training	Alternate activity program
Significant local pain	NSAIDs
Local tenderness, crepitus, and swelling	Splinting
Grade 5	
Pain interferes with sport and activities of daily living	Prolonged rest from activity
Symptoms often chronic or recurrent	NSAIDs
Signs of tissue damage and altered associated muscle function	Steroids
	Surgery Cast/splint

TABLE 32-4 Indications for Surgery

3 to 6 months of unsuccessful rehabilitation program
Quality of life altered
Night pain with or without sports
Objective signs
Persistent weakness
Positive diagnosis

7. Spinal (Facilitated Segment or Spinal Pathology) Mechanism

Injuries to the spine that affect the vertebrae and result in rotational or side-bent abnormal positions or damage the invertebral disk can set up pathology in the dermatome, myotome, sclerotome, or viscera served by that segment. These disk or vertebral problems can cause weakness in the muscles served by that segment and may make them vulnerable to injury. For example, a C6 problem may cause weakness to the wrist extensors, which then develop lateral epicondylitis. Segmental problems should be tested by assessing the spine that serves the lesion site. Motions of forward bending, extension, side bending, and rotation will determine the vertebral restriction, while neurologic testing will help determine the vertebral cause. If the segment is suspected as part of the cause or all of the cause, treatment should involve the lesion site in the distal tissue, but the spine also should be addressed. Manual traction, mobilization, and manipulation will help the segment. The intervertebral disk pathology is best treated with McKenzie exercises as well as clear postural advice.

Summary

Chronic injuries that are a result of an indirect mechanism are characterized by a slow, insidious onset of signs and symptoms. This subthreshold structural damage may last for months or even years and is distinguished by persistence of symptoms without resolution. Chronic injuries may involve a chronic inflammatory response as a result of tissue deformation. It is the therapist's role to determine the cause of the chronicity through a very complete assessment that looks at the arthrology of the joints of the entire kinetic chain, tests the spinal segment and neurology of the segment, tests the muscles for strength and length, looks for myofascial restrictions, investigates the athlete's training procedure, understands differential diagnoses, and can recognize systemic pathology. Sometimes there is more than one cause, and there is an interplay of several causes. Only a thorough assessment of all these details will ensure that the treatment and rehabilitation program will treat the cause and not just the symptoms.

Terminal Goals:

1. Joint range is full and equal bilaterally to meet the requirements put on it by the athlete's sport. All-over quadrant and body flexibility.
2. Muscle strength is full (strength/power/endurance) and equal bilaterally (concentric/eccentric) and meets the requirements of the sport needs (slow/fast speed) (open/closed chain).
3. Overall cardiovascular fitness meets the athlete's and sport requirements.
4. The athlete's biomechanical function is normal and not conducive to reinjury.
5. The athlete's training schedule is altered to prevent reinjury.
6. The athlete is psychologically, emotionally, and physically ready to return to sport.
7. The athlete has an off-season, preseason, or on-season program to prevent reinjury.
8. There is no pain or instability for the athlete when returning to play (if instability is present, he or she should be protected or braced).
9. Test the athlete with sport-related drills (i.e., on skates, court, etc.)

RECOMMENDED READING

Visner C, Colby LA: *Therapeutic Exercise: Foundations and Techniques*, 3d ed. Philadelphia, FA Davis, 1996.

Reid D: *Sports Assessment and Rehabilitation*. New York, Churchill-Livingstone, 1992.

Prentice W: *Rehabilitation Techniques in Sports Medicine*. St Louis, Mosby, 1994.

Andrews J, Harrelson G: *Physical Rehabilitation of the Injured Athlete*. Toronto, Saunders, 1991.

Griffin L: *Rehabilitation of the Injured Athlete*, 2d ed. St Louis, Mosby, 1995.

Hartley A: Practical joint assessment: Upper quadrant, in *A Sports Medicine Manual*, 2d ed. St Louis, Mosby, 1995.

Hartley A: Practical joint assessment: Lower quadrant, in *A Sports Medicine Manual* St Louis, Mosby, 1995.

Hartley A: *Therapeutic Ultrasound*, 2d ed. Toronto, Anne Hartley Agency, 1993.

Hartley A: *Neuromuscular Electrical Stimulation*, 2d ed. Toronto, Anne Hartley Agency, 1997.

33 | Endurance Training

R. Charles Bull   Hugh Cameron

The ancient Greeks stressed athletics because their religious beliefs revolved around the "whole man." Second, athletic competitions closely paralleled activities of war, and although the Olympic Games were a time of peace, the amnesty was over when the games were over.

Long-distance events are 3000 m (2-mile equivalent), 10,000 m (6 miles), and 3000-m steeplechase. Cross-country races vary from 3, 4, to 6 miles. They are often run as a team event with seven participants on each team, and the goal is to have the top five finish well. Marathons cover 26 miles and 385 yards and also can be run as a team event with five runners covering a 5-mile or greater segment each.

MECHANICS

The triathlon is the ultimate individual test of endurance. The most important aspect of long-distance running is pacing. Good runners read their bodies so well that they know their pace to within 15 s every mile. They also know when to speed up and break away from their competitors.

The runner should run naturally and not try to stride out too much. If the foot lands in front of the body's center of gravity, it can cause a deceleration with each step.

The arms are just allowed to swing naturally and lightly at the lower rib cage level, and long-distance runners do not need to pump.

In training, even a half-minute mile difference in pace can be quite fatiguing, i.e., $6\frac{1}{2}$-min mile versus a 7-min mile pace. Remember, *"Train, don't strain!"*

The most important aspect of running is a relaxed pace. Most joggers land on the lateral heel, and you can check this with their shoe wear. The elite marathoners dance along like little birds, landing on the ball of the foot, and then the heel touches instantly afterwards.

Running is the best cardiovascular endurance sport, but everyone cannot run. Team Canada's hockey team encourages aerobic exercise in training camp. They allow the players to do touch football, ride bikes, spin, or run. Gretzky would not make the team if the sole criterium was running prowess.

ANATOMY

Runners obviously have a varying anatomy, and with impact, the foot is slightly supinated as the heel strikes and then pronates for between 50 and 60 percent of the support phase. Excessive pronation can be a problem when it transmits too much force into the ankles, legs, knees, and hips (see Chap. 24).

If the runner's anatomy is less than ideal (i.e., pronated feet and valgus knees), he or she tends to transfer the weight improperly and hit hard. He or she then has to flip the foot to get into the proper running mechanic, and this contributes to excessive mobility of the patella in particular and chondromalacia or patellofemoral syndrome.

Also, long-distance runners have a preponderance of slow-twitch fibers, and it is interesting that long-distance runners can have a fast finishing kick and thus can do sprinting to a certain extent, but sprinters have major trouble running long distances. The odd sprinter that will do a 10-km race often suffers a significant injury following that type of long run.

The red fibers are the slow-twitch fibers, and they are usually sturdy and dependable. They have an excellent mitochondrial system for combustion and supplying energy. They can constantly supply this energy and are an abundant source of exogenous circulating material.

The white fibers are the streamlined fast-twitch fibers with rapid contractility. They are the high-performance fibers with a well-developed sarcoplasm. They have a rapid response and reaction to their nervous input. They have to have a full gas tank and an abundant supply of stored energy to work most efficiently. This is determined to a great extent at birth, but individuals can change a certain percentage of their fibers by training.

MECHANICS

The average recreational runner makes approximately 1500 foot plants per mile, and this varies between 800 and 2000. His or her foot strikes approximately 60 times a minute. There is an impact of two times his or her body weight, and it can be up to four times the body weight with hard sprinting or rapid downhill running.

Joggers are classified as doing an 8-min mile pace or slower and running 3 to 20 miles per week. Runners are classified as doing less than an 8-min mile pace and running 40 to 70 miles per week.

The average recreational runner can compete satisfactorily at 7 miles a day 6 days a week, but he or she should mix up that type of training and not just grind out 7 miles on the pavement each morning.

There are many variations of training, from long slow distance (LSD) to repetitive sprints (speed work). All athletes need a 2-mile a day base; they also have to do pace work and anaerobic fast-twitch workouts, and only after they have this base can they subspecialize into their more frequent speed or endurance workouts (Fig. 33-1).

DIAGNOSIS

The runner should be instructed to bring his or her running log. He or she should have input from the coach and parents, and ideally, the doctor should see him or her run. Thus he or she should bring his or her shoes and running gear.

When a runner comes in for the first time, make sure you set aside an extra half hour to take the history. Look at the running log, go over the schedule, and check the shoes. If you cannot pinpoint the injury, get the runner to go out and run and then come back.

A *good history* sometimes can take up to two or three visits because the runners are naturally academic and reticent. It takes time to get to know the runner. You also have to do a thorough *past history*. Some runners come from other sports such as hockey, and they will have more of a wide-track type of gait.

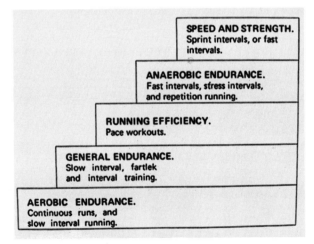

FIG. 33-1   Anaerobic/aerobic training schedule. All athletes from the 1000-m runner to the marathoner need to have some aerobic endurance and a base. They also have to do pace workouts and some anaerobic fast-twitch workouts. Only after they have this base, can they subspecialize into their more frequent speed or endurance workouts.

Runners also should have a good *family history* regarding cardiac problems, and a personal history should be taken regarding drinking, smoking, bulemia, etc. A dietary history is important because a lot of runners are vegetarians, and some put the majority of their food in a blender. They also tend to accept the latest fad diets.

A history of lack of sleep, psychological problems, and other spare time activities is important. It is interesting that the competitive personality of the runner has its own running addiction side effect. Ask about the use of weights and weight training; cross-training such as aerobics is also important.

The runner's work history is also essential. Some elite runners get up at three in the morning and stretch and train in order to be at work by 7 A.M. Other runners who are not working can train three times a day.

It is important to be prepared to counsel runners psychologically right when you are taking the history. You should emphasize their personal best rather than winning, and we always tell them that Gretzky does not score every night and does not win every game.

Runners tend to be their own coaches and be individuals in their training to a certain extent, and this is where running clubs are good. They can get coaches outside their school, and running camps are also good. They can have video analysis studies and learn the habits and training routine of other runners.

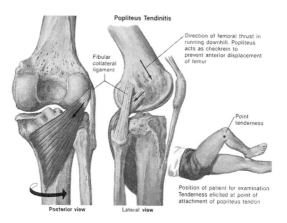

Popliteus Tendinitis

Fibular collateral ligament

Direction of femoral thrust in running downhill. Popliteus acts as checkrein to prevent anterior displacement of femur

Point tenderness

Position of patient for examination. Tenderness elicited at point of attachment of popliteus tendon

Posterior view   **Lateral view**

FIG. 33-2   Popliteus tendinitis. Be careful to differentiate this from the iliotibial band syndrome. In iliotibial band friction syndrome the pain is more diffuse.

Physical examination is extremely important, and it has to be a head-to-toe examination (see Chap. 32). You have to be very specific anatomically, since just a few millimeters can make the difference between diagnosing iliotibial band syndrome or a popliteus syndrome (Fig. 33-2).

Feet

The feet are probably most important, and thus we actually make the examination toe to head. You should emphasize proper foot care to runners right away. Some of them should tape their feet to prevent blisters and use lamb's wool between the toes. You have to emphasize a proper foot plant, and you can gauge this to a certain extent by having the patient run on the spot. We then have them stand with their feet parallel, 1 ft apart, and see if they have pronated feet or valgus knees.

We usually see runners with a *physiotherapist* in our clinic, and we put our heads together and try to devise plan of treatment right away. In younger runners, we make sure that a parent or the coach is with them so that they know the diagnosis and follow the treatment regime.

Legs

Check for shin splints (leg pain), palpate the tibialis posterior area, then the bony tibia, and then the anterior compartment (Figs. 33-3, 33-4). Squeeze firmly and tap the tibia; very sharp pain and withdrawal suggest a stress fracture. Patients then hop, jump, kneel, and jump back to a standing position. All these agility exercises are used to provoke discomfort in the foot, ankle, and knee, for instance.

The quadriceps and calves should be measured, and leg length also should be measured (anterosuperior spine to medial malleo-

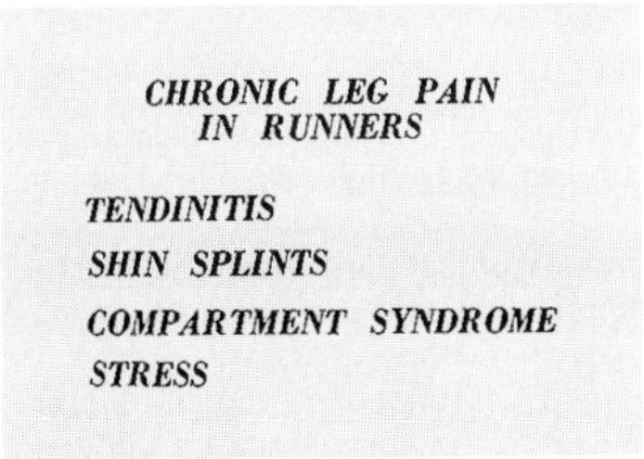

**CHRONIC LEG PAIN
IN RUNNERS**

TENDINITIS

SHIN SPLINTS

COMPARTMENT SYNDROME

STRESS

FIG. 33-3 Shin splints can be divided into four categories: 1. Tib posterior tendinitis. 2. Pretibial periostitis—the classical shin splint. 3. Anterior compartment syndrome. 4. A stress fracture.

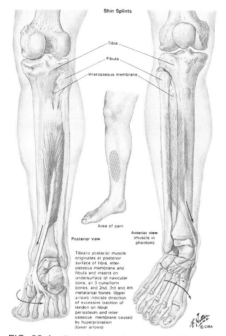

Shin Splints

Tibia

Fibula

Interosseous membrane

Area of pain

Posterior view

Anterior view
(muscle in
phantom)

Tibialis posterior muscle
originates at posterior
surface of tibia, inter-
osseous membrane and
fibula and inserts on
undersurface of navicular
bone, all 3 cuneiform
bones, and 2nd, 3rd and 4th
metatarsal bones. Upper
arrows indicate direction
of excessive traction of
tendon on tibial
periosteum and inter-
osseous membrane caused
by hyperpronation
(lower arrows)

FIG. 33-4 One of the most common problems we see in runners is leg pain. I classify this into four categories; the first is usually tib posterior tendinitis occurring in the lower medial portion of the shin. The second is periostitis over the body of the tibia. The third is an anterior compartment syndrome on the outer aspect of the lower leg. The fourth is true stress fracture.

lus). Adduction and abduction power and hip flexion and psoas power should be gauged. Estimate the Q-angle (see Fig. 33-6) and patellar tracking.

You want to know the flexibility of the runner's hips and the mobility of his or her back. The runner should perform a sit-up and a sloppy push-up.

The runner's *upper body, neck, and shoulders* should be examined carefully. A lot of runners do not concentrate on the upper body. Theoretically, they should lift some light upper body weights because the repetitive movement of the arms in the long races requires good strength.

Runners then should do *quick drills*, side stepping, back stepping, quick stepping on and off a stool, backwards running, stool jumping, and plyomorphics. If possible, *body fat* can be measured with calipers.

If a specific area such as the ankle is lax, stress x-rays can be done, and these should be done by the doctor himself or herself if possible so that he or she knows that an equal stress is placed on each ankle. Bone scans are often ordered in runners, particularly if the doctor suspects a stress fracture.

Also, a *gait analysis and treadmill test* are important if you are considering orthotics. A computed tomographic (CT) scan and/or magnetic resonance imaging (MRI) for back pain should be considered, and we emphasize that an accurate diagnosis in a runner is very important because they are the most dedicated athletes regarding their training. They will not stop training unless they have confidence in you and confidence in your diagnosis.

Associated injuries can be provoked by the psychological deprivation of having to give up running. A lot of runners have bowel trouble and gastric upset when they suddenly have to stop running their 60 to 70 miles per week. Running clubs are good in counseling runners to avoid injuries, as well as emphasizing that runners come back slowly from an injury.

TREATMENT (ACUTE INJURY)

The principle of treatment for the acute injury in particular is rest. This does not mean "stop"; it means cross-train and avoid torque and pressure on the affected area.

Remember that ordinary walking will put a force equivalent to your body weight through your lower extremity joints. Kicking a football can put a force of 1000 lb through those same joints, and any type of fast running can at least double your weight. Sprinting can put forces of up to 640 lb through your knee joint.

Thus rest means *rest from anything that causes pain*. *Anti-inflammatories* usually help, and they can be used steadily for the first week to 10 days and then intermittently depending on the pain. The athlete can take them for 2 or 3 days and then stop for 3 or 4 days. Continue with ice as long as there is significant pain. The old rule of icing for 48 h has gone by the board. You can *ice for 10 days if the pain persists*. More *stretching*, and this should be done scientifically through the advice of a physiotherapist or athletic therapist. Cut down the interval, cut down on the hills, go back to walking, and as soon as the runner can walk quickly, i.e., 4 miles in an hour, he or she can progress to walk/jogging. *Steroid injections* are questionable in a runner and particularly dangerous in the Achilles tendon area and the knee.

Once the runner goes back to running, he or she has to *stretch significantly and warm up* before running. The runner should not compete until he or she is well warmed up. Any injury also should turn on a red light, and the runner should do significant *strengthening* to correct muscle imbalance so that the injury does not recur. This is particularly important in young people, and you have to watch the epiphyses. Certainly, if such young runners have severe pain, one should think of an apophysitis or inflammation of the epiphysis. Such runners have to lay off until the pain goes, or they will sustain permanent damage.

Initial Management

In all the brochures that we give runners, there is the word *rest*. We emphasize that this is *judicious* rest; it does not mean stop running. They should be encouraged to cycle, swim, rollerblade, cross-country ski, and use the Nordic Track, Stair Master, and treadmill. The treadmill can actually be different from running on the track or road. That is so because runners can walk/jog and jog and stop the jogging right away if they have discomfort. The elliptical trainer also simulates running without impact.

Definitive Management

Definitive management is most often physiotherapy, and it is crucial that runners go to a sports clinic or a runner's clinic where they can be counseled on the effects of the injury and the effects of ignoring the injury. Gradual progression through stages 1 to 4 of physiotherapy is extremely important. The management of shin splints leg pain is typical of the treatment of most running injuries (Fig. 33-5). Runners should not start to run until both the physiotherapist and the doctor give them the "green light." Nonsteroidal anti-inflammatory drugs (NSAIDs) are important, and there are seven families of NSAIDs (Table 33-1).

The runner with tendinitis can be given naproxen, for instance, for 1 week consistently and then intermittently, i.e., 2 days on, 2 to 3 days off. If it is effectual, stay on this intermittent dose until the problem completely subsides. If the medication is ineffective, go to another family, i.e., Tylenol. If the medication is effective but the benefit wears off after a few weeks, try another family, i.e., Voltaren. Do not mix two medications from different families, i.e., Tylenol and Anaprox.

Alter the Cause of the Injury

Altering the cause of the injury is important. This can be done by changing the shoes, ordering orthotics, altering the warm-up, mus-

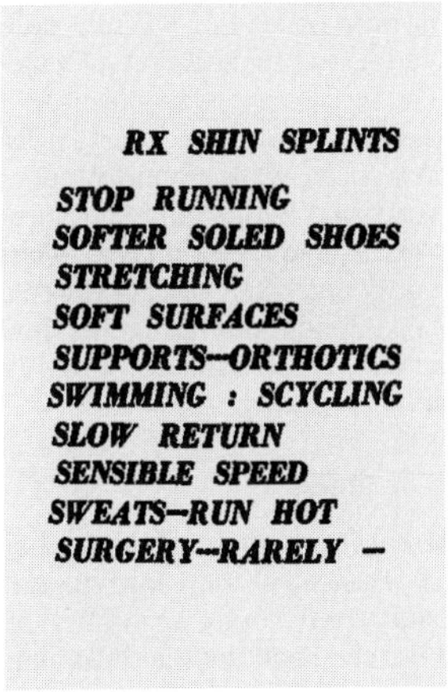

RX SHIN SPLINTS

STOP RUNNING
SOFTER SOLED SHOES
STRETCHING
SOFT SURFACES
SUPPORTS--ORTHOTICS
SWIMMING : SCYCLING
SLOW RETURN
SENSIBLE SPEED
SWEATS--RUN HOT
SURGERY--RARELY --

FIG. 33-5   Prescription for shin splints.

cle strengthening, and changing the training schedule. It could well require a session with the coach and runner together.

Progress is sometimes one step forward and one step back. We emphasize that at times a runner's progress can be slow, slow, slow! Patients will almost invariably try to run and reaggravate the problem. At this stage, a Cybex or Kincom test or $\dot{V}_{O_2max}$ test can emphasize to them that they are just not ready to return so quickly.

With regard to the *anticipated time frame of the return*, it is important to learn their schedule; e.g., cross-country starts on September 3 and indoor track starts on January 3.

Return to Competition

Return to peak competition is variable. A lot of elite runners will peak only two or three times a year. They should run at half a

TABLE 33-1 Nine Families of NSAIDs

Salicylates	Aspirin, dolobid
Acetaminophen	Tylenol
Propionic acids	Naproxen, Anaprox, Motrin, Orudis
Acetic acids	Diclofenac, Voltaren, Indocid, Clinoril
Oxicams	Feldene
Naphthylackanones	Relafen
Fenamic acids	Meclomen
Etodolac	Pyroxicam-β-cyclodextrin
Ultradol	Brexidol

minute off their pace, i.e., a $7\frac{1}{2}$-min mile instead of a 7-min mile, and they should feel loose and relaxed. Good runners feel as if they can run forever.

When runners return to their full schedule after an injury, it has to be a slow return that incorporates speed walking and running. They should run hot and wear sweats and avoid hills and speed work. You have to aim for realistic goals, and we emphasize that it takes 6 weeks to heal a soft tissue injury and often another 6 weeks to get back to normal performance, i.e., 3 months. During this time, patients have progressive physiotherapy, cross-train, and progress slowly on a running return schedule.

Return to Running After an Injury or Illness

Competitive runners are much different from other athletes in their motivation and training dedication. Basically, they love to run; *nothing replaces running*. Thus their philosophy regarding resumption of running is, "Just head out the back door and run until you are tired out."

This is where track clubs can help. Advice by more experienced colleagues will ensure moderation. Runners will listen to their doctor if he or she has their respect. But it takes ages of discussion and counseling to gain that respect.

The return is intangible too. You cannot and should not apply exact times, as you tend to do in other sports, i.e., 6 weeks after a second-degree torn knee ligament. Research by Dr. Saltin, reported by Gledhill, studied untrained and moderately trained subjects. They studied aerobic capacity after 3 weeks of bed rest, followed immediately by 8 weeks of retraining. The retraining consisted of 30 min of continuous and interval running with a heart rate of 170 to 180 beats per minute 6 days a week.

Following the bed rest, there was a 25 percent decrease in aerobic capacity (we tell people they lose 10 percent a week). In the untrained group, subjects got back to pre-bed rest jogging activities in 12 days. In the moderately trained group, it took 29 days to regain the pre-bed rest running activities.

The authors recommended that if the illness lasts for longer than 3 to 4 weeks, return to training is the same as initiating a new training program. If the illness lasts for 3 weeks or less, consider it an interruption in training and start back more rapidly.

Thus, projecting this work to elite or well-trained athletes, you can estimate that they require *2 to 3 weeks of training* for each week of bed rest to attain complete recovery (3 weeks of rest requires 9 weeks of recovery). Moderately active individuals require 1 to 2 weeks for each week of inactivity (3 weeks rest requires 3 to 6 weeks of recovery).

Return after an injury is often too rapid, as you can see from the case histories. Runners must have a goal (the Boston Marathon in April), but it should be very realistic. *Most athletes do not get their endurance back until they attain full muscle bulk.* If their quads are down by an inch, they cannot train for a marathon properly. Isokinetic (Cybex, Kincom) testing is also important to give them a tangible, accurate assessment of their lack of power. This reinforces their own estimate of their lack of endurance.

Team Approach

It is important to

1. See the running log (notebook)
2. Talk to the parents and coach
3. If necessary, talk to the head coach
4. See the patient run on the track or the road in front of your office
5. See the patient with the physiotherapist or trainer or at least speak with them
6. See a video of the patient walking or running on a treadmill if possible. The coach can video the patient running toward him or her, running away from him or her, and he or she can pan the runner with a lateral video to see if he or she is favoring the affected limb or running with an uncoordinated style.

Then in conjunction with the athlete and coach, you can supervise the return to competition.

Runners can split their workouts, i.e., 2 to 3 miles in the morning, 3 to 4 miles in the evening. We use 7 miles per day as a maximum if there are any residual problems after an injury. The ultimate goal is to return the runner back to competition in better shape than he or she was in prior to the illness or injury.

Clues

Think of runner's anemia, particularly in women and vegetarians. Runners usually have a lower hemoglobin level due to dilution. Do a serum ferritin determination for iron deficiency (less than 12 mg/dL is diagnostic). Treatment is oral iron pills for up to 6 months or more.

SUDDEN DEATH IN RUNNERS

Most runners recall Jim Fixx, who dropped dead suddenly while running in July of 1984. Until his death, it was suggested that runners had some type of immunity to coronary infarction and sudden death if they had run a marathon. Jim Fixx proved this theory wrong. It also was suggested that you could run through angina and not suffer any problems. We always used to tell people that it was all right if it was not *our* angina.

Jim Fixx was noted as the running guru, and he wrote a book called *The Complete Book of Running* and published this in 1977. He followed it later with *The More Complete Book of Running*. It was debated in running circles, as documented by David Blaikie, whether Fixx's running actually prolonged his life or caused his death. Fixx's father had recurring heart problems and died of a heart attack at the age of 43 years. Fixx himself began running in his middle thirties when he was overweight and out of shape and smoked two packs of cigarettes a day. After he started running, his weight went from 220 to 159 lb, and he became a very dedicated marathon runner.

Thus the question is, with bad heredity and conditioning, would he have survived the 17 years if he had not taken up the marathon running. He used to consistently run 10 miles a day.

Runners World columnist and noted cardiologist and philosopher, Dr. George Sheehan,[1] states:

1. Preexisting heart disease exists in all cases of runner's sudden heart death.
2. Running does not protect individuals from coronary artery disease.
3. Most cardiac runners have symptoms that warn them not to run.
4. Sudden heart deaths are unlikely to occur in supervised training programs such as cardiac rehabilitation programs. (These excellent programs, run by Dr. Terrence Kavanagh of Toronto and Dr. Kenneth Cooper of Dallas, have had excellent results.)

Dr. Sheehan preached that exercise prolongs life in most people with coronary artery disease, and he felt that running was the preferred exercise.

All practitioners should be prepared for a sudden collapse in sports and have their cardiopulmonary resuscitation techniques up to snuff (CPR). Dr. Dave Reid, in his sports injuries book,[2] emphasizes that one rescuer can do four groups of 15 chest compressions per minute and do two quick lung inflations between each group (sequence 15 to 2); two rescuers can do five chest compressions at a rate of 60 per minute and one lung inflation between each set of 5 (sequence 5 to 1).

HEAVY SWEATING AND FLUID REPLACEMENT

A runner often may lose between 5 and 10 lb during a long-distance run or marathon in a hot environment. Perspiration can account for 6 to 8 percent of the body weight and 13 to 21 percent of the plasma volume in a marathoner.

The first mechanism that signals you to drink and replenish your body water is a delayed one and thus not reliable. This is especially important when the tension and anxiety that go with competition are increased by the elevated epinephrine level.

Water is the mainstay of sweat replacement. The faster water leaves the stomach, the faster the absorption of fluids from the intestine occurs. Gastric emptying can be delayed by sugar content. Larger volumes of water empty more rapidly, but larger volumes can cause cramps, and runners do not like water sloshing around in their stomach.

Thus you are best to take 4 to 8 oz of water at 10- to 15-min intervals, and this minimizes gastric filling. Water should be cooled to 40 to 50°F because cold fluids empty more quickly from the stomach than warm fluid due to increased gastric motility. Cold drinks also aid in stabilizing the core temperature of the body.

Gatorade and other similar replacement drinks have a low glucose level, but they should be diluted. Grab a cup of Gatorade and water at the same time.

Also, 10 to 15 min prior to competition, a runner can drink 10 to 20 oz of cool water. This fluid will not get through to the kidneys, since exercise reduces the production of urine.

The use of coffee prior to a run is debated. Coffee is usually not recommended because it alters fat metabolism during endurance runs. Recently, caffeine and ephedrine (5 mg, i.e., 3 cups of coffee, and 1 mg of ephedrine) have shown benefit in enhancing endurance.

In the ironman competitions in the heat, the competitors are weighed. A 10 percent weight loss from dehydration can result in heat stroke and circulatory collapse, and runners should weigh themselves daily to make sure that they are not getting into a chronically dehydrated state.

PREVENTION OF RUNNING INJURIES

Prevention of running injuries is most successful if the runner is academic and takes a keen interest in reading running books and studying the sport itself. Runners have to have a conditioning base, and a long-distance runner should have the equivalent of 7 miles a day. Sprinters also should have a base of 2 to 3 miles a day. Competitive runners should train 6 days a week.

It is best to train on grass, but modern footwear does allow runners to do a lot of work on roads. Speed work on the track, i.e., repeat 200 m and then walk 200 m and repeat it again, can be done under the direction of the coach but should only be done twice a week. If runners are stiff and do not feel loose, they should warm up again and stretch and then warm up again and stretch. They will have their good days and bad days.

Warm-Ups

We cannot emphasize the warm-up too much. Runners should always warm up a good 15 to 20 min prior to a training run and prior to a race and then warm down. If you do not feel loose, warm up again. Warm-ups should consist of stretching, calisthenics, bounding, and light running until you are in a light sweat.

Agility Drills

Runners also should be able to do agilities tests, backward running, sideways running, sideways running on a treadmill, strength tests on the Hydragym (20 repetitions in 20 s), and endurance test running of a steep hill 6, 8, 10, and 12 times.

Overtraining

An index of overtraining is often fatigue and tiredness, insomnia, temperamental personality and crankiness, and loss of appetite. The average endurance runner can eat three sandwiches for lunch. Excessive sweating and excessive colds and flu often herald overtraining and overuse.

Training errors and excessive mileage are the main cause of the running problems and overuse. Too much too soon is the cause of the initial problem and the cause of recurrences. A guide for increasing mileage, particularly when the runner is coming back after an injury, is 10 percent a week, i.e., 10 miles the first week, 11 miles the second week, 12 miles the third week, etc.

We tell the recreational runner to walk 4 miles in an hour consistently for a week and then start picking it up by walking a half, running a half, and gradually increase. We emphasize that if he or she is training for an upcoming race, he or she should do one-third to two-thirds of the race distance on a daily basis and one longer run a week. If he or she cannot do this, he or she will not do well in the race.

Running Equipment

Shoes

The most important aspect of the running equipment is the shoes and shoe selection. The first running shoes were made in 1920, and the first Adidas shoe was used in 1936 in the Olympics by Jesse Owens. The first three-striper was made in 1947 when the two brothers split up and one started Puma.

The basic shoe should emphasize sound foot support and a good, comfortable fit. It is most important to go to a specialty shoe store and be fitted and to try several different types of shoes. You can have both a training shoe and a racing shoe, but for the beginner or recreational runner, a training shoe is satisfactory for the race.

Also, you "get what you pay for," although some of the specialty stores have phenomenal sales.

Some shoes come in widths, such as New Balance, and others have additional support for hard cross-country running or for use on rough terrain, such as the Adidas shoe with the torsion bar.

Shoes denature over time, and although they might look all right, they will lose up to one-third of their shock absorption after 100 to 150 miles. This depends on the weight, impact, and style of the runner, of course.

Singlets and Shorts

The singlets and shorts should be loose fitting to avoid chafing. You can wear a long-leg girdle beneath the running shorts, which is available commercially, to prevent chafing. Liberal use of Vaseline on the nipples and in the groin in both males and females helps stop chafing and is suggested.

Dehydration and Fluid Replacement

The major factor in the endurance workouts is rehydration. The best fluid is just plain water. However, the different elite athletes vary in their choices from water with sugar or fruit juice to diluted Gatorade, defizzed Coke, or gingerale. At one stage there was a substance called Gluconaid prepared by Bill Glucon, a pharmacist, which was reconstituted sweat. It did not catch on because it tasted so salty. It also contained potassium, which tended to give some runners diarrhea.

Runners' Diets

Runners also have varying diets. A lot of them like to put their food in a blender and blend up various concoctions of fruit and vegetables and take multiple small meals of liquid or soft, easily digested material. They like apricots, papaya, mangos, carrot juice, honey, and ice cream. A lot of runners are vegetarians, and some are strict vegetarians and will not even take meat sauce on their spaghetti.

They tend to like a pasta dinner prior to a race, and some do carbohydrate loading. This requires them to go on a protein diet 1 week prior to the marathon race. At that time they will do their long run, i.e., 20 miles, and then have strict protein for 3 days. Following this, they will load up on carbohydrates. This does give them increased performance and carbohydrate reserve, but it tends to make some of them feel loggy and bloated during the race.

Dietary Aids and Performance Enhancement

Runners are apt to take all sorts of vitamin concoctions, probably with little benefit, but the latest work suggests that ephedrine 1 mg with caffeine 5 mg (3 cups of coffee) does enhance performance up to 10 percent at the marathon distance. Creatine phosphate, 5 g four times daily for 4 to 5 days, followed by 1 g twice daily, may increase muscle size and strength and may improve high-intensity exercise performance.

Body Fat Content

The key to continuing to have significant aerobic capacity to age 70 is to continue to work out and stay lean. Most people gradually increase their body fat as they age and decrease their physical activity.

Aerobic Capacity

A study from the Johnson Space Center in Houston noted that the NASA workers who stayed lean and continued to train lost only 7 percent of their aerobic capacity by age 70. Sedentary people, however, lost at least 30 percent, and the majority lost 55 percent. A lot of this is mental, and George Sheehan, the famous running guru, said it best: "Everyone should run 30 minutes each day, and this will alter your body. After that, you must proceed with great caution, because the next 30 minutes will alter your life."[1]

Longevity

With regard to the amount of running needed to attain longevity, the National Runners Health Study found that benefits improve in a linear fashion all the way to 50 miles a week. This study appeared in the *Journal of the American Medical Association* on February 1, 1995. Thus, in essence, for the average athlete, the motto is, "The more you exercise, the better."

Cancer Immunity

In addition, a study from *Medicine and Science in Sports Exercise* from May of 1995 concluded that runners who had completed an average of 24 marathons had a greater natural killer cell activity than nonexercisers and thus more immunity to disease and malignancy.

Peaking

Elite runners have to be very careful not to peak too frequently or too quickly. Certain individuals can peak more frequently, but usually the high-quality long-distance runner can only peak two or three times a year.

Strength Training

Runners should do strength training. A study from the University of Wisconsin Biodynamics Laboratory compared three groups of runners over a 10-week period. The first group was strength only (S). They lifted weights three times a week. The second group was endurance only (E). They rode stationary bikes at 70 percent of $\dot{V}_{O_2max}$ three times a week. This was equivalent to a moderately paced running workout. The third group (SE) did both cycling and weight training three times a week. This group matched the strength gain of the S group and equaled the $\dot{V}_{O_2max}$ gain of the E group.

Thus, if you want to reach maximum fitness, you have to do both strength training and running. Aim for 7 to 10 repetitions per exercise, and every week or two increase this by lifting more weights more frequently at each station.

The Fitness Institute has a gold card for the fittest athletes, and an individual who only runs cannot get this gold card. Similarly, an individual who only does weight training cannot get the gold card. You have to have an overall fitness level of cardiovascular health, strength, flexibility, endurance, and agility to get the gold card.

SPECIFIC RUNNING INJURIES (OVERUSE)

The most common cause of running injuries is overuse. The second is inflexibility, and the third is inappropriate shoes. Also, inappropriate surfaces and episodic training are important.

Severity of Overuse Syndromes

Grade I: Pain after running but does not impede performance.
Grade II: Pain during a run but does not impede performance.
Grade III: Pain during a run that restricts distance and speed.
Grade IV: Pain so severe that it prevents running.
Grade V: Pain that is continuous during activities of daily living.

Runners can continue and sensibly work through grade I. Grade II merits a medical consultation. Grade III requires time off and cross-training. Grades IV and V restrict the athlete to water running and upper body work only.

Achilles Tendinitis, Bursitis

Achilles tendinitis and bursitis constitute a major problem. This can be extrinsic bursitis or Achilles tendinitis per se, with a tenosynovitis and inflammation and swelling of the tendon sheath. Achilles tendon rupture can be missed. Remember that it is almost never partial. Feel the gap! Squeeze the calf and see the foot plantarflex. Refer the athlete with any doubt.

The deep or retrocalcaneal bursa can be inflamed, and this can be due to impingement of the Achilles tendon and bursa on a prominent calcaneus. This is most often treated by elevation of the heel at all times, and as noted in some of the case histories to follow, the runner should not go barefoot even in the house. The runner should always wear some soft, clean running shoe in the house with heel lifts. Cowboy boots or the equivalent with a good heel are satisfactory at work.

Higher-heeled running shoes are often the answer. This often can be associated with plantar fasciitis or a compartment syndrome of the foot or tarsal tunnel syndrome.

When the runner returns, a more flexible, resilient running shoe with an air absorption factor such as the Nike Air shoe can be advantageous. However, a shoe in widths such as New Balance may be necessary or a lighter shoe such as a Sauconey is also needed at times. We tell people to go to a good running store and see a knowledgeable shoe person and to try on several pairs to get the best fit and comfort.

Patellofemoral Syndrome, Chondromalacia

Patellofemoral syndrome is due to maltracking and an abnormal gait. It often occurs in runners with pronated feet and valgus knees. Orthotics are beneficial in some cases, and the maltracking problem can be changed by altering the gait. It probably should be called *patellofemoral syndrome*, and this is a better term than chondromalacia, which is really an arthroscopic diagnosis.

Abnormal mechanics and patellar tracking are lateral subluxation, abnormal and poor quad girth and power, vastus medialis weakness, hip flexor weakness, and tight quads and hams. To counteract this, you have to alter the stresses, and you should check the Q-angle, which is normally 14 degrees in males and can be as far off as 20 degrees in females (Fig. 33-6). You correct the vastus medialis hypoplasia with intensive physiotherapy and muscle stimulation. Also, you have to examine the whole leg and concentrate on a total lower body program including the hip flexors and even the back.

The differential diagnosis includes jumper's knee, which is an inflammation right at the patella and patellar tendon junction; patellar tendinitis; Osgood-Schlatter's disease; torn meniscus; and plica

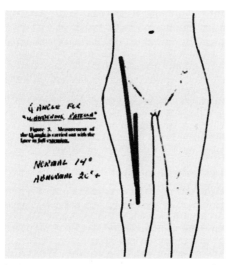

FIG. 33-6 The Q-angle is used to differentiate significant patellar and mechanical imbalances. Normal is 14 degrees, in males and 20 degrees in females. It is one indication of imbalance, and orthotics and osteopathic treatment will often help (see Chaps. 32 and 40).

syndrome. You also can have various types of bursitis around the patella, a prepatellar bursitis, superficial infrapatellar bursitis, pes tendon bursitis, and deep infrapatellar bursitis. In the case of pes tendon bursitis, for instance, this often responds well to cortisone injection, but some even need to be operated on.

Patellofemoral syndrome also can be operated on arthroscopically, and about 10 percent of these people need a lateral release. This is usually for grades III and IV clinical chondromalacia with associated inflammation. However, remember, "time, time, time!" Youngsters usually grow out of patellofemoral problems at full maturity. Thus there is no reason to rush to do a lateral release. Also, patellar shaving or arthroscopic debridement alone is probably not totally worthwhile without realignment. As a principle, you should not do a repeat arthroscopy before 12 months have elapsed in the cases that fail.

Popliteus Tendinitis (see Fig. 33-2)

Popliteus tendinitis is another problem that has a very localized lateral point tenderness. This tendinitis is much more common in the female athlete, due to body habitus and overtraining.

FEMALE RUNNERS

We want to emphasize that the first female athlete allowed in the Boston Marathon was Kay Switzer in 1974. She snuck in using the name K. Switzer, and Jock Semple, who used to run the marathon, tried to pull her out of the race when he realized she was a woman. The first women in the U.S. Military Academy joined in 1976, and the first women's marathon was won by Joan Benoit in 1984.

Now women train as well as men and are closing the gap when it comes to marathon times. Remember that it takes 7 years to train your body to reach a peak for marathon running, and it takes a lot of mental discipline and maturity. It can take amazing endurance, and some marathoners run 150 miles a week consistently.

THE YOUNGER RUNNER: SHOULD CHILDREN RUN A MARATHON?

Think back to your own childhood, and you can probably remember playing hockey, football, or just hide-and-go-seek for hours on end. You might have gone home for supper a little tired, but by the next morning you were ready to do it all again.

Children are well suited for endurance activities. We cherish such happy childhood memories as these, but we also can remember some of the tougher workouts on the lacrosse team while our coach, Lloyd Percival, put us through the paces. Lloyd's motto was "force yourself," and the memory of having to run 8, 10, or even 12 windsprints in a state of almost total exhaustion at the end of a session will stay with us a lifetime.

After all this exercise, we were none the worse for wear physically and mentally; it probably did us good. We ended up having a pretty decent lacrosse team too.

Let's turn the clock forward and change sports. After retiring from years of strenuous, mind-wrenching workouts in the pool, many top competitive swimmers would not even want to put their toes in the water again. Will the same thing happen to our young marathoners? I certainly hope not, but there are a lot of children who have been taken along too quickly and who eventually have tired of running. To avoid this pitfall, parents must always try to keep the sport interesting, fun, and progressively challenging. The American Academy Pediatrics Committee on Sports Medicine recommends children be allowed to participate in distance running as long as the child enjoys the activity and is asymptomatic.

CASE HISTORIES

We have selected some case histories of running injuries from our distance running group called the Etobicoke Huskies Strider Track and Field Club. This club has evolved over 26 years and consists of beginning runners and school runners, and there are special competitors who have gone on to the National Championships and even the Olympic Games. The key to understanding the injuries of these distance runners is to listen to your body and monitor the body responses during both training and races.

Cross-Training

We have found that cross-training complements regular running, and this is especially true as advanced age becomes a factor, i.e., over the age of 30 years. A guide to the amount of training gives running one unit, swimming two units, and cycling half a unit. Thus, if you were running 60 miles a week, i.e., 10 h a week, you would have to swim or run in the water for 5 h a week or cycle 120 miles a week. This would give you the same level of fitness.

Case 1 (Stress Fracture, Tibia)

A 29-year-old female marathoner, national champion, best time: 2.32 min.

Injury 1

Chief complaint: Sudden onset of shin pain. Tried to run through it, but soreness persisted. After running on and off for weeks, she could not run anymore.

History: The bone scan shows a positive stress fracture of the tibia.

She was completely off running for 6 weeks but did swimming and ran intervals in the pool and used an elliptical fitness cross-trainer. The legs move quickly, but they avoid the pounding.

Then she started light weights to strengthen the lower leg and foot and continued weights on an every-other-day basis.

After 6 weeks, she started running slowly on level grass, and after 10 days, the pain went away. After another 4 weeks, easy running was resumed, and then the normal training schedule was resumed. Experienced best cross-country season ever.

Authors' Comment: We usually tell patients that a stress fracture takes 6 to 8 weeks to heal and another 6 to 8 weeks to get back to full competitive running. This young woman was ahead of schedule.

Injury 2 (Plantar Fasciitis)

Arch of right foot was tight during season and ran a hilly 8-km course in High Park. Tore plantar fascia on one of the downhills. Could not walk after the race and had a lot of pain and swelling.

No running for 3 weeks. Maintained cardiovascular status by running in water every day.

Started running after 3 weeks, but it was too early. Continued to run with pain for about 4 months. Finally got new orthotics with good arch support, and this helped.

The pain finally went away 6 months after the cross-country race in High Park.

Authors' Comment: Plantar fasciitis can be quite tenacious. In this case, she started back too early, as she states. The motto is, "Let pain be your guide. If it hurts, back off." The old adage, "No pain, no gain" refers to cardiac endurance, not musculoskeletal problems.

Injury 3 (Hamstring Tendinitis)

Hamstring and buttock area extremely tight. After 1 week developed shooting lower back pains. Pain not manageable and had to stop in middle of next run.

Treatment: Received immediate chiropractic manipulation as well as massage therapy. Back pain went away quickly, although hamstring and buttock pain lasted for a longer period. Continued hamstring stretching and chiropractic care for another 3 months, and at that stage was running normally.

Authors' Comment: We believe in chiropractors, but regular maintenance visits have no proven scientific benefit. In this runner's case, the response was quite gratifying.

Case 2 (Calcaneal Fasciitis)

A 30-year-old female marathoner, national champion, best time: 2.28 min.

Injury 1

Chief Complaint: Calcaneal fasciitis.

Some awareness in right heel during a normal base training run. Doing high mileage (100+ miles per week) on hard surfaces. This training included some intense interval sessions.

Authors' Comment: The amount of training individuals need and can tolerate varies widely. Some individuals benefit from 60 miles a week and others can do up to 150 miles a week, and they each do well in the races.

The interval sessions are usually limited to 2 days per week. Use fatigue as your guide. The runner who is tired, irritable, cranky, and cannot sleep is overdoing it.

Initial Response: Competed in half marathon wearing racing flats that could not accommodate orthotics. Was concerned prior to the race that she was quite tired because of the high mileage.

Authors' Comment: She should *not* have run this race. Since she could not warm up well and be comfortable, she should have listened to her body.

If she had significant pain during the race, she should have stopped. Following the race, severe pain in the heel, even with walking. Stiff and very painful in early part of the day.

Treatment: No running, icing, stretching, anti-inflammatories. Naprosyn (naproxen) was ineffective, took Voltaren (diclofenac) and did foot exercises. Cortisone injections by three. Wore good support shoes all the time, right from the time of getting out of bed in the morning. No walking barefoot.

She said she was almost ready to opt for surgery, but fortunately, the doctor was more patient.

Authors' Comment: Only 5 to 10 percent of calcaneal spur patients need surgery. Removal of the spur and fascial release are usually a good operation. Nerve decompression is also needed in some patients and is 80 percent successful (see Chaps. 10 and 31).

Injury 2 (Multiple Stress Fractures)

Stress fractures, various types: First metatarsal, 3 times; third metatarsal, 1 time; calcaneus, 1 time; navicular, 1 time; multiple ribs posterior, 4 times; pubic arch, 2 times.

Stress fractures were all left-sided except for two pubic arch fractures that occurred during the last year of career, both times after an orthotic change. They were right-sided.

Cause: Stress fractures usually occur when training quite intensely and quite fatigued and tending to be too aggressive in training. Would resume weight-bearing activities too quickly, before the skeletal system was prepared for a rigorous sudden increase in weight-bearing activity.

Treatment: No running, depending on fractures. Rib fractures, approximately 3 weeks; pubic arch, 12 weeks; navicular, 10 to 12 weeks; other, 7 to 8 weeks.

Amenorrhea and Osteoporosis

Authors' Comments: This runner probably had amenorrhea and has the potential for osteoporosis if she does not have it already. She had a low body fat and body weight and persisted with increased physical stresses on her bones. This decreased bone density could not handle it, and thus the repeat stress fractures.

Bone density studies should be done, and treatment with calcium supplement 1200 to 1500 mg/day (two-thirds as food) and vitamin D is suggested. Whether she takes Fosamax or Didrocal depends on the individual doctor's recommendation. However, she should have 600 mg of elemental calcium and vitamin D. The role of estrogen replacement in young women has been controversial, but the recommended dose to protect against bone loss in menopausal women is 0.625 mg of conjugated estrogens daily. In amenorrheic athletes after 16 years of age, low-dose oral contraception and monitoring are suggested.

She also should have her serum ferritin measured and possibly be studied by an internal medicine metabolic specialist.

Case 3 (Stress Fracture of Foot)

A 19-year-old female junior 5000-m and 10,000-m national champion.

Injury 1

Stress fracture of left foot, fifth metatarsal. Felt like a bone bruise. Kept running on hard surfaces. X-rays did not show anything. Three weeks later a bone scan confirmed the fracture.

Treatment: No running for 6 weeks, anti-inflammatories, ice, massage, and electric stimulation. Swimming and running in water, timed intervals, stationary bike and cycling, light weight training.

After 6 weeks, started running 20 min every other day and increased gradually. After 4 months, started interval training and returned to normal running.

Injury 2 (Piriformis Syndrome)

Piriformis syndrome, right leg. School gym flexibility test without proper warm-up. After race could still train in a limited way and ran on grass as much as possible.

Continued to have tightening up in the buttock after hard workouts. Continued to run and competed in the world championships. After this race, proper rest followed, and the condition gradually settled, with cross-training and 2 months of rehabilitation.

Case 4 (Achilles Tendinitis)

A 31-year-old male national champion

Chief Complaint: Achilles tendinitis. Running and wearing variable heel heights. Shoes used for training, normal heel. Racing flats had low heels. Normal street shoes had higher heels. When standing for long periods following training in low heeled shoes, a greater strain was felt.

Authors' Comment: Make sure your shoes have a good heel. The old flats or negative "earth shoes" provoked Achilles tendinitis. A heel lift in normal street shoes and in the racing flats would help here.

Initial response: extreme pain and no response to treatment.

Operation: Split tendon sheath and remove bone spurs. Eventually, he ran well after 6 months and never had problems for the next 11 years.

Operative Treatment of Achilles Tendinitis

Authors' Comment: The operation he had is fairly major, requiring a general anesthetic and tourniquet and a long recovery.

If the Achilles tendinitis is less severe, it can be operated on under local anesthesia. This procedure removes the thickened synovial scar tissue from the back of the tendon. It changes the tunnel of the sheath and scar to a canal and effectively decompresses the tendon. The overall recovery is more rapid than with the more extensive operation under general anesthesia. If the procedure under local does not work, you can go to the larger operation.

THE GOOD DOCTOR'S PRESCRIPTION FOR FITNESS

From the best of past *Fitness Bulletins*, here's advice from Dr. Charles Bull, a member of the advisory panel of the Fitness Institute. He offers "ten commandments" to keep in mind about your fitness program:

1. If you're just starting, expect that daily fitness will alter your lifestyle, introducing you to different stresses, friends, values, priorities, and habits.
2. Train at your own level. Slow work does little to improve fitness, and fast work can cause pain, injury, and burnout.
3. Don't ignore injury. It could get worse. Heed pain. It's a safety valve.
4. If you're injured, don't rush back into action. Remember, you have the rest of your long life to get fit again.
5. Don't try to be your own doctor. If in doubt about a medical problem, ask your doctor. Don't rely on published advice.
6. Always warm up. Even to the point of being bored with it. And always do a cool-down at the end of your training session.
7. Train every day, and do it sensibly. Train hard one day and lightly the next.
8. Do more than one fitness activity. For instance, runners should do flexibility, strength, and stomach exercises and maybe swim, cycle, or try some yoga.
9. Whatever fitness discipline you pursue, seek out experts now and again for instruction and inspiration.

10. Have fun. Your workout should be the best, most exhilarating part of your day!

RECOMMENDED READINGS

1. Sheehan G: *Dr. Sheehan on Running*. Mountainview, CA, World Publications, 1975.
2. Reid DC: *Sports Injury: Assessment and Rehabilitation*. New York, Churchill-Livingstone, 1992.
3. Drez D Jr: Running. *Clin Sports Med* 4(4): WB Saunders, Philadelphia Oct, 1985.
4. Peterson L: *Sports Injuries: Their Prevention and Treatment*. St Louis, Mosby–Year Book, 1986.
5. Torg J: *Current Therapy in Sports Medicine*, 3d ed. St Louis, Mosby–Year Book, 1995.
6. Zachazewski JE, Magee D, Quillen B: *Athletic Injuries and Rehabilitation*. Philadelphia, Saunders, 1996.
7. Kostrabula T: *The Joy of Running*. Philadelphia, JB Lippincott, 1976.

Rick Zarnett   *R. Timothy Deakon*

The goal of surgery on the athlete is to return the athlete to his or her sport. The athlete, coach, and other members of the team are interested in as early a return to the sport as possible. It is the duty of the physician and therapist to make sure that when the athlete returns to sport, he or she does so without risk of further injury. Guidelines on return to sport following injury and specifically following surgery are vague. We will attempt to provide guidelines on return to sport following specific surgeries.

KNEE

Medial Collateral Ligament Injury

The medial collateral ligament (MCL) is the primary restraint to valgus load of the knee. An MCL injury can be difficult to differentiate from a torn medial meniscus. Often the history will suggest a ligamentous injury rather than an injury to the meniscus. The MCL is commonly injured by a valgus stress. On examination, pain is located at the MCL origin, either on the femoral epicondyle or at the insertion on the tibial metaphysis. It is unusual for the knee to develop an intraarticular effusion. In contrast, the meniscus is usually injured by a twisting or torsional force. The tenderness is located over the joint line, and the knee usually will develop an intraarticular effusion. Often in the acute injury it may be difficult to differentiate whether the MCL or the meniscus is injured. It may be necessary to examine these athletes on more than one occasion. If difficulty still exists, then a magnetic resonance imaging (MRI) can be helpful.

Rehabilitation and Return to Sports

The goals of treatment are to decrease pain and swelling and increase the knee range of motion, strength, and proprioception. Grade I injuries require only symptomatic treatment. Grade II injuries are treated with a hinged brace to prevent valgus strains on the healing ligament. The brace is worn for 4 to 6 weeks. Full range of motion and full weight bearing are permitted. Local modalities are used to treat pain and swelling. These include cryotherapy and systemic anti-inflammatory medication. In grade III injuries, the athletes are placed in a hinged knee brace that restricts motion. Initially, we allow 30 to 90 degrees of motion. As healing progresses, the restrictions on the range of motion are gradually decreased over a 6-week period. Manual treatment includes massage, active assisted

717

range of motion, and patellar glides. Modality treatment includes ultrasound, laser, iontophoresis, compression pump, muscle stimulation, interferential current, and cryotherapy (see Chap. 33).

Patients are allowed to return to sports when they have a full painless range of motion and strength has been restored. In the grade III MCL injuries, especially in the athlete involved in contact sports, we often recommend a functional knee brace for the remainder of the season.

Patellar Dislocation

In the athlete who has had an acute patellar dislocation, it is important to x-ray the knee to rule out intraarticular loose bodies secondary to an osteochondral fracture. If an osteochondral loose body is present, the patient will require an urgent arthroscopy. The vast majority of acute patellar dislocations do not require surgery.

Rehabilitation and Return to Sports

Our treatment protocol starts with local modalities to reduce pain and swelling and early range of motion. We no longer immobilize these patients but instead treat them with a functional patella-stabilizing brace. Early quadriceps exercises are initiated with attention to strengthening the vastus medialis obliquus (VMO), gluteus medius, hamstrings, and hip abductors. Muscle stimulation is often used to increase the VMO in functional activities. Patients can return to sport when (1) the knee swelling has resolved, (2) they have a full painless range of motion, and (3) they have maximized the strength around the knee. We usually recommend a brace for at least the remainder of the season and possibly longer. It is not unusual for the patient to have further episodes of patellar instability. If this occurs or the patient has significant patellar malalignment, he or she may require surgical intervention.

Knee Arthroscopy

The meniscus plays an important role in load transmission, shock absorption, joint stability, joint lubrication, and joint proprioception. Twenty years ago it was not uncommon to remove the entire meniscus, but as we now know, meniscectomy results in increased stress through the joint. These increased stresses result in degeneration of the articular cartilage and ultimately lead to degenerative osteoarthritis.

Arthroscopic partial meniscectomy or meniscal repair is now the standard of care in the athlete with a torn meniscus. Many factors determine whether the meniscus can and should be repaired. These include the age of the patient, the location of the meniscal tear, the type of tear, and the status of the anterior cruciate ligament. If meniscal repair is not indicated, then a partial meniscectomy is the treatment of choice.

The diagnosis usually can be made with a good history and physical examination. The meniscus is usually injured in a torsional type of injury. Characteristically, a knee effusion develops, and the athlete has tenderness over the joint line. In the athlete with a bucket-handle tear, the knee may be locked (a mechanical inability to fully extend the knee). Gold and Rose[1] and Miller[2] compared the accuracy between clinical examination and MRI. Both concluded that in patients with suspected meniscal tears, a careful history and clinical examination are at least as good as or better than MRI. While the use of MRI has gained popularity in recent years, in the majority of patients it is not necessary, nor is it cost-efficient, and therefore, it is not used routinely.

Arthroscopic Meniscectomy

With the advent of arthroscopic surgery in the 1960s and 1970s, the medical team has been able to return the athlete to sport much sooner. The goals of arthroscopic meniscectomy are to remove the torn portion of the meniscus, leaving as much of the normal meniscus as possible. It is important to leave the capsular rim. This is particularly important at the popliteal bridge in the lateral meniscus.

Rehabilitation and return to sports Following arthroscopic meniscectomy, the patient is allowed full weight bearing. We do not use crutches routinely postoperatively and do not feel that they are necessary. The athlete is allowed full weight bearing and unrestricted range of motion and is allowed to begin isometric exercises immediately postoperatively. The goals of postoperative therapy are to reduce joint swelling, regain full range of motion, and regain muscle strength. Cryotherapy immediately following surgery decreases pain and swelling. We routinely prescribe a nonsteroidal anti-inflammatory drug (NSAID) for a period of 10 to 14 days. This has been shown to decrease pain and swelling in the postoperative period. The athlete is allowed to start impact-type activities as soon as he or she is pain-free and has regained full range of motion. Generally, athletes can return to their sport 4 to 6 weeks postoperatively if all goals have been achieved.

Meniscal Repair

Preservation of the meniscus is preferred, if technically possible. The success rate of meniscal repair depends on several factors. These include the location of the tear, the size of the tear, and the presence of an anterior cruciate ligament (ACL) injury. Repairs in the "red zone" (within 3 mm of the periphery) will heal in 90 to 95 percent of patients. Meniscal repair in association with ACL reconstruction has a higher success rate than the isolated meniscal repair. A meniscus that has been repaired in an unstable knee is subject to increased shear forces, and subsequently, those repaired in this setting will fail in up to 50 percent of patients. The tears that have the greatest chance of healing are acute vascular tears in young patients with an intact anterior cruciate ligament.

The meniscus can be repaired through an arthrotomy (open repair) or arthroscopically. Arthroscopic repair has many advantages over open repair. These include the morbidity associated with a knee arthrotomy as well as improved access and visualization, especially in posterior horn tears.

Arthroscopic techniques include the inside-out technique, the outside-in technique, and the all-inside technique. Recently, bioabsorbable implants (meniscal arrows) have allowed the meniscus to be repaired in an all-inside technique without the need to tie sutures intraarticularly. Although this method is promising, the long-term results are not yet available.

Rehabilitation and return to sports In the past, postoperative protocols protected the meniscal repair to allow for collagen healing. More recently, Shelbourne and Nitz[3] has shown that an accelerated rehabilitation program that allows immediate full weight bearing and unrestricted range of motion does not adversely affect the success rate of meniscal repair. In patients who have undergone an ACL reconstruction in addition to a meniscal repair, we do not rehabilitate them any differently than if they had undergone only an ACL reconstruction.

In the athlete who has undergone a meniscal repair, we allow immediate postoperative full weight bearing, unrestricted range of motion, and immediate quadriceps and hamstring strengthening. Once adequate strength has been obtained, the athlete is pain-free, and the knee has a full range of motion, we allow the patient to return to jogging and running. This usually occurs at the 3-month mark, and we allow the athlete to return to full activity at 6 months.

ACL Reconstruction

ACL injury is becoming increasingly common in the athlete. Once considered a career-threatening or career-ending injury, now over 95 percent of athletes will be able to return to the sport following ACL reconstruction.[4]

The athlete who is involved in pivoting sports and those with high-grade instability are at high risk for further injury. Further episodes of instability will place the meniscus and articular surface in jeopardy. In addition, recurrent instability can lead to chondral damage and in the long term to arthritis. For the athlete to return to sport, a stable knee is a must.

There still remains a role for nonsurgical treatment in the athlete with an ACL tear. Most athletes, though, especially those involved in pivoting-type sports and those playing sports at a competitive level, will not tolerate a knee that is not almost "perfect." Many will not tolerate a functional knee brace, and in some sports (i.e., rugby, wrestling, martial arts) they will not be allowed to participate with an ACL brace. Athletes are becoming increasingly educated about the various aspects of ACL reconstruction.

The two most common mechanisms for ACL injury are either a valgus, external rotation injury or a hyperextension injury. The athlete often will report that he or she felt a "pop" or a "snap" in the knee or that the knee "dislocated." The athlete will be unable to continue playing the sport, and swelling usually starts 4 to 6 h following the injury. The knee will feel unstable, and it is not uncommon for the athlete to report that the knee buckles as he or she attempts to walk. In the athlete with a chronic injury, the history is almost diagnostic. The athlete will report recurrent episodes of instability, usually associated with twisting or pivoting sports.

In the athlete with an acute injury, the diagnosis can be difficult. Often the patient will have to be reexamined once the initial pain and swelling have subsided. The history should make the examiner suspicious. It is important to examine the uninjured knee to have a reference point. What appears to be an abnormal amount of anterior translation in an injured knee may be normal for that patient. Tenderness over the posterolateral corner of the knee is suggestive of an ACL injury. This is due to a lateral capsular avulsion, which is the soft tissue equivalent of the Segond fracture. The Segond fracture is an avulsion from the lateral corner of the tibia and is said to be pathognomonic for an ACL tear if present. The Lachman test and the pivot-shift test are the best tests for determining ACL integrity. Patient relaxation is essential but, as mentioned previously, may be difficult in the acute setting. When performing the Lachman test, both the amount of translation and the feel of the endpoint are important. In the patient with a locked knee, it can sometimes be very difficult even in the most experienced hands to assess the status of the ACL. In the chronic setting, it is much easier to examine the knee, and a positive pivot-shift test is diagnostic for ACL insufficiency (see Chap. 8).

MRI is rarely needed to diagnose a tear of the ACL. The MRI is most useful in assessing the status of the meniscus in an acute knee injury. This may influence the timing of surgery, especially if the MRI indicates a reparable meniscus.

The three most common tissues used for ACL reconstruction are autogenous patellar tendon, hamstring, or allograft. A major advantage of patellar tendon, either autogenous or allograft, is the strength of immediate fixation obtained with interference screws. Although the fixation technique for hamstring tendons continues to improve, this technique does not offer the same immediate strong fixation offered by interference screws (see Chap. 8).

Allograft tissue offers several theoretical advantages in ACL reconstruction. These include less graft-site morbidity and decreased risk of postoperative complications, including patellar fracture, patellar tendinitis, and postoperative patellofemoral syndrome. Unfortunately, the long-term results of allograft ACL reconstruction are not as good as those in which autogenous tissue has been used. Despite careful donor selection, there still remains the possibility of disease transmission (i.e., hepatitis C, HIV, etc.). We believe that autogenous tissue is the preferable and superior tissue, and it is used in almost all our primary reconstructions. We reserve allograft tissue for revision ACL reconstructions and posterior cruciate ligament (PCL) reconstructions.

In the acute injury, surgery should be delayed until the patient has achieved full range of motion. This may take up to 6 weeks to obtain but can occur in as few as 2 to 3 weeks. Failure in adhering to this principle will subject the athlete to an increased risk of developing postoperative stiffness (arthrofibrosis).

Rehabilitation and Return to Sports

Our rehabilitation protocol allows for immediate full weight bearing and unrestricted passive range of motion. We protect the knee with crutches until the patient has adequate quadriceps control. This generally takes 10 to 14 days. In the first 6 weeks the goals of therapy are to maintain full extension, increase knee range of motion, and improve muscle strength. Once these goals have been achieved, the objectives are to achieve full range of motion, increase muscle strength, and start proprioceptive retraining. It is during this period that we allow the athlete to begin running and jogging, provided that he or she is pain-free and does not have any joint swelling. At 3 months we start isokinetic training and sport-specific rehabilitation. At 6 months we will allow the athlete to return to competitive sport if the following criteria are met: (1) the patient is pain-free, (2) there is no swelling, and (3) the quadriceps/hamstring ratio is greater than 90 percent. We protect the athlete for 1 year in a functional knee brace. It is important that the rehabilitation of each athlete be individualized.

SHOULDER

Shoulder Instability

Open Repairs

The various risks and benefits of arthroscopic versus open repair for recurrent traumatic anterior instability are beyond the scope of this chapter. Both the open and arthroscopic repairs have proponents. Many procedures have been developed to treat patients with recurrent instability. These can be divided into those which restore the normal anatomy (repair the avulsed inferior glenohumeral ligament, Bankart repair) and those which do not (Putti-Platt, Magnuson-Stack, Bristow, etc.) (see Chap. 6).

We prefer to do an anatomic repair. The goal is to reconstruct the inferior glenohumeral ligament complex (IGHLC). The Bankart lesion is repaired directly into the glenoid neck using suture anchors, and then, if necessary, a capsular shift is performed to address the capsular laxity.

Rehabilitation and return to sports We usually immobilize the shoulder for 3 to 4 weeks. Patients remove their elbow and wrist from the immobilizer twice a day for range-of-motion exercises to prevent stiffness. The patients then start a program of active range of motion. As the range of motion improves, a program of progressive strengthening is started.

Arthroscopic Stabilization Procedures

The indications for arthroscopic stabilization procedures and their long-term success are controversial. The success rate in the literature varies widely for a number of reasons. Many of the studies are not homogeneous. The surgical method varies (suture anchors, transglenoid sutures, staples, etc.), and the patient populations vary (in age), as does the pathology (subluxation versus dislocation). When one analyzes the results, one must look closely at all these variables.

Postoperative treatment A shoulder immobilizer is worn for 4 weeks. As in the open repair, the immobilizer is removed twice a day to allow elbow and wrist range of motion. At 4 weeks we start a program of pendulum exercises and passive assisted range of motion. The shoulder immobilizer is worn at night for a further 2 weeks. Our goal is to have a full range of motion by 12 weeks. A program of resistance training, proprioceptive retraining, and isokinetics is then advocated. Most patients are allowed to return to their sports at 6 months.

Rotator Cuff Surgery

The athlete with shoulder pain, especially the overhead athlete, continues to be a challenge to the physician and therapist. The etiology of rotator cuff tendinopathy is controversial. The causes of pain are certainly not one-dimensional and include both intrinsic and extrinsic factors. The intrinsic causes include the blood supply to the rotator cuff and specifically the supraspinatus tendon insertion and age-related degenerative changes (angiofibroblastic hyperplasia) to the tendon itself. The extrinsic causes include the morphology of the acromion, the coracoacromial ligament, and the acromioclavicular (AC) joint. Neer[5] has described three stages of rotator cuff tears. Stage I is dominated by edema and hemorrhage, but this is reversible. Treatment includes rest, anti-inflammatory medication, subacromial cortisone injections, and exercise. Stage II, fibrosis and tendinitis, results in a partial rotator cuff tear. In this stage recurrent pain with activity develops, and surgery is often necessary. Stage III is characterized by a full-thickness tear of the rotator cuff. The treatment is surgery.

Subacromial Decompression

The indications for subacromial decompression (SAD) are failure of conservative treatment and inability to return to the sport or to perform at the usual level. It is important, especially in the overhead athlete, for the physician to rule out shoulder instability as a cause of rotator cuff tendinitis. If instability is present and not addressed, then subacromial decompression will fail. Subacromial decompression is rarely performed in patients with symptoms of less than 6 months' duration.

Subacromial decompression can be open or arthroscopic. The advantages of performing this arthroscopically include (1) the ability to assess and treat intraarticular pathology, (2) less pain and surgical morbidity than in the open procedure, and most important, (3) the ability to perform the acromioplasty without violating the deltoid insertion. The results of arthroscopic subacromial decompression are as good as or superior to those of the open procedure, but the operation is technically demanding and should not be done unless the surgeon is a proficient arthroscopist who is familiar with arthroscopic SAD. The success rate of SAD done either arthroscopically or open is approximately 80 percent. In the high-demand athlete, especially one involved in overhead activity, the success rate can be even lower.

The goal of surgery is to (1) remove the thickened bursa, (2) debride the frayed and torn rotator cuff, (3) decompress the space by removing the anterior hook of the acromion, and (4) resect the coracoacromial ligament.

Rehabilitation and Return to Sports

The primary advantage of arthroscopic SAD is that the deltoid has not been violated, and therefore, rehabilitation can be started earlier and the athlete can return to sport earlier. Immediately following surgery, range-of-motion exercises are started. Pain control is achieved with adequate analgesia. Cryotherapy has been found to be extremely useful in decreasing pain and postoperative inflammation. We routinely place the patient on a minimum 2-week course of NSAIDs. The rehabilitation program first restores range of motion and then concentrates on strengthening the shoulder. Strengthening exercises are kept below shoulder level until the shoulder is completely pain-free. Isokinetic strengthening using surgical tubing is started in the second postoperative week. The athlete can progress to resisted exercises and eccentric strengthening at the 4- to 6-week mark. Sport-specific exercises start when the athlete has a full range of motion, normal scapular and thoracic muscular rhythm, and a minimum of 90 percent strength compared with the opposite side. If the athlete is not involved in overhead sport, then he or she generally can return to competition in 4 months. In the overhead athlete, return is usually not before 6 months. The two criteria for return to sport are a pain-free shoulder through a full range of motion and strength equal to the opposite shoulder.

Rotator Cuff Repair

Partial-Thickness Tears

Partial-thickness tears can be on the bursal side of the rotator cuff or on the undersurface of the rotator cuff. Articular-side cuff tears can be caused by anterior shoulder instability and have been termed *inside impingement*. These patients should undergo a sports-specific rehabilitation program before surgery is contemplated. If this is unsuccessful, then surgery may be necessary. In this type of patient, the rotator cuff pathology can be treated by arthroscopic debridement and either an arthroscopic stabilization procedure or an open instability repair. The postoperative rehabilitation and return to sports are the same as described for the athlete with primary shoulder instability.

Our treatment of choice for partial-thickness rotator cuff tears secondary to subacromial impingement is arthroscopic debridement of the tear and a subacromial decompression. There is a role in selected athletes for debriding the articular-side tears and not performing an SAD. In the throwing athlete, one must look carefully for underlying shoulder instability. If an SAD is performed and the shoulder instability is not addressed, a poor result may be seen.

Full-Thickness Tears

Indications for rotator cuff repair in the athlete are to relieve pain and improve function. Small rotator cuff tears may be treated with a "minirepair." This consists of an arthroscopic SAD in combination with a 3-cm deltoid splint to repair the rotator cuff into the humerus. Large tears require an open acromioplasty and tendon repair. The obvious advantage of the "open minirepair" as in an arthroscopic SAD is that the deltoid is not detached from the acromion and an early aggressive rehabilitation program can be started. A complete rotator cuff tear in the athlete carries a guarded prognosis. The rate of return to sport is in the range of 50 to 60 percent and is lower in the overhead athlete.

Rehabilitation and Return to Sports

The goals of rehabilitation are (1) to achieve a full range of motion, (2) to eliminate pain, and (3) to return full strength and function. Postoperatively, whether the repair is an open minirepair or a full open repair, we only allow passive range of motion for the first 6 weeks. The arm is held in a sling, and active assisted and active range of motion is initiated at 6 weeks. Resisted exercises are usually not started until 3 months postoperatively. Throwing is not allowed for 9 months. Sports-specific rehabilitation is continued for up to 2 years.

Labral Injuries

The labrum is a triangular structure in the shoulder made of fibrocartilage. The function of the labrum is (1) to deepen the glenoid, (2) to provide attachment to the anterior glenohumeral ligaments, and (3) to provide attachment superiorly to the biceps tendon. The labrum contributes to the stability of the glenohumeral joint. The labrum can be injured from either compressive, shearing, or deceleration forces. Labrum tears can be classified as flap tears, degenerative tears, bucket-handle tears, and those secondary to traction of the biceps tendon (throwing tears). Synder and colleagues[6] described the SLAP (superior, labrum, anterior, posterior) lesion involving the superior anchor of the biceps tendon into the labrum. Synder and colleagues have classified the SLAP lesion into four types. In type I, the superior labrum is markedly frayed, but the biceps tendon remains intact. In type II, the superior labrum is degenerative as in type I, but in addition, the labrum is detached from the bone, making the biceps-labrum complex unstable. In type III, the superior labrum has a bucket-handle tear, but the biceps tendon and the attached labrum remain intact. In type IV, in addition to the bucket-handle tear of the labrum, the labral tear extends into the biceps tendon, allowing it to sublux into the joint. Treatment of flap, degenerative, and bucket-handle tears involves arthroscopically debriding the tissue back to a stable rim. Often these lesions are associated with instability, which may not become apparent until the labral tears have been debrided. Treatment of SLAP lesions depends on the specific lesion present. Type I lesions are treated by debridement. The labral attachment to the biceps anchor must be left intact. In type II lesions, the labral tear is debrided back to stable tissue, and then the superior labrum is attached back to the bony glenoid with either a suture anchor or a bioabsorbable tack. In type III lesions, the bucket-handle tear is resected. In type IV lesions, the labral and biceps tissue are resected, and if the biceps tendon is adequate, then nothing further need be done. If the biceps tendon is inadequate, it is either repaired or a biceps tenodesis is performed (see Chap. 6).

Rehabilitation and Return to Sports

In the athlete who has had a simple arthroscopic debridement, treatment goals are to eliminate pain and swelling and restore joint motion and strength. In the athlete who is not involved in overhead sports, recovery is usually complete in 6 to 8 weeks. Postoperatively, patients are placed on NSAIDs for 14 days. Cryotherapy has been very useful to control swelling and decrease postoperative pain. An active exercise program including strengthening is started immediately and progressed as the athlete becomes more comfortable and pain-free. Early isokinetic and resistive exercises are encouraged.The athlete can return to sport when he or she is pain-free, has a full range of motion, and muscle strength has been restored. In the overhead athlete, the recovery and return to throwing should not be rushed. Often these patients will have an instability problem that will require a rehabilitation program that is specifically designed for that particular athlete.

In the athlete who has undergone a procedure to repair the labrum to the glenoid, the shoulder is immobilized for a period of 4 to 6 weeks. A program is then initiated to regain motion and strengthen the shoulder. At 2 months, eccentric and concentric strengthening is started. Isokinetic strength training is started at 3 months, and as the athlete becomes pain-free, range of motion is full, and shoulder strength normalizes, gentle throwing is allowed. Generally, full-speed throwing is not allowed until 6 to 7 months.

REFERENCES

1. Rose NE, Gold SM: A comparison of accuracy between clinical examination and magnetic resonance imaging in the diagnosis of meniscal and anterior cruciate ligament tears. *J Arthroscopy* 12:398–405, 1996.

2. Miller GK: A prospective study comparing the accuracy of the clinical diagnosis of meniscus tear with magnetic resonance imaging and its effect on clinical outcome. *Arthroscopy* 12:406–413, 1996.

3. Shelbourne KD, Nitz P: Accelerated rehabilitation after anterior cruciate ligament reconstruction. *Am J Sports Med* 18:292, 1990.

4. Wojtys EM (ed): *The ACL-Deficient Knee*. American Academy of Orthopaedic Surgeons Monograph Series. New York, AAOS, 1994.

5. Neer CS: Impingement lesions. *Clin Orthop* 173:70, 1983.

6. Synder SJ, Karzel RP, DelPizzo W, et al: SLAP lesions of the shoulder. *Arthroscopy* 6:274, 1990.

High Performance and the Treatment of the Elite Athlete

Mike Clarfield

John Brown injured his leg badly in the game last night. He will be having a MRI tomorrow and MRI can tell us if he can play the game next week.

The sports medicine physician is trained to treat athletes, ultimate or *elite* althletes. They are fine-tuned machines; they demand the most from their bodies and therefore the most from the people who surround them, including their medical care providers. The most challenging aspect of being a sports medicine physician is treating elite athletes, as they demand so much of themselves and of you. The gratifying part is that their performance, which you become a part of, will be seen by thousands of people. Although the athlete derives most of the fame, the medical people involved in dealing with these athletes also derive fame from being involved. Treating the elite athlete can therefore be very stressful. On the other hand, it can be fun, as you are involved in high-exposure events.

It takes years of experience to develop the expertise to understand the elite athlete's body and mental state. These are finely tuned athletes, both mentally and physically, and it is important to be in touch with both factors in order to treat them effectively. These athletes must have full confidence that you understand the nature of their injuries, and the nature of the sport or activity they are participating in, in order for them to trust you to prescribe treatment. There must be a thorough understanding of the biomechanics and the physical demands that the sport places on these patients. It is important in treating these elite athletes that their goals are paramount in both their and your mind. Then, and only then, can you develop a relationship with an elite athlete of mutual trust and admiration.

Elite athletes, whether professional players, Olympic athletes, or prima ballerinas, all place high physical and mental demands on themselves. Nonetheless, different athletes may have different approaches to their bodies. It is important to understand the adherent differences in the activity they are doing to understand how to treat their injuries. The recovery and expectations may be quite different for athletes in various sports, and you must adjust your treatment appropriately.

Elite athletes are the most demanding of all your patients; to accept the challenge and reap the benefits in treating elite athletes you must be prepared to devote yourself to these individuals.

INJURIES OF THE ELITE ATHLETE

The most important part of dealing with an elite athlete is dealing with injuries. The athlete will depend on you to understand the injuries and treat them to get the athlete back to participation as soon and as safely as possible. The athlete will demand that he or she returns to the activity at the same if not at a higher preinjury level. When an athlete pushes to the limits of high performance there is a fine line between that and the point at which the body breaks down and becomes injured. Therefore, all athletes at the elite level sustain injury. The goal of the sports medicine physician is to act proactively to prepare them so they can avoid as many injuries as possible. When an athlete does get injured, it is important that the athlete be rehabilitated to the level where he or she can go back to the activity with the least risk of injury and maintain a high performance. The true challenge in dealing with an elite athlete is to play that fine line between high performance and risk of injury.

The injuries sustained by the elite athlete are no different than any other injuries sustained by any other person. It is simply the demands and pressure on the athletes that makes treating these injuries so different. It is only when you actually treat elite athletes that you understand this difference. As in all sports injuries, there are two types of injuries, acute and chronic.

It is important, if not mandatory, to be in attendance during the elite athlete's participation in the sport or dance. While present at the event you can understand what the athlete does and the level of the competition. This allows for a closer bond between the athlete and the physician, and allows the physician to treat the athlete with more confidence. Over time the athlete will become more comfortable with the physician and will develop a relationship that will facilitate treatment. One of the most important things in treating an elite athlete is to develop the athlete's respect. By making him- or herself available to the athlete and watching the event, a trusting, respectful relationship develops. The medical person will learn to respect the elite athlete's commitment to the sport, while the elite athlete will respect the physician for dedicating time to him or her.

Perhaps the most challenging aspect in dealing with an elite athlete is dealing with acute injuries. Most athletic injuries occur during an event as opposed to practice. This is particularly true for acute and traumatic injuries. Once an acute injury has occurred the physician is immediately called into play. The medical personnel at an event must be prepared for all emergencies. Not only must he or she be capable of treating the acute injury, but also of being watched by the many thousands of spectators present at the event and possibly millions more watching at home. The treatment on the field level almost always will be captured on film. The medical personnel covering elite athlete events should practice and train for emergencies before they actually happen. It is only with these practice sessions that the physician will be efficient and smooth in the care of these athletes.

As in any acute injury that is life-threatening, whether it be a head, cervical, or other injury, the ABCs of acute medical care are paramount. The athlete must be secure and stabilized on the field before he or she is evacuated. If there is a risk of spinal injury the athlete must be properly back boarded and protected before being taken off the playing area. Once off the playing area and in the privacy of a medical room, more efficient medical care can be administered if needed. The medical room must be equipped to deal with these emergencies; again, practice of operation ensures that these athletes are well taken care of. Protocols must be set up and maintained to ensure that the athlete is transported efficiently to the hospital and the appropriate medical care is available.

Sometimes luck is on your side. In a professional hockey game I was attending several years ago, one of our players suffered a ruptured spleen. Fortuitously, when we paged the general surgeon he just happened to be in the stands observing the game. There was obviously immediate care available and the surgeon performed smoothly and efficiently to save this player's life.

Fortunately, we do not see a lot of emergency-type injuries in athletics, but we do see a lot of other acute injuries. These can obviously affect any joint, and certain sports have a predisposition to certain injuries. The doctor must be aware of the common injuries in that sport and the mechanics that cause an injury. A classic lateral inversion sprain is very common in a sport such as basketball and volleyball. In sports, when an athlete wears a more rigid boot, such as in skating, hockey, or skiing, we rarely see a typical lateral inversion sprain. A rotational syndesmodic injury is much more common, and the physician must be aware of this to treat the injury appropriately. As the injury occurs the athlete, coach, and management immediately want to know the nature and severity of the injury and most importantly when the athlete can return to play. This is perhaps the most stressful and challenging part of dealing with elite athletes. An athlete will more often get injured in competition and therefore can be seen immediately to determine whether he or she can return to the field. The great fun and satisfaction in treating athletes is becoming part of the athlete's performance and the team. Obviously, the team physician wants the team or athlete to do well. The most important part of being a team physician is being able to disassociate yourself from the level of excitement and the pressure from the team to win at all costs. The most important concept is that the physician–patient relationship be maintained. You must always treat the athlete considering his or her short-term career and long-term life situation. Whether it is a recreational athlete or the Super Bowl, the athlete must be protected from long-term injury or even a life-threatening situation. In a very short period of time, usually without the aids of any other investigations, the physician must decide if the athlete can continue. At this point almost the sole decision is up to the physician.

Even if the athlete does return, you must watch the performance carefully to make sure the athlete is performing up to the level you expect. If he or she does not, then you may have to consider withdrawing the athlete again and reconsidering your decision. The player will rarely mention deficiencies if the urge to play is high.

Once the decision is made that the athlete cannot play, then a definitive diagnosis must be made and the appropriate treatment plan carried out. Often, further investigations, such as MRI, must be done to help classify and make the diagnosis definitive. With the elite athlete these investigations must be obtained expediently to allow the athlete to deal with the injury. Although the media will sometimes think an MRI or further investigations tell the diagnosis and allow the physician to determine if the athlete can return to play, these investigations should only be used as adjunct to your own clinical impression. When dealing with elite athletes you soon learn that these fine-tuned bodies respond to injuries in a somewhat different manner than the other patients you see in your office.

Communication is of paramount importance in dealing with an elite athlete. Everyone must be kept abreast of the athlete's injury and progress. Obviously the athlete's consent must be obtained to give this information to the coach or management. Again, physician–patient confidentiality must be maintained. The general time line concerning when the athlete can expect to return to certain levels of activity and eventually play should be given to everyone involved. This allows everyone to plan for the duration of time that the athlete will not be available to compete. The athlete, physician, and therapist must all work together to help the athlete return as soon and as safely as possible.

If you follow the preceding guidelines and maintain the patient–physician relationship you will very soon gain your patients' respect. As in any situation, it is very tough to gain respect and very easy to lose that respect. Therefore, it is important to maintain professionalism at all times. If you in fact lose the respect of the players and/or the management you will not be dealing with elite athletes much longer. For the most part the treatment of the elite athlete's injuries is not any different than the treatment of any other person. The difference lies in the intensity of the treatment.

Whereas a recreational athlete may receive therapy a few times a week for an injury, the elite athlete may receive therapy three times a day to treat the same injury. Not only that, the difference in recovery is quite incredible if the injury is treated immediately and thoroughly, as opposed to being left for even 24 to 40 h. Many secondary problems are avoided with immediate treatment. Functional rehabilitation is the key to allowing the injury to heal and then to training the athlete to go back into "playing shape" and have the strength to prevent further injury.

There are a lot more mitigating factors to deal with concerning when the elite athlete can return to play than there are with weekend or even high-level recreational athletes. The decision of when to return to play involves a lot more people and a lot more stress on the athlete when he or she returns. The ultimate decision of when the athlete returns to play is the athlete's. Medical personnel are there only to advise and provide guidance, although the athlete usually follows the medical personnel's guidelines.

You will see many different kinds of athletes under many different situations. The two extremes are the athlete who wants to return to play too soon and the athlete who wants to delay return as long as possible. The player has a lot of people advising him or her. Other factors will affect the athlete's decision. Most athletes have a lot of pride and want to return as soon as they can. They want to prove to themselves they can go back to their own form. They want to show support to their team. An athlete does not feel comfortable watching his or her team or opponents compete when he or she is on the sidelines. Nonetheless, there are other factors that may effect the decision. One of the most important factors is the athlete's contract. The athlete may have to return to play as soon as possible to prove that he or she can play in order to renegotiate a new contract. On the other hand, if a contract dispute with management exists, then the athlete may want to delay return, as he or she may not feel the team is supportive. An athlete may have bonus clauses in the contract that can have financial implications. Without play he or she may not reach these bonuses. Often an athlete has a lot of fear going back to play. The longer the athlete is away from playing, the more fear there is of going back to play. There is a fear the injury may inhibit the ability to play. The athlete may feel that he or she has lost some of the skills or speed needed to participate at the previous level. The athlete may have been performing poorly before the injury, which will only escalate this fear. The athlete will get a lot of advice from the people involved around him or her. All these people may try to influence him or her to either play too soon or delay recovery too long. When the athlete should be focusing all of his or her energy on recovery, other factors may affect recovery, mentally as well as physically. It is important for the physician to be aware of all these other factors and try to deal with them appropriately. Often there will be factors that the physician may not be aware of, such as marital problems. The physician must keep all channels of communication open and explore all possibilities to give the athlete every opportunity to express feelings and cope with the decision of returning to play. In most cases this happens very smoothly, and the athlete returns within the appropriate time lines. It is only under unusual circumstances that there is a more serious problem that has to be dealt with. Most athletes you may treat are recreational and do not depend on their bodies to make a living for them; elite athletes, on the other hand, depend on their bodies to perform as a financial means to an end.

It is for this reason that many athletes request a second opinion. This happens now more than ever. If the athlete's concerned or the injury is complicated I will often encourage a second opinion. You want to do anything possible to facilitate the second opinion, such as talking to the physician the athlete wants the second opinion from and sending along all clinical notes and investigations that have been done thus far. The second opinion will help the athlete deal with the injury, knowing that more than one physician has been consulted. This also will appease all the other people involved in the athlete's decision. Sometimes a second opinion is necessary as there may be a limited number of physicians who have dealt with a unique or specific injury that occurs in their sport. There are only a limited number of physicians who see the volume of certain injuries such as a couple of physicians in the United States who see shoulders and elbows of professional baseball players. These athletes have unique injuries from the stress and want to see a physician who has the most experience in dealing with these injuries. As a physician who treats elite athletes it is important to ignore your ego and allow the athlete to seek a second opinion if needed. This in fact may make your job somewhat easier, as it takes some of the pressure off of you. In the rare case where there is a discrepancy or the injury is very unusual, a third opinion may even be required.

MEDICAL LEGAL

Medical legal issues may come into play. Since athletes may have contracts and endorsements worth over $100 million, there may be a very large lawsuit if an athlete is mistreated. It is important for physicians treating elite athletes to ensure that they have enough insurance coverage through their personal insurance or through the team to cover them in the case of a lawsuit. Although lawsuits involving elite athletes are not common, it is important to act appropriately. The most important thing is maintaining the physician–patient relationship. The athlete must be treated as an individual. The athlete cannot be placed at risk so he or she can return to sport to help the team if the athlete is not ready to return to the sport. It is important that communication be maintained at all times. Proper communication between the athlete and physician will ensure that everyone understands the problem fully. At an event on the road it is more difficult to maintain proper clinical notes. It is of paramount importance to maintain clinical notes to ensure that you document everything clearly and legibly. If there is a situation where an athlete returns to play without your consent, it is important that it is well-documented and that a release has been signed.

There is also a question of treating athletes from other countries. In Canada, where physicians are covered under the Canadian Medical Protection Association (CMPA), they are not protected if the jurisdiction of the lawsuit is out of Canada. The CMPA recommends that the physician have the athlete sign a consent form before treatment, so that, if there is a later lawsuit, the jurisdiction will take place in Canada, where the physician is covered. The physician covering elite athletes should check the insurance if they want to treat athletes from another country, even if it is in their home locale. The physician treating elite athletes must be aware that any lawsuit may create media coverage as well, which can affect him or her personally and financially.

MEDIA

The sport and often the main sections of newspapers focus on the elite athlete. Sports journalists make their career writing about elite athletes. Therefore, anything that happens to an elite athlete will be portrayed in the media. Because injuries or medical problems greatly affect the athlete's career, the media want to know exactly what is going on with the athlete. The media will often approach the physician to find out the exact nature of the medical problem and the implications for the athlete.

As stated previously, the most important thing is to maintain physician–patient confidentiality. If you are going to talk to the media it is important that the athlete knows exactly what you will say and that you have the athlete's permission to do so. Athletes are like any other patient; you must not freely disclose their medical problems. If, for some reason, the athlete does not want the injury disclosed, you must respect his or her wishes. If you are involved in team sports, it is important to communicate with the management. The management of the team may have a certain protocol for releasing information to the media. Often the information does not go through the medical personnel but through a press release from the front office. If a release of your information is going through the front office it is important that you declare exactly what they want to say, so there is no confusion about the diagnosis.

It is important to learn how to deal with the media. The media are by nature always looking for an angle or controversy, and medical issues are no exception. Although media personnel can be good friends, they can also work against you. If there is a message you want to portray through the media, you must learn to allow the media to receive the appropriate information you want to give them. The media can then be used to advantage to deliver a message to the public.

DRUGS

Prescription medications are frequently used to treat illnesses and injuries sustained by the elite athlete. Special care must be given so drugs are not prescribed that will adversely affect the athlete's performance. Side effects of the medication must be weighed against the potential benefits of the medication. It is important to document all medications given to the athlete as you would with any patient. Medications must be explained to the individual athlete so he or she understands what is being taken. If you are going to give an athlete an injection such as cortisone the procedure and the implications must be fully explained.

If you are treating athletes competing at an international level you may have to consult a banned list to ensure that the athlete is not taking a banned substance. All over-the-counter and prescription medications must be reviewed to ensure the athlete is not ingesting a substance that may provide a positive test during an international competition and disqualify him or her not only from the event but also future competition. Medical personnel treating athletes should have a list of banned substances readily available. Although athletes are generally aware of the need to check medications, it is prudent to be proactive and advise your athlete to check any medications he or she is taking.

Athletes at the elite level may take performance-enhancing drugs. To an athlete competing in international events, such as the Olympics, these are banned substances. Most professional sports either do not test at all or do random testing for performance-enhancing drugs such as anabolic steroids. It is important for medical personnel to train elite athletes to be aware of what drugs the athletes may be ingesting and their implications. The physician must be aware of possible side effects of the medications. The physician must be available to counsel these athletes about the pros and cons of taking performance-enhancing drugs. An elite athlete may approach a physician to help him or her monitor the use of performance-enhancing substances. This places the physician in a significant ethical dilemma. On the one hand, the physician would seem to condone these actions if he or she agrees to monitor these banned substances. On the other hand, if the physician knows the situation, the athlete may well take the substances anyway and not gain the respect and confidence of the physician to come to him or her if the athlete develops complications. This is one of the toughest ethical dilemmas the physician has in dealing with elite athletes.

Elite athletes have also been known to take mind-altering recreational drugs. This may include alcohol as well as any other drug available on the black market. Medical personnel should keep their eyes open to evidence of a problem with any of these drugs. Certain sports may have more abuse of one substance over another. The physician must be open-minded—if an athlete approaches him or her with a problem, the physician should be able to deal with it on a professional and nonconfrontational level in order to help the athlete. Many professional sports now have set protocols to help an athlete with a substance abuse problem.

If an athlete has a problem with substance abuse it may not only affect the ability to perform at the level required but also it may be life-threatening. If the physician suspects there is a problem, he or she must confront the problem and deal with it in the best interests of that individual.

PERSONAL PROBLEMS

The media will have you believe that the elite athlete is prone to substance abuse, promiscuity, and infidelity, whether or not in fact this is true. Certainly, athletes today are much more educated in all these issues. Nonetheless, the team physician may be called on to deal with such issues. The physician must deal with these problems discreetly and without judgment. A medical personnel dealing with elite athletes will hear and see more than is known by the general public. Maintaining confidentiality is crucial.

Athletes' personal problems may affect how they respond to an injury. The stress of a personal problem, such as divorce or family illness, will affect performance as well as how they respond to injury. Medical personnel must be aware of this and deal with it appropriately. On the other hand, the physician or medical personnel may not even be aware of personal problems that may be affecting the athlete's recovery. Often it is months later that you gain clarity. At times, medical personnel must be part physician and part psychologist. At times, the part of psychologist greatly outplays the part of physician.

IMPORTANCE OF THE TEAM PHYSICIAN

The physician treating elite athletes has a very important part in the athlete's success. Athletes rely on their physician and medical personnel to keep them healthy and performing at the highest level. They trust the medical personnel to do the utmost for them. They demand the most from themselves and thus demand the most from those working with them, including their medical personnel. Treating the elite athlete requires a great deal of time, patience, and commitment. Although your role is crucial to the athlete it is important to maintain your professionalism. It is important not to take too much credit when they perform badly and not to take too much credit when they perform well. The key to survival in treating elite athletes is to maintain professionalism. The athletes are truly the great stars, especially judged by their financial rewards. To maintain their respect and confidence in you as a trained medical person, it is vital to maintain your professionalism. If you can do this, the satisfaction of treating elite athletes makes all that time and dedication worthwhile. The longer you treat these athletes the longer you learn to respect and understand what drives them to perform at such a high level.

TESTING AND TRAINING

Since the ancient Greeks, humankind has striven to be the best it can be in athletic pursuits. The exceptional performance of today's athletes can be attributed to many factors. Genetic endowment, motivation, nutrition, skill development, and coaching are but a few of the complex blend of qualities needed to create a star. Another factor that has a profound effect on performance is the amount and the suitability of the training that precedes competition.

Today through training, as in ancient times, the athlete prepares him- or herself for a definite goal. In physiologic terms, the goal is to improve the body's systems and functions in order to optimize athletic performance. There are many more aspects of a good training program that will allow for these improvements. These include general physical development, sport-specific physical development, technical factors, tactical factors, physiologic aspects, health, and theoretical knowledge. We now concentrate on the methods for creating physiological adaptations in the body, including exercise-testing techniques, an overall plan for training, aerobic capacity, anaerobic power, speed, specific strength, flexibility, movement, and reaction time.

EXERCISE TESTING

Before beginning an exercise program it is prudent to determine the athlete's fitness level, goals for development, and which training techniques will be of most use for the particular sport.

For the healthy athlete, the exercise test is considered a primary training aid. There are two types of assessments used to determine an athlete's strengths and weaknesses, laboratory and field tests. A laboratory test is a measurement that is conducted in a controlled environment and that uses protocols and equipment that simulate the sport or activity. A field test is a measurement that is conducted while the athlete is performing in a simulated competitive situation.

An effective testing program follows:

- Evaluate variables that are relevant to the athlete's specific sport.
- Include tests that are valid and reliable.
- Be repeated at regular intervals.
- Report results directly to the athlete and coach.
- Include training programs designed on the basis of the results.

The ultimate concern in high-performance sport is the final performance, and final performance is dependent on a number of factors, some of which can be measured with appropriate assessments. The five major physiologic characteristics that fitness testing measures are strength and power, aerobic power, anaerobic power and capacity, flexibility, and kinanthropometry.

The relevance and relative importance of these five factors varies widely in different sports. An appropriate testing protocol chooses specific measurable factors applicable to each individual sport; for example, a vertical jump test is very sport-specific for a basketball player but is not an applicable measure for a swimmer. The following list summarizes the basic tests that are available to assess these five areas.

1. Strength and power
     Weight lifting
     Isometric testing
     Isokinetic testing
     Isotonic testing
     Stretch shortening cycle testing

   (Common protocols include: one repetition max for bench press and squat, calisthenics [push-ups, sit-ups], vertical jump, grip strength, isokinetic [i.e., Cybex Norm, Kincom], isotonic, and isometric testing equipment.)

2. Aerobic power
     Direct $\dot{V}_{O_2}$ max
     Lactate threshold
     Predicted $\dot{V}_{O_2}$ max

   (Common protocols include: discontinuous treadmill, cycle ergometer tests, step test, and the 12-min run.)

3. Anaerobic power and capacity
     Short-term anaerobic performance capacity ATP-CP system (0–10 s)

Intermediate-term anaerobic performance capacity, lactic
acid (0–30 s)
Long-term anaerobic performance capacity, lactic acid
(0–90 s)

(Common protocols include: 30-s Wingate test, Margaria stair-
case test, Quebec 10-s test, and the 60-s vertical jump test.)

4. Flexibility
   Range of motion at a joint or at a series of joints
   Static flexibility
   Dynamic flexibility

(Common protocols include: direct methods such as the
Leighton Flexometer and Goniometer and indirect methods
such as the sit and reach test and head to floor touch test.)

5. Kinanthropometry
   Percent body fat
   Height
   Weight
   Body girths and breadths
   Body mass
   Muscle typing
   Somatotype

(Common protocols include: [for body fat percent] Harpenden
calipers, hydrostatic [underwater] weighing, and bioelectrical
impedance.)

PERIODIZATION

The concept of periodization is not new. In many ways, it is as old
as athletic competition, having been used by the ancient Greeks to
organize training into 3- and 4-day cycles. In modern times,
coaches use periodization to divide the training into off-season,
preseason, and in-season periods.

Peroiodization is based on the concept that each individual
body is highly adaptable and, if it is given the proper training
stress at the appropriate time, will accommodate the training stimulus to attain new levels of fitness. Coaches will focus on recovery periods as well as the training periods to allow the body a
chance to adapt to the stress of training. It is important to understand that each athlete is different and will have different training
goals for different sports. The basic plan must be adapted to fit the
individual.

The Off-Season Program

By breaking down the off-season into three 4- to 6-week segments, you can provide a periodized program that will bring the athlete to peak physical form.

General Preparation Phase

The general preparation phase is the first 4- to 6-week period and has the objective of developing a high level of physical conditioning. During his or her competition, the athlete must emphasize a high volume of training that reflects the energy systems used. For example, a swimmer or runner emphasizes training the aerobic system, where the wrestler or weight lifter emphasizes general and maximum strength development. The intensity of training is of secondary importance during this phase, the emphasis must be made on volume.

Long slow distance characterizes the aerobic training portion of the program. The strength-training program involves three to four sets of 10 to 15 repetitions for upper body and 20 to 30 repetitions for lower body using a fairly light weight (60 to 70 percent of 1 RM).

Specific Preparation Phase

The specific preparation phase is the second 4- to 6-week period and represents a transition toward the competitive season. The volume of training remains high, but most of the work is directed toward the specific exercises related to the skill patterns of the sport. Toward the end of the phase, the volume drops as intensity increases.

During this phase the emphasis is on developing sport-specific strength and training the energy systems used in each different activity.

The athlete by now has developed a base aerobic and strength level, which can be added to. For example, hockey players work on interval training (biking, running, or Stairmaster) to train the lactic acid system used in a game. Hockey shifts usually consist of 30 to 45 s of all-out effort, with a 2- to 3-min rest (on the bench) in between. The aerobic–anaerobic training program will reflect these parameters. The strength-training program should target any imbalances found in the athlete and the muscles used in hockey. Multijoint lifts, such as cleans, deadlifts, and squats, are more reflective of the actions of hockey and thus should be selected for the training program.

It is important to note that young athletes who have not developed fully may start with exercises involving their body weight (push-ups, chin-ups, etc.) and should be cautioned against maximal lifts. Any young athlete participating in a strength program should be fully supervised by a qualified instructor.

The weight program should focus now on strength development, with higher weights being used (75 to 90 percent of 1 RM) in conjunction with less repetitions; 6 to 8 repetitions for upper body and 10 to 15 repetitions for lower body.

Precompetition Phase

The final phase of this program is the precompetition phase. This phase is the most fun for the athlete, but it may also be the most taxing physically. The intensity of the training program peaks during this phase, as the actual volume of training decreases. The focus of this phase is on developing sport-specific power, agility, and targeting the high-end ATP energy delivery system that works in the first 6 to 8 s of effort. By building the base through the first two phases of training, the athlete can focus on training this high-end system two to three times per week. The power development involves the use of pliometric exercises. These exercises involve hopping, bounding, and jumping with resistance and require a solid muscular base before being attempted.

In-Season Training

The underlying principle for in-season training is to use exercises that are sport-specific and can emulate the vertical and lateral movements of the specific sport. Explosive, multijoint weight training exercises that are ground-based tend to reinforce the movement patterns of basketball and enhance the overall coordination and timing.

Exercises, such as lateral squats, split squats, and power cleans, are examples of these types of exercises. It is important to note that an underlying base of weight training must be acquired (usually through the off-season) before attempting these more advanced lifts. The volume and intensity of training in-season vary from one athlete to another and are dependent on playing and practice schedule, travel, and age.

Heavy loads and low repetitions allow most athletes to maintain a large percentage of acquired strength; one to two sets of four to six repetitions for five to six exercises are recommended. The idea is to keep the volume of training low, but maintain a high game-like intensity. A typical workout may be scheduled for a practice involving light skill acquisition or an off day.

Some sports involve sprints and quick movements that utilize the alactic and lactic acid energy delivery systems. An aerobic base is required for these systems to perform at their peak; however, during the season it is best to simulate the actual game situations for your aerobic and anaerobic workouts. Sprint interval training is the best way to improve these systems. Sprint lengths include baseline to foul lines, half court and full court, or sprinting on a high-speed treadmill. The movements may include sprinting and backpedaling. The completion of each repetition requires from 6 to 45 s of high-intensity work followed by a brief rest. This time period is equivalent to the amount of time during which the ATP-PC/lactic acid energy system is being utilized. The recovery may be from 1 to 3 min, depending on the intensity of effort.

Interval training should be performed at least twice a week either during a practice or on the athlete's own time. It is a great way to develop sport-specific speed and quickness. Remember, the more you put into it, the more you will get out of it.

PLIOMETRICS

One of the components that forms the off-season training program is pliometric training. Pliometrics refer to the exercises characterized by powerful, muscular contractions in response to rapid dynamic loading or stretching of the involved muscle.

The Russians are said to have invented pliometrics; however, kids of all countries have been skipping and playing hopscotch for years. Basically, that is what pliometrics is—skipping, hopping, bounding, and jumping. The key in all these movements is the slight lengthening of the muscle fibers in the muscle groups responsible for generating the power. This slight stretch activates the muscle spindle reflex that sends a very strong stimulus via the spindle cord to the muscles, causing them to contract powerfully.

Pliometric exercises are thought to stimulate various changes in the neuromuscular system, enhancing the ability of the muscle groups to respond more quickly and powerfully to slight and rapid changes in muscle length.

There are many different types and levels of pliometric exercises, ranging from quick hops and pattern jumps, to depth jumps and medicine ball work for the upper body. The intensity of the pliometric exercise varies with the amount of overload employed to forcibly stretch the muscle and bring about a rapid rise in the firing frequency of the muscle spindle.

Pliometrics are classified into beginner, intermediate, and advanced level exercises. An athlete who is relatively unskilled and just starting a fitness program should progress slowly and with supervision into a low-intensity pliometric program involving skipping, cone hops, and box drills from 6 inches. The medicine ball work should be simple movements using the 4- or 6-lb ball.

Athletes who have been exposed to weight-training programs can benefit from moderately intense programs, and accomplished athletes with strong weight-training backgrounds should be able to perform ballistic-reactive, high-intensity exercise with no problem.

Before designing a pliometric program there are a number of points to consider.

- *Age of the participant.* Because of the potential risk of injury to growth plates, it is recommended that athletes who have not reached pubescence do not perform advanced level pliometrics.
- *Body weight.* Large athletes, 220 to 250 lb, are not able to perform the same drills, volumes, and intensities as smaller athletes.
- *Strength ratio.* The National Strength and Conditioning Association recommend an athlete squats 1.5 times his or her body weight before attempting advanced level pliometrics.
- *Experience.* Athletes with low skill levels have a higher risk of injury.
- *Surface.* Ideal surfaces are gym-like sprung floors for ease of landing. Natural grass is an ideal surface.
- *Safety considerations.* Pliometrics requires an emphasis on correct technique. A coach should be present at all times to monitor and correct the exercise technique.

Pliometric Exercise Prescription

When looking at the prescription for pliometric exercises a coach should think in terms of foot contacts—that is, every time a foot or feet together contact the surface per workout. Volumes for beginners should be 100- to 150-foot contacts in the preseason program. Intermediates would perform 150 to 300 foot contacts, and advanced athletes would perform 150 to 450 foot contacts.

The intensity of the exercises is low moderate in the off-season and moderate to high in the preseason. The frequency of the pliometric training workout usually ranges from one to three sessions per week. Recovery between sets is recommended, 15 to 30 s between repetitions and 3 to 4 min between sets. Pliometric exercises have to mimic as much as possible the key movement patterns, the dominant skills of the athlete's sport. This is vitally important and makes the difference in enabling the athlete to take his or her performance to the next level.

The training of athletes has progressed quite significantly (especially in the past 25 years) as the science of human movement becomes more and more refined in terms of the specific effect on the athlete. Coaches and trainers are now armed with a myriad of techniques. The challenge is selecting the appropriate method of training for the individual. What works well for one athlete may not work as well for the next. Each sport also has different physical demands for strength, aerobic capacity, anaerobic power, flexibility, and speed. It is important to individually design each program and make constant adjustments for the continually adapting body.

36 Drugs and Ergogenic Aids

Andrew Pipe

RESPONSIBILITIES OF THE SPORTS MEDICINE PRACTITIONER

All sports medicine professionals should be aware of the problems posed by drug use in sport. Fundamental concerns about the well-being of athletes entrusted to our care and a consideration of the side effects, potential and real, of many drugs abused in sport have led to regulations against their use. Of equal significance is the degree to which the integrity of sport is eroded by the perception that athletic achievements are now the product of biochemistry or pharmacology rather than the result of talent, dedication, and training. The discipline of sports medicine is itself threatened by the belief that sports medicine professionals are practitioners of a murky science in which victory is pursued at all costs and by all means. The provision or prescription of banned drugs to athletes is antithetical to the practice of good medicine and a violation of professional ethics at the most basic level.

For more than three decades, sports medicine organizations and sports authorities have sought to address the problems posed by "doping" through the development of rules and regulations concerning the appropriate and inappropriate uses of drugs and other compounds in sport. At times, such rules prove frustrating for those with responsibilities for the care of athletes with specific medical conditions. All sports medicine practitioners should advocate anti-doping rules that are cogent, fair, grounded in science, and have been developed in accordance with an understanding of sports and the special circumstances of athletes. Such rules also should protect the rights of athletes to drug-free sport but also to interpretation and decisions reached in accordance with commonly accepted principles of justice and fair play. To the extent that antidoping regulations or their application does not meet these criteria, sports medicine professionals must campaign for their change.

A knowledge of the relevant rules regarding doping is essential for the practitioner. Unfortunately, the rules may vary between and among sports organizations. This places added responsibilities on sports medicine professionals. Athletes assume that health professionals working in sports are familiar with the rules and that they will not provide medications or other compounds that might cause the athlete to run afoul of the regulations. It may be argued that athletes ultimately must be responsible for what they consume (including medications and supplements); it can be argued equally

745

that those who profess special expertise in the care of the athletic patient have a greater responsibility to ensure that such patients do not receive care that would violate the antidoping regulations. This latter argument is all the more compelling when dealing with young athletes or considering the relative degree of sophistication that might be necessary for an athlete to distinguish between banned and permitted medications.

THE IOC MEDICAL CODES

Most regulations regarding doping in sports are based on the Medical Code of the International Olympic Committee.[1] While this code has several shortcomings, it does provide an appropriate template for the development of internationally consistent rules and regulations. A review of the list of the code's categorizations (Table 36-1) demonstrates the range of substances and practices the document addresses. It would be impossible in these pages to attempt a comprehensive discussion of the code and its implications for the sports medicine professional. What follows is an attempt to review the categories and provide specific, practical advice for the practitioner.

PROHIBITED CLASSES OF SUBSTANCES

Stimulants

Notwithstanding the problems posed by the ingestion of medicinal mushrooms, herbal preparations, and the various "tonics" that were reported in association with the early Olympic games, the contemporary concern with doping in sports began earlier in the twentieth

TABLE 36-1 IOC Medical Code (Prohibited Classes of Substances and Prohibited Methods as of January 31, 1998)

I. Prohibited classes of substances
A. Stimulants
B. Narcotics
C. Anabolic agents
D. Diuretics
E. Peptide and glycoprotein hormones and analogues
II. Prohibited methods
A. Blood doping
B. Pharmacologic chemical, and physical manipulation
III. Classes of drugs subject to certain restrictions
A. Alcohol
B. Marijuana
C. Local anesthetics
D. Corticosteroids
E. Beta blockers

century when it became clear that amphetamines were being used in cycling races. The sudden deaths during competition of riders who had taken amphetamines spurred the development of rules against such use and were instrumental in the development of the IOC Medical Commission. An understandable concern for the protection of athletes' safety and health was coupled with a desire to ensure that competitors were not cheated by those whose performance was artificially accentuated. Sadly, the perverted ingenuity of some competitors and their handlers, then as now, seemed to know no bounds, and it soon became clear that it was necessary to forbid the use of a variety of stimulating compounds.

The list has now grown significantly and concludes with the now ubiquitous phrase ". . . and other related compounds." Included within the list are such products as caffeine and the sympathomimetics. The latter products are found all over the world in an almost endless list of over-the-counter cough, cold, sinus, and allergy medications and pose special problems for athletes and their medical advisors. Great care must be taken to ensure that athletes do not inadvertently consume such compounds at a time when competition is imminent.

Cases of "inadvertent doping" occur frequently and can cause considerable pain for athletes and their physicians. Perhaps more important, the degree to which athletes are sanctioned in such circumstances erodes the confidence of athletes in antidoping measures and undermines support for programs that seek to eliminate doping from sports. The situation could be improved considerably if the rules were changed so as to declare a "doping violation" only when certain realistic urinary thresholds for specific compounds were exceeded. There is hope that this might be the case in the future. In the meantime, vigilance is required of practitioners and athletes alike. Physicians should know that the use of nasal decongestants containing xylometazoline is permitted. These agents are commonly available in North America. When in any doubt about the status of any product or medication, it is important that practitioners verify the same by contacting an appropriate authority (in Canada, the Canadian Centre for Drug-free Sport: 1-800-672-7775; in the United States, the U.S. Olympic Committee: 1-800-233-0393).

Caffeine is also a controlled stimulant. A threshold has been established for the detection of this compound, and a urinary concentration of less than 12 μg/mL will not be reported as a positive result. Athletes and physicians should be advised, however, that it is possible, given individual circumstances and patterns of caffeine use, for athletes to approach this level in the course of ingestion of caffeine-containing beverages and foods.

A sad reality of modern sports has been the degree to which certain patterns of drug use have become more common within certain sports subcultures. A number of deaths, for instance, have been associated with cocaine use in basketball and result, in part, from cocaine's capacity to produce marked coronary vasoconstriction. Its use is banned in sports. Such phenomena underscore the sports physician's responsibility to provide clear, nonjudgmental advice to athletes about the use of "recreational" drugs and other health-related behaviors in addition to the obvious need to address the issue of the ethics and safety of the use of performance-enhancing products.

The beta-agonist medications salbutamol and salmeterol, commonly used in the treatment of asthma and the prevention of exercise-induced bronchospasm, are considered stimulants in the IOC Medical Code—but they are permitted, provided that notification of their use is given to the relevant authorities prior to competition. Antidoping regulations may prove particularly vexing for asthmatic athletes or those involved in their care. Given the increasing prevalence of this disorder worldwide and the rise in mortality associated with this condition, regulations that stipulate that athletes must have been reviewed by a respirologist or other consultant in order for their asthmatic status to be verified place a burden on athletes, physicians, and health care systems. It is hoped that such regulations will be revised in the future.

Narcotics

Narcotics have been banned in sports in order that such products are not used to eliminate the pain and discomfort associated with injury or overexertion. In this way an athlete's health might be safeguarded. Commonly used and more "benign" narcotics such as the analgesic codeine and the cough suppressant dextromethorphan are permitted.

Anabolic Agents

A product of the German chemical industry, anabolic steroids were first developed in the hope that they might have military application. In the late 1950s their use became apparent in the athletic community, and by the 1960s, they had been introduced to North America. Sharing the basic structure of the fundamental male hormone testosterone, all synthetic agents possess both anabolic and androgenic capabilities. Modifications of anabolic products influence the anabolicity and androgenicity of a particular compound and determine whether it can be ingested orally. Although the use of these compounds exploded in the athletic community in the 1970s and 1980s, scientists and sports medicine practitioners were reluctant to attest to their effectiveness because of the lack of evidence for such in the scientific literature. That evidence was not available largely because ethical considerations precluded the administration of the large quantities of a variety of anabolic agents typical of the doses used by many athletic users. Clear evidence about the effectiveness of anabolic steroids in improving performance did not become available until 1996, when Bhasin and colleagues[2] demonstrated an increase in muscle size and strength following the administration of anabolic steroids.

Anabolic agents are also androgenic, given that they are all essentially modifications of the male sex hormone testosterone. Consequently, the administration of exogenous anabolics can lead to the development of masculine features in the female and an accentuation of the normal effects of anabolic activity in the male (Table 36-2). It is important to understand that there is as yet no body of information reflecting long-term experience with those known to have administered large quantities of anabolic-androgenic agents. It may take decades before the consequences of such self-administration become clear. The tragic revelations of widespread, systematic use of anabolic steroids throughout the sports system of the former German Democratic Republic (East Germany) represent the first glimpses of the implications of the sustained use of the these products in athletes.[3] It is known that the use of anabolics may cause problems in a variety of the organ systems of certain unfortunate users. Such problems may involve the cardiovascular, hepatic, hematologic, endocrine, and reproductive systems.[4] Case reports are appearing with increasing frequency describing the more lurid complications associated with steroid use in sport.[5,6] It is probably correct to assume that such complications are underreported.

TABLE 36-2 Side-Effects of Anabolic Steroids

Premature closure of the epiphyses in adolescents
Distortion of lipid profiles
Disruption of liver enzyme activity
Cholestasis
Jaundice
Peliosis hepatis
Hepatoma
Gynecomastia
Acne
Virilization of females:
   Male-pattern baldness
   Deepening of the voice
   Development of facial hair
   Clitoral hypertrophy
Accentuation of secondary sexual characteristics in males
Testicular atrophy
Reduction in sperm count
Changes in mood states

The sports clinician may at times be approached by athletes or their coaches with a request that anabolic use be "monitored" in order that the athlete's health might be safeguarded. Physicians contemplating such a strategy should consider that to participate in such practices is to become caught up in doping activity.[7] Such conduct, in the first instance, is not in keeping with the ethical practice of sports medicine; second, it may expose the physician to a range of problems and liabilities both within and outside the sports community. Nevertheless, such requests should produce a response that is constructive and nonjudgmental, recognizing the significant opportunity for the provision of objective advise and counseling. Many would argue that such patients should be managed in the same way as those with other drug or alcohol problems.

The extent to which anabolic steroid use is common in sports is not clear. No reliable data exist. Sadly, there is evidence that the use of anabolics has spread to nonathletic youths, who administer such drugs in attempts to develop a certain muscular appearance.[8]

In many nations, programs of year-round, out-of-competition testing of athletes have been implemented; they are seen as the only appropriate way to deter and detect anabolic steroid and other drug use.[9] Sports physicians must be familiar with the procedures and protocols in use in the environments in which they practice.

Diuretics

Diuretics are banned in sports because they have been used to accelerate the excretion of other banned drugs or to facilitate weight loss in sports in which competition is arranged by weight categories (e.g., rowing, wrestling, judo, and other combatives). Most health professionals understand the hazards of the electrolyte disturbances that can accompany the use of diuretics; such hazards may be accentuated when other bizarre strategies are applied in attempts to lose weight. Despite such knowledge, the use of diuretics and laxatives has been commonplace in wrestling in North America. A number of deaths of collegiate wrestlers in late 1997 may focus more attention on the practice of "making weight" and the unfortunate consequences that sometimes follow. There is a need for sports medicine professionals to speak out about such practices and to ensure, to the extent possible, that athletes for whom they have responsibility are not involved in such practices.

Peptide and Glycoprotein Hormones and Analogues

This category includes a variety of hormones that have been used in attempts to produce anabolic effects. They include human chorionic gonadotropin (HCG), corticotropin (ACTH), human growth hormone (HGH), and the respective releasing factors for such products. Such compounds are not used commonly in the treatment of athletes, and their provision in the absence of a documented clinical indication for their use betrays a sinister intent on the part of a physician and/or athlete. HGH is now available as a genetically engineered product.

Erythropoietin (EPO), the hormone that stimulates the production of red blood cells, is also now available as a product of genetic engineering. Among the unscrupulous, its use has superseded the practice of "blood doping" (see below), a tactic in which the red blood cell mass is artificially increased in order to accentuate the blood's oxygen-carrying capacity and, as a consequence, aerobic performance.[10] There are growing concerns that an associated increase in blood viscosity may induce a hypercoagulable state or otherwise potentiate the risk of cardiovascular or cerebrovascular collapse in those using EPO.

A number of deaths are alleged to have occurred in cycling attributable to EPO use.[11] Officials in all sports in which aerobic capacity is fundamental to success are understandably concerned about the use of this product. There are no currently reliable means to detect its use with urine or blood tests. In some sports (notably cycling, track and field, and cross-country skiing), blood tests are being applied in an attempt to identify athletes with levels of hemoglobin or a hematocrit greater than an arbitrarily developed threshold. Such athletes are then denied permission to compete on the basis of a concern for their health. This approach is not without problems and undoubtedly will spawn controversy in the future.

PROHIBITED METHODS

The IOC has tried in the development of its rules to ensure that unusual practices or techniques designed to enhance performance or assist in evading the detection of doping are specifically banned. In this respect, IOC addresses a series of issues beyond the provision or consumption of a banned drug.

Blood Doping

Blood doping refers to a practice that first appeared in the 1980s. It was noted several years ago that the reinfusion, after a certain period of time, of previously withdrawn red blood cells would increase the red cell mass and increase aerobic performance. This led to the practice of blood doping athletes in a variety of sports. These approaches often involved physicians and exercise scientists who cast their ethical and clinical responsibilities to the wind. In 1984, members of the U.S. cycling team at the Los Angeles Olympics practiced blood doping using unmatched blood under the supervision of a physician and with the encouragement of a prominent exercise physiologist! Predictably, some athletes became ill and required hospitalization. Others won gold medals. Following the discovery of this incident, the IOC developed rules specifically prohibiting this practice. Blood doping, it has already been noted, has largely been replaced by the use of erythropoietin among those seeking to surreptitiously enhance red blood cell mass and aerobic capacity.

Pharmacologic, Chemical, and Physical Manipulation

Attempts to manipulate physiology or tamper with urine samples so as to reduce the likelihood of the detection of doping practices are banned by the IOC. By way of example, the use of probenecid to reduce the excretion of anabolics and the substitution of "clean" urine via catheterization or other techniques are specifically prohibited.

CLASSES OF DRUGS SUBJECT TO CERTAIN RESTRICTIONS

The IOC recognizes that individual international sport federations may wish to add to the banned list because of concerns particular to their sport. Thus alcohol and marijuana are noted as falling into a special category; "drugs that are subject to certain restrictions." In certain shooting sports, for example, there exist obvious concerns about safety and hence a concern with the use of alcohol. Similar concerns are said to underlie the addition of marijuana to the banned list of certain sport federations. Neither of these drugs can be said to be capable of enhancing performance (although the use of alcohol might eliminate tremor, again of significance in shooting or target sports). There is a view that these drugs were added to the banned list because of concerns not only for safety but also to attempt to protect the integrity or image of the sport itself and to control the social behavior of athletes. In this respect, the use of an antidoping policy to address social drug issues may be shortsighted. There is the danger that sanctions applied under these rules will erode support for antidoping programs in general. It also can be argued that there are far more effective ways to encourage responsible behavior among athletes and other members of the sporting community.

In an attempt to ensure that the legitimate treatment of illness or injury is not impaired by the antidoping regulations, the IOC has developed a category of medications whose use is permitted under certain circumstances. *Local anesthetics*, with the exception of cocaine, are permitted, as is the concurrent administration of vasoconstrictors. However, notification of the use of such medications and their clinical justification must be provided to the relevant competition authorities. The use of the commonly prescribed *beta-agonist medications* salbutamol, salmeterol, and terbutaline is permitted by inhalation, but their oral administration is not permitted. Athletes must obtain written authorization for their use in advance of doping control tests. This administrative requirement can produce problems.

A perception that the nontherapeutic use of *corticosteroids* has been increasing has led to the development of stronger restrictions on the use of these drugs. Their systemic administration is banned; topical, inhalational, intraarticular, or local use is permitted. *Caffeine*, a compound whose use is widespread in almost all cultures, is regulated by the provision that a urinary level of more than 12 μg/mL will be interpreted as a doping infraction. *Betablockers* are subject to the rules and regulations of particular international federations; their ability to lower anxiety, heart rate, and tremor has resulted in their being banned in target sports. Similarly, the regulations also permit international federations to test for the presence of *alcohol* and *marijuana* and to apply appropriate sanctions. Alcohol is banned only in shooting sports (as a consequence of its ability to reduce tremor and also as a safety measure).

The IOC list could be simplified. (It would be helpful, for instance, to remove the onerous requirements for sports physicians, sports organizations, and national antidoping agencies to document and certify the diagnosis of asthma and the use of salbutamol and salmeterol—this is a requirement that is poorly followed, and most sports organizations do not have the capacity to administer it.) It is also important for sports medicine professionals to be familiar with the list of restricted substances and the various "notification" requirements that surround it. Failure to adhere to these rules could, unfortunately, lead to problems for athletes and their medical advisers. Confusion surrounds this list; many practitioners are unaware of the notification requirements. The notification rules exist to protect athletes and to facilitate the review of drug testing results.

Sadly, it is sometimes the case that the authorities responsible for the interpretation and administration of such rules (or even the results of positive doping tests) are themselves either inexperienced, nonclinicians, or thrust into such circumstances as well-meaning but ill-equipped volunteers. The development and administration of antidoping rules and regulations are an unfortunate but essential component of contemporary elite sports. It is essential that all phases of antidoping activities be managed in a thoroughly professional manner. This has obvious financial and administrative implications for sports organizations, implications that they ignore at their peril.

Implications for the Health Professional

All health professionals involved in sports have a responsibility to be familiar with the rules relating to doping. More important, they have a responsibility to ensure that their own practices reflect a commitment to drug-free sport. In this respect, there is a need to ensure that athletes, their coaches, and other members of the sporting entourage understand their roles in addressing this unfortunate issue. All need clear, reliable information, and sports scientists and physicians are its logical source. Special care must be taken to ensure that athletes and others understand the problems that can develop in association with the use of supplements, nostrums, herbal preparations, and nutritional supplements (see below). Physicians have particular obligations to ensure that in treating or advising athletes, they do not produce a situation in which athletes run afoul of antidoping regulations. Finally, all should serve as advocates not only for drug-free sport but also for the development of appropriate, relevant regulations and their intelligent administration.

ERGOGENIC AIDS

Athletes and their advisors have for centuries sought access to foods or compounds that might dramatically accentuate their athletic performance.[12] Hundreds of such products have been used in the past, and a preoccupation with the pursuit of a nutritional "Holy Grail" continues apace! Surprisingly, in this supposedly sophisticated and scientific age, athletes and their coaches frequently fall prey to the exhortations of those whose accomplishments are in marketing rather than in maximizing performance. The list of products that have been touted as capable of enhancing athletic performance seems endless and cannot possibly be dealt with here. Each year it seems, another diet "guru" appears on the scene whose approach (and heavily marketed book and/or products) makes extravagant promises of new levels of energy, endurance, and accomplishment. Sadly, among many athletes and their coaches, nutrition has become a religious movement rather than a scientific discipline. Ironically, in the pursuit of the ergogenic panacea, many proven, well-documented approaches to performance enhancement are often ignored.

A well-balanced diet, carefully designed with the particular needs of an athlete's specific sports is a foundation of successful athletic performance. Its utility is often derided by those who promote more exotic approaches to nutrition. The specific needs of female athletes may merit the use of supplementary iron. Those with unusual dietary requirements or preferences will benefit from professional nutritional counseling.

For female athletes experiencing amennorrhea or preoccupied with minimizing caloric intake, a reduction of training load and an increase in iron, calcium, and caloric intake may enhance performance and accentuate health. Simple attention to adequate rest, the provision of appropriate hydration, and the ongoing replacement of energy stores can be profoundly "ergogenic" for all athletes. The training cultures of many sports have come to emphasize prodigious training loads that often may be counterproductive in terms of nutritional status, health, and performance. "Success," it has been said, "consists of doing ordinary things extraordinarily well." Nevertheless, there are certain techniques or approaches that have been shown to be capable of enhancing performance. A brief discussion follows.

Mental Preparation

The recognition that psychological factors can significantly constrain or increase performance has led to the development of an entire discipline—sports psychology.[13] Mental skills including visualization, other forms of mental rehearsal, self-arousal techniques, focusing, and disassociation strategies have all become part of the repertoire of many successful athletes and might be described as "psychoergogenics." They are beyond the scope of this discussion but are an important element in the scientific preparation of the modern athlete.

Nutritional Strategies

As noted earlier, the provision of an appropriately designed diet is central to the optimization of performance. The provision of a diet high in complex carbohydrates in the period before endurance events lasting more than 1 h is now commonplace; it serves to ensure an optimal supply of muscle glycogen and is commonly known as carbohydrate loading. Evidence continues to accumulate of the value of replacing small amounts of carbohydrate during the course of an athletic event.

The beneficial effects of fluid replacement during competition are also clear. It is not that long ago, however, that coaching techniques in some sports stressed fluid restriction! In certain sports played in hot, humid conditions, rules actually *forbid* the provision of fluids to athletes during breaks in play!

NUTRITIONAL SUPPLEMENTATION

A number of specific products have been used in the belief that they can enhance performance. It is not possible to discuss them all, nor any in detail, in this brief review. Additional information may be found elsewhere.[14–16] The sports medicine practitioner has a special responsibility to try to ensure that athletes understand the problems that may surround the use of certain supplements: problems that may follow from the lack of evidence of their efficacy; that there are no regulations concerning their preparation, purity, labeling, and marketing; and concerns relating to their safety. Sir William Osler once observed that "it is the responsibility of the physician to persuade the public not to take medicines." His advice was intended for a population fascinated by nostrums and "snake oil"; it may be equally appropriate for those intent on the pursuit of a nutritional panacea. Athletes, too often it seems, place their faith in nutritional supplements of dubious or no value. A brief discussion of commonly touted or consumed supplements follows.

Branched-Chain Amino Acids

These constituents of protein-rich foods are touted as being helpful in overcoming the central nervous system component of fatigue. There are theoretical grounds to support this contention, but research findings in this regard are inconclusive.

Beta-Hydroxy-Beta-Methylbutyrate (HMB)

It is speculated that HMB, a metabolite of the amino acid leucine, is capable of decreasing protein breakdown, thereby exerting an anabolic effect of sorts. Animal research has shown increased lean muscle mass and decreased levels of body fat in association with HMB supplementation. Limited human research conducted by the developers of this product has supported the animal findings. The safety of this compound is unknown at this point. [It is very important to distinguish this product from gamma-hydroxybutyrate (GHB); this latter compound is claimed to facilitate sleep and weight control. It has been marketed particularly to bodybuilders, and it has been implicitly suggested that it can affect growth hormone release. Its actual effects in this regard are unknown. What is clear is that its use was associated with many cases of poisoning in the United States in 1990. No deaths resulted, but hospitalization and respiratory support were required for several unfortunate individuals).[17]]

Caffeine

Caffeine is present in an abundance of commonly ingested food and beverages. Caffeine's use is controlled in sports (see above), urinary levels of more than 12 μg/mL being considered as doping. It is known to improve performance in a variety of tasks, particularly in those accustomed to regular caffeine intake.[18] Athletes should understand that a small increase in normal caffeine intake may cause the development of "caffeinism," in which anxiety, nervousness, and irritability will all contribute to a diminished performance. This is particularly true of those unaccustomed to regular caffeine ingestion.

Carnitine (L-Carnitine)

Formed in the body from several amino acids, carnitine, it is suggested, might enhance aerobic power by facilitating the use of fatty acids in energy production, thereby sparing glycogen (the principal energy source in aerobic activity) consumption. It is also theorized that carnitine might enhance the delivery of pyruvate (produced by the breakdown of glucose) to the mitochondria and accentuate energy production. There is little evidence to support either view.[19]

Choline (Lecithin)

Perhaps more popular several years ago, choline was promoted as having the ability to maintain adequate levels of acetylcholine, a neurotransmitter, during periods of prolonged aerobic exercise. The research evidence to support this view is inconclusive.[20] Dietary choline is found in egg yolks, organ meats, spinach, and wheat germ.

Chromium

An essential mineral, chromium is claimed to enhance the development of lean muscle mass and to reduce body fat. Interest in this mineral increased when it became apparent that exercise causes chromium loss. It has been suggested that chromium supplementation will improve insulin sensitivity, promote the transfer of amino acids into the muscle cell, and thereby stimulate protein synthesis. Recent well-designed investigations have failed to support the contention that chromium supplementation will improve lean body mass or strength.[21] In addition, concerns exist about the potential hazard of excess chromium intake above that recommended as a daily requirement.[22]

Creatine

Creatine is a compound that exists normally in the body and is found in the normal diet in animal protein. Creatine is normally found in muscle, where it is combined with phosphate to form creatine phosphate (CP). Creatine phosphate is responsible for providing and replenishing muscle energy in situations involving the rapid production of maximal effort. Many laboratory investigations have confirmed that the addition of supplemental creatine increased performance in repetitive tasks of maximal effort.[23,24] Whether this translates into increased performance capacity in the course of an actual athletic event is more difficult to prove. Several other investigators have shown no evidence of increased performance in athletic situations. More studies are necessary to resolve these contradictory findings. At this point, evidence does exist to support the use of creatine to enhance repeated explosive muscular activity, and thus it may assist in accentuating training intensity. Its use in other situations cannot, at present, be supported by the scientific literature. This has not prevented the development of a thriving market in the sale of this supplement to athletes at every level of ability in a variety of sports.

Ginseng

The allure of ginseng as a supplement is perhaps explained by the traditional use of this product in Oriental medicine and the degree of marketing that surrounds its use. While there is little doubt that the ginsenosides (the constituents of ginseng) are biologically active, there is no clear evidence that they are capable of enhancing performance.[25] Many of the commercial preparations of ginseng are blends of a variety of ginsenosides of differing quality and potency; this makes evaluation of their properties more difficult.

As with all so-called natural supplements, there are no regulations that control the ingredients, purity, or accuracy of labeling of these products. It is not unknown for such supplements to be deliberately or inadvertently contaminated with other pharmacologically active substances. Athletes must be aware of such unfortunate realities and, to the extent possible, assure themselves of the quality and purity of any products they may be considering purchasing or consuming.

FINAL THOUGHTS

Sport is a powerful and normally positive cultural force in our community and in the modern world. Unfortunately, there are those who would cheat to secure sporting success. There are others who would exploit athletes and their trust by manipulating their training practices or programs. The artificial enhancement of athletic training or athletic accomplishments by pharmacologic means is both irresponsible and unethical. Health professionals involved in sports have a central responsibility to care for athletes in the most complete sense and to protect and preserve the integrity of any sporting experience. This may seem a naive or hopelessly optimistic perspective. However, the true magic of sports is that it is a place where seemingly naive or hopelessly optimistic aspirations often can become reality!

ACKNOWLEDGMENTS

The assistance of Ms. Dina Bell and Drs. Tony Galea and Robert Stalker who graciously reviewed this chapter is gratefully acknowledged.

REFERENCES

1. International Olympic Committee: *The IOC Medical Code.* Lausanne, Switzerland, IOC, 1995.
2. Bhasin S, Storer TW, Berman N, et al: The effects of supraphysiologic doses of testosterone on muscle size and strength in normal men. *N Engl J Med* 335:1–7, 1996.
3. Franke WE, Berendonk B: Hormonal doping and androgenization of athletes: A secret program of the German Democratic Republic government. *Clin Chem* 43(7):1262–1297, 1997.
4. Bagatelli CJ, Bremner WJ: Androgens in men: Uses and abuses. *N Engl J Med* 334:707–714, 1996.
5. Yoshida EM, Karim MA, Shaikn JF, et al: At what price glory? Severe cholestasis and acute renal failure in an athlete abusing stanozolol. *Can Med Assoc J* 151(6):791–793, 1994.
6. Menkis AH, Daniel JK, McKenzie N, et al: Cardiac transplantation after myocardial infarction in a 24-year-old bodybuilder using anabolic steroids. *Clin J Sports Med* 1:138–140, 1991.
7. Pipe AL: Sport, science and society: Ethics in sports medicine. *Med Sci Sports Exerc* 25:888–900, 1993.
8. Melia P, Pipe A, Greenberg L: The use of anabolic-androgenic steroids by Canadian students. *Clin J Sports Med* 6:9–14, 1996.
9. Bahr R, Tjornhom M: Prevalence of doping in sports: Doping control in Norway, 1977–1995. *Clin J Sports Med* 8:32–37, 1998.
10. Ekblom B, Berglund B: Effect of erythropoietin administration on maximal aerobic power. *Scand J Med Sci Sports* 1:88–93, 1991.
11. Ramotar J: Cyclists' deaths linked to erythropoietin? *Phys Sportsmed* 18(8):48–49, 1990.
12. Mottram DR: Drugs and their use in sport, in Mottram DR (ed): *Drugs in Sport.* Champaign, Ill, Human Kinetics, 1988, pp 1–31.
13. Weinberg RS, Gould D: *Foundations of Sport and Exercise Psychology.* Champaign, Ill, Human Kinetics, 1995.
14. Clarkson PM: Nutrition for improved sports performance: Current issues on ergogenic aids. *Sports Med* 21:293–401, 1996.
15. Armsey TD, Green GA: Nutrition supplements: Science versus hype. *Phys Sportsmed* 25, 1997.
16. Williams MH: *The Ergogenics Edge: Pushing the Limits of Human Performance.* Champaign, Ill, Human Kinetics, 1998.
17. Multistate outbreak of poisonings associated with illicit use of GHB. *JAMA* 265:447–448, 1991.

18. Graham TE, Spriet LL: Caffeine and exercise performance. *Sports Sci Exch* 9(1):1–5, 1996.
19. Vuchovich MD, Costill DL, Fink WJ: Carnitine supplementation: Effect on muscle carnitine and glycogen content during exercise. *Med Sci Sports Exerc* 26(9):1122–1129, 1994.
20. Spector SA, Jackman MR, Sabounjian LA, et al: Effect of choline supplementation in trained cyclists. *Med Sci Sports Exerc* 27:668–673, 1995.
21. Clancy SP, Clarkson PM, DeCheke ME, et al: Effects of chromium picolinate supplementation on body composition, strength, and urinary chromium loss in football players. *Int J Sports Nutr* 4(2):142–153, 1994.
22. Wasser WG, Feldman NS: Chronic renal failure after ingestion of over-the-counter chromium picolinate (letter). *Ann Intern Med* 126(5):410, 1997.
23. Greenhaff PL, Bodin K, Soderland K, et al: The effect of oral creatine supplementation on skeletal muscle phosphocreatine resynthesis. *Am J Physiol* 266(5 pt 1):E725–E730, 1994.
24. Maughan RJ: Creatine supplementation and exercise performance. *Int J Sports Nutr* 5(2):94–101, 1995.
25. Bahrke MS, Morgan WP: Evaluation of the ergogenic properties of ginseng. *Sports Med* 18:229–248, 1994.

37 | Computers in Medicine

Don Johnson

INTRODUCTION

We are currently living in interesting times. The information revolution is the third major revolution, after the agricultural and industrial revolutions. It is affecting everyone today, especially the physician. The computer provides the physician immediate access to educational resources through the World Wide Web and from free medline searches (available at http://www.medscape.com). The physician has improved communication with colleagues through email. Computerizing billing and patient accounts enhances office practice. The patient benefits through improved educational information available on the World Wide Web. The major use of computers in medicine still remains in the area of practice management, where a good computer system can improve the efficiency and cost-effectiveness of your practice. Communication is the future of the Internet, and computers are the tools to connect to the internet.

What Hardware Do You Need?

The basic computer should be a 486 PC, with a modem of 28.8. You can improve the efficiency with a Pentium loaded with Windows 95 and a ISDN line or a cable modem. Most people have to be satisfied with the 28.8 modem for home use.

What Software Do You Need?

You need to have a TCP/IP connection with PPP. The connection to the net is made with a browser, either Netscape or the Internet Explorer from Microsoft. If you buy a new Pentium computer, with Windows 95 loaded, and an internal modem, you will only have to get an Internet service provider. Even that used to be difficult, but with Windows 95 you use the built-in TCP/IP found in the dial up networking, sign on with the Microsoft network and you'll be up and running in a few hours.

Access to the Internet

The access to the net can be made with a local service provider, a national service provider (e.g., sympatico from Bell telephone), or by a commercial provider. The main commercial providers are AOL (America Online), CompuServe, The Microsoft Network, and

Prodigy. The advantage of the commercial providers is that they are very easy for the novice. I initially started with a commercial provider and then switched to a local provider, to obtain unlimited connection at a fixed cost. It sometimes can be difficult to stop your service to some of the companies without actually cutting up your Visa card! Be sure that your phone connection is a local call, and not long distance, or you will quickly run up a large phone bill.

WORD PROCESSING, BILLING, AND ACCOUNTING

Every country in the world has a different system of billing and accounting, but everyone can benefit from computerizing this aspect of practice. Word processing is essential in orthopedics for patient documentation and consultants' referrals. Most orthopedic surgeons still prefer to dictate their notes, and have their secretary transcribe the note on a word processor. The typewriter is used only occasionally for filling in forms.

The holy grail of the paperless office is still unrealistic at present. In fact, I think that we have increased our paper use and not decreased it with the current state of computerization in our office. The next steps in arriving at the computerized medical chart are so far very expensive and difficult to justify in our cost containment atmosphere.

Voice recognition software is available now, but is still slower than normal typing. The best program is Dragon—Naturally Speaking (www.dragonsys.com). When this improves then the dictation will go directly into the work processor. The current speed is about 100 words per minute, at 95% accuracy. This needs to be 99.9% accurate before it becomes widely used in business, and that may take 5 years. Accounting and billing software greatly reduce the amount of time required for the secretary to process the data. In Ontario all our bills are submitted by codes on a floppy disc twice a month to one central billing office. In our sports medicine clinic, one secretary does all the billing for two orthopods, and five family physicians in 8 h per week. Software is available for appointments and scheduling, but works only in low-volume practice with appointments booked in advance.

PATIENT DATABASES

The more exciting area for future development is with *patient databases*. At present there are several available that allow the physician to record the history and physical examination on a hand-held computer, such as the Apple Newton, and have this data immediately entered on the main computer by infrared transfer. From this information the consultants note may be composed and printed. This is mailed to the appropriate source (emailed in the future).

SPORTS MEDICINE APPLICATIONS

An onfield reporting version of Apple Newton software is available from Aristar.com. This allows you to enter the history, physical examination, and initial treatment plan on the sidelines. The standard injury reporting form that the NHL and CFL uses can be adapted to this software. Documenting the examination and treatment at the time of injury is much more accurate than recording it after the fact. More practical is the use of a regular laptop with the documentation software loaded and ready to enter data in the training room. This is one area for concern in sports medicine, the documentation of injuries when traveling with sports teams. With the laptop and appropriate software this task is easy and accurate.

INTERNET

The use of the Internet to search for information is hampered at present by slow speed connections. With the cable modem (100× faster than a 33-phone modem) and other faster connections, this may become a more important means of obtaining medical information during the working day. The current statistics are that one in three Canadians is online in 1997 (Angus Reid survey, 1997). The medical community online rate is probably higher.

Email

Communication has been revolutionized by email. This form of asynchronous communication is the best thing to happen since sliced bread. You can send a note to your colleague that can be answered later. This is similar to the fax, but with no ongoing expense.

The use of email for list serves, or mailing lists, has also extended our communication of medical problems. The problem case is posted on a orthopedic or arthroscopy list (a mailing list of interested members), the case appears when I open my email. I then can send a reply back to the individual who sent it, or to the list for everyone to read. The outcome is a little like grand rounds, but with 250 members from around the world giving an opinion on the case.

Examples of these mailing lists are:

- orthopedic@weston.com
- arthroscopy@aana.org
- sport-med@mailbox.ac.uk
- AMSSMNET@msu.edu

World Wide Web Sites

The best method of searching is to use Yahoo, found at yahoo.com. At this site all the web sites are categorized according to topics. You can search down through the categories or you can go to search and enter the topic. Yahoo searches the titles of the web pages. If you use Excite or Alta Vista, then you can search into the pages of the sites. If you want to narrow the search further, enter quotes around the words. For example "anterior cruciate ligament" searches for the three words used together.

The *web sites* of orthopedic organizations offer their members various services; members directories, abstract forms for the next meeting, educational books and materials, and summaries from previous scientific meetings. When faster connections become available, then it will be possible to view video of operative procedures, and the complete slide and audio digital capture of the previous scientific meeting. This will be especially important for the instructional courses. The problem of how to charge for this service will be solved by secure credit card transactions or by a secure member's password.

Examples of some sites of orthopedic and sports medicine intrest are:

- http:///www.aana.org, the Arthroscopy Association of North America
- http://www.aaos.org, The American Academy of Orthopedic Surgeons
- http://www.sportsmed.org, The American Association of Orthopedic Sports Medicine

There are numerous other web sites of orthopaedic information. The best summary of all the major sites may be found at http://www.virtualkamloops.com/cloughs/orthlink.html. This lists all the sites that are related to orthopedics. The Wheeless online orthopedic textbook is available to read online at http://www.medmedia.com. There is a sports medicine button to connect to sports medicine articles. If you want to do a medline search then go to http://www.medscape.com/ and use the free online search. You have to pay to receive photocopies of the articles mailed out to you. There is a button on the home page of medscape that connects to orthopedics and sports medicine. An orthopedic web site that has some PowerPoint presentations and case examples with x-rays and clinical photos is http://www.bonehome.com. Another interactive sports medicine site is "sports doc" at http://www.medfacts.com. The *Journal of Arthroscopy* has abstracts of the latest journal at www.arthroscopyjournal.org. The sports science site is at: www.sportsci.org. The commercial newsletter "Orthopedics Today" is at www.slackline.com/bone/ortoday/othome.htm. A good site on ACL reconstruction with drawings and photos of the operation is www.datacomm.ch/~kruzli. An orthopedic and trauma site from the UK is www.worldortho.com. An online sports medicine journal is at www.cewl.com. The Hughston Orthopedic and Sports Medicine Clinic is at www.hughston.com. The home page of Dr. Rick Hammesfahr is www.arthroscopy.com. Dr. Kevin Stone's web site is at www.stoneclinic.com.

ELECTRONIC PRESENTATIONS

PowerPoint has proven to be an excellent software package for presentations. Now the presentation can be projected from the laptop by an LCD projector to a large audience. There is no need to make slides. Images and video may also be incorporated into the project. The multimedia may be saved as html and put up on the web site for later viewing and downloading.

ELECTRONIC PUBLISHING

Journals, newsletters, and books are all available in multimedia format on CD-ROM. The *Journal of Bone and Joint Surgery* is now available for the past years, and now even the current editions are on a CD-ROM. The *Journal of Arthroscopy and Sports Medicine* is also available on CD.

The *Sports Medicine Digest* is available in traditional paper format from Lippincott-Raven publishers. *Practical Arthroscopy* is available in traditional paper format from Sports Medicine International, PO Box 15043, Sarasota, FL 34277. *Practical Arthroscopy* is also available online at http://www.newsltr.com/arthro.

Macromedia is a complex and powerful authoring tool for electronic publications. In many respects this is far superior to books for learning. Think how much more vivid a video of the pivot shift examination is, rather than a textbook description of the same. The textbook of *Operative Arthroscopy* is available on a CD-ROM with video of arthroscopic ACL reconstruction techniques.

Electronic publishing is certainly much easier and faster than the traditional methods. Instead of the text and prints having to be submitted separately, you can edit the layout on your own desktop publishing program, such as Microsoft Publisher or Adobe PageMaker. This is then immediately available to print or to change to html and put on the web site.

Many of these programs are expensive, and beyond the reach of the busy practitioner to become proficient.

Vivatexte is an alternate program, based on a Windows help file. I have opted to use this program because it may be mastered in a few hours and allows me to publish my information on a floppy disc or CD-ROM. This can be read by any computer running Windows (including Windows 3.1). The cost of writable CD-ROM drives has dropped to about $500.

With this technology most university departments or individuals can put out their own educational material in a very cost-effective way. Some of the projects that we have authored electronically on Vivatexte are:

• Technique of joint and soft tissue injections
• Technique of ACL reconstruction with semitendinosis and Bio-screw fixation
• Clinical examination of the knee
• Osteoarthritis of the medial compartment of the knee

FUTURE

Education and the Internet

Will the Internet revolutionize the process of teaching, and replace the current methods? I do not think so. I still believe that medical teaching will be done with a teacher, a student, and a patient. Even in 10 years there will be no substitute for this one-on-one, live, real-time, hands-on experience. So, where will the Internet fit in? I think that it will add to our experience, especially in quickly searching for information, and discussion of interesting cases. The latter may be one of the greatest benefits. An interesting case, with images and even video, will be presented and hundreds of comments from around the world will be posted. This is much like a grand rounds format.

The standard forms of communication by peer review articles and hard copy magazines will continue. The Internet will only provide that information faster. However, there is no substitute for lounging around home in your favorite chair reading a journal.

Voice Recognition

Voice recognition programs are still in the developmental phase. When they become faster and easier to use they will open up the capabilities of the computer to many more people. There are many physicians who would use the computer more, but their typing skills are lacking enough to make the experience painful. When they are able to talk into a microphone and see the words appear at 60 words per minute, then it will make sense to dictate letters and patient notes, avoiding the extra expense of a transcriptionist.

Now with a software program we can use the computer for long distance phone calls without paying long distance rates. I think the phone companies will probably not let this software develop too much farther!

Video Conferencing

With the addition of an inexpensive videocamera ($100 black and white) you can send video and voice to another computer with the same software. Once we have higher-speed modems and more bandwidth, this may become more popular. We keep hearing that next year everyone will be using this, but so far it is limited by the bandwidth of the services.

Cable modems are 100× faster than the 28.2 that we now use. Bill Gates seems to be banking on this, since he bought controlling shares in Comcast, one of the large U.S. cable companies, last year. This technology would eliminate some of the traveling to meetings for information that we now have to do. There is, however, no substitute for the one-on-one interaction that occurs during the meeting or over dinner. This may be most helpful for committees to plan meetings and conferences.

IMAGE AND VIDEO INTEGRATION
IN DOCUMENTS AND COMMUNICATION

The next logical step is the integration of the digital video of patient's clinical examination, digital capture of arthroscopy images, x-rays, and videos of operative procedures into the patient's chart. This is then stored in medical records and available on hospital Intranets. This information is then accessed with a secure password, when the patient makes a postoperative visit to your office. Some parts of the record would be available to print, such as the operative record and the arthroscopy image, to give the patient or send to the referring physician.

In summary, in the medicine of the future, you are either going to drive the bus or be waiting at the bus stop wondering if this is the right bus line. Or, it is going to be like the Middle Ages—you will be either a peasant or a landowner. In this digital age of information, you had better know how to access and use the information available.

38 | Heat and Cold Injuries

Kris D. Stowers

Exercise in the extremes of the environment creates special problems for the body as it attempts to maintain normal internal body temperature. Exposure to the heat and cold, wind, humidity, and rain can lead to severe and permanent injury, even death. Since our bodies are actually over 50 percent water, maintenance of temperature is influenced greatly by our fluid status.

Our body temperature is impacted through conduction, convection, radiation, and evaporation. Air is a poor conductor of heat, while water is a very good conductor of heat. Therefore, in warming or cooling the body the temperature can be greatly affected by exposure to water. Convection depends on wind to remove the heat or cold from the skin while radiation picks up or removes heat through electromagnetic waves. Evaporation releases heat at a rate of 0.58 kcal/mL. At temperatures less than 35ºC, we lose 75 percent of heat through convection and radiation. At temperatures greater than this we rely almost exclusively on evaporation.

Evaporation is directly affected by a combination of temperature and humidity commonly called the heat index. It is critical, therefore, to evaluate the environment for heat stress by determining the heat index. This is commonly done through the use of a wet bulb thermometer. Even at mild temperatures when the humidity is elevated the heat index can be elevated significantly enough to cause severe physical injury during exercise. Guidelines are frequently given in charts such as in Table 38-1. However, they become difficult to follow in certain areas of the country. In some regions the heat index is always at a very high-risk status and practice or competition could not take place for months at a time if the athlete were to avoid the higher risk days. Therefore, consideration must be given to many factors, including previous acclimation, fitness status, physical condition, and medication usage.

Heat production during exercise can be extremely high, producing muscle temperatures 15 to 20 times that of muscles at rest. This increase can generate 1000 kcal/h which the body must eliminate. The radiant activity of the sun during outdoor sporting events can increase the body temperature an additional 150 kcal/h. Other difficulties of cooling the body during exercise are created by the cooling mechanism itself, as the evaporation of fluid creates a potential deficit in fluid balance. A 1 percent loss of fluid from the body will increase the body core temperature another 0.1 to 0.4ºC and increase the heart rate eight beats per minute.

769

TABLE 38-1 Temperature Cascades for Activity Modification Based on Wet Bulb Globe

Temperature (°C/°F)	Flag	ACSM Road Race	MSHSL Heat & Cold Guide	Youth Soccer Guide	Military Guide (Barthell 1990)
<10/50	White	Increased hypothermia risk	Hypothermia risk		
10/50 to 18/65	Green	Low risk hyperthermia and hypothermia	Normal activity	Normal play	
18/65 to 23/73	Yellow	Caution (moderate hyperthermia risk)	Decrease intensity	Add quarter breaks and allow free access to fluids	
23/73 to 28/82	Red	Extreme caution (High hyperthermia risk)	Heat sensitive participants withdraw, others slow pace and decrease intensity	Shorten games or allow unlimited substitution; add quarter breaks and allow free access to fluids	Caution for heat stroke

		Extreme high hyperthermia risk Cancel or postpone	No competition or practice recommended	Establish alternate schedule in advance to move mid-day games to early and late hours; and all of above or cancel	Discretion Unseasoned—no heavy exercise
>28/82	Black				
>30/85				Cancel	Suspend exercise <3 weeks training
>31/88					Curtail <12 weeks hot weather training
>32/90					Suspend all training and exercises

Heat injury includes many types from skin damage to brain injury and even death. Unfortunately the most severe, heat stroke, can lead to death and occurs without warning in approximately 80 percent of the cases. Much more common is heat fatigue, which may even go unnoticed.

Heat fatigue is associated with mild dehydration and poor acclimation to the environment. This produces a generalized malaise and fatigue and may lead to a mild decrease in performance both mentally and physically. This is often noticed in early training or can be associated with seasonal changes in the springtime or summer as temperature and humidity increase producing a greater heat index.

Early Signs of Heat Injury
Weight loss
Diarrhea
Irritability
Cramping
Nausea/Vomiting
Confusion
Headaches
Don't rely on skin changes (i.e., redness) or the presence or absence of sweat

The skin injury mentioned above is secondary to solar radiation and is commonly known as a sunburn. There are many reports of increasing frequency of skin cancer felt to be directly related to skin solar injury. Therefore, it is imperative to protect the skin from chronic exposure, as well as acute exposure resulting in skin injury and blistering. The majority of sun exposure during our lifetime occurs in the first two decades of life including blistering sunburns which may be related to melanoma. Skin can be protected through limiting exposure by clothing, use of sunscreen (with SPF greater than 15), and limiting time in the sun. It is important to apply sunscreen several minutes before sun exposure as well as to reapply after exposure to water (swimming or perspiration). Not only is the skin damaged by solar radiation, but the skin injury and inflammation decrease the ability to exchange heat, thus increasing the difficulty of eliminating body heat during exercise.

Heat cramps receive a lot of attention during competition and can have a major impact on the athletic performance of teams and individuals. In my experience, cramps are not only related to heat and conditioning of the individual athlete but are multifactorial. Cramping may vary from a solitary muscle cramp in the hands or particularly the calf muscle to entire body cramps, removing an individual from athletic competition. Certainly fluid status plays a very powerful role, but I have seen well-hydrated, well-conditioned athletes cramp even in cool, dry environments. I have found that electrolyte status, glycogen stores, anxiety, and acclimation all impact cramping as well. Electrolyte replacement appears to be very significant in the first few weeks of acclimation when cramping appears to be most frequent and is often associated with dehydration. I have recommended that athletes increase their sodium intake by salting their food the first few weeks of practice and it has appeared to reduce the frequency of cramps. I have not seen a significant change in cramping through supplementation with potassium or the intake of bananas. However, I have had several athletes and even elderly patients who have eliminated their cramping with magnesium supplementation. Carbohydrate replacement following strenuous exercise has also reduced the incidence of cramping, again particularly in the first few weeks of increasing strenuous activity. The first few hours after exercise are the most valuable in replenishing utilized glycogen stores.

In spite of appropriate acclimation and fluid and electrolyte status, some athletes continue to cramp during competition, even when the competition is much shorter in duration than a typical practice session. Therefore, I began using low-dose anxiolytics in some athletes who cramped on a repetitive basis. Through the use of this very low dose, cramping has been almost completely eliminated during competition with no adverse effect on competition.

It must be remembered, however, that fluid status is critical and must be maintained not only to reduce cramping but to maintain the ability to eliminate heat produced during activity. A simple rule to follow is to drink approximately 8 oz of water for every 15 min of athletic competition. When athletes wait until they are thirsty to drink fluid, there is already a very large fluid deficit. Fluid that is flavored and cooled is usually tolerated better for replacement and is therefore more likely to be consumed during competition. It is not necessary to consume the electrolyte/carbohydrate replacement fluids during competition as water is an excellent source. Although most athletes prefer a flavored drink, it is important to remember that fluids with high carbohydrate concentrations like carbonated sodas and fruit drinks are slowly absorbed and therefore make poor replacements during competition. During prolonged activity (greater than 1 h), electrolyte/carbohydrate fluid replacements have been demonstrated to improve performance. When appropriate fluid is available, the rate limiting step is oral intake, so it is critical to encourage athletes to continue to consume fluids throughout competition.

Dehydration
___
1 lb = 1 pint of fluid
2% weight loss impairs mental and work performance
Replacement fluids are tolerated best when:

1. Cooled
2. Flavored
3. Low carbohydrate

Do not wait for thirst.
Do not restrict fluids during activity.
___

When cramping is isolated to a solitary muscle, stretching appears to resolve this most of the time. When cramping involves multiple muscle groups, it is best managed with IV fluid replacement. I usually use lactated ringers initially, then if cramping persists (or if there is felt to be a significant fluid deficit), I add another liter of d5 normal saline as persistent cramping may elevate potassium levels secondary to muscle injury. If cramping persists in spite of fluid replacements, low doses of IV valium usually eliminate them.

Acclimation to extremes of environment takes several exposures. During this time several physiologic exchanges need to occur. Included among them is an increase in vascular fluid volume to accommodate the large fluid loss associated with perspiration increases. The rate of perspiration markedly increases with conditioning. The intestinal tract can be trained to absorb more fluid by drinking during exercise and may absorb 1 to 2 L per hour. Heart rate and core temperature decrease as exercise tolerance increases. At a minimum, 8 to 10 exposures are required over a 1-week period. Each exposure should be a minimum of 30 min. An athlete can lose the level of acclimation during periods of no training, therefore during injury it is important to continue some of the rehab in the extremes of heat before returning athletes to their previous level of activity.

Scheduling practice time is also helpful during acclimation. It is best to begin practice periods when the extremes of the environment are minimized, particularly in the early morning and later evening when possible. This helps avoid practicing in the extremes of the heat index. Scheduling frequent breaks initially for cooling and fluid replacement are also very important. The breaks can be manipulated depending on the heat index and the acclimation level of the athletes. It is extremely important to never withhold fluids and a very good practice to have fluid replacement available at all times during practice.

Maintain adequate hydration
Monitor heat index
Get adequate sleep
Increase salt intake first few weeks of exercise
Eat carbohydrates after exercise
Schedule time for breaks, acclimation and fluid replacement
Monitor weight before and after practice
Wear appropriate clothing
Be aware of medications and illness if possible

Heat exhaustion is another form of heat illness characterized by fatigue and malaise but also by dizziness, nausea, and headache. Heat exhaustion is a serious medical problem and may be the only warning sign prior to heat stroke. Heat exhaustion is associated with increasing core body temperature and dehydration of 1 to 2 percent or greater. Mental performance and physical ability are definitely reduced with even mild levels of dehydration. The main difference between heat stroke and heat exhaustion is the absence of mental status changes. As core temperature continues to rise, heat exhaustion leads to heat stroke and potential brain injury. There is confusion over the presence of dry skin versus continued perspiration with heat stroke. In athletes heat stroke is very frequently associated with continued perspiration. Therefore do not wait to be concerned until the skin is hot and dry, waiting to do so will lead to serious complications. An interesting study on Israeli soldiers demonstrated that sleep deprivation was a very significant factor in the frequency of heat stroke.

The incidence of both of these illnesses, heat exhaustion and heat stroke, is directly related to body temperature and fluid status. Therefore in treating these individuals, the critical thing is to cool and replace the fluid deficit as quickly as possible. The first step is to monitor the respiratory and cardiac status. As quickly as possible, move the athlete to a cool area. Fluid replacement is best if it can be administered orally, however if there is any neurologic impairment, the intravenous route needs to be used. Since air does not have great conductive capacity compared to water, fluid immersion is much more effective at reducing body temperature than fans, mysts or ice packs. Placing a childs swimming pool in a cool shaded place is a simple thing that can allow rapid cooling in an emergency. Removing the clothing quickly on the field can improve some heat loss as well.

Treatment
Initiate emergency CPR if necessary
Contact EMS if necessary
Removal from heat
Initiate fluid replacement
Oral if alert
IV if severe
Immersion in cool water

Heat exhaustion and heat stroke are both serious medical illnesses and therefore require several days of rest before returning to the playing capacity in order to allow the body time to recover. Practicing will be limited following heat exhaustion. All cases of heat stroke need to be carefully monitored and evaluated before returning to competition.

Remove From Activity When
Hallucination
Visual disturbance
Loss of coordination
Severe cramping
Persistent vomiting

Preparation
CPR training
Telephone
Sunscreen
IV setups
Lactated Ringers/D5 normal saline
IV Valium
Cool water immersion (kiddie pool)

Although heat illness is frequently said to be a preventable illness, even with extreme caution and preparation it still may occur. It is important to have a plan to reduce the frequency and severity of injuries as well as a plan to treat as quickly as possible. As mentioned in the discussion on cramping two of the most important factors in prevention are acclimation and maintaining appropriate fluid status. One way of monitoring the fluid status is to weigh the athletes before and after practice. This way an athlete who is developing a fluid deficit can be detected, corrected, and monitored more closely. As an athlete becomes more dehydrated urine color may become darker and have a stronger odor.

Clothing and equipment have an impact on the ability of the body to exchange heat. Maintaining maximum skin exposure to allow for perspiration helps heat exchange, but solar radiation can damage the skin. Therefore it is best to wear loose-fitting, light-colored clothing. Lighter colors decrease the heat absorbed from solar radiation. Hats also decrease the solar radiation on the face and head. Athletes with extra tape and equipment decrease the exposed surface area for heat exchange. During breaks in the shade it is helpful to remove head gear.

Other factors to consider as preventative measures include health status, medication, obesity, and age. Obesity is not only a demonstration of decreased conditioning but also represents a decrease in surface to mass area making it more difficult to eliminate heat. This represents a high-risk group, especially if there is limited acclimation. An unconditioned athlete produces more heat for the same activity than a conditioned athlete. Even a conditioned athlete who is only acclimated to a cool environment tolerates heat better than an unconditioned athlete from an adverse environment.

Health status and medication create several problems which impact heat injury. First of all, a recent febrile illness can reset the set point that regulates body temperature, increasing the risk of heat injury for the next several days after the illness has resolved. Recent gastroenteritis with nausea, vomiting, or even decreased carbohydrate or fluids can greatly impact the frequency of heat injury and the tolerance of exercise. Nausea and diarrhea have a very significant influence on the frequency of cramping and intensity of cramps in my experience. Not only does the loss of fluids create a problem but the absorption may be affected for the next several days.

Medication during acute illness impacts heat tolerance. Antihistamines and decongestants can impact the body's responsiveness. Chronic illnesses and the medication required to treat these problems can also make heat regulation more difficult. Diuretic use poses a special problem by eliminating fluid and altering the electrolyte status. Medications that affect vascular tone, fluid status, cardiac output, and mental status affect thermoregulation. Alcohol not only affects the fluid status but can impair the mental response and the ability to make appropriate decisions.

Diabetes not only affects the sugar/glycogen status, but also affects autonomic controls which can decrease the tolerance to heat exposure. Anemias can obviously make a difference in cardiac output and fluid status and response to stress. There are also some studies that place at increased risk athletes who have sickle cell trait secondary to sudden death associated with heat exposure.

Children are more at risk than their adult counterparts. They are more dependent on convection for removal of heat and in higher temperatures absorb more heat from the environment. Children perspire at a slower rate for the same amount of work as an adult.

Therefore it is especially important to include more frequent breaks, increase fluid intake, and avoid the heat of day with practice.

COLD INJURIES

Cold weather exposure can also pose serious risks. Not only is exposed skin at risk, but the lungs, and the entire body can be injured by cold environments. Athletes of all kinds can have difficulty breathing in cold weather. Bronchospasm is frequently experienced with the decrease in humidity and cold air irritation. Bronchial irritation can produce burning pain, wheezing, coughing up blood and may last several weeks. This is sometimes called frozen lung. When the diaphragm is irritated, shoulder and stomach pain may also result. This is treated by warm humidified air, rest, and increased fluids.

Cold Injuries

Skin
Chilblains
Frostnip
Frostbite
Lungs
Bronchospasm
Frozen lung
Hypothermia

Skin exposure can be mild or very destructive leading to permanent injury and death. Skin injury is frequently described as chilblains, frostnip, and frostbite. Areas at greatest risk include the ears, nose, hands, fingers, feet and toes. Chilblains occur to exposed skin at temperatures below 60°F. They do not actually result from freezing of the tissue, but possibly from histamine release. The result is erythema, swelling, and pruritis. Treatment is warming and application of ointments like Vaseline. Frostnip is freezing of the skin surface only and can be treated immediately as long as frostbite has not occurred. Warming must take place for treatment and can be done with hand warmers, covering the nose, and blowing air onto the hands. Covering ears with warm hands and warming feet by placing them next to a heat source or simply moving them inside shoes may help restore heat and circulation. Frost nip may cause surface numbness, skin whiteness, and may go unnoticed.

Frostbite is freezing deeper than the surface and involves the thickness of the tissue. This requires outside temperatures below freezing. Damage can be severe with ice crystals forming and damaging the cells. As skin freezes, it initially feels cold, then becomes painful and finally numb. Thawing the skin causes pain and burning, and should only be done when there is no risk of refreezing. Blisters may develop but should not be opened because of the risk of serious infection. The best way to thaw is hot water immersion (104 to 133°F). Do not rub snow or anything else into the skin for thawing or you may damage the tissue. Frozen tissue may develop a black eschar which should also be left alone. Eventually this eschar will fall off.

Prolonged cold exposure (greater than 1 h) to exposed skin reduces the blood flow and decreases the sensations of touch and pain. Manual dexterity and agility are also decreased. The skin is more sensitive when exposed to moisture and/or wind. Therefore it is imperative to keep skin covered and dry in wet high wind exposure.

Treatment of Skin Injuries
Chilblains and frostnip
Rapid warming
Protection from reinjury
Frostbite
Thaw in hot water (104 to 133°F)
Thaw only if no risk of refreezing
Use pain medicine liberally as rewarming is very painful
Do not:
Remove blisters or blackened skin
Rub with snow
Warm with water greater than 133°F

Hypothermia is a result of a reduction of core temperature below 35°C (95°F). As with heat injury, severity of injury increases as the body temperature varies from normal. When the body temperature decreases below 36°C, the athlete should be removed from exposure. Hypothermia can have a powerful role in athletics, reducing ability and removing atheletes from competition. In the military, for example, 10 percent of casualties in World War II were secondary to cold injuries.

Signs of hypothermia are usually gradual and progressive, including confusion, drowsiness, slowed slurred speech, frequent stumbling, trembling hands, withdrawn bizarre behavior, shallow breathing, decreased blood pressure, weak pulse, removal of clothing, decreased coordination, unconsciousness and altered vision. Hypothermia often occurs between 30 and 50°F as people underestimate the impact of being wet and the impact of the wind. This nonfreezing cold injury can occur particularly when the hands and feet cannot be kept warm and dry.

Body heat loss occurs through several mechanisms. Respiration can produce heat losses of up to 10 to 20 percent. This can be reduced by covering the mouth and nose area with wool or other material. This depends on air humidity, the drier the air, the greater the evaporative loss. Heat loss also occurs through evaporation, conduction, radiation, and convection.

Evaporation of perspiration leads to heat loss. Wet clothing next to the skin greatly enhances the removal of heat from the skin and lowers body temperature. Therefore, the ability to keep dry clothing next to the skin is of utmost importance in maintaining core body temperature by reducing evaporation.

Conduction occurs through contact with cold surfaces, of particular importance during cold water immersion, as water increases conductive capacity up to 25 times. Therefore clothing that provides insulation and limits water absorption is excellent. Wool and synthetic fabrics (pologuard, polypropylene, fiberfill, quollofil) have good wet characteristics.

Radiation heat loss occurs through the skin into the cold environment and can be decreased by covering exposed areas, especially the head and hands. Convection occurs when the body heat is removed by wind (wind chill factor). The air warmed next to the skin can be maintained by protecting the skin with wind resistant clothing on the outer layer.

As with heat illness, cold tolerance is greatly dependent on hydration status. Maintaining adequate hydration remains critical to thermoregulation in both hot and cold weather extremes. Dehydration reduces circulation and leads to increase of risks to injuries of the extremities. Adequate nutrition is also necessary in order to generate the energy required to maintain core temperature.

When core temperature is maintained by exercise or any physical activity, an athlete who stops to rest or is unable to continue secondary to fatigue is at high risk of hypothermia. Temperature may drop rapidly following competition as heat production from activity is decreased. In the field away from medical care, particular concern is necesssary when a person is fatigued. This person should be removed from cold and warmed as quickly as possible to prevent the rapid fall in temperature that can occur.

Hypothermia

Type	Body Temperature	Recovery
Mild	Less than 90°F	Good
Moderate	80 to 90°F	Fair, permanent injury possible
Severe	Less than 80°F	Poor, permanent injury probable

Do not forget that mental status can quickly be impaired with even mild hypothermia.

Hypothermia can be classified as mild, moderate, and severe. Mild hypothermia is present when body temperature is reduced but maintained above 90°F. The person will feel chilled with numb like sensation in the skin, stiff, clumsy fingers and slowed and improper responses will develop. If core temperature is below 93.2°F temporary amnesia may occur. Shivering will develop as the body attempts to maintain adequate core temperature. Shivering can increase basal heat production by up to three times. Shivering is a warning sign that basal temperature is decreasing and should never be ignored. When your body begins to lose heat faster than it produces heat, you may spontaneously exercise to increase heat production. When this fails to maintain the temperature, shivering begins.

What To Watch For:

Shivering and the cessation of shivering
Poor judgment
Exercising to keep warm
Skin discoloration

Moderate hypothermia represents a drop in core temperature to between 80 to 90°F and is associated with decreasing muscular coordination, stumbling, confusion, decreased cooperation, and lethargy. Cardiac arrhythmias may also begin to occur at temperatures below 90°F. Difficulty standing usually indicates core temperature of less than 90°F.

Severe hypothermia occurs when core temperature is below 80°F. Shivering stops as there is depletion of energy, progressive mental deterioration, incoherence, and irrational behavior. Exposed skin may be blue.

As mentioned above, hypothermia, even in mild and moderate cases, can produce impaired mental performance and decision making. Therefore prevention is best performed by preparation. Prevention begins with adequate nutrition, fluids, clothing, and companions.

Prevention

Maintain hydration status
Wear appropriate clothing
Keep hands, feet, head all well protected
    Protect all exposed areas
Get to warm environment at 1st sign of cold injuries
Keep dry and protected from wind
Have a companion with you
Avoid alcohol

Clothing is a critical factor in preventing hypothermia. Clothing should be worn in layers. Ideally the layer closest to the skin will wick away moisture from the body. When clothing is wet, approximately 90 percent of the insulating value is lost. Cotton and down provide little thermal protection when wet. Wearing a wet shirt is less effective than wearing no shirt at all. It is wise to bring extra clothing to change into after activity to decrease the amount of heat loss from evaporation. Wool is much better closer to the skin, or a synthetic material that wicks away moisture like polypropylene covered by another layer of wool would be much more effective. Wind quickly removes the moisture and heat from the body so an outer wind resistant layer, such as nylon or Gortex, is very helpful. A tremendous amount of body heat is lost from the head, so it is important to protect the head as well. The thermoregulatory system is greatly influenced by the hands and feet, so appropriate socks, footwear, and gloves need to be considered with the same principles mentioned above. It is imperative that shoes and socks fit appropriately and not minimize insulation. Clothing that is too tight can decrease the blood flow and greatly increases the risk of skin injuries. This is often seen with elastic that is too tight around the wrists and ankles, causing damage to the hands and feet.

Clothing
Wear synthetic "wicking" material next to skin
Insulating middle layer (wood is excellent)
Outer wind and water resistant layer
Wear a hat that covers exposed areas well
Wear well-fitted shoes, boots, and socks
Wear gloves
Do Not:
Allow wet clothing next to skin
Use elastic compression that decreases blood flow to the extremities

In emergency situations when a person is unprepared for cold weather, it is wise to take advantage of surrounding material and sources of heat. For example, insulation can be removed from car seats in an accident or a vehicle trapped in severe weather. Sharing a sleeping bag with another person can help minimize heat loss. Creating a shelter to avoid wind and water exposure also cuts down on risk of hypothermia. Do not encourage people to exercise after hypothermia as a means of increasing body temperature. This may result in cardiac arrythymias as the cold blood rapidly returns to the heart.

As with heat injury, risk of cold injury increases with medical illness. Included are those with thyroid abnormalities, stroke, or paralysis who experience decreasing awareness of cold injuries. Arthritis and prolonged immobilization, as well as circulatory problems that decrease blood flow may contribute to cold injuries.

Many medications which may impact circulation or judgment can also make a difference. Alcohol consumption increases blood flow to the skin enhancing heat loss and decreases awareness of skin surface temperature changes in addition to impairing decisions. Children and the elderly are also at increased risk. The elderly can become hypothermic in temperatures as low as 65°F. In contrast to heat injury, increased body fat is somewhat protective. Larger, fatter people are less affected by cold exposure: the thicker the fat, the greater the insulation.

Diuretics and vasoconstriction of any kind can decrease available fluids to the skin and increase the risk of hypothermia and skin injuries. Smoking increases the risk of cold injuries because of the vasoconstriction. Training or traveling alone in severe weather is risky as injuries can occur that may prevent further travel and lead to hypothermia. At least let another person know the route of travel and expected duration of activity.

The keys to treatment are drying and warming. It is important to remember, however, to thaw frozen tissue only if there is no chance of refreezing. In the field, remove the injured individual from cold and dry the skin. Do not rub the skin with snow or anything else as this may further damage the tissue. It is critical to remove all wet clothing and then begin rewarming. If the individual is mentally aware, drinking warmed fluids can be helpful, as well as warm packs next to the skin, particularly next to the major arteries. Sharing body contact with another person can increase body temperature if other sources are not available. To thaw frozen skin, hot water immersion is most effective with temperatures between 40 and 45°C. Do not use water any warmer than this without risk of more severe injury.

Treatment

Remove person from cold and wet environment and clothing
Warm and dry body as rapidly as possible
Hot water immersion is best for extremities
Give warmed fluids IV or oral depending on mental status
Use other heat sources as available for warming (other body heat)

Do Not:
Use exercise to rewarm a hypothermic patient

If a person is suffering from cold exposure and mental status is affected, try to keep the person awake. Warm IV fluids if available can be very helpful to rewarming. The chance of permanent injury greatly increases with decreasing core temperatures. With mild hypothermia, recovery is usually very good with little permanent risk. However moderate hypothermia commonly produces some permanent injury and in cases of severe hypothermia, most people do not survive.

Cold water immersion is also important to consider. Water at temperatures below 60°F can have a rapid effect on body temperature. Obviously, body temperature can best be improved by removal from the exposure. Do not try to swim, however, unless you can reach safety as this will increase body temperature loss. Keep your head out of water as much as possible and huddle with others if present.

In summary, exercise does take place in the extremes of our environment from sub-zero temperatures to stifling heat, dry to sticky humidity, and potentially wet and windy days. As this is out of our control, we must learn to adapt and prepare ourselves to maximize performance and prevent severe injury. Treatment begins with prevention as much as possible and then with a plan to manage as quickly and effectively as possible.

39 | Knee Braces

R. Timothy Deakon   Rick Zarnett

Despite the tremendous advances in the knowledge of knee-ligament biomechanics, injury, and treatment, the indications and efficacy of the practice of knee bracing remain less clearly defined. A lack of compelling research on the subject and lack of consensus among the orthopedic community led the Sports Medicine Committee of The American Academy of Orthopaedic Surgeons to hold a symposium on knee bracing in 1984. The committee categorized braces as either prophylactic, rehabilitative, or functional.

Prophylactic braces are those used to decrease the incidence or severity of knee injuries during sport without impairing the athlete's performance.

Rehabilitative braces are used postoperatively to protect the healing tissues from further injury or to control knee motion during the rehabilitative period. Rehabilitative braces are also used following an injury when nonsurgical treatment is selected.

Functional knee braces are used to provide stability to a knee following a ligamentous injury. A functional knee brace should reduce or eliminate instability but should not deter the athlete from carrying out normal activities or participating in their desired spot. The brace should be comfortable and easy to apply, and should not increase the risk of injury to the athlete.

Prior to the late 1960s, attempts at bracing the unstable knee usually involved modifying an orthosis which had been used in the treatment of neuromuscular disease. Braces specifically designed to stabilize an injured athlete's knee gained higher profile in the late 1960s when Nicholas and Castaglia of the Lenox Hill Hospital developed a brace to support football player Joe Namath's unstable knee. This functional knee brace was designed to control anterior and lateral instability. Later designs of the brace employed derotation straps to address the rotary component associated with anterior cruciate ligament deficiency.

Throughout the 1970s and 1980s a proliferation of functional knee brace designs occurred. Various designs, using both hinge-post strap and hinge-post shell design concepts were marketed. Today there are more than 30 nationally and internationally marketed brands of braces.

PROPHYLACTIC KNEE BRACING

Prophylactic knee bracing remains the most controversial aspect of knee bracing and support. Despite growing enthusiasm for prophylactic knee bracing in the sports of American football and motocross racing a definitive study showing its efficacy has yet to be conducted.

In 1979 Anderson et al.[1] described the use of a lateral hinged knee brace to prevent further injury in an athlete who had suffered a medial collateral ligament injury. They termed this brace "the stabler" and since then the use of prophylactic lateral hinged braces to prevent the knee injuries in American football has become increasingly popular. Studies to determine the effectiveness of this type of bracing have failed to show conclusively a reduction in the number, incidence, or severity of injuries. Hansen et al.[2] found an the incidence of injury to be 11 percent in a nonbraced group versus 5 percent in a braced group and thus concluded that bracing was effective. In contrast, Hewson et al.[3] found no difference in the knee injury rate using a prophylactic knee brace in intercollegiate-level football players. Grace et al.[4] found that players wearing single hinged braces had a higher incidence of injury, as well as an increased number of injuries of the ankle and foot. Dr. Robert Jackson[5] published a retrospective study on professional football players using a prophylactic knee brace and found that the proportion of injuries to be considered major was significantly reduced in those players wearing a prophylactic knee brace although injuries to the anterior cruciate ligament and meniscus were not affected.

A 2-year study of a major college football team by Rovere, Haupt, and Yates[6] found a significant increase in the rate of knee injuries in players wearing prophylactic knee braces. They also found an increase in the number of anterior cruciate ligament injuries in the braced group. They reported increased episodes of muscle cramping and complaints of brace slippage in the braced group. Garrick and Requa,[7] in a statistical analysis of the retrospective studies performed on prophylactic knee bracing in the 1980s, determined that there existed no strong evidence to either support, or recommend against, prophylactic knee bracing in American football. In 1990 Michael Sitler et al.[8] published a prospective randomized study on the efficacy of prophylactic knee bracing in American football from The West Point Military Academy, New York. These authors detected a significant decrease in the incidence of medial collateral ligament injuries and knee injuries in general in defensive players wearing prophylactic knee braces. This finding was not borne out in players in offensive positions. This study was continued in the 1990 and 1991 football seasons at West Point, and again a decreased incidence of all knee injuries and medial collateral ligament injuries was noted.

More recently a multi-center study by Albright and Powell[9] on NCAA Division One college football players, demonstrated a decrease in injury incidence for all offensive and defensive positions during practice situations and for line positions, line backers, and tight ends during both practices and game situations. They also noticed an increase in the incidence of injury rate in players in skilled positions (backs and kickers) during game situations.

Cadaveric studies have not demonstrated any significant protective effect using a single upright lateral hinged knee brace. Lonnie Paulos'[10] group looked at a surrogate limb, braced with a protective knee brace, and showed a significant reduction in the degree of injury force transmitted to the medial collateral ligament by one brace.

Thus it would appear that prophylactic knee bracing can only be recommended for defensive line positions and linebackers in American football.

When contemplating the use of prophylactic knee bracing, it is important to consider the effect the brace may have on the performance of the player and the possible harmful effect the brace may have on an opposing players.

REHABILITATIVE BRACING

Rehabilitative braces are used in the post-injury and post-surgical period primarily to control knee motion and to protect healing tissues. These braces are designed for temporary use and have hinges with easy to adjust motion stops. Anderson et al.[1] were the first to report the use of a single hinge knee brace to more rapidly return athletes with MCL injuries to sport.

As the routine treatment of the ruptured MCL is now nonoperative, a rehabilitative brace is commonly used to protect the medial collateral ligament from repetitive reinjury. Knee extension can be limited in the first 2 to 3 weeks to aid in complete healing of the ligament. Some surgeons prefer to cast a high-grade MCL injury for the first 2 weeks to absolutely prevent recurrent injury. Cawley et al.[11] has investigated the effectiveness of rehabilitative braces in controlling motion and determined that these braces allowed 6 to 18 degrees more motion than the stops would indicate. To accurately limit range of motion the stops should be set at least 10 degrees short of the desired amount.

FUNCTIONAL KNEE BRACING

The first functional knee brace designed for the anterior cruciate ligament deficient knee occurred in the early 1970s when Nicholas and Castaglia of the Lenox Hill Hospital in New York developed the derotation brace. The popularity of this brace among the sports medicine community led to the development and marketing of a wide variety of functional knee braces. Despite the popularity of knee bracing for ligamentous instability research in the area remains incomplete, and in many cases anecdotal. Functional knee braces have been purported to stabilize the unstable knee by means of reducing anteroposterior translation, by reducing rotational instability, and by reducing varus and valgus stresses. Furthermore, functional knee braces have been hypothesized to affect the afferent neural impulses from the injured knee, thereby modifying the muscular control of the unstable knee. Functional knee braces have also been recommended for use in the knee with a partial ligament tear and for protection in the athlete with a reconstructed anterior cruciate ligament.

Literature on the subject can be divided into three groups: (1) general review papers; (2) specific brace type reviews; and (3) biomechanical studies.

General review articles are particularly helpful in providing an overview of the existing literature. Millet and Drez[12] have classified braces into two basic designs (1) hinged post strap and (2) hinged post shell brace. The authors believe that this basic description is too confining and there now exist numerous variants of these two basic design types.

Cawley[13] addresses the current state of functional knee bracing research and the use of knee bracing for skiing and Butler et al.[14] provides a very detailed analysis of the biomechanics of functional brace use, as well as addressing the limitations of using an external orthosis to control abnormal motion of the injured skeletal structure. Ott and Clancy[15] published a review of functional knee braces with a concise documentation and interpretation of bracing studies to date.

Review articles describing specific types of braces are unfortunately largely composed of anecdotal and interpretive data. These articles often recommend specific brace designs without good objective data.

Biomechanical analyses of functional knee bracing can be divided into those involving the use of cadaver models and those involving in vivo analyses of brace function.

Cadaver studies constitute a large body of the present knowledge of the effect of functional knee bracing on knee stability. However cadaver studies do have significant limitations. Cadaver tissues tend to be far less compliant than normal human tissue and a greater variability exists between specimens depending on age and preservation techniques employed, leading to difficulty in reproducing an accurate soft tissue interface between the brace and the underlying bony structures. Furthermore, the involvement of muscle action in knee stability and brace function has been difficult to reproduce in the cadaver setting. Early studies involved non-weightbearing constructs. Baker et al.[16] studied the effect of prophylactic and functional knee braces on strain in the MCL and ACL during application of a valgus force to the foot and found that functional knee braces are more effective than prophylactic braces in resisting abduction and rotational stresses in both flexion and extension.

Wojtys[17] tested cadaveric specimens under axial load near full extension and Mortensen et al.[18] incorporated simple quadriceps muscle action when he tested the effect of functional knee braces on knee stability under anteroposterior and rotational forces during axial loading in higher degrees of flexion. These studies demonstrated that the braces were effective in constraining knees to anteroposterior and rotational forces, but at force levels that must be considered subphysiologic. Some of the braces tested actually appeared to overconstrain the knee when tested in axial rotation and one must be aware of the possible negative effect this could have on an athlete's performance in the in vivo setting.

Another group of studies employed the use of instrumented knee ligament testing, or radiographic stereophotogrammetric techniques in evaluating tibial translations and rotation during applied external forces. Jonsson and Karrholm[19] assessed the constraint afforded by functional knee orthoses in the anterior cruciate ligament deficient knee using these radiographic techniques. Their analyses revealed that these braces did reduce anterior tibial translation but not to normal levels. Their studies also showed a reduction in external tibial rotation but not internal tibial rotation. However, the loads exerted on these braced limbs did not approach physiologic levels. Cawley[13] has commented on the use of knee ligament arthrometers when assessing the effectiveness of functional knee braces, and has pointed out that the loads exerted by these devices are subphysiologic and has concluded that the data obtained from these studies is of little clinical use. Nonetheless, studies of this type continue to be performed and published.

Of greater validity in determining the effect of knee bracing on the unstable knee are studies performed in the in vivo setting. Knutzen et al.[20] assessed the effect of a functional knee brace on a reconstructed anterior cruciate ligament deficient knee. He found no statistical difference between the braced and unbraced knees when tested for tibial rotation at 90 degrees of flexion but stated that there appeared to be a slight trend towards reduction of internal rotation in the braced subjects. One can debate the validity of this study to the normal brace user as most athletes spend little time with the knee flexed 90 degrees and encounter minimal ACL instability at this degree of flexion.

A number of authors have investigated the effect of functional knee bracing on the athlete's performance and endurance. Houston[21] found that there was an increased energy expenditure for endurance type of activities and an increase in blood lactate levels while wearing a functional knee brace. Houston further found that there was a reduced angular limb velocity in the braced, versus the unbraced, limbs. Zetterlund et al.[22] found a similar increase in energy expenditure during an endurance type event, showing an increase in O_2 consumption and heart rate of approximately 5 percent in the braced group. In contrast, Inglehart[23] studied athletes undergoing short-duration speed events and found that the brace had no effect on performance. One can deduce from these studies that the type of activity has a significant impact on whether or not an athlete will benefit from the use of a functional knee brace in the presence of an unstable knee.

Some authors postulate that a knee brace may affect improvement of functional knee stability by altering the afferent input from a proprioceptively altered ACL deficient knee. Using EMG techniques, Branch et al.[24] found knee braces had no effect on muscle firing patterns, amplitude, or duration of muscular activity. They also found a decrease in quadriceps and hamstring activity while performing cutting maneuvers. This may indicate that the braced ACL deficient knee requires less muscular activity to maintain adequate stability and this, in turn, may be a benefit of brace use.

Nemeth et al. studied the electromyographic activity in expert downhill skiers using functional knee braces after anterior cruciate ligament injuries and found increased activity in the hamstrings during certain phases of the skiing motion. These authors suggested that the brace caused an increased or altered afferent input from proprioceptive nerve endings resulting in an adapted motor control pattern which secondarily modified muscle activity and timing.

Beynnon and coworkers[25–27] have contributed greatly to our knowledge of the normal strains on the anterior cruciate ligament during daily activities and the effect of functional knee braces on these strains. This group assessed strain in the anterior cruciate ligament with arthroscopically implanted Hall-effect transducers. Subjects were then examined during daily activities and the activities involved in the rehabilitation of ACL reconstructed knees. They also studied the impact of brace wearing on these strains in both weightbearing and non-weightbearing conditions. These studies demonstrated that functional knees braces reduce strain in the anterior cruciate ligament with internal/external torque forces up to 6N and anteroposteriorly directed forces up to 140N in a non-weightbearing limb. Forces exceeding these values appear to be beyond the constraint of a functional knee brace in the non-weightbearing setting. However they did find that a functional knee brace was more effective in protecting the ACL against excessive strain with higher applied loads in the weightbearing state. These authors also examined the effect of different brace strap tensions on the strain in the ACL under loading conditions and found no difference between the low (22N) and high (45N) strap tension settings indicating that high strap tensions are apparently not necessary to produce the desired constraining effect.

With this information in hand the authors have attempted to provide some practice guidelines to the use of functional knee braces in the clinical setting.

THE PRACTICAL ASPECTS OF FUNCTIONAL KNEE BRACING

Proper brace fit is essential for adequate brace performance. The brace fitter should be aware of the different techniques used by various brace manufacturers to obtain proper brace fitting information. It is important to mark the bony landmarks and to pay attention to existing scars, or future surgical incisions. The brace fitter should familiarize her- or himself with the recommended techniques for a particular brace model. If the recommended technique is a negative cast mold the preferred material for that cast is fiberglass. A fiberglass mold is less likely to be damaged in shipment and it holds the asperities of the limb more rigidly, in turn producing a brace with a more intimate fit. Where the recommendation of the brace manufacturer is for a measurement system to obtain the dimensions of the limb, the brace fitter should become familiar and proficient in using this system.

Most braces are suspended by the superior calf strap. The adequate function of this strap is in turn dependent on an adequate superior calf muscle definition. Instances of poor muscle definition in this area, and the presence of the inverted conically shaped leg, presents a particularly difficult fitting problem for the orthotist. Under these circumstances braces are prone to slippage and malrotation. Caution should be exercised in undertaking fitting of patients with these types of limbs.

Adequate brace performance also depends on the proper application of the brace. It is incumbent on the brace fitter, or orthotist, to instruct the patient in appropriate application of the brace and the appropriate tensioning of the brace straps. Careful attention should be paid to the bony landmarks and the positioning of the hinge(s) of the brace.

Use of a functional, or prestressed, knee brace can lead to loss of muscle strength and the brace wearer should be encouraged to maintain muscle strength in the quadriceps, hamstring, and surrounding muscles by the performance of daily muscle strengthening exercises.

The timing of brace fitting is important. Most braces will accommodate 10 to 15 percent changes in thigh girth, and less than 5 percent changes in calf girth while still functioning adequately. It is important at the time of time brace fitting to take into account adequate rehabilitation of thigh and calf musculature.

New symptoms of instability or pain in a braced individual may be an indication that: (1) the brace hinges or other moving parts have worn out, or the straps are no longer adequately fitting; (2) the patient's musculature may be deficient and the patient may need a further rehabilitation program; (3) the patient has developed new intraarticular pathology; (4) the patient's degree of instability has increased due to these meniscal lesions or loosening of the secondary constraints about the knee, or (5) the patient is noncompliant with use or application of the brace.

PATIENT SELECTION FOR FUNCTIONAL KNEE BRACING

In general bracing is more effective in stabilizing a knee with a low-grade linear instability rather than high-grade rotational instability. A brace is most effective in stabilizing against varus and valgus instabilities and stresses and is less effective against abnormal anterior or posterior motion. It is least effective in stabilizing against rotational instability. When deciding between conservative (physiotherapy and bracing) and surgical management of the unstable knee the ideal brace candidate is one with a mild to moderate, predominantly linear, instability. The patient should have minimal laxity of the secondary constraints, intact menisci and chondral surfaces, a slim build, compliant in use and application of the brace, and participates in sports that involve little pivoting or those in which the knee remains flexed during the activity (i.e., skiing or skating). Patients with high-grade rotational instabilities with significant meniscal or chondral damage and with significant secondary constraint laxity with large difficult-to-fit legs may be better surgical candidates.

Certain sports usually do not require the use of a brace as they do not involve pivoting or lateral movement. These sports are cycling, running on level ground, swimming, and cross-country skiing.

Some sports-governing bodies prohibit the use of braces fabricated with rigid material as they feel this may constitute a danger to the other participants in the sports (e.g., rugby, soccer, and wrestling). Certain sports are ideally suited to brace use as they involve participation with the knee in a flexed position; sports such as downhill skiing, skating, and hockey are examples.

A brace, particularly one fitted with a patellar cup, may also provide a protective function in contact sports such as football, hockey, or motocross racing.

In sports where considerable pivoting occurs with the knee in an extended position and the foot fixed on a rigid surface such as basketball or volleyball, performance of the brace may be enhanced by the use of an extension stop to block or limit the extension. In most cases a 10-degree extension stop will allow knee extension to 0 degrees and a 20-degree extension stop will stop the knee from extending approximately 5 to 10 degrees short of full extension. Extra care should be exercized in fitting of the brace utilizing an extension stop as this will put increased stresses on the pretibial area and may lead to irritation and skin breakdown.

It is always important for the physician and brace fitter to emphasize to the athlete the limitations of a functional knee brace in providing normal stability to an injured knee and allowing the athlete to return to his or her sport of choice.

REFERENCES

1. Anderson G, Zeman SC, Rosenfeld RT: The Anderson knee stabler. *Phys Sports Med* 7:125, 1979.
2. Hansen BL, Ward JC, Diehl RC: The preventive use of the Anderson knee stabiliser in football, *Phys Sports Med* 13:75, 1985.
3. Hewson GF, Medini RA, Wang JB: Prophylactic knee bracing in college football. *Am J Sports Med* 14:262, 1986.
4. Grace TG, Skipper BJ, Newberry JC, et al: Prophylactic knee braces and injury to the lower extremity. *J Bone Joint Surg* 70A: 422, 1988.
5. Jackson RW, Reed SC, Dunbar F: An evaluation of knee injuries in a professional football team—risk factors, type of injuries, and the value of prophylactic knee bracing, *Clin J Sport Med* 1:1, 1991.
6. Rovere GD, Haupt HA, Yates CS: Prophylactic knee bracing in college football. *Am J Sports Med* 15:111, 1987.
7. Garrick JG, Requa RK: Prophylactic knee bracing. *Am J Sports Med* 15:471, 1987.
8. Sitler M, Ryan J, Hopkinson W, et al: The efficacy of a prophylactic knee brace to reduce knee injuries in football. *Am J Sports Med* 18:310, 1990.
9. Albright JP, Powell JW, Smith W, et al: Medial collateral ligament knee sprains in college football. *Am J Sports Med* 22:12, 1994.
10. Paulos LE, France EP, Rosenberg TD, et al: The biomechanics of lateral knee bracing. *Am J Sports Med* 15:419, 1987.
11. Cawley PW, France EP, et al: Comparison of rehabilitation knee braces. *Am J Sports Med* 17:141, 1989.
12. Millet C, Drez D: Knee braces. *Orthopaedics* 10:1777, 1987.
13. Cawley PW, France EP, Paulos LE: The current state of functional knee bracing research. *Am J Sports Med* 19:226, 1991.
14. Butler PB, Evans GA, Rose GK, et al: A review of selected knee orthoses. *Br J Rheumatol* 22:109, 1983.
15. Ott JW, Clancy WG: Functional knee braces. *Orthopaedics* 16:171, 1993.
16. Baker BE, Van Hanswyk E, Bogosian S, et al: A biomechanical study of the static stabilizing effect of knee braces on medial stability. *Am J Sports Med* 15:566, 1987.
17. Wojtys EM, Goldstein SA, et al: A biomechanical evaluation of the Lenox Hill knee brace. *Clin Orthop* 220:179, 1987.
18. Morteson WW, Foreman K, et al: An in vivo study of functional knee orthoses in the ACL disrupted knee. *Orthop Res* 13:520, 1988.

19. Jonsson H, Karrholm J: The stabilizing effect of the knee braces after ACL rupture. *Acta Orthop Scand* 231:29, 1989.

20. Knutzen KM, Bates BT, Hamil J: Knee brace influences on the tibial rotation and torque patterns of the surgical limb. *J Orthop Sports Phys Therap* 6:116, 1984.

21. Houston ME, Goemans PH: Leg muscle performance of athletes with and without knee support braces. *Arch Phys Med Rehab* 63:431, 1982.

22. Zetterlund AE, Serfass RC, Hunter RE: The effect of wearing the complete Lenox Hill derotation brace on energy expenditure during horizontal treadmill running at 161 meters per minute. *Am J Sports Med* 14:73, 1986.

23. Inglehart TK: Strength and motor task performance as effected by the C Ti knee brace in normal healthy males. Innovation Sports, Irvine, CA, 1985.

24. Branch TP, Hunter R, Donath M: Dynamic EMG analysis of anterior cruciate deficient legs with and without bracing during cutting. *Am J Sports Med* 17:35, 1989.

25. Beynnon BD, Flemming BC, Johnson RJ, et al: Anterior cruciate ligament strain behavior during rehabilitation exercises in vivo. *Am J Sports Med* 23:24, 1995.

26. Beynnon BD, Pope MH, Wertheimer CM, et al: The effect of functional knee braces on strain on the anterior cruciate ligament in vivo. *J Bone Joint Surg* 74A:1298, 1992.

27. Beynnon BD, Johnson RJ, et al: The effect of functional knee bracing on the anterior cruciate ligament in the weightbearing and nonweightbearing knee. *Am J Sports Med* 25:353, 1997.

40 | Orthotics

Lloyd Nesbitt

INTRODUCTION

The successful use of an orthotic device to control the abnormal biomechanics of the foot in the past 20 years or so, has opened up a new area in the field of sports medicine, namely, podiatric sports medicine.

However, in recent years there has been increasing overutilization in the use of orthotics. Often orthotic devices are being recommended unnecessarily when other treatment modalities may be all that is required. Overutilization also seems to be owing to the fact that many allied health personnel and even retailers have jumped on this orthotics bandwagon. Indeed, many people are dispensing inserts for a shoe and calling it an "orthotic," when it is simply no more than a basic arch support. The difference is that arch supports, which have been around for over 50 years, simply push up against the arch during static stance. However, a biomechanical orthotic, when properly prescribed and fabricated, precisely controls the gait cycle from heel contact through midstance, to toe-off.

The key to understanding the effective use of orthotics and why they will or will not work lies in the basics of podiatric biomechanics. An overview of clinical biomechanics in this chapter will help the reader to ascertain which problems can best be treated with orthotics and the preferred methodology to use in their fabrication.

HISTORY OF PODIATRIC BIOMECHANICS AND ORTHOTICS

Prior to 1970, mechanical foot problems such as flat feet were commonly addressed from a static point of view. That is, arch supports were commonly used to provide support for the foot. They pushed up against the arch when a patient was standing, and in some cases would provide some degree of relief of common problems such as foot fatigue. Shoe modifications were commonly used, such as "arch cookies," heel wedges, and metatarsal pads, all of which were nonspecific from a biomechanical point of view, but did alter the position of the foot slightly. The treatment was basically hit-and-miss. Common advice for flat feet in the 1950s was to "wear good shoes."

In the late 1960s, researchers at the California College of Podiatric Medicine in San Francisco were analyzing the gait cycle and

795

breaking it down into its various segments to better understand the forces that were affecting the foot. Motion of the foot during heel contact, midstance, and toe-off were analyzed with emphasis on subtalar and midtarsal joint function during the weightbearing phases of the walking and running cycle. The researchers discovered that by controlling the abnormal subtalar and midtarsal joint function during weight bearing, they could successfully treat many foot problems. The subtalar joint, which is the talocalcaneal joint, has triplane motion of adduction and abduction, inversion and eversion, dorsiflexion and plantarflexion.[1] The subtalar joint acts to allow the foot to be a mobile adaptor to the supporting surface. Therefore, during the first 25 percent of the gait cycle, pronation was found to be a normal and necessary component of walking. That is, the subtalar joint allows the foot to absorb shock by adducting, everting, and dorsiflexing all at the same time—called pronation.

At the midstance phase, the foot resupinates to become a rigid lever for propulsion. The subtalar joint then adducts, inverts, and plantarflexes. The podiatrists researching biomechanics of the foot had realized that the subtalar joint, when held in its neutral position, would allow for normal foot stability during the midstance phase of the gait cycle.[2] The "neutral position" is that position where the subtalar joint is neither pronated nor supinated. From this position, the subtalar joint can supinate twice as much as it can pronate. Furthermore, they had discovered that forefoot imbalances led to rearfoot compensation. For example, forefoot varus was found to be a common problem that resulted in subtalar joint pronation. Forefoot varus is an inverted relationship of the forefoot (metatarsals 1 to 5) in relationship to the vertical bisection of the calcaneus. Therefore, when the heel is vertical, the forefoot would be inverted and basically off the ground. The foot then compensates as the patient bears weight, and the forefoot comes down to the ground and the subtalar joint pronates (Fig. 40-1).[3]

Researchers realized that if the forefoot and rearfoot imbalances can be corrected, then the subtalar joint remains neutral and, hence, more stable. This was accomplished with a non-weightbearing plaster case of a patient's foot that could accurately capture the inherent angular imbalances between the forefoot and rearfoot. With the subtalar joint placed in a neutral position with the patient sitting supine, a loading force could then be applied to the plantar surface of the fourth and fifth metatarsal heads in a dorsal direction that would fully pronate the forefoot at its oblique midtarsal joint axis and basically represent the reactive force of gravity.[4] This would provide an optimum stable position of the foot.

The cast would then be slipped off the patient's foot and sent off to a podiatric biomechanics laboratory along with the orthotic pre-

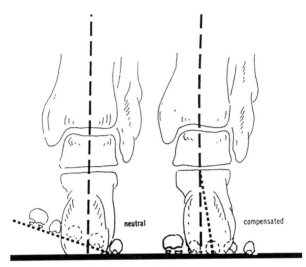

FIG. 40-1   Forefoot varus and compensation. (Reprinted with permission from Subotnick S: *Podiatric Sports Medicine.* Mt. Kisco, NY: Futura, 1975, p. 40.)

scription. The laboratory would fill the cast up with additional plaster, peel off the original cast, and a mold of the patient's foot would be available to the laboratory technicians. A line would then be drawn on the posterior aspect of the heel to bisect the heel vertically. The forefoot varus in the cast would be seen when the heel was vertical, representing forefoot varus of the patient's foot (Fig. 40-2). Following an additional twenty steps or so, an orthotic device could be fabricated that would be molded exactly to the patient's corrected foot position. It would be balanced or angulated with forefoot or rearfoot varus posts. These posts or elevations would basically bring the ground up to meet the foot so that the forefoot or rearfoot would not compensate (Fig. 40-3). Subtalar joint motion would then be controlled and the foot would be maintained in its most stable structural position. Result: normal adaptation to the supporting surface at heel strike followed by re-supination of the foot at midstance as it becomes a rigid lever for toe-off. In the early 1970s, Rhoadur, a rigid plastic material, was being used for orthotic devices. Biomechanical problems that were previously unresponsive to treatment were responding to correction with orthotics.[5]

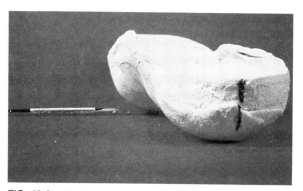

FIG. 40-2 Forefoot varus as seen in neutral cast. Note that when heel is vertical, forefoot is inverted causing compensation at subtalar joint with weightbearing.

RUNNING BOOM

By the mid-1970s, more and more Canadians and Americans were taking up running for fitness. The field of sports medicine seemed to grow rapidly since runners were not willing to accept the commonly prescribed "aspirin and rest" as a treatment. Physicians who were developing an interest in sports medicine found that the typical treatment modalities for the common overuse syndromes that they were seeing in runners seemed in many cases to be short-lived. That is, after rest, anti-inflammatories, ice, stretching, or strengthening exercises as well as many physiotherapy treatments, those overuse problems in runners were recurring. Articles in running magazines were steering runners to podiatrists for the treatment of running-related foot and leg overuse syndromes.

In 1975, Dr. George Sheehan, a prominent cardiologist and runners' guru, wrote in his book that it was not until he came under the care of a podiatrist that he was able to run for prolonged periods, thanks to the use of orthotic devices.

It seemed that his anecdotal report was enough to convince thousands of runners to try a visit to a podiatrist. Following Dr. Sheehan's advice, many patients reported back to their family physician that their symptoms had improved with podiatrists' orthotics and that they were back into their running program. Word eventually spread and podiatrists were seen to be an integral part of the sports medicine team.[6]

Over time, more shock absorbing materials as well as more flexible plastics were used in the fabrication of orthotic devices for

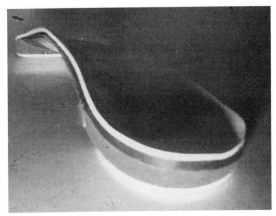

FIG. 40-3 Forefoot varus on orthotic matches forefoot varus of cast. Rearfoot varus post also shown which prevents pronation but allows 4 degrees of motion at heel strike for normal shock absorption.

enhanced comfort. By the 1980s, orthotics were well established as an effective treatment modality for biomechanically related foot problems.[7]

ORTHOTICS OVERUTILIZATION

In the late 1980s, there were many people taking an interest in foot care. Often chiropractors, physiotherapists, athletic therapists, occupational therapists, nurses, and others were recommending and selling orthotics to patients. Obviously, some practitioners were more skilled than others in assessing and treating the athlete's biomechanical problems. As a result, the efficacy of treatment was quite varied. In fact, many people thought that orthotics were useless since they did not work for them. The question in these cases would then arise as to just how the orthotic devices were fabricated. For example, many people outside of the podiatry profession will take a foam impression of the foot to have an orthotic device fabricated. However, a weight-bearing foam impression of a pronated foot will capture the foot in its deviated, unstable position. Instead, a plaster cast of the foot in its neutral, subtalar joint position would be preferred in order that the corrected or neutral position of the foot be made available for the laboratory. Usually, orthotics made from a foam impression of the foot are based on off-the-shelf, stock items. Those using this type of orthotic, who have had some cursory courses on biomechanics may have elected to add some forefoot or rearfoot varus posting to the devices. This helps somewhat, but foam "casting" should be avoided if true biomechanical correction is to be achieved.

Although some patients may have symptoms improve with various types of inserts placed in their shoes, it should be noted that even stuffing tissue paper under the arch could perhaps offer some temporary relief. Problems invariably recur, however.

The key is optimum control of the biomechanics of the foot through each phase of the gait cycle, to a precise degree. The orthotics that most closely control the biomechanics of the foot are the more effective. Therefore, the more training and knowledge in biomechanics the clinician has, the better end result that can be expected for the patient. If you are going to change the function of the 26 bones of each foot for the thousands and thousands of foot strikes that will take place, there should be no room for guesswork.

INDICATIONS FOR THE USE OF ORTHOTICS

Doing Your Own Biomechanical Analysis

The simplest way for the clinician to determine whether or not the patient has a biomechanical imbalance of the osseus structure of the feet starts off with visual inspection. If the patient has calluses inferior to the second and third metatarsal heads, this is indicative of shearing forces owing to pronation taking place during the gait cycle. As the foot pronates, the metatarsal heads undergo valgus rotation, resulting in friction and hyperkeratosis.[8] The patient rolls off the medial aspect of the hallux and calluses may be present there as well, which is also indicative of pronation.

If, however, the patient has callus formation inferior to the first metatarsal head of first and fifth metatarsal heads, this will usually indicate the opposite foot type or a rigid pes cavus foot. The first metatarsal is plantarflexed and the weight-bearing areas are inferior to the first and fifth metatarsal heads as well as the heel.[9,10]

Stance

By having your patient stand up, you should be able to easily determine whether he or she has a normal foot, or an excessively pronated foot; or the opposite, a rigid pes cavus foot type.

With pronation, the arches are flattened and the ankles tend to roll in medially toward each other. Looking at the patient from the posterior aspect, a vertical bisection of the calcaneus would appear everted with a pronated foot. To see this more clearly, you can draw a line on the posterior aspect of the patient's heels when they are prone, then have the patient stand up. Also with pronation, the hallux is often in abduction and in valgus rotation.

A rigid pes cavus foot type can be easily demonstrated as well. You could simply look at the medial aspect of the foot and see if there is quite a high arch and a prominent first metatarsal head, plantarly (Fig. 40-4A). The posterior view demonstrates inverted heels. Casts of a pes cavus foot type would reveal this as well (Figs. 40-4B,C).

Gait Analysis

By watching the patient walk back and forth, you can see eversion of the calcaneus with a pronated foot (Fig. 40-5). The talus is adducted and prominent medially. The patient usually has an apropulsive gait where he or she rolls off the medial aspect of the hallux and the arch is flattened.

Conversely, with a pes cavus foot type, the patient has an inverted position to the rearfoot and excessive supination results in him or her appearing to have an inverted forefoot in relation to the rearfoot. The first metatarsal is plantarflexed and as the forefoot bears weight, the plantarflexed first metatarsal throws the rearfoot into eversion. The first metatarsophalangeal joint area seems quite prominent plantarly.

Patients demonstrating these abnormal foot types would benefit with an orthotic device designed to specifically control each phase of the walking cycle.

Computerized gait analysis is becoming quite popular. It should confirm your diagnosis and although it is a nice tool, a computerized gait analysis seems to be used more to impress patients than anything else. As a research tool it is excellent, but it is certainly no substitute for biomechanical knowledge when it comes to treating foot imbalances.

CLINICAL ENTITIES REQUIRING THE USE OF ORTHOTICS

There are a number of clinical entries that are directly related to abnormal biomechanics of the foot that will respond to proper biomechanical control. Correcting the foot mechanics will often eliminate the *cause* of the problem. At the same time, *symptoms* can be treated with traditional therapeutic modalities that may include stretching and strengthening exercises, massage therapy, application of ice, rest, compression and elevation, and possibly non-steroidal anti-inflammatories (NSAIDs). Wearing soft-soled, laced walking shoes or running shoes may enhance comfort. Modification of activity, such as a runner shortening the stride, eliminating hills or speed work, or reducing running mileage may help. Often some lessons or coaching in a sport will help to offset improper techniques that can contribute to overuse syndromes.

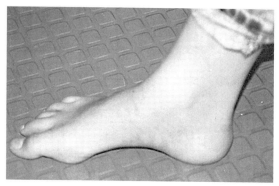

A

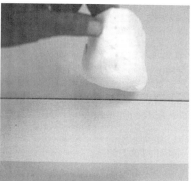

B

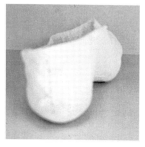

C

FIG. 40-4 *A.* Rigid pes cavus foot type. Excessive pressure inferior to first metatarsal head which is plantarflexed, can be easily visualized when patient is standing. *B.* Forefoot valgus/plantarflexed first ray as seen in neutral case. When heel is vertical, medial side of this left foot is plantarflexed or in valgus. This cannot be accurately captured in a foam box impression. *C.* When above cast is placed on a table one can see how the compensated or weightbearing position of forefoot causes rearfoot to invert. Therefore forefoot valgus posting is required on orthotic along with 0-degree rear foot post.

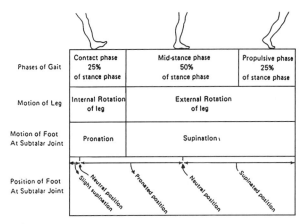

Phases of Gait	Contact phase 25% of stance phase	Mid-stance phase 50% of stance phase	Propulsive phase 25% of stance phase
Motion of Leg	Internal Rotation of leg	External Rotation of leg	
Motion of Foot At Subtalar Joint	Pronation	Supination	
Position of Foot At Subtalar Joint	Slight supination / Neutral position	Pronated position / Neutral position	Supinated position

FIG. 40-5 (Reprinted with permission of the author from Hlavac HF: *The Foot Book.* World Publications, 1977, p 90.)

Many problems that have been treated traditionally in the past would demonstrate a decrease in symptoms but only on a temporary basis. Often when patients would return to running or sports, the problem would recur.

When treating patients' symptoms, consider addressing the cause of the problem if it is biomechanical in nature.

Patellofemoral Pain Syndrome (PFPS)

When a patient presents with chronic symptoms in the peripatellar area with no history of trauma and you are considering patellofemoral pain syndrome in your differential diagnosis, take a look at the feet when the patient is standing. A pronated foot will result in internal rotation of the lower leg and therefore increasing the Q-angle of the knee. Abnormal patellar tracking is often associated with pronated feet.[11,12]

Along with this is often weakness of the vastus medialis or a tight vastus lateralis. Your recommendations may include the use of ice, strengthening exercises, NSAIDs, and physiotherapy, but should also include biomechanical treatment of the feet if pronation is present.

Shin Splints

Shin splints are usually a combination of periostitis, myositis, and tendonitis. The anterior and posterior tibial muscles and tendons act to supinate the foot. If the foot is pronated, then ongoing stretching of these tendons and muscles results. Although physiotherapy is of course indicated for patients with these complaints, a look at the foot mechanics may be in order. Stretching exercises for tight Achilles may lessen the forces required to dorsiflex the foot during the swing phase of the gait cycle. At the same time strengthening exercises for the lower leg muscles anteriorly are helpful, particularly in runners whose calf muscles overpower the anterior muscles. Rest, ice, and modification of activity are helpful. However, if the pronated foot is not addressed, then the reduction of symptoms with therapy will likely result in a resumption of symptoms with activity if the foot remains pronated. It should be noted also that excessive use of the posterior tibial muscle necessitated by supinating or elevating the foot into its proper position can play a role in compartment syndrome.[13]

There are also patients with shin splints who exhibit a rigid pes cavus foot type. In this case there's not much shock absorption at heel strike and the continual jarring that is taking place with a rigid pes cavus foot type requires enhanced shock absorption. Usually in this case, a flexible, well-cushioned type of orthotic device that redistributes the weight-bearing areas would be beneficial for the patient, along with physiotherapy.

Heel Spur Syndrome/Plantar Fasciitis

Heel pain is one of the most common foot complaints seen in athletes. Typically these patients have pain on weightbearing first thing in the morning. Their foot has been at rest, but as soon as they stand up, there is a sudden pulling of the plantar fascia. Abnormal foot mechanics definitely play a role. A rigid pes cavus foot type has a high calcaneal inclination angle to the calcaneous and there is quite a bit of jarring that takes place at heel strike. There is not the normal 4 degrees of motion at heel strike and therefore shock is transmitted to the plantar posterior aspect of the heel. At the same time, there is quite a bit of tension on the plantar fascia during the midstance phase of the gait cycle.

The pronated foot is an even more common cause of heel pain. The ongoing stretching of the plantar fascia may result in the development of a calcaneal spur over many years as the heel basically deposits more bone at the site where the plantar fascia is pulling away, usually at the medial tuberosity at the calcaneus.[14]

Controlling the abnormal biomechanical forces with a neutral position orthotic device will go a long way in treating these heel problems.[15] Using enhanced cushioning in the orthotic will help the cavus foot, and a more controlling type of orthotic is beneficial for the pronated foot. In the meantime, patients would benefit with the use of well-cushioned heel pads, the application of tape in a low-dye fashion, along with some ice and massage as well as the wearing of soft-soled shoes. Stretching exercises for the plantar fascia are best left until the patient is asymptomatic, since stretching can aggravate the problem.

An anti-inflammatory injection can be used when these heel spur syndromes are not responding or when they are in an acute stage. In podiatry, we prefer a medial approach to the heel rather than a plantar approach. A 27-gauge, 1.25-in. needle can be used with this medial approach that is far less painful for the patient.

In adolescence, calcaneal apophysitis should be differentiated from plantar fasciitis. In these cases, ice, rest, heel pads, and taping are usually all that is required and the symptoms settle down.

Neuromas

Physicians can usually suspect a neuroma based on a patient's history. That is, the patient typically gets a burning pain in the forefoot, which will sometimes radiate to the toes. Often he or she will have to stop and take the shoe off and massage the foot. The pain of a neuroma can come and go. Indeed, sometimes patients can experience pain while they are non-weightbearing for no apparent reason. Neuromas result most commonly from a pronated foot. With pronation, there is valgus rotation of the metatarsals resulting in impingement of the intermetatarsal nerve, most commonly between the third and fourth metatarsal heads, although they are also seen between the second and third metatarsal heads as well.[16] Ice is helpful, along with the wearing of soft-soled shoes. Some people recommend a metatarsal pad to be placed proximal to the affected metatarsal head area, and although this usually does not do a great deal, it may be worth a try.

Correcting the foot mechanics with orthotics will work quite dramatically in reducing symptoms associated with a neuroma. In fact, those patients who wear orthotics and have neuromas often will find that if they go without their orthotics, their symptoms recur. Putting the orthotics back into their shoes frequently is all it takes to calm down the symptoms. If the neuromas are quite painful, an anti-inflammatory injection works well. Podiatrists prefer a dorsal approach with a 27-gauge, 1.25 in. needle, and in so doing, it is less painful for the patient than a plantar approach. Also incorporated into the injection along with the steroid are xylocaine, marcaine, and also cyanocobalamin (vitamin B_{12}), which seems to have a sclerosing effect on the neuroma. In most cases a series of three injections spaced 2 to 4 weeks apart (maximum of three injections in a year) along with orthotics is enough to circumvent surgery about 95 percent of the time.

Hallux Abducto Valgus and Associated Bunion Deformity

You will see patients present with bunions in various stages. Mild to moderate bunion deformities are often asymptomatic, but are worth treating on a preventive basis to avoid progression of the deformity. In most cases, patients will have pronated feet and may demonstrate forefoot varus (inverted relationship of the metatarsals 1 to 5 in relation to the vertical bisection of the calcaneus). As the forefoot bears weight in its inverted position, compensation of the subtalar joint results so that the forefoot gets to the ground, and hence pronation results. The patient rolls off the medial aspect of the hallux, and the hallux is forced into abduction. This rolling off the medial aspect of the forefoot increases the pressure to the first metatarsal head area and eventually a bursitis develops over the first metatarsal head.[17] If left untreated, continual pressure increases and an exostosis develops at the medial aspect of the first metatarsal head as the hallux is forced into abduction. The first metatarso-phalangeal joint becomes deviated in a bunion deformity, and in an advanced stage, becomes more subluxed. Bunions in mild to moderate stages respond well to orthotics. Mild symptoms often subside and the problem no longer progresses.

Severe bunion cases demonstrate a hallux in a great degree of abduction. A retrograde force of the hallux tends to push the first metatarsal more medially, increasing the deformity.[18] Although orthotic devices will allow a patient to propel off the plantar aspect of the hallux rather than the medial aspect, advanced bunion cases will not be resolved with orthotic devices. Therefore, surgical correction is necessary where often an osteotomy has to be performed on the first metatarsal and the proximal phalanx of the hallux in order to realign the deformity. Certainly, orthotic devices would allow for speedier recovery postoperatively in terms of allowing the patient to propel off the plantar aspect of the hallux, which reduces pressure to the surgical site. Preferred, however, is the correction of the foot mechanics in the early stage of the bunion development so that it does not progress in the first place.

Stress Fractures

Stress fractures, a common overuse syndrome, are most often caused by excessive, repetitive trauma to a specific area of the foot or lower leg. Faulty foot mechanics often contribute to the development of this condition. Frequently, tibial stress fractures are associated with a rigid pes cavus foot type. A stress fracture in the foot is commonly found in the second, third, or fourth metatarsals. Abnormal foot mechanics will place excessive strain on the metatarsals, as pronation will result in an increase in valgus rotation of the metatarsals. Depending on the nature of the patient's activity, this repetitive trauma tends to progress unless the foot mechanics are treated. A rigid pes cavus foot type can also be associated with stress fractures in the foot because of excessive jarring. X-rays are initially normal, but bone callus will be demonstrated on the metatarsals with healing—usually 6 weeks after onset. Rest, ice, compression, elevation, soft-soled shoes, and orthotics will help.

OTHER PROBLEMS ASSOCIATED WITH ABNORMAL FOOT MECHANICS

Tarsal Tunnel Syndrome

This is a less common condition involving pain, numbness, or tingling at the medial aspect of the foot inferior to the medial malleolus and is often associated with a pronated foot. As the foot pronates, the tibial nerve will be compressed inferior to the laciniate ligament. Pain or paresthesias may radiate proximally or distally from the site. Nerve conduction studies may be in order. Surgical releases are rarely necessary. Anti-inflammatory injections are sometimes used, although often simply treating the mechanics of the foot is enough to reduce symptoms. Using a rearfoot varus post on the orthotic will help to limit the compression taking place as a result of pronation.

Calluses

Calluses inferior to the metatarsals 2, 3, or 4 are owing to shearing forces during pronation, or they are owing to plantarflexed metatarsals. Also a rigid cavus foot demonstrates calluses under the first or fifth metatarsals. Debridement of the calluses works temporarily, but unless the foot mechanics are treated, calluses recur as a protective mechanism for the underlying structures. Pads and cushioning help temporarily.

Sesamoiditis

Inflammation of the sesamoids inferior to the first metatarsal head is not uncommon. Pinpoint tenderness to palpation may reveal whether the tibial or fibular sesamoid is involved. Frequently, a rigid plantarflexed first metatarsal is associated with sesamoiditis. Also, pronation can increase pressure to the tibial sesamoid during the toe-off phase. Orthotics can accommodate the area of excessive pressure, provide enhanced cushioning, as well as limit the biomechanical force that creates the problem.

IN THE ABSENCE OF TRAUMA

Generally speaking, when patients present with orthopedic complaints of their feet or lower extremities when there has been no history of trauma, think in terms of abnormal biomechanics. Have a look at their stance and gait, put the ankle and subtalar joints through their ranges of motion, as well as the first metatarsal to see whether or not the first metatarsal is dorsiflexed or plantarflexed in relation to the other metatarsals. By routinely examining the biomechanics of the foot, you may be able to determine the cause of the patient's problem. The end result should be that in addition to resolving their symptoms, you can prevent recurrence of their problem by eliminating abnormal biomechanical forces. Weightbearing x-rays would reveal abnormal biomechanics as well (Fig. 40-6).

TYPES OF ORTHOTICS

When orthotics were first used in the early 1970s, they were primarily a Rhoadur material. This was a rigid plastic that worked well in maintaining the foot in the neutral subtalar joint position. These orthotics allowed 4 degrees of motion at heel strike, which is the necessary amount of pronation required to be a mobile adaptor to the supporting surface. They worked well, and despite their rigidity, patients were able to run marathons with them. However, over time, a number of newer materials have been designed that allowed for more flexibility and shock absorption.

Today, a number of materials can be used to best suit the patient and activities. It should be kept in mind that if an orthotic device is too well-cushioned, then it bottoms out and the foot will pronate

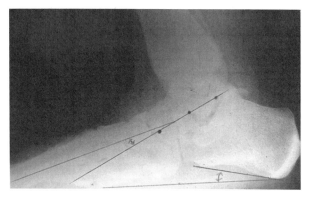

FIG. 40-6 Pronated foot as seen on weightbearing x-ray. Bisection of talus should normally bisect long axis of first metatarsal, but with pronation, this bisection falls plantarly. Also not decrease of calcaneal inclination angle. (This demonstrates why weightbearing x-rays should always be taken of the foot.)

over the orthotic. Hence, it would not provide the degree of support required. Podiatrists find that a flexible, polypropylene plastic works well. Often a 1/16-in. PPT or Poron top cover works well for added shock absorption.

For patients with shin splints or a rigid pes cavus foot type, a Spenco top cover works well in providing additional cushioning. In some cases, the entire orthotic can be quite thick and be made with more PPT, for example, in order to provide that much more cushioning.

SPORT-SPECIFIC ORTHOTICS

Often one orthotic can be used for a number of activities and will work well in controlling the mechanics of the foot. However, the needs of the patient have to be accurately assessed and the end-product orthotic should satisfy the patient's requirements in terms of sport. For example, a patient with a rigid pes cavus foot type who is playing basketball, tennis, or other lateral motion sports requires orthotics with deep heel cups and 0-degree rearfoot posts. This enhances stability and would prevent an inversion sprain when they come to a sudden stop. One should be careful when using rearfoot varus posting (the raised medial aspect of the rear segment of the orthotic). Although rearfoot posts will control pronation, too much rearfoot posting may result in a propensity toward an unstable ankle in sports such as tennis, squash, racquetball, basketball, or soccer, when there are sudden stops with lateral motion.

If a patient is a long distance runner and has a rigid cavus foot type, he or she requires maximum shock absorption at heel strike.

If the patient experiences a lot of pain at the ball of the foot or has a neuroma, calluses, or a plantarflexed metatarsal, then accommodative extensions distal to the orthotic can balance the forefoot and allow for more cushioning. This is especially helpful for those sports where a lot of time is spent on the ball of the foot, such as tennis.

WHEN ONE PAIR OF ORTHOTICS
CAN BE USED AT ALL TIMES

Often patients can use the same orthotics for their sport shoes and dress shoes. The orthotics can be made with a shallow heel cup, with no top covers and they can allow for good control in sport shoes and at the same time they will fit easily into dress shoes. Intrinsic forefoot or rearfoot posting can be used so that the orthotic is not bulky and so that the patient's heels do not flip out of the shoe (a common problem with posted or bulky orthotics). Some people recommend orthotics specifically for sport shoes and others for dress shoes; however, in many cases one pair of orthotics will work for both (unless the patient is a female wearing dress pumps or similar shoes).

ASSESSING YOUR PATIENT'S ORTHOTICS

If a patient presents to you saying that he or she already wears orthotics that are not working, you could determine whether or not the orthotics are suitable for the patient. If the patient complains that the orthotics are uncomfortable or painful, or causing knee, hip, or back problems, you can expect that there has been over correction with the orthotic.[19] You can take a look at the device and see if it seems excessively high under the arch or at the medial aspect of the device. If this is the case, then the patient should be directed back to the person who made the orthotics so that the correction can be decreased. Often posting has to be reduced or flexibility enhanced in order that the patient can tolerate the orthotic device. Four degrees of motion has to be available at heel strike; therefore, the orthotic should rock slightly or tilt medially when placed on a table and downward pressure is exerted on it.

If the patient presents with orthotics saying that they do not work at all, you can have him or her stand on the orthotics and see if the feet pronate over them. It may be that the orthotics do not have enough correction and the height of the arch has to be increased, or the posting has to be increased as well. This is a common problem with orthotics made from a foam impression.

Another clue may be to simply ask the patient how the orthotics were made. If a plaster cast was taken of the foot non-weight-bearing, then chances are the proper technique was used. However, the cast may have been too supinated or too pronated, depending on the positioning of the subtalar joint during the casting procedure.

If, however, the patient indicates that he or she stepped into a foam box, then this may be all you need to know that the orthotics are inaccurate and not providing proper biomechanical control. If the orthotics were "made from a computer," they may not be providing precise correction. Likely, a computerized gait analysis was done, but the orthotics are probably a prefabricated, stock, standard size.

COMPUTERIZATION AND ORTHOTICS

In recent years we have seen the development of some very sophisticated gait analysis machines. Patients can take a few steps over a pressure pad and a digital readout of the pressure points on their feet can be seen in color on a screen. This appears very impressive to the patient and indeed it is interesting to show points of excessive pressure on the foot. However, as a clinician, you should be able to easily determine where the pressure points are on the foot by simple examination as indicated earlier in this chapter. If the calluses are inferior to a particular metatarsal head, then you know that that segment of the foot is bearing more than its share in weight, and basically the gait analysis readout would confirm this. Therefore, you should be able to come up with a diagnosis without a computerized gait analysis.

What is misleading and a disservice to the patient, is that the orthotic devices that are dispensed after a high-tech computer analysis, are often no more than off-the-shelf devices. In many cases, those that are using computerized gait analysis machines wind up selling orthotics that are basically prefabricated with varying arch heights for each size of the foot. This will not specifically control the biomechanics of the gait cycle. Often these devices do not have heel cups, which therefore cannot control the calcaneal eversion that takes place with pronation. Patients feel that they are getting "computerized orthotics," when in fact, they are just simply getting a computerized gait analysis, followed by less than precise orthotics.

In some cases, there may be the option of having varus or valgus posting placed on these prefabricated devices, but the end result is still less effective than the plaster casting method.

HOW TO AVOID USING EXPENSIVE ORTHOTICS

If your patient has a mild biomechanical imbalance demonstrating slight pronation, and presents with fairly mild symptoms, then your routine therapeutic modalities may be all he or she needs. You may want to suggest to the patient that he or she try an over-the-counter arch support found at a local drugstore or sporting goods shop. This bit of support may suffice. If you suspect that a mechanical imbalance is causing the problem, then try simply using a rearfoot varus pad that you can fabricate out of various materials. For example, by taking a 1/4 in. piece of felt, you can skive it or thin it down laterally so that it raises the heel at the medial side. This may reduce the amount of calcaneal eversion taking place by a few degrees. PPT materials can be used with adhesive felt placed along the medial segment to provide temporary support.

Patients with a rigid cavus foot type may respond simply with a well cushioned sports insole such as Spenco, Viscoped, or Sorbathene. By having a look at their running shoes for excessive wear, you may recommend more supportive or new shoes. Soft-soled, laced dress shoes may be all they need if they are wearing leather soled slipons, for example. Reducing pressure points on the plantar aspect of the foot with 1/8th adhesive felt pads used in a biplane fashion can often accommodate a sore spot by placing pressure around the sore spot.

DOING WHAT'S BEST FOR THE PATIENT

When it comes to foot problems, often there are multiple, complex factors taking place. There are 26 bones in each foot and considering the average person walks over 100,000 miles in a lifetime, our feet do an amazing job of getting us from place to place. Very often, biomechanical abnormalities are associated with orthopedic or structural problems that may then produce dermatologic manifestations of the underlying pathology. Neurologic or vascular involvement can further complicate the picture.

Orthotic devices are not a panacea for the treatment of foot problems. When indicated, however, they work well in reducing symptoms and treating the cause of problems as well as preventing further deforming forces. Unfortunately, there is such a broad range of inserts being placed in patient's shoes that are being referred to as "orthotics" that often the patient or practitioner does not know where to turn to achieve desirable results. If orthotic devices are indicated for a patient, then a plaster casting technique is the preferred method for optimum results. There's a combination of flexible plastics and shock absorbing materials that can be used to provide optimum foot function and comfort for the patient.[20] It should be emphasized that follow-up visits are of paramount importance to evaluate how the patient is progressing with orthotics. Often on a follow-up visit, it becomes clear that modifications or adjustments have to be made to the orthotic to enhance patient compliance or to improve correction.

One should not depend on orthotics alone to correct patients' foot problems as often consideration has to be given to other therapeutic modalities as well as the nature of the spots the patients are participating in.

For those patients who have had unsuccessful results with orthotics in the past, the key would be to determine whether or not the orthotic devices were made properly in the first place, and if they are controlling the mechanics of the foot to a precise degree. Unfortunately, too many patients are advised to get orthotics when in fact what they are getting is no more than an overpriced and disguised, over-the-counter arch support by an individual with little or no training in podiatric medicine.

The entire area of orthotic therapy needs a "shaking out" so that patients are assured proper treatment and follow-up by individuals who understand the biomechancis of the foot and the clinical entities associated with these foot imbalances.

REFERENCES

1. Sgarlato TE: *A Compendium of Podiatric Biomechanics.* San Francisco, College of Podiatric Medicine, 1971, pp 60–66.

2. Hlavac HF: Differences in x-ray findings with varied positioning of the foot. *J Am Podiatry Assn* 57:465, 1967.

3. Root ML, Orien WP, Weed JH: *Normal and Abnormal Function of the Foot*. Los Angeles, Clinical Biomechanics, 1977, pp 313–314.

4. Kominsky J, Jay RM, Silvani SM, et al: *Advanced in Podiatric Medicine and Surgery*. St. Louis, Mosby, 1996, pp 1–2.

5. Subotnick SI: *Podiatric Sports Medicine*. Mt. Kisco, NY, Futura, 1975, pp 87–88.

6. Rinaldi RR, Sabio ML: *Sports Medicine 1980: Part I*. Mt. Kisco, NY, Futura, 1980, pp 19–20.

7. Donatell R, Hurlbert C, Conaway D, et al: Biomechanical foot orthotics: A retrospective study. *J Orthop Sports Phy Ther* 10(6):205–212, 1988.

8. Root ML, Orien WP, Weed JH: *Normal and Abnormal Function of the Foot*. Los Angeles, Clinical Biomechanics, 1977, pp 319–321.

9. Root ML, Orien WP, Weed JH: *Normal and Abnormal Function of the Foot*. Los Angeles, Clinical Biomechanics, 1977, pp 344–345.

10. Sgarlato TE: *A Compendium of Podiatric Biomechanics*. San Francisco, College of Podiatric Medicine, 1971, pp 237–245.

11. Valmassy RL: *Clinical Biomechanics of the Lower Extremeties*. St. Louis, Mosby, 1996, pp. 75–76.

12. Gordon GM: Knee, ankle, and foot problems in the preadolescent athlete. *Clin Podiatric Med Surg* 3(4):742–744, 1986.

13. Subotnick SI: *Podiatric Sports Medicine*. Mt. Kisco, NY, Futura, 1975, pp 79–81, 181–187.

14. Fu FH, Stone DA: *Sports Injuries*. Baltimore, Williams & Wilkins, 1994, pp 573–574, 994–995.

15. Valmassy RL: *Clinical Biomechanics of the Lower Extremeties*. St. Louis, Mosby-Yearbook, 1996, pp 67–68.

16. Kominsky J, et al: *Advances in Podiatric Medicine and Surgery*. St. Louis, Mosby, 1995, pp 1–13.

17. Gerbert J, Sokoloff TH: *Textbook of Bunion Surgery*. Mt. Kisco, NY, Futura, 1981, pp 46–54.

18. Gerbert J, et al: *The Surgical Treatment of the Hallux Abducto Valgus and Allied Deformities*. Mt, Kisco, NY, Futura, 1973, pp 19–28.

19. Subotnick SI: Foot orthoses: An update. *Phys Sportsmed* 11(8): 108, 1983.

20. Hunter S, et al: *Foot Orthotics in Therapy and Sport*. Champaign, IL, Human Kinetics, 1995, pp 76–80.

Role of the Physician, Trainer, and Coach

Derek Mackesy

THE SPORTS MEDICINE TEAM

Time has documented humanity's ability to call on our physical capacity for survival. The skills and strength needed for survival were transformed into games of skill during times of peace. Historians claim that the first sports physician was Herodicus. During the fifth century BC, he treated athletes and other injured Athenians with therapeutic exercises and diet. His most famous pupil was Hippocrates, who later wrote of the value of exercise in both the treatment of injuries as well as the prevention of illnesses.

As civilization progressed and athletic contests became more organized, more highly trained and skilled athletes competed in teams and as individuals. Retaining fitness and recovering from injuries proved increasingly important as the sophistication and popularity of sport grew. The need for physicians, trainers, and therapists knowledgeable in the formal care and rehabilitation of athletes progressed simultaneously. Injury prevention through regulation, equipment, and playing rules, as well as pertinent research became extremely important in the realm of athletic medicine.

The success of an individual athlete or collective team is not only measured in wins and losses, but also in how effective the sports medicine team has been in preventing injuries and effectively treating those that invariably occur. The care of the athlete is a team effort in which members of the sports medicine team support each other for the benefit of the athlete and the team. Depending on the level of participation, the medical support team might consist of a single individual (i.e., trainer, physiotherapist, paramedic, or physician). In such situations, the individual practitioner must develop a network of support personnel who can assist when and where additional professional management is needed.

Professional, national, university and, to a certain extent, high school teams often have a medical support team consisting of a number of different sports medicine personnel. Both clinical and nonclinical support may be utilized. The individual responsible for assembling the team must serve as the pointman or quarterback, and ensure that not only do all members of the support team have high professional standards, but also that they work well together in a team situation. Availability and communication are the hallmarks of a successful sports medicine team. Individuals who may be part of the sports medicine team include the following:

1. Primary care sports medicine physician
2. Orthopedic surgeon
3. Coach
4. Athletic trainer
5. Physiotherapist
6. Sports psychologist
7. Nutritionist
8. Dentist
9. Internist
10. Equipment manager
11. Strength coach
12. Fitness advisor
13. Ophthalmologist
14. Gynecologist
15. Urologist
16. Other sport-specific specialists

Specific areas of responsibility for diagnosis and treatment of injuries need to be defined to avoid conflict between various members of the team. Daily, one member of the team should be the "quarterback," taking ultimate responsibility for availability, event coverage, and any problems that may be encountered.

THE TEAM PHYSICIAN

Dr. Morris Mellion deems the role of the team physician to be "a special privilege and an awesome challenge."

Team physicians have a unique responsibility for important decisions. They are expected by parents, coaches, and management to make decisions about athletes' health, qualifications to join the team, and ability to participate safely. These decisions are often made in a setting of intense time pressure. They may affect the success of the team, not to mention the future of the athlete. They often influence the athlete's mental and economic, as well as physical well-being.

The team physician has a vital position that entails multifaceted responsibilities to the athlete, the team, and the medical profession.

The health and well-being of the participating athlete begins at the preseason assessment. A comprehensive history and examination should be done prior to the start of organized training. A review of past injuries, current medication, allergies, and a full physical examination must be conducted. Ancillary fitness testing, blood and urine analysis, and sports-specific tests are discretionary and dependent on time and budgetary constraints.

Each athlete should have an up-to-date chart detailing current injury status, treatment plan, and current medication. Confidentiality is of the essence. The team physician must be sensitive as to how freely information is provided to the coaching staff and management. Information on the athlete's medical status should be divulged to the media only after having been cleared by all involved parties.

It is essential to maintain good medical records for patient care and medical-legal purposes. It becomes particularly important when more than one member of the medical team is involved in the treatment of the patient.

The team physician must be readily available for his or her team. A well-organized coverage system with other members of the medical team should provide for care during games, practices, and travel.

The physician should be available on the sidelines, in the training room, in the office and at home.

The team physician also has responsibilities to the coach, management, and to the ethics of the medical profession.

As an integral part of any sporting team, the team physician cannot simply do his or her job from the stands. During participation, he or she should be as close to the action as possible. By watching the play in a vigilant manner, the team physician can note the injuries as they may happen in an attempt to understand the mechanism. He or she should be "more than just a privileged spectator." The suggested contents for a medical bag for a team physician are listed in Table 41-1.

THE ATHLETIC TRAINER

Athletic training is the "front line" discipline in sports medicine. Its practitioners are the most closely involved with the day-to-day care of the modern athlete. Today's athletic trainer must have a working knowledge of virtually every aspect of sports medicine to successfully treat, rehabilitate, and condition athletes. He or she must be familiar with basic medical procedures to communicate well with physicians and coaches as well as understand the implications of medical treatment.

The sports medicine team may have the best of all practitioners, but if the trainer is not competent, then they will have a poor program.

The primary athletic training team consists of the coach, the athletic trainer, and the team physician. A highly educated and well-trained professional athletic trainer is most valuable. An athletic trainer's responsibilities include the following:

TABLE 41-1 Suggested Contents of Team Physician's Bag

Equipment	Medication
Diagnostic Tools	**Injection**
Stethoscope	Atropine, 0.4 mg/mL, four 1-mL vials
Otoscope/ophthalmoscope (Check batteries: if recharge-	Betamethasone, 6 mg/mL, one 5-mL multidose vial
able, periodically discharge and recharge fully)	Epinephrine (1:1000) 1 mg/mL, four 1-mL, ampules
Sphygmomanometer (aneroid)	and/or 0.3-mg autoinjector
Clinical thermometer	Meperidine 100 mg/cc, two 1-mL ampoules
Reflex hammer	Morphine sulfate 15 mg/cc, two 1-mL ampoules
Safety pins	Lidocaine (1% without epinephrine), one 20-mL vial
Tongue depressors	Bupivacaine hydrochloride (0.5%) one 50-mL vial
Latex examination gloves	Glucagon, one 1-mg vial with diluent
Tape measure	Promethazine 50 mg/mL, two 1-mL ampoules
Mini-Maglite	Diazepam 5 mg/mL, two 2-mL ampoules
Resuscitation Tools	Naloxone 0.4 mg/mL, one 1-mL vial
Oral airways	Sodium bicarbonate (8.4%) one 50-mL vial
Pocket resuscitation mask	Sodium chloride (0.9%) two 30-mL vials
Oral screw	**Inhalation**
Tongue forceps	Albuterol inhaler
Laryngoscope	Oxymetazoline (0.05% nasal spray), one 15-mL bottle
Ambu bag	**Oral**
Endotracheal tubes, one 6.5 mm, one 7.5 mm	Amoxicillin capsules, 250 mg
Surgical Tools	Diphenhydramine capsules, 25 mg or 50 mg
Bandage scissors (large, sturdy, sharp)	Erythromycin capsules, 250 mg
Syringes	Ibuprofen tablets, 600 mg
Needles, three each: 18 gauge × 1.5 inch	Antacid tablets
three each: 25 gauge × 1.5 inch	Sublingual nitroglycerin tablets, 0.4 mg
Steri-Strips, two packets, 1/8 inch, 1/4 inch	Chlorzoxazone caplets, 500 mg

Sterile latex gloves
Minor surgical set:
  Scalpel handles, three: (BT3) with
  Detachable blades (10, 11 and 15)
  Iris scissors
  Thumb forceps
  Splinter forceps
  Nylon suture, two each: 4-0, 5-0, and 6-0
  Drape
Disposable suture set:
  Needle holder
  Hemostat
  Scissors
  Drape
Suture removal scissors
Rubber tourniquet

Acetaminophen caplets, 500 mg
Acetaminophen tablets with codeine, 30 mg
Loperamide capsules, 2 mg
Propoxyphene napsylate tablets with acetaminophen, 650 mg
Dextrometorphan liquid, 100-mL bottle
Topical
  Proparacaine (0.5%) (eye anesthetic)
  Polymyxin-neomycin-garamycin ophthalmic solution
  Colymycin-hydrocortisone otic solution
  Nitrofurazone cream
  Mupirocin ointment
  Corticosteroid cream
  Ketoconazole cream (2%)

1. Preventing and managing injuries
2. Communication
3. Management of the training room
4. Education and research
5. Professional certification

Injury Prevention and Management

The preventative approach within sports medicine has yielded significant reduction in injury rates for all sports. Dr. Tom Pashby's recommendation for protective eyewear during racquet sports has led to significant diminution in eye injuries and associated health-care costs.

The health of each athlete must be continually monitored before, during, and after the competitive season. A complete history and physical is essential prior to the start of each sport's season. Many teams require a post-season evaluation as well.

Athletic trainers should know how to create effective conditioning programs to assist the athlete in gaining and maintaining maximum performance. The trainer must monitor playing surfaces, environmental conditions, and hazardous structures that may inadvertently cause injury.

The day-to-day burden of the athletic trainer is early recognition and evaluation of athletically related injuries. He or she must have a thorough knowledge of the sports medicine sciences, as well as confidence in his or her ability to respond skillfully in an emergency situation.

The athletic trainer is often the first provider of treatment to the injured athlete regardless of whether he or she is acting on personal initiative or executing the direct instructions of a physician. After evaluating an injury and rendering first aid (when no physician is present), the athletic trainer must decide the appropriate treatment and determine whether medical attention is necessary. With direction from the physician, the athletic trainer organizes a treatment regimen, using a variety of therapeutic methods, supportive procedures, or other techniques to aid in recovery.

Injury rehabilitation is often one of the most challenging of the profession. The athletic trainer must be able to establish goals and the criteria for recovery. He or she should be able to assess by objective measurement when the goals have been achieved, as well as the athlete's readiness to return to participation.

Communication

The athletic trainer requires a constant and timely flow of oral, written, and electronic communication in order to facilitate these decisions. When communicating with the athlete's parents, physicians, coaches, students, and other professionals, the athletic trainer must be precise, intelligent, and professional.

Management of the Athletic Training Room

The purchase of supplies and equipment is of prime importance to the athletic trainer. Maintaining appropriate records on all the athletes is time-consuming but essential. With regard to prescription medication, athletic trainers cannot dispense these medicines to athletes without direct physician supervision. Moreover physicians may not lawfully delegate prescriptive drug dispensing acts to trainers.

A library of books, publications, and articles on sports medicine, physical education, athletics, and recreation, as well as first aid, should be available for those who are interested.

Education and Research

Athletic trainers often instruct athletes in all aspects of the injury, including the nature, condition, and procedures to be followed for rapid recovery. They provide information about their profession to coaches, parents, and the community. They also provide ongoing instruction to assistant trainers, students, and volunteer personnel. The athletic trainer may counsel the athlete on emotional problems, substance abuse, or personal problems. At the first sign of serious psychosocial difficulties with an athlete, the athletic trainer must make proper professional referrals.

Professional Certification

Both the National Athletic Trainers' Association and the Canadian Athletic Therapists' Association provide certification examinations that evaluate clinical competence. Certification ensures that proper educational preparation and clinical experience has been obtained prior to passing a written and practical examination.

It is the trainer's responsibility to maintain his or her active certification status as well as working toward improvement of personal knowledge and skills within the profession.

THE COACH

The coach is directly responsible for teaching individual sport-specific skills as well as the strategy necessary for competitive team participation. As a member of the sports medicine team, he or she should impart a proper game philosophy, and an overall safety awareness. Coaches must show concern for safety by meeting with team members to inform them of potential injuries, and outlining an approach to prevention. The "win at all cost" attitude can be extremely dangerous.

Coaches are responsible for orchestrating effective and safe conditioning programs that ensure endurance, strength, flexibility, and agility necessary for that particular sport.

The coach must also provide, or delegate to a competent aide, emergency care of athletic injuries and application of first aid in the absence of the trainer or team physician. At least one member of the coaching staff should have CPR training and basic first aid knowlege.

Unfortunately, some coaches have a distrust of medical and paramedical practitioners. The coach often feels, rightly or wrongly, that the main role of the sports medicine clinician is to prevent the athlete from practicing or playing. The coach must understand that the team physician and trainer are all part of the same team, aiming to maximize the performance and health of the athlete (Fig. 41-1).

It is imperative that the coach is involved in the health care decision-making process. Many coaches overestimate their limited medical knowledge and often demand that an injured star player be put back into the game against the advice of the physician. Involving the coach in the decision-making process and explaining the rationale behind any recommendations increase the chance of the athlete's total compliance.

The author has worked for many years with one of the world's most successful hockey coaches. Whenever he was told that one of his best players had to miss the remainder of the game, he would say, "Take good care of him. We'll be alright." That is a knowledgeable and and ethical coach!

Once that good rapport with the coach has been established, all parties will benefit. The coach will have a better understanding of

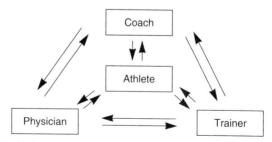

FIG. 41-1   The sports medicine team.

what the clinician has to offer. He or she is more likely to seek help for minor problems that, if managed properly, will prevent subsequent major problems. Conversely, the clinician will benefit from an increased understanding of the demands of a specific sport and may have an opportunity to institute preventative measures, which will ultimately help to reduce health care costs.

Although game officials enforce rules during competition, coaches are responsible for teaching game regulations and insisting that they be followed. Often injuries result from blatant violations of rules that are designed to keep a sport safe. Coaches must severely discipline any team member guilty of attitudes and practices that place both teammates and opposition members at risk. A team should play to win, but always within the rules of the sport.

THE ATHLETE

The health and performance of the athlete are the main focus of the sports medicine team. Many people contribute to the athlete's optimal performance and provide specific treatment should the athlete become injured (Fig. 41-2). It behooves the athlete to be cognizant of the professional expertise that can be provided by members of the sports medicine team and its secondary support system.

Injury prevention strategies such as appropriate warmups, stretching, and use of protective equipment, are necessary for the athlete to perform well. The athlete must know the importance of early reporting of injuries as well as following the instruction of definitive treatment. It is required that all players report any other treatment being received for their injuries. Athletes must play an active role in their own physical conditioning, such as participating in off-season, preseason, and in-season programs.

Athletes should refrain from the ingestion of alcohol or drugs. One would hope that today's athlete is aware of the detrimental effects that narcotics, hallucinogenic drugs, anabolic steroids, and alcohol have on the body. Team members must be advised that it is essential that they do not take any medication without informing the medical staff. Seemingly benign over-the-counter medications can render a drug test positive.

Athletes are also responsible for the proper care, fit, and maintenance of their own equipment. Examination of personal equipment should be routine before and after each practice and game.

The sports medicine team should have the confidence and respect of the athlete so that athletic as well as social problems may be discussed openly and honestly without fear of condemnation or reprisal.

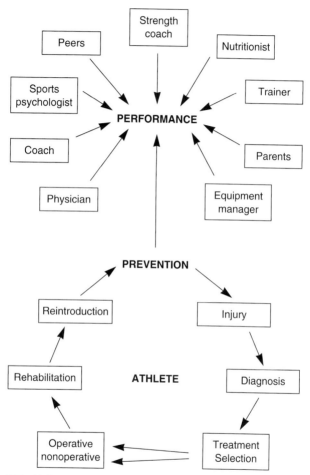

FIG. 41-2 The health and performance of the athlete are the main focus of the sports medicine team.

AVOIDING DANGEROUS PITFALLS

1. The team physician should be appointed because he or she is the best-trained and qualified physician to treat the majority of injuries that a particular team may encounter, NOT because he or she has an interest in sports or is a friend of the coach or manager.
2. The team physician is NOT just a privileged spectator, but an integral member of the sports medicine team who must be available and who should lead by example.
3. The team physician must NOT allow an athlete to compete in his or her chosen sport without having a complete history and medical examination.
4. Do NOT hesitate to obtain a second opinion in a case where the diagnosis is not clear.
5. Do NOT hesitate to elicit consultation from an appropriate member of the sports medicine team. Do NOT be pressured to provide care beyond your personal sense of expertise and skill.
6. The athlete's physical and emotional welfare always come first, NOT the outcome of the game. The team physician must NOT be a party to win-at-all cost mentality.
7. Do NOT wait for a catastrophic on-field event to take place to see if the appropriate emergency response plan works. Practice to ensure that it will work.
8. The use of radiographic imaging techniques is NOT to be neglected when diagnosing and treating sports-related injuries.
9. The competent team physician does NOT belittle the benefits rendered by teaching, continuing medical education, and sports-related research.
10. A physician should NOT agree to provide care for an athletic team without first carefully reviewing his or her professional liability insurance. As in all medical practice, it is essential to maintain accurate records, especially when more than one member of the sports medicine team is involved in treating the athlete.
11. There is NO "i" in team.
12. Do NO harm! Do everything within your professional capacity to identify, treat, and prevent injuries to members of your team.

SUGGESTED READINGS

1. Arnheim DD: *Modern Principles of Athletic Training.* St. Louis, Times Mirror/Mosby, 1989.
2. Brukner P, Khan K: *Clinical Sports Medicine.* Roseville, New South Wales, McGraw-Hill, 1993.
3. Duff JF: *Youth Sports Injuries.* New York, Macmillan, 1992.
4. Mellion MB, Walsh WM, Shelton GL: *The Team Physician's Handbook.*

Philadelphia, Hanley and Belfus, 1990.
5. Mellion MB: *Sports Medicine Secrets*. Philadelphia, Hanley and Belfus, 1993.
6. Snider RK: *Essentials of Musculoskeletal Care*. Rosemont, IL, American Academy of Orthopaedic Surgeons, 1997.

SPORTS MEDICINE RESOURCES

American Academy of Family Physicians Sports Committee
8880 Ward Parkway
Kansas City, MO 64114
(816)333-9700

The American Academy of Orthopaedic Surgeons Sports Medicine
   Committee
6300 North River Road
Rosemont, IL 60018
(708)823-7186

American Academy of Pediatric Sports Medicine
1729 Glastonberry Road
Potomac, MD 20854
(301)424-7440

American College of Sports Medicine
P.O. Box 1440
Indianapolis, IN 46206-1440
(317)637-9200

American Medical Society for Sports Medicine
11639 Earnshaw
Overland Park, KS 66210
(913)327-1415

American Orthopedic Society for Sports Medicine
2250 East Devon Avenue
Suite 115
Des Plaines, IL 60018
(708)803-8701

Canadian Academy of Sport Medicine
1600 James Naismith Drive
Gloucester, ON, Canada K1B 5N4
(613)748-5851

Canadian Athletic Therapists Association
4825 Richard Road, S.W.
Calgary, AB, Canada T3E 6K6
(403)240-7228

Disabled Sports USA
451 Hungerford Drive
Suite 110
Rockville, MD 20850
(301)217-0960

National Athletic Trainers' Association
2952 Stemmons Freeway
Suite 200
Dallas, Texas 75247
(214)637-6282

Sport Physical Therapy Section of the American Physical
  Therapy Association
220 Grand View Drive
Suite 150
Fort Mitchell, KY 41017
(606)341-6654

Sports Physiotherapy Canada
1600 James Naismith Drive
Gloucester, ON, Canada K1B 5N4
(613)748-5794

Index

Page numbers in *italics* refer to illustrations; those ending in the letter "t" to tables.

READING LIST

ISBN 0-07-008993-0

90000

9 780070 089938